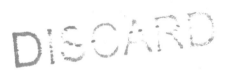

Atlas of Pediatric Emergency Medicine

Atlas of Pediatric Emergency Medicine

Editors

Gary R. Fleisher, M.D.
Thomas Morgan Rotch Professor and Chairman
Department of Pediatrics
Harvard Medical School
Pediatrician-in-Chief
Department of Medicine
Children's Hospital
Boston, Massachusetts

Stephen Ludwig, M.D.
Professor
Departments of Pediatrics and Emergency Medicine
The University of Pennsylvania School of Medicine
Associate Physician-in-Chief
John H. and Hortense Cassel Jensen Endowed Chair
Division of Pediatric Emergency Medicine
The Children's Hospital of Philadelphia
Philadelphia, Pennsylvania

Marc N. Baskin, M.D.
Assistant Professor
Department of Pediatrics
Harvard Medical School
Attending Physician
Division of Emergency Medicine
Children's Hospital
Boston, Massachusetts

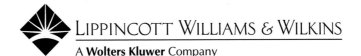
LIPPINCOTT WILLIAMS & WILKINS
A **Wolters Kluwer** Company
Philadelphia • Baltimore • New York • London
Buenos Aires • Hong Kong • Sydney • Tokyo

Acquisitions Editor: Anne Sydor
Developmental Editor: Tanya Lazar
Project Editor: Erica Woods Tucker
Manufacturing Manager: Benjamin Rivera
Cover Designer: David Levy
Compositor: Maryland Composition
Printer: Walsworth Publishing

© 2004 by LIPPINCOTT WILLIAMS & WILKINS
530 Walnut Street
Philadelphia, PA 19106 USA
LWW.com

Printed in the USA

Library of Congress Cataloging-in-Publication Data

Atlas of pediatric emergency medicine / editors, Gary R. Fleisher, Stephen Ludwig, Marc N. Baskin.
      p. ; cm.
      Includes bibliographical references and index.
      ISBN 0-7817-3918-7
      1. Pediatric emergencies—Atlases. I. Fleisher, Gary R. (Gary Robert), 1951- II. Ludwig, Stephen, 1945- III. Baskin, Marc N.
      [DNLM: 1. Emergencies—Child—Atlases. 2. Emergencies—Infant—Atlases. 3. Wounds and Injuries—Child—Atlases. 4. Wounds and Injuries—Infant—Atlases. 5. Critical Care—methods—Child—Atlases. 6. Critical Care—methods—Infant—Atlases. WS 17 A8788 2003]
      RJ370.A85 2003
      618.92′0025—dc22

                                                                          2003058810

                                                                 10 9 8 7 6 5 4 3 2 1

To the thousands of children, who by trusting our care, came to our Emergency Departments in Philadelphia and Boston. In allowing us the privilege of trying to help them, they have helped us and our readers.

Contents

Section I. Medical and Surgical Emergencies

Section II. Trauma

Section III. Psychosocial Emergencies

Section IV. Procedures

Preface

"Once you have **seen** this, you'll never forget it." "If there are any medical students around today, they should definitely **see** this." "Let's get the attending, he may have **seen** this before." "**See** one, do one, teach one." "The only thing wrong with every other night on call is that you don't **see** half of the good cases." Although we do not want to admit it, most of us have used one or more of the phrases above. All of which are linked by the use of the word, "**see**" or "**seen**," which helps to convey the idea that visual memory plays an important part in medicine. For this reason, some residents even joke that having seen a procedure once qualifies them to perform it, and that their failure to see half the good cases (caused by an occasional need to sleep every other night) may compromise their education.

Truth be told, no one can work 24 hours per day, 7 days per week. Nor would they be allowed. Additionally, no matter how much time one spends in training or practice, the reality of clinical experience is somewhat erratic. One intern may diagnose two patients with herpes zoster and never see an abused child while the next intern may encounter three cases of abuse and none of zoster. Often physicians train in areas of the country where diseases common in other regions are rarely seen due to geographic factors or the ethnic mix of the population. In an effort to smooth out these inequalities in exposure to various conditions, we have culled our files of images to assemble this atlas, which will be uniquely helpful to both practitioners and trainees.

Thus, this book is an atlas of acute and emergent pediatric illness and injury. We refer to it as an atlas to highlight the prominent role played by the images, even though they are supplemented by a substantial amount of informative text. In general, we have concentrated on acute illness and injury, although we have included a few patients with more chronic conditions that may show up with complications or as diagnostic dilemmas. All of our patients are in the pediatric age range and are suffering from an illness or injury. Thus, we have directed our efforts to students, residents, and physicians learning or refining the approach to the practice of acute and emergency pediatric care.

Rather than limit the text to the surface of the body as in a dermatology atlas, we travel visually down orifices, incise through the integument, and employ various types of probes to provide you with diagnostic specimens, radiographs, CT scans, electrocardiograms, and photographs of the body illustrating more than just lesions of the skin. These additional illustrations are either specimens or images routinely viewed by primary practitioners or are used, in a few cases, to explain clinical findings in more depth.

We focus on acute disease rather than normality. Although we cover findings that are elicited by physical examination, we do not review the methods for examining children of various ages along the expected normal variations. Instead, we emphasize both abnormal findings and the process for weaving these clues together to diagnose various diseases and injuries. In most cases, we move beyond diagnosis to management, covering procedures when applicable.

As authors of the *Textbook of Pediatric Emergency Medicine*, *Synopsis of Pediatric Emergency Medicine*, and the *Pictorial Review of Pediatrics*, we feel that there is still new ground to be covered. While the textbook and the synopsis relied primarily on the written word, the atlas will use a large number of images to convey the precepts of acute care and emergency pediatrics by evoking visual learning. Therefore, this book provides an overall approach across the gamut of the subspecialty for the reader.

Gary R. Fleisher, M.D.
Stephen Ludwig, M.D.
Marc N. Baskin, M.D.

Acknowledgments

First and foremost, we acknowledge the support of our wives, Elayne, Jan, and Zelda, and our children, Emily, Michael, Daniel, Carl, Madeline, Susannah, Michael, Elisa, and Aubrey. Additionally, we thank our staff for their tireless work in the creation of this book. Cindy Chow, in Boston, showed incredible creativity in cataloging the images and endless dedication in retrieving and matching slides and figures. She served as a critical liaison between the publisher and the editors, coordinating communication and the submission of the completed materials. In Philadelphia, Carolyn Trojan, served as Dr. Ludwig's unfailing assistant, and Mona Mahboubi, a premedical student, also provided additional help.

As the textual material for many of the chapters in this Atlas derive from the Textbook of Pediatric Emergency Medicine and the Synopsis of Pediatric Emergency Medicine, we wish to also acknowledge the many authors who contributed to these publications.

Atlas of Pediatric Emergency Medicine

SECTION I

Medical and Surgical Emergencies

CHAPTER 1

Abdominal Emergencies

Editor: Marc N. Baskin

DISEASES THAT PRODUCE PERITONEAL IRRADIATION

Acute Nonperforated Appendicitis

Clinical Manifestations

Usually the child with appendicitis complains initially of poorly localized midabdominal pain. Unfortunately, this symptom is common to many other intraabdominal, nonsurgical problems. Anorexia, nausea, vomiting, and a low-grade fever often occur soon thereafter. Characteristically, the pain then migrates to the right lower quadrant (Table 1.1). Because the position of the appendix may vary in children, the localization of the pain and the tenderness on examination may also vary. Motion aggravates peritoneal irritation, and a child with appendicitis typically prefers to lie still.

On examination, palpation is usually reliable for demonstrating focal peritoneal signs at the site of the inflamed appendix. If the appendix is in the pelvis or retrocecal area, however, typical anterior peritoneal signs may be absent. The physician can confirm his or her impression of point tenderness by pressing gently in each quadrant and asking the child to indicate which area is most tender. This impression of focal tenderness can sometimes be confirmed by shaking the child's abdomen or getting him or her to cough, which often produces a wince of pain at the involved area.

A complete blood count in a child with appendicitis usually shows an elevated white blood cell (WBC) count in the range of 11,000 to 15,000/mm^3 in the first 24 hours of the illness. As the appendix becomes more gangrenous, the WBC count increases further, and the differential demonstrates an increasing number of neutrophils. If the inflamed appendix lies over the ureter or adjacent to the bladder, a few WBCs may be found in the urinary sediment.

Many consider the abdominal radiograph a peripheral study valid only for the demonstration of a fecalith or free air. Abdominal radiographs are normal in most cases of acute appendicitis, although in fewer than 10% of cases, a calcified appendiceal fecalith can be identified (Fig. 1.1). Today, to evaluate appendicitis, Doppler ultrasonography or computed tomography (CT) is preferred. Routine chest radiographs are not indicated unless the symptoms and signs are atypical right and/or splinting respirations or other pulmonary findings are present. A chest radiograph in such a case may reveal evidence of a right lower lobe pneumonia.

Management

When appendicitis is suspected, surgical consultation should be obtained. The patient should receive nothing by mouth, and intravenous fluids should be started, with emphasis on replacing the child's deficits. A complete blood count, a blood specimen to hold for cross-matching, and possibly electrolyte, blood urea nitrogen, and creatinine levels should be obtained. The emergency physician must keep in mind the many ways in which appendicitis can present. As a good rule of thumb, a patient should at least be admitted for observation if there are positive findings in two of the three classic modes of assessment: history, physical examination, and laboratory tests.

Perforated Appendicitis

Clinical Manifestations

In most cases, within a few hours after perforation has occurred, the child begins to develop increasing signs of toxicity. The abdomen becomes rigid with extreme tenderness. Bowel sounds become sparse. There are signs of prostration such as pallor, dyspnea, grunting, tachycardia, and high fever. Rarely, the patient may develop septic shock from the overwhelming infection caused by bowel flora. Occasionally, however, a perforation remains contained and the patient presents with signs of a localized abscess.

Initially, the findings may be confused with those of pneumonia because the extreme abdominal pain may cause rapid, shallow respirations. In infants and toddlers, the findings may also be confused with meningitis because any movement of the child (even flexion of the neck) produces crying. If the spinal fluid analysis is found to be normal, perforated appendicitis should be suspected.

TABLE 1.1. *Progression of symptoms and signs of appendicitis*

Nonperforated appendicitis
  Poorly defined midabdominal or periumbilical pain
  Low-grade fever
  Anorexia
  Vomiting that usually starts after the onset of
    abdominal pain
  Tenderness in right lower quadrant
  Localization depends on position of appendix
  Pain on coughing or hopping on right foot
  Rectal examination: pain on palpation of right rectal wall
  WBC count: 10,000–15,000/mm³
Perforated appendix
  Increasing signs of toxicity
  Rigid abdomen with extreme tenderness
  Absent bowel sounds
  Dyspnea and grunting; tachycardia
  Fever: 39°–41°C (102.2°–105.8°F)
  WBC count: >15,000/mm³ with shift to left
  Eventual overwhelming sepsis and shock

WBC, white blood cell.

The laboratory findings in the child with perforated appendicitis may support the diagnosis. The WBC is significantly elevated, usually more than 15,000/mm³, with a marked shift to left.

The radiographic evaluation of suspected perforated appendicitis should include both plain abdominal radiographs and abdominal ultrasonography or CT. The plain film of the abdomen may show free air. Ultrasonography or CT may show a complex mass with or without a calcified fecalith or free fluid within the abdominal cavity.

Management

Initially, the focus of therapy should be on resuscitation. There must be careful attention to airway, breathing, and circulation. The severely septic child may need positive-pressure ventilation with high concentrations of oxygen to overcome ventilatory insufficiency. Hypovolemia should be corrected with 5% dextrose in either normal saline or Ringer lactate solution. The child should receive broad-spectrum antibiotics (e.g., 200 mg/kg ampicillin per day, 6 to 7.5 mg/kg gentamicin per day, and 25 mg/kg clindamycin per day). A nasogastric tube should be placed to evacuate the contents of the stomach and to drain ongoing gastric secretions. Several units of blood or packed red cells must be prepared for the operative procedure.

Peritonitis

Peritonitis may be primary due to a bacterial infection of the peritoneal cavity, usually secondary to a bloodborne or lymphborne infection. It can occur in children with nephrosis, cirrhosis, ascites, or other underlying conditions and may mimic appendicitis. Primary peritonitis is usually caused by pneumococci, group A streptococci, or gram-negative organisms. It is important to remember that children with nephrosis or cirrhosis may have appendicitis unrelated to their underlying disease.

Secondary peritonitis may occur due to fecal soilage from a perforated intestinal viscus. Patients have generalized peritoneal signs similar to those described for appendicitis. Radiographs may show pneumatosis intestinalis or pneumoperitoneum. Pneumatosis cystoides intestinalis, or gas within the wall of the intestine, is usually associated with bowel necrosis or perforation from necrotizing enterocolitis in premature neonates. Older patients may develop intramural gas from mucosal lesions (e.g., ulcerations or Crohn disease, infection, infarction in compromised patients) (Fig. 1.2). Pneumoperitoneum can originate from any ruptured viscus (Figs. 1.3 and 1.4).

Pancreatitis

Acute pancreatitis is rare in children. The most common causes are abdominal trauma, sepsis/shock, associated systemic illness (e.g., diabetic ketoacidosis, cystic fibrosis, hyperlipidemia), or structural disease of the pancreatobiliary tree. Pancreatitis causes vomiting and upper abdominal pain, often radiating to the back. Serum amylase and lipase levels are usually elevated, and serum calcium level may be decreased. When pancreatitis occurs in a child without a history of trauma, the physician should evaluate the patient for possible congenital abnormalities of the biliary tree or pancreatic ducts, such as abnormal insertion of the main pancreatic duct or the presence of a choledochal cyst.

Acute Intestinal Obstruction

In any child who vomits persistently, particularly if the vomitus becomes stained with bile, the diagnosis of acute intestinal obstruction must be considered. If the obstruction is high

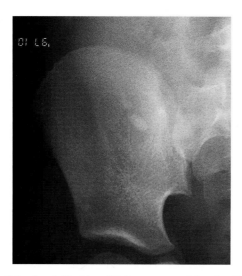

FIG. 1.1. A calcified fecalith is seen overlying the ilium.

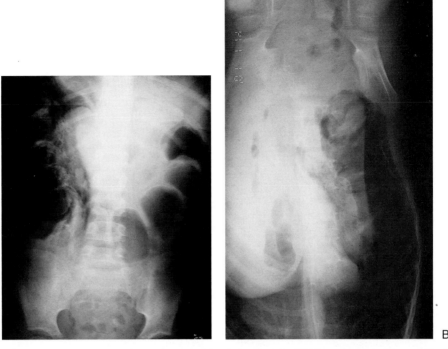

FIG. 1.2. A 4-year-old child with Acute Lymphoblastic Leukemia (ALL) presented with constipation and abdominal pain. **A:** A plain frontal supine radiograph shows pneumatosis cystoides intestinale of ascending colon and probable retroperitoneal air outlining the kidney. **B:** The decubitus view shows pneumoperitoneum. (Courtesy of Dr. Mark Waltzman.)

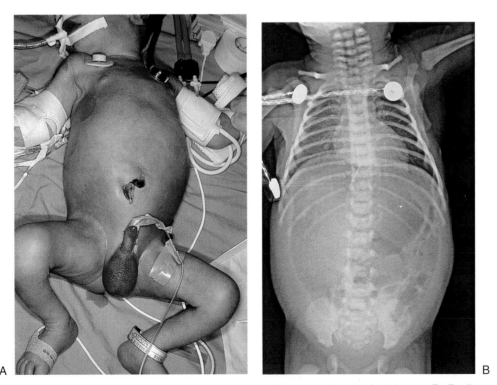

FIG. 1.3. A: A 3-day-old newborn with vomiting and a discolored distended abdomen. **B:** Radiograph demonstrates free intraabdominal air laterally and adjacent to the falciform ligament. *(Continued on next page.)*

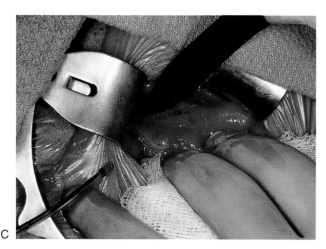

C

FIG. 1.3. *(continued)* **C:** Intraoperative view of the perforated duodenal ulcer. (Courtesy of Dr. Dennis Lund.)

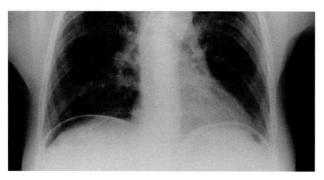

FIG. 1.4. A 17-year-old with a history of multiple gynecologic reconstructive surgeries presented with vomiting, abdominal pain, tachycardia, and a rigid abdomen. A plain frontal supine radiograph showed air under the diaphragm, and an emergency laparotomy revealed a ruptured hemosalpinx.

in the intestinal tract, the abdomen does not become distended; however, with lower intestinal obstruction, there are generalized distention and diffuse tenderness. Only if the bowel perforates or vascular insufficiency occurs will signs of peritoneal irritation be found. All patients with suspected bowel obstruction should have radiographs of the abdomen with supine, and either upright, or prone cross-table lateral views. In patients with acute mechanical bowel obstruction, multiple dilated loops are usually seen. Fluid levels produced by the layering of air and intestinal contents are seen in upright or lateral decubitus radiographs (Fig. 1.5).

Intussusception

Background

Intussusception occurs when one segment of bowel telescopes into a more distal segment, occurring most commonly between 4 and 24 months of age. The most common intussusception is ileocolic, but the small bowel may intussuscept into itself. Typically, the small bowel intussusception then prolapses through the ileocecal valve. The intussusception continues through the colon a variable distance, occasionally as far as the rectum, where it can be palpated on rectal examination. In children older than 2 years of age, a specific lead point, such as a polyp, Meckel diverticulum, or tumor may be found.

Clinical Manifestations

The main manifestation of intussusception is crampy abdominal pain. Gradually, the child becomes more irritable and may vomit. The pain is usually episodic and may cause the infant to cry out with intermittent spasms. The child may

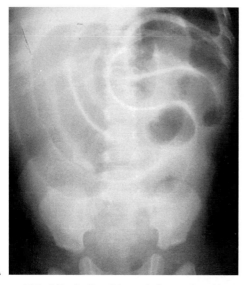

A

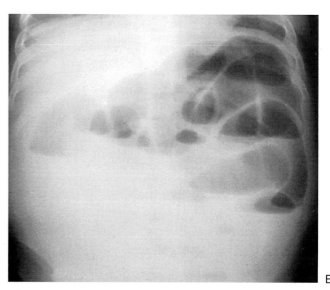

B

FIG. 1.5. A: Small bowel obstruction. Numerous dilated small bowel loops occupy the mid abdomen and have a stepladder configuration. Minimal air is seen in the rectum. **B:** Same patient as in **A.** The upright abdominal radiograph shows numerous dilated loops in the small bowel with differential fluid levels in one loop indicating mechanical bowel obstruction.

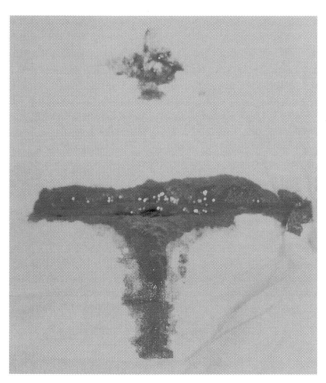

FIG. 1.6. This 14-month-old child had vomiting without diarrhea and progressive lethargy until he passed this dark red stool.

appear to be perfectly comfortable or only slightly irritable between these episodes. More often, the patient becomes lethargic between the episodes of pain. The infant may become still and pale and exhibit an almost shocklike state because of the intense visceral pain.

In some cases, the intussuscepted mass can be palpated as an ill-defined, sausage-shaped structure in the right upper quadrant. More often the abdomen is either soft or minimally tender on the right side.

Over time, the mesenteric veins become compressed, whereas the mesenteric arterial supply remains intact. This leads to the production of the characteristic currant jelly stool, which may be passed spontaneously or found on the rectal examination (Fig. 1.6). However, development of melena may occur quickly, which fact reinforces the need for a rectal examination in a child with unexplained abdominal symptoms. Once the intussusception has become tight, even the arteries are occluded by the pressure of entrapment and the bowel can become gangrenous and even perforate, leading to peritonitis.

Plain film radiographic findings of intussusception are variable and depend primarily on the duration of the symptoms and the presence or absence of complications. In early cases, a normal gas pattern is seen. In the patient with symptoms lasting longer than 6 to 12 hours, flat and upright films often show signs of intestinal obstruction, including distended bowel with air–fluid levels, a soft-tissue mass in the right abdomen, or even the actual head of the intussusceptum outlined by intraluminal bowel gas (Fig. 1.7). In many centers, ultrasonography is used to help to diagnose intussusception.

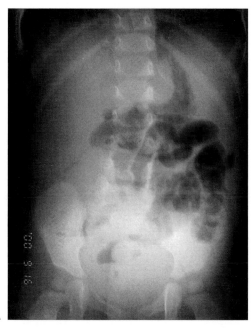

A

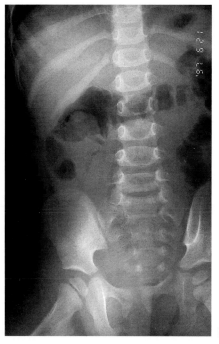

B

FIG. 1.7. A: A plain frontal supine radiograph shows no obstruction but a soft-tissue density in the right lower abdomen. **B:** A plain frontal supine radiograph shows the head of the intussusceptum outlined by intraluminal air in the right upper quadrant.

Management

An intravenous line and a nasogastric tube should be inserted to prepare the patient. Intravenous fluids should be given to correct dehydration.

In recent years, hydrostatically controlled barium enema reduction or reduction by air insufflation has been a successful therapy in more than 60% of cases. If this is unsuccessful, surgical intervention will be necessary.

Incarcerated Inguinal Hernia

Approximately 60% of incarcerated hernias occur during the first year of life. Incarceration occurs more often in girls than in boys but usually involves the ovary rather than the intestine. Incarceration does not necessarily mean that the nonreducible portion of intestine is compromised or gangrenous. However, necrosis of the bowel can occur within 24 hours of a nonreduced incarcerated hernia because of progressive edema of the bowel caused by venous and lymphatic obstruction.

The clinical presentation of a child with an incarcerated hernia is usually irritability and vomiting. A firm, discrete mass can be palpated in the inguinal region and may or may not extend into the scrotum. Occasionally, the testicle may appear dark blue because of pressure on the spermatic cord causing venous congestion. An abdominal radiograph may show gas-filled loops of intestine in the scrotum.

Unless the child is extremely ill with signs of intestinal obstruction or toxic from gangrenous bowel, a manual reduction of the incarcerated hernia should be attempted. If necessary, the child should be sedated with 0.1 mg/kg morphine intravenously. Mild pressure should be exerted at the internal ring with one hand while the other attempts to squeeze gas or fluid out of the incarcerated bowel back into the abdominal cavity. If the reduction is unsuccessful, the child should be taken promptly to the operating room. After the hernia has been reduced manually, the child may be admitted for observation but not immediate repair or may be sent home, if the parents are properly informed concerning signs of recurrence or intestinal obstruction and they are thoroughly reliable.

Malrotation of the Bowel with Volvulus

Background

Malrotation of the bowel is a congenital condition associated with abnormal fixation of the mesentery of the bowel. Therefore, the bowel has a proclivity to volvulize and obstruct at these points of abnormal fixation.

Clinical Manifestations

Bile-stained vomiting and abdominal pain (manifested by irritability in an infant) usually occur in malrotation with volvulus, which presents in 70% to 80% of cases during the first 2 months of life. The pain is usually constant. Blood may appear in the stool within a few hours, which suggests

the development of ischemia and possible necrosis of the bowel. Malrotation most commonly presents with the sudden onset of abdominal pain and bilious vomiting with no history of gastrointestinal (GI) problems. Less commonly, the patient has a history of "feeding problems" with or without transient episodes of bilious vomiting.

On physical examination, there may be only mild distention of the abdomen with only mild diffuse tenderness and no clear signs of peritonitis. On rectal examination, the presence of blood on the examining finger is an alarming sign of impending ischemia and gangrene of the bowel.

Management

The key to management is to be suspicious of malrotation and to obtain flat and upright radiographs of the abdomen immediately. The films may be normal or only show gastric and/or duodenal dilation with a paucity of distal air. The presence of loops of small bowel overriding the liver shadow is suggestive of an underlying malrotation. When complete volvulus has occurred, there may be only a few dilated loops of bowel with air–fluid levels. Distal to the volvulus, there may be little or no gas in the GI tract (Fig. 1.8).

Unless a plain frontal supine radiograph of the abdomen demonstrates another obvious cause for bilious emesis, an upper GI series should be obtained immediately. The ligament of Treitz is absent in the malrotation anomaly, so the C loop of the duodenum is not present, the duodenum lies to the right of the spine, and the jejunum presents a coiled-spring appearance in the right upper quadrant (Fig. 1.9). A barium enema is not a reliable study to rule out malrotation.

Any child with a possible volvulus should be prepared for immediate surgery.

Pyloric Stenosis

Narrowing of the pyloric canal as a result of hypertrophy of the musculature often occurs in the first-born male of a fam-

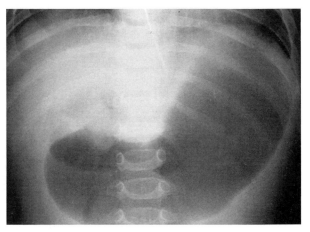

FIG. 1.8. Malrotation of the bowel. A plain supine radiograph of the abdomen shows distended stomach and proximal duodenal loop.

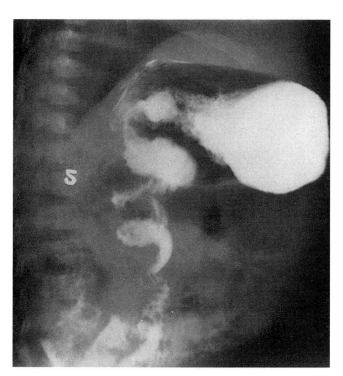

FIG. 1.9. Malrotation. Upper gastrointestinal study shows absence of the ligament of Treitz and coiled-spring appearance of jejunum.

ily. A familial incidence has been shown, particularly if the mother had hypertrophic pyloric stenosis as an infant. There is a male:female ratio of 5:1. The age at onset is usually 2 to 5 weeks. Rarely, the onset may be late in the second month of life. The cause of the muscle hypertrophy is unknown, but the symptoms, diagnosis, and therapy are well defined.

Clinical Manifestations

Characteristically, the infant does well, without vomiting, for the first few weeks of life and then starts regurgitating, at either the end of feedings or a few minutes later. The infant is hungry and will eat heartily immediately after such a regurgitation. The vomiting becomes more prominent and eventually becomes more forceful, called projectile vomiting. The vomitus ordinarily contains just the feeding that has been given and does not contain bile or blood. If not recognized, the patient may present with failure to gain weight and cachexia (Fig. 1.10).

The examination of an infant is best accomplished after the infant's stomach has been emptied. With the child lying on his or her back, the examiner holds the infant's ankles and flexes the thighs at a right angle to the trunk as the mother feeds some sugar water. Once the infant starts to suck, the upper abdominal musculature will relax and the examiner's opposite hand can then gently palpate the upper right abdomen. By palpating under the edge of the liver in an up-and-down direction, the physician may discern a firm mass in the shape of an olive.

Serum electrolyte levels may be abnormal because of gastric losses. This hypochloremic hypokalemic alkalosis may be profound with serum chlorides in the range of 65 to 75 mEq/L.

Management

Infants should be hospitalized and rehydrated with appropriate fluid and electrolyte replacement.

If a pyloric "olive" or mass is palpable, radiographic confirmation of the diagnosis is not needed. A plain frontal supine radiograph often shows a dilated gastric air bubble (Fig. 1.11). If the history of vomiting is not typical and a mass cannot be felt, ultrasonography is the first study to confirm the diagnosis. The hypertrophic pyloric muscle is seen as a thick hypoechoic ring surrounding a central echogenic mucosal and submucosal region. If ultrasonography does not show a hypertrophic pylorus, an upper GI series should then be considered to eliminate gastroesophageal reflux, malrotation, and antral web as diagnostic possibilities.

Chronic Constipation

Chronic constipation is probably one of the most common causes of abdominal pain in children. The history may attest to chronic constipation or encopresis; however, occasionally, such a child is diagnosed only by palpating a large fecaloma through the intact abdominal wall or a hard fecal mass blocking the anal outlet on rectal examination. Chronic constipation may also cause rectal prolapse, which may be gently reduced using manual pressure. In children 2 to 11 years old, the impaction may be relieved by instilling a 2.25-oz pediatric enema. Often, a gloved finger is necessary to break up a hard fecal mass and allow its evacuation.

Aganglionic Megacolon (Hirschsprung Disease)

In patients with Hirschsprung disease, the parasympathetic ganglion cells of the Auerbach plexus of the colon are absent. The effect of this absence of ganglion cells produces spasm and abnormal motility of that segment, which results in either complete intestinal obstruction or chronic constipation. The involved segment varies in length, from less than 1 cm to involvement of the entire colon and small bowel.

These children have a lifelong history of constipation, so it is important to obtain an accurate account of the child's stool pattern from birth. A child with Hirschsprung disease typically has never been able to stool properly without assistance (e.g., suppositories, stimulation with the finger or thermometer). Normal stooling is not possible because of the failure of the aganglionic bowel and interval anal sphincter to relax. These children have chronic abdominal distention and are often malnourished. Table 1.2 summarizes the pertinent diagnostic features differentiating functional constipation from Hirschsprung disease.

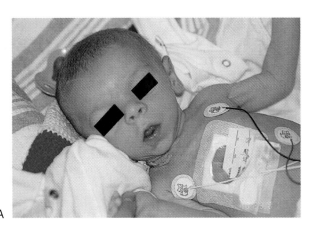

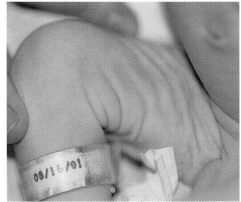

FIG. 1.10. A, B: This 10-week-old, 2.6-kg infant presented with a 6-week history of vomiting. Note the decreased subcutaneous fat over the face and skull and prominent skin folds of the upper and lower extremities. **C:** The same infant 10 weeks after surgical repair.

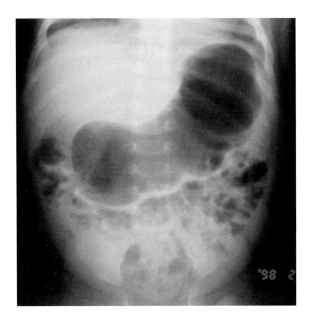

FIG. 1.11. A 6-week-old infant with a 1-week history of vomiting. A supine radiograph demonstrates a dilated gastric air bubble with the "caterpillar sign" suggesting active peristalsis.

TABLE 1.2. *Differential diagnosis of functional constipation and Hirschsprung disease*

	Functional constipation	Hirschsprung disease
Onset	≥2 yrs	Birth
History	Coercive training	Enemas necessary
	Colicky abdominal pain	No abdominal pain
	Periodic volume stools	Episodes of intestinal obstruction
Encopresis	Present	Absent
Abdominal distention	Absent or minimal	Present
Rectal examination	Feces-packed rectum	Empty rectum
Barium examination	Dilated rectum	Narrow segment
Motility	Normal	Abnormal
Biopsy	Ganglion cells	No ganglion cells

After flat and upright abdominal radiographic studies have been obtained, a properly performed barium enema is the best initial diagnostic procedure. The key to diagnosis is seeing a "transition zone" between the contracted aganglionic bowel and the proximal dilated ganglionated bowel. Anorectal manometry to determine the presence or absence of relaxation of the internal anal sphincter is helpful in establishing the neurogenic dysfunction of the bowel. Barium enema studies and manometry are clearly complementary in the diagnosis of Hirschsprung disease. However, rectal manometric studies are more reliable than radiographic methods for short aganglionic segments that are usually not apparent on barium enema studies. Because of the complicated evaluation and management of this disease, referral to a pediatric surgeon is recommended.

Inflammatory Bowel Disease

The older child or adolescent may develop either Crohn disease or ulcerative colitis, and these entities must be included in the differential diagnosis of chronic intestinal obstruction. Usually, the child has a history of changing bowel habits, with mucus or blood in the stools, chronic abdominal pain, and weight loss.

DISEASES THAT PRODUCE RECTAL BLEEDING

It is important to determine the quantity of bleeding and whether the blood is on the outside of the stool or mingled with it. A "tarry" stool suggests a source of bleeding in the proximal portion of the GI tract and bright red blood suggests a more distal origin (Fig. 1.12). All patients with rectal bleeding should have a rectal examination. Those with significant hemorrhage require flexible colonoscopy and a contrast enema.

Fissures

An anal fissure is probably the most common cause of bleeding, especially in infants. The child usually has a history of passing large, hard stools with anal discomfort. If bleeding occurs, it usually involves streaking of bright red blood on the outside of the stool, or red blood on the toilet tissue. The diagnosis can easily be made by inspection or anoscopic examination.

Juvenile Polyps

Older infants and children can develop polyps. Polyps bleed but rarely cause massive hemorrhage. They may intermittently prolapse at the anus or on occasion come free and be passed as a fecal mass associated with bleeding (Fig. 1.13). Colonic polyps may be lead points for intussusception. Usually, however, polyps are asymptomatic except for the associated bleeding. These are not premalignant lesions, and they tend to be self-limiting.

Meckel Diverticulum

Two percent of the population is born with a Meckel diverticulum, the most common omphalomesenteric duct remnant. The most common complication of a Meckel diverticulum is a painless bleeding ulcer.

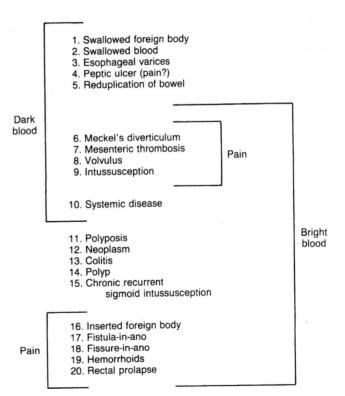

FIG. 1.12. Causes of rectal bleeding in children.

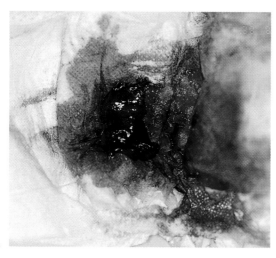
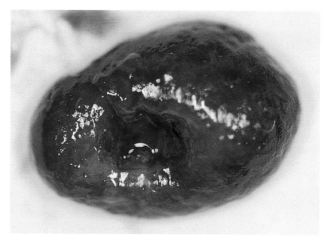

A

B

FIG. 1.13. A: An asymptomatic 17-month-old child passed a "bloody stool" and was referred to the emergency department due to currant jelly stools. **B:** This necrotic juvenile polyp was found in the stool.

Barium studies usually fail to outline a Meckel diverticulum. The imaging modality of choice for the detection of ectopic gastric mucosa in a bleeding Meckel diverticulum is nuclear scintigraphy. A duplication cyst with gastric mucosa shows the same focal accumulation of radionuclide. The accuracy of scintigraphy in the detection of ectopic gastric mucosa in Meckel diverticula is approximately 95%. False-negative results may rarely occur with rapidly bleeding Meckel diverticula and with those diverticula that do not contain gastric mucosa.

Henoch–Schönlein Purpura

Henoch–Schönlein purpura (see Chapter 17, Renal and Electrolyte Emergencies) is a vasculitic disorder that can produce a purpuric rash, joint pain, abdominal pain, or rectal bleeding. Usually there is visible evidence of vasculitis on the skin surface, but a patient initially may have only abdominal pain (Fig. 1.14). Occasionally, a child will develop

a small bowel intussusception from a submucosal hemorrhage that is acting as a lead point.

Intraabdominal Masses

Sacrococcygeal Teratoma

The presacral sacrococcygeal teratoma is the most common tumor of the caudal region in children and is more common in females than in males (4:1 ratio). Tumors in patients beyond neonatal age have a higher incidence of malignancy. Radiography often shows calcifications and a soft-tissue mass. Ultrasonography confirms whether teratomas are cystic, solid, or mixed. Tumors with more solid components are more often malignant than those with more cystic components.

Fecaloma

A lower abdominal mass, particularly one on the left side, is often related to retained stool and is more often associated with

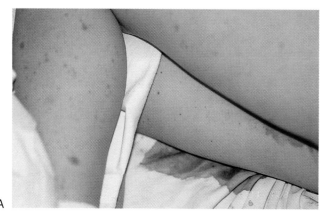
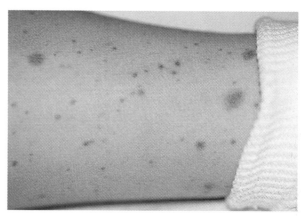

A

B

FIG. 1.14. Henoch–Schönlein purpura. **A:** A 6-year-old boy with mild abdominal pain and rectal bleeding seen here on the bedsheets. **B:** His ankle demonstrates the typical purpuric rash.

functional constipation than with Hirschsprung disease. If a mass is found, a careful review of the bowel habits is important. If an abdominal mass is a fecaloma, a large bolus of stool usually can be felt on rectal examination just inside the anus.

Ovarian Masses

Simple ovarian cysts and solid teratomas are not uncommon and may be asymptomatic even though they have reached a large size. Granulosa cell tumors of the ovary produce precocious puberty because they are hormonally active tumors. They may be malignant. The sudden onset of severe abdominal pain may indicate a torsion of an ovarian mass with resultant infarction. Most ovarian masses are smooth and nontender. Radiographs may show calcification in approximately half of patients with teratomas. Because an occasional ovarian tumor is malignant in children, children with ovarian masses should be promptly evaluated and prepared for surgery.

Omental Cysts

Omental cysts are rare and usually asymptomatic and can reach gigantic size. It is often difficult to differentiate an omental cyst from ascites. Smaller cysts are more mobile and can be pushed freely into all quadrants of the abdomen. If a cyst volvulizes on its pedicle or has bleeding within it, it may cause abdominal pain or tenderness.

Mesenteric Cysts

Mesenteric cysts can occur anywhere in the mesentery but are most common in the mesentery of the colon. They tend to be multilocular and are often discovered during a routine examination or after an episode of abdominal trauma with enlargement from bleeding.

Duplications

GI duplications within the abdomen can occur anywhere along the greater curvature of the stomach, the lesser curvature of the duodenum, or the mesenteric side of either the small or large intestine. Duplications that produce abdominal masses are either noncommunicating (and hence gradually enlarge) or communicating in that their secretory lining has a distal communication with the true lumen of the bowel. Except for the rare occurrence of massive rectal bleeding in a child with a communicating duplication, most duplications do not present as emergencies. Instead, they present in children either as unexplained abdominal masses or with symptoms of intermittent colic resulting from partial obstruction of the true lumen of the adjacent bowel.

Neuroblastoma

Neuroblastoma most often occurs as a tumor in the left or right adrenal gland, but it can develop anywhere along the sympathetic chain or in the pelvis. It has the ability to grow extensively, often crossing the midline of the abdomen and enveloping key vascular and visceral structures. CT is superior to ultrasonography for clearly defining the morphologic details of neuroblastoma, such as calcifications, and the precise extent of tumor by direct spread or lymphatic metastasis.

Wilms Tumor

Wilms tumor is the most common intrarenal tumor seen in children. The tumor can reach a gigantic size before its discovery. Wilms tumor should be considered in any child who has hematuria even if he or she has a history of trauma. A solid renal mass demonstrated by ultrasonography in infants and children is usually a Wilms tumor. Pediatric surgical consultation should be obtained immediately.

Rhabdomyosarcoma

Rhabdomyosarcoma can occur anywhere in the abdomen or pelvis where there is striated muscle. Tumors are particularly common in the pelvis, involving the prostate, uterus or vagina, and retroperitoneal structures. These tumors can reach a large size before they become symptomatic. Modern selective therapy has greatly improved the survival rate of this highly malignant tumor.

Neoplasms of the Liver

Hepatoblastoma is the most common malignant liver tumor, usually presenting in infancy as an asymptomatic abdominal mass. Liver function tests and radiographs can be normal, and CT is necessary for diagnosis. Hepatocellular carcinoma is more rare and presents in older children with abdominal distention, pain, and nausea. Survival depends on both complete resection of the primary tumor before metastases have occurred and intensive prolonged chemotherapy postoperatively.

ABDOMINAL WALL DEFECTS

Inguinal Hernias and Hydroceles

Many infants and children manifest the classic bulge in the inguinal canal that occurs during straining or crying. This is caused by a loop of intestine distending into the hernia sac. Usually, the hernia sac contents reduce into the abdominal cavity when the straining ceases. If the prolapsing loop of intestine becomes entrapped in the hernia sac, an incarceration has occurred. This is a true emergency that could eventually lead to intestinal obstruction and possibly strangulation of the bowel. Elective herniorrhaphy should be done shortly after the hernia is diagnosed.

Epiploceles (Epigastric Hernias)

If a discrete mass occurs intermittently approximately one-third of the distance from the umbilicus to the xiphoid, it is usually the result of a weakness of the linea alba through

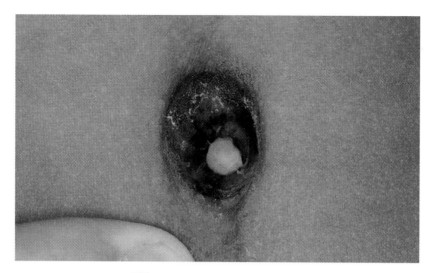

FIG. 1.15. Umbilical granuloma.

which properitoneal fat protrudes. This defect is called an epiplocele. If it becomes excruciatingly tender, it is a sign that fat has become incarcerated in the hernia.

Umbilical Hernias

Umbilical hernias are common in small infants, particularly in African Americans. Fortunately, most of the hernias tend to close spontaneously and only rarely does incarceration occur. Umbilical hernias can be large and unsightly, and families need reassurance that watchful waiting is the best course. However, if the umbilical hernia fails to close by 5 to 6 years of age, surgical repair is indicated. Hernias that have a supraumbilical component tend not to close spontaneously and may be operated on at an earlier time of life.

Other Umbilical Defects

Omphalomesenteric duct remnants may persist in either of two forms. When the duct is patent from the ileum to the umbilicus, there is a release of small bowel contents via an opening in the umbilicus. A second form involves a remnant of the omphalomesenteric duct that contains a secreting mucosal patch that is attached to an opening in the center of the umbilicus. Passage of a sterile blunt probe or instillation of contrast dye under fluoroscopy via the umbilical opening will usually confirm either of these conditions. Once identified, these remnants must be excised surgically. By contrast, some infants present with umbilical granuloma in which an excessive amount of granulation tissue has built up after separation of the umbilical cord (Fig. 1.15). In these patients, no opening in the granulation tissue can be seen or felt by means of a probe. These granulomas are usually best treated by careful application of silver nitrate to the granulation tissue.

If the urachus persists after birth, it can form a urinary fistula that drains at the umbilicus. This problem is ordinarily noted in the newborn period. Older infants or children may present with drainage at the umbilicus caused by persistence of part of the urachus even though connection with the bladder may be obliterated.

Foreign Bodies of the Gastrointestinal Tract

Most swallowed foreign bodies move through the GI tract without complication. Occasionally, a foreign body lodges in the esophagus, necessitating removal. Plain film radiography for a suspected foreign body should focus on the suspected area initially but then expand to include the base of the skull to the anus if the object is not seen. Once an esophageal foreign body has been identified, it should be removed promptly to prevent complications such as ulceration, aspiration, and perforation.

Foreign bodies that reach the stomach, whether pointed or sharp edged, usually pass completely through the intestinal tract and are evacuated. Occasionally, a long, thin foreign body such as a bobby pin may not be able to traverse the turn where the duodenum joins the jejunum at the ligament of Treitz. If a foreign body is trapped in this area, perforation with local or generalized peritonitis may occur. When entrapment occurs anywhere beyond the pylorus, surgical removal is indicated to either prevent or treat local perforation.

SUGGESTED READINGS

Buonomo C. Neonatal gastrointestinal emergencies. *Radiol Clin North Am* 1997;35:845–864.

Forman BP, Leonidas JC, Kronfeld GD. A rational approach to the diagnosis of hypertrophic pyloric stenosis: do the results match the claims. *J Pediatr Surg* 1990;25:262–266.

Garcia Pena BM, Mandl KM, Krauss SJ, et al. Ultrasonography and limited computed tomography in the diagnosis and management of appendicitis in children. *N Engl J Med* 1999;282:1041–46.

Harrington L, Connolly B, Hu, X, et al. Ultrasonographic and clinical predictors of intussusception. *J Pediatr* 1998;132:836–839.

O'Neill JA, et al., eds. *Pediatric surgery.* St. Louis: Mosby. [Chapters on Disorders of rotation and fixation, Hirschsprung disease, Inguinal hernia, Intussusception, and Wilms tumor.]

CHAPTER 2

Allergic/Rheumatologic Emergencies

Editor: Stephen Ludwig

ASTHMA

Clinical Findings

A general guide to several parameters useful for estimating the severity of the episode can be found in Table 2.1. The history should include the duration of the current episode and rapidity of onset, the parent's or patient's subjective assessment of severity, other associated symptoms, and the suspected trigger. The child's current medications should be determined, including details of when the medications were started, the dose, the route, the timing of the last dose, and a history of missed doses from noncompliance or emesis. A history of medications, particularly oral or inhaled steroids in the past 6 months, should be elicited. For children with their first episode of wheezing, the possibility of a foreign body aspiration or another cause of wheezing should be explored.

The physical examination begins immediately with an overall assessment of the child's degree of respiratory distress. Severe retractions, accessory muscle use, nasal flaring, cyanosis, decreased muscle tone, and altered mental status all are indicative of impending or existing respiratory failure and require prompt intervention. The respiratory rate and heart rate should be noted and compared with age-appropriate normals (Table 2.1). The remainder of the respiratory examination includes auscultation for decreased breath sounds, wheezing, rhonchi, and crackles. Crackles can occur and are most often caused by focal areas of atelectasis.

Peak expiratory flow rate can serve as a simple, quantitative, reproducible, and inexpensive measure of airway obstruction in the child with mild to moderate distress. A flow rate of less than 80% of predicted or personal best is considered abnormal, and less than 50% indicates moderate to severe obstruction. Pulse oximetry provides a noninvasive, continuous, and generally valid measure of arterial hemoglobin oxygen saturation (Sao_2). Confirmation of adequate oxygenation is reassuring and obviates arterial blood gas analysis in most mild to moderate exacerbations. Arterial blood gas sampling provides an objective measure of ventilation and oxygenation. It is essential in the evaluation of any child in whom impending or existing respiratory failure is suspected clinically, although it should never delay the initiation of therapy. It should be emphasized that a normal $Paco_2$ of 40 mm Hg in a child with tachypnea or significant respiratory distress may be a sign of impending respiratory failure and requires aggressive management and close monitoring. The role of chest radiographs in the emergency management of acute asthma is not well defined. Typical findings on routine films such as hyperinflation, atelectasis, and peribronchial thickening do not correlate with severity and rarely alter management. Patients for whom a chest radiograph may be of a higher yield include those with failure to respond to therapy, persistence of focal findings after bronchodilator therapy, reduced oxygen saturation after therapy, or clinical suspicion of a complication or a cause of wheezing other than asthma. Radiographic evaluation of the sinuses may be helpful for the child with chronic, persistent wheezing in whom sinusitis is suspected (Fig. 2.1).

The uncommon child taking theophylline may benefit from a theophylline level to help to determine further management. The level should be obtained early in the course of therapy. Serum potassium measurement should be considered in children at risk of hypokalemia secondary to receiving frequent β-agonist therapy.

Complications

The most common pulmonary complication is atelectasis secondary to mucous plugging (Fig. 2.2A). Air leaks that lead to a pneumomediastinum and/or a pneumothorax are potentially life threatening (Fig. 2.2B, C). A pneumothorax should be suspected in any child with a sudden deterioration associated with chest pain, asymmetry of breath sounds, or a shift of the trachea. Cardiac arrhythmias are associated with both adrenergic agents and theophylline. Frequent β-agonist therapy can cause hypokalemia. The syndrome of inappropriate antidiuretic hormone secretion (SIADH) also is a potential, although rare, complication of acute asthma.

TABLE 2.1. *Estimation of severity of acute asthma exacerbation*

Sign/symptom	Mild	Moderate	Severe
Respiratory rate[a]	Normal to 30% increase	30%–50% increase	>50% increase
Alertness	Normal or agitated	Normal or agitated	Agitated to decreased level of consciousness
Dyspnea	Absent or mild; speech normal	Moderate; speaks in phrases; difficulty feeding	Severe; single words or short phrases; refuses feeding
Accessory muscle use	None to mild IC retractions	Moderate IC with TS retraction; use of sternocleidomastoid muscle; chest hyperinflation	Severe IC and TS retraction; nasal flaring; chest hyperinflation
Color	Normal	Pale	Possibly cyanotic
Wheeze	Often end expiratory only	Throughout exhalation	Throughout inhalation and exhalation; breath sounds markedly decreased
Oxygen saturation (in room air)	>95%	91%–95%	<91%
Peak expiratory flow rate[b] (% predicted or personal best)	>80%	50%–80%	<50%
$Paco_2$	<42 mm Hg	<42 mm Hg	≥42 mm Hg

Note: Within each category, the presence of several parameters, but not necessarily all, indicates general classification of exacerbation. Many of these parameters have not been systematically studied, so they serve only as general guides.

[a] Normal rates of breathing (per minute) in awake children of ages 2 to 12 months. Normal pulse rates (per minute) in children ages 1 to 2, 1 to 5, 2 to 8, and 6 to 8 years.

[b] For children at least 5 years of age or older.

IC, intercostal; TS, tracheosternal.

Adapted from Expert Panel Report of the National Heart, Lung, and Blood Institute, 1991 and 1997.

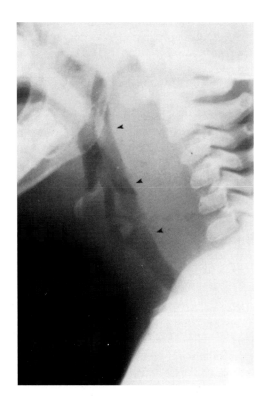

FIG. 2.1. Sinusitis. Bilateral mucosal thickening is noted in both maxillary sinuses (*arrowheads*). This configuration frequently is seen in allergic children. In addition, the ethmoid sinuses, located just along the medial aspect of the orbital rims, also are partially obliterated and involved by inflammatory change. (From Swischuk L. *Emergency radiology of the acutely ill or injured child*, 2nd ed. Philadelphia: Lippincott Williams & Wilkins, 1986:148, with permission.)

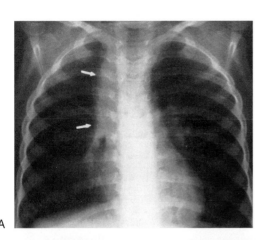

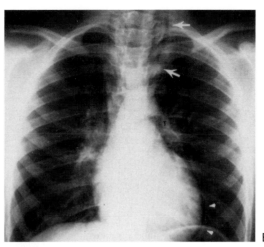

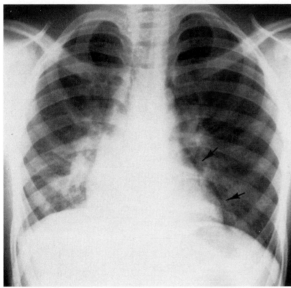

FIG. 2.2. Pulmonary complications. **A:** Sublobar atelectasis. Asthmatic child with acute asthma attack. Note area of apparent consolidation in the right paratracheal region (*arrows*). This represents collapse of one portion of the right upper lobe. A subtler finding assisting interpretation is that the minor fissure is slightly elevated. **B:** Pneumomediastinum. Asthmatic child with pneumomediastinum with air surrounding the small triangular thymus gland (*T*), extending as linear sheaths into the neck and superior mediastinum (*upper arrows*) and extending along the lower left cardiac edge (*lower arrows*). **C:** Medial pneumothorax. Note the thin strip of free air along the left cardiac border (*arrows*). The finding represents a medial pneumothorax and should not be confused with pneumomediastinum or pneumopericardium. (From Swischuk L. *Emergency radiology of the acutely ill or injured child*, 2nd ed. Philadelphia: Lippincott Williams & Wilkins, 1986:63,77,79, with permission.)

Management

Initial Approach

The primary goals in the acute management phase of an asthma exacerbation are to correct hypoxemia and to rapidly reverse airflow obstruction. Supplemental oxygen, repetitive β_2-agonists, and the early addition of systemic corticosteroids achieve this. For children who are discharged, the emergency physician should prescribe an intensified regimen for a minimum of 3 to 5 days and recommend appropriate follow-up so that long-term management issues can be addressed. This section of the chapter presents a stepwise ap-

proach that is summarized in algorithm form in Figure 2.3, with specific dose recommendations in Table 2.2.

All children with acute asthma can be assumed to be hypoxemic unless SaO_2 is measured immediately and indicates otherwise. Hence, unless SaO_2 is greater than 90%, humidified oxygen should be administered immediately. It should be delivered at a flow rate sufficient to eliminate cyanosis and, ideally, to maintain SaO_2 levels higher than 90% (95% in infants).

Repetitive, inhaled β_2-agonists are the mainstay of initial bronchodilator therapy in children. Frequent (every 15 to 30 minutes) doses of nebulized albuterol appear to be effective

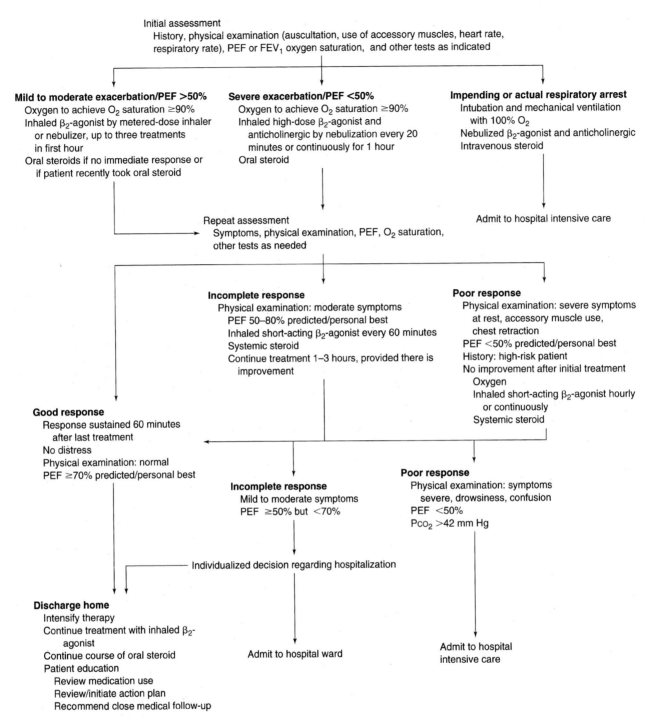

FIG. 2.3. Approach to acute asthma in children. PEF, peak expiratory flow; FEV$_1$, forced expiratory volume in 1 second. (Modified from NHLBI. Highlights of the expert panel report 2: guidelines for the diagnosis and management of asthma. NIH publication no. 97-4051A, 1997, with permission.)

in reversing airway obstruction. Although the ideal dose of albuterol (0.5%) has not been determined, the Expert Panel 2 (National Institutes of Health) recommends 0.15 mg/kg per dose. From a practical standpoint, patients older than 1 year who weigh less than 30 kg should be given 2.5 mg (0.5 mL) and those who weigh more than 30 kg should be given 5 mg (1 mL). A minimum of 1.25 mg (0.25 mL) is used for infants younger than 1 year old. Recent evidence suggests that an albuterol metered-dose inhaler and chamber may be just as effective as nebulized treatments.

Subcutaneous injection of epinephrine or terbutaline remains an acceptable alternative in settings in which nebulized therapy is unavailable or delayed or for the toddler resisting an inhalation treatment. It also may be indicated as initial therapy for the child with severe obstruction, hypoventilation, or apnea in whom the delivery of nebulized medication to the airways is believed to be inadequate. Under these circumstances, the injection can be given simultaneously with the initial aerosol and, if indicated, by mask ventilation during preparation for intubation.

Early treatment of asthma exacerbations with steroids has been shown to prevent progression of airway obstruction, to decrease the need for emergency treatment and hospitalization, and to reduce morbidity. As a rule, almost all children who have had a significant exacerbation ultimately receive steroids. An exception is made for children with mild symptoms who require either no nebulizer treatments or, at worst, one treatment that immediately produces adequate resolution. Exposure to chickenpox in the susceptible host is one of the rare instances in which steroids may need to be avoided acutely. Depending on the level of distress and the child's ability to tolerate oral medications, the dose of corticosteroid is given either intravenously (2 mg/kg methylprednisolone or equivalent; maximum, 125 mg) or by mouth (2 mg/kg prednisone or prednisolone; maximum, 80 mg). Recent studies suggest that nebulized steroids may have a role in the management of acute asthma exacerbations. Children taking inhaled steroids with minor exacerbations may sometimes be adequately managed by doubling their inhaled steroid dose.

TABLE 2.2. *Emergency department acute asthma therapy*

Therapy	Dose	Maximum	Comments	
Oxygen	Maintain Sao2 >90% (>95% of infants)			
Adrenergic agents				
Aerosolized albuterol (0.5%) nebulizer solution	Intermittent; 0.15 mg/kg q 15–20 min in 2 mL normal saline solution × 3, then 0.15–0.3 mg/kg q 1–4 hr	5 mg/dose	2.5 mg minimum Usual dose: <30 kg 2.5 mg 30 kg 5 mg	Continuous: 0.5 15 mg/hr mg/kg/hr
Metered-dose inhaler	4–8 puffs q 20min × 3, then q 1–4hr as needed		Use spacer/holding chamber	
Subcutaneous epinephrine 1:1,000	0.01 mL/kg SC q 15–20 min	0.3–0.5 mL	See text for indications	
Terbutaline (0.1%)	0.01 mL/kg SC q 15–20 min	0.25 mL	See text for indications	
IV terbutaline (0.1%)	Loading dose: 10 μg/kg over 10 min; initial maintenance: 0.4 μg/kg/min		Titrate up by 0.2 μg/kg/min Usual effective range: 3–6 μg/kg/min	
Anticholinergics Ipratropium bromide nebulizer solution (0.25 mg/mL)	0.25 mg q 20 min × 3, then q 2–4 hr as needed	0.5 mg	May mix with same nebulizer as albuterol; should not be used as first-line therapy, should be added to β2-agonist	
Corticosteroids Methylprednisolone	2 mg/kg IV bolus	125 mg		
Prednisone	2 mg/kg orally	80 mg		

q, every; SC, subcutaneously; IV, intravenous.

Ipratropium may be mixed with albuterol and delivered simultaneously. Recommendations vary, but the National Institutes of Health's guidelines suggest 0.25 mg for children (0.5 mg in adolescents and adults) every 20 to 30 minutes mixed with the first three albuterol treatments, then every 2 to 4 hours as needed.

After 2 to 4 hours of frequent bronchodilator treatments and the initiation of corticosteroid therapy, the limit of emergency department management has been reached and a disposition decision should be made. If appropriate resources are available, continued management of the patient in an observation unit or clinical decision unit for as long as 24 hours may avoid the need for hospital admission.

Approach to the Child with Respiratory Failure

The options include continuous nebulized albuterol, intravenous (IV) β_2-agonist therapy, and/or mechanical ventilation. The use of continuous nebulized therapy is well established in the intensive care unit setting and currently is under study in emergency departments. Continuous terbutaline and albuterol have been demonstrated to reverse respiratory failure and to eliminate the need for mechanical ventilation. Albuterol is administered as 0.5 mg/kg per hour (maximum, 15 mg/hr). IV β_2-agonist therapy is an option for children who fail continuous nebulized therapy. In the United States, terbutaline is administered as a 10-mg/kg loading dose over 10 minutes followed by an initial infusion of 0.4 mg/kg per minute. The infusion is titrated up to effect in increments of 0.2 mg/kg per minute while the child is monitored for unacceptable tachycardia. The usual effective range is 3 to 6 mg/kg per minute. If the child continues to deteriorate, intubation and mechanical ventilation should be considered. Many authorities consider ketamine (1 to 2 mg/kg IV) to be the induction agent of choice because of its bronchodilating effects. Agents that may increase bronchospasm through histamine release such as meperidine, morphine, d-tubocurare, and atracurium are best avoided. Volume-controlled ventilation is preferred using larger than average tidal volumes (10 to 20 mL/kg), normal respiratory rates for age, and high flow rates to ensure long expiratory times.

Although IV magnesium sulfate has been studied extensively in adults and appears to improve pulmonary function, there is no consensus regarding its role in the management of asthma exacerbations. A recent study of children with moderate to severe exacerbations showed that the group treated with magnesium (25 mg/kg IV; maximum, 2 g) had greater improvement in forced expiratory volume of 1 second, were less likely to require admission, and had no significant adverse effects compared with the group treated with placebo. This study suggests that IV magnesium may have a role as an adjunct in treatment of children with moderate to severe acute asthma exacerbations.

Disposition

Admission should be considered for children who meet any of the following criteria: (1) persistent respiratory distress, (2) SaO_2 of 91% or less in room air, (3) PEFR less than 50% of predicted levels, (4) inability to tolerate oral medications (i.e., vomiting), (5) previous emergency treatment in the past 24 hours, (6) underlying high risk factors (e.g., congenital heart disease, bronchopulmonary dysplasia, cystic fibrosis, neuromuscular disease), (7) evidence of air leak. Children who also meet the criteria listed in Table 2.3 should be admitted to an intensive care unit.

Discharge Management

In general, if a child already on a regimen of medication has had an exacerbation that required emergency management, this regimen must be intensified, at least for the next 3 to 5 days. Short-course, high-dose oral steroids (i.e., 2 mg/kg prednisone per day to as much as 80 mg per day for 3 to 5 days) should be prescribed and administered for essentially all children who present to the emergency department with a significant exacerbation. In addition, all patients currently taking or who have recently been taking oral or inhaled corticosteroids must be given steroids as part of the acute management of their exacerbation. Children who experience frequent acute exacerbations, nocturnal symptoms, or multiple absences from school may also benefit from the addition of a systematic or inhaled corticosteroid to their regular regimen.

For children who experience their first episode of wheezing or who are not receiving long-term therapy, inhaled albuterol is generally well tolerated in the subacute phase after the acute episodes. Children younger than 5 years old should use a metered-dose inhaler with a spacer and mask or a nebulizer. The use of a spacer device in all children will improve delivery of medications in metered-dose inhalers. If the child is receiving other long-term therapy, such as cromolyn sodium or inhaled steroids, it is important to continue it during acute exacerbations. Table 2.4 lists outpatient treatment options.

TABLE 2.3. *Criteria for admission to the intensive care unit*

Severe respiratory distress
Estimate in severe range after therapy[a]
PaO_2 <60 mm Hg or SaO_2 <90% in 40% O_2
$PaCO_2$ <42 mm Hg
Significant complications
Pneumothorax
Arrhythmia
Theophylline toxicity

[a] See Table 2.1.

TABLE 2.4. *Outpatient asthma therapy*

Medication	Dose	Maximum	Comments
Quick relief β_2-agonists MDI			
Albuterol	2 puffs q 4–6 hr	q 4 hr	Use spacer; may double dose for mild exacerbations; encourage consulting with physician if more frequent use required
Nebulized albuterol	0.05–0.1 mg/kg q 4–6 hr in 2 mL normal saline solution	5.0 mg	1.25 mg minimum; may mix with cromolyn or ipratropium solutions; may double dose for exacerbations
Long-acting β_2-agonists Salmeterol MDI	1–2 puffs q 12 hr		Should not be used for symptom relief or exacerbations
DPI 50 μg/blister Corticosteroids	1 blister q 12 hr		
Oral prednisone, prednisolone	2 mg/kg/d × 3–5 d	60–80 mg/d	May require taper
MDI Beclomethasone Budesonide Flunisolide Fluticasone Triamcinolone	Doses vary greatly depending on severity of chronic asthma; consult with primary care physician or asthma specialist		May consider doubling usual daily dose for minor exacerbation in lieu of systemic steroids; long-term use has adrenal suppressive effect; use spacer to limit local adverse effects
Cromolyn sodium MDI	2 puffs q 6–12 hr		
Nebulized	20 mg q 6–12 hr		
Leukotriene modifiers Zafirlukast, 20-mg tablet	20 mg PO b.i.d.		Age, 12 yr
Zileuton, 300- or 600-mg tablet	600 mg q.i.d.		Age, 12 yr

MDI, metered-dose inhaler; q, every; DPI, dry powder inhaler; PO, orally; b.i.d., twice daily; q.i.d., four times daily.

ANAPHYLAXIS

Clinical Findings

The time between exposure to the inciting agent and onset of symptoms can vary from minutes to hours, although most reactions occur within 1 hour. Although uncommon, some patients experience a biphasic reaction in which symptoms may recur as long as 12 hours after the initial reaction. The signs and symptoms of anaphylaxis vary in both the spectrum and severity of involvement. Reactions may be limited to the skin, as in a mild urticarial reaction, or catastrophically involve multiple systems, leading to shock and death (Fig. 2.4).

In general, systemic reactions include cutaneous involvement such as pruritus, flushing, erythema, urticaria, and, in more severe cases, angioedema (Fig. 2.5). A more detailed discussion of urticaria is found at the end of this section. Mucous membrane involvement may be limited to pruritus and congestion of the eyes, nose, and mouth (Fig. 2.6). Swelling of the lips or tongue can potentially impair swallowing and ventilation.

An immediate life-threatening feature of anaphylaxis is upper airway obstruction that results from edema of the larynx, epiglottis, and other surrounding structures. This may be experienced as subtle discomfort of the throat or as obvious stridor and respiratory distress. Anaphylaxis also can cause lower airway disease secondary to bronchospasm. This leads to findings similar to acute asthma, such as a sense of chest tightness, cough, dyspnea, wheezing, and retractions.

Another potential life-threatening feature of anaphylaxis is cardiovascular collapse and hypotensive shock. Although the mechanisms are not fully understood, these cardiopulmonary manifestations are thought to result from profound vasodilation, increased vascular permeability, capillary leak, and intravascular volume depletion as well as a possible direct toxic effect of circulating mediators. Arrhythmias and electrocardiographic evidence of myocardial ischemia also may be seen.

Gastrointestinal symptoms are relatively common and include nausea, vomiting, diarrhea, and crampy abdominal pain.

Urticaria is a common manifestation of immediate hypersensitivity reactions and several other disease processes (Fig. 2.7). In the patient with acute urticaria from an immunoglobulin E–mediated process, the urticaria may be localized to the area of exposure, such as the area around a sting.

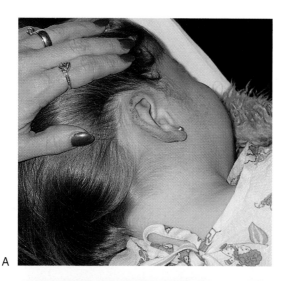

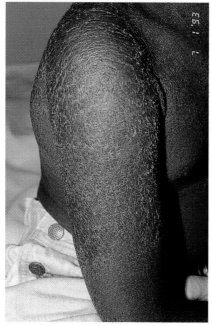

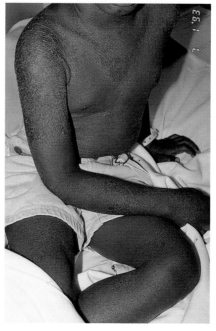

FIG. 2.4. Drug related allergic reactions. **A:** Petechia on ear, a reaction from carbamazepine (Tegretol). **B, C:** Allergic reaction to griseofulvin.

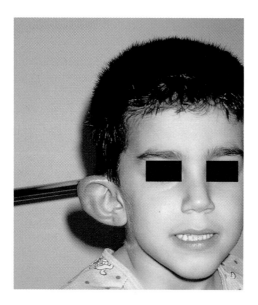

FIG. 2.5. Cutaneous allergic example. Allergic edema/insect bite.

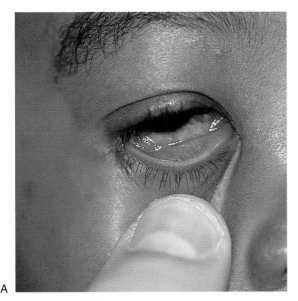

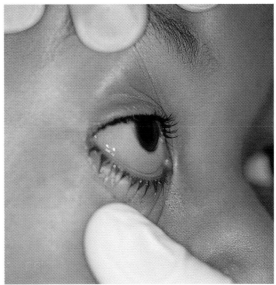

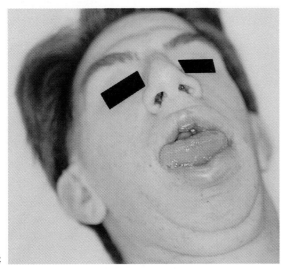

FIG. 2.6. A: Conjunctivitis. **B:** Chemosis. **C:** Facial swelling caused by an allergic reaction.

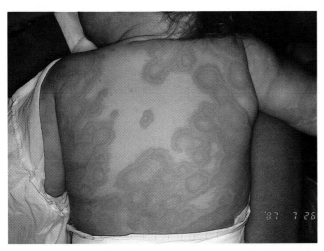

FIG. 2.7. Urticaria.

In addition to the localized urticaria, there may be a systemic reaction. Urticaria may be associated with angioedema, i.e., swelling of the lower dermis and subcutaneous tissues. The angioedema associated with urticaria is pruritic. Angioedema without pruritus usually is secondary to processes other than immediate hypersensitivity. The physical urticarial reactions may be life threatening and should be included in the differential diagnosis of anaphylaxis.

Management

Maintenance of the Airway and Oxygenation

The physician should administer 100% oxygen and/or bag-valve-mask ventilation, as indicated. If there is complete airway obstruction, immediate endotracheal intubation should be attempted. If intubation is unsuccessful, cricothyrotomy is indicated. Rapid administration of epinephrine may lessen the difficulty of airway management. Epinephrine can be administered subcutaneously in the patient with reasonable perfusion (1:1,000, 0.01 mL/kg epinephrine to a maximum of 0.5 mL). If the patient is hypotensive or hypoperfused or if the initial subcutaneous dose is ineffective, the epinephrine should be administered intravenously or through an intraosseous needle as a 1:10,000 solution, 10 g/kg (0.1 mL/kg) over 1 to 2 minutes. In severe cases, this may need to be followed by a continuous epinephrine infusion of 0.1 g/kg per minute, which can be titrated to effect to a maximum of 1.0 g/kg per minute (6 mg epinephrine should be added to 100 mL D5W normal saline solution; 1 g/kg per minute = 1 mL/kg per hour). Bronchospasm should be treated aggressively with supplemental oxygen, β_2-agonists such as albuterol or epinephrine, and corticosteroids, as outlined in the previous section on asthma.

Maintenance of the Circulation

Hypotensive patients should be placed in the Trendelenburg position, and a rapid bolus of 20 mL/kg of a crystalloid solution should be administered immediately and repeated as necessary. Because plasma volume may fall precipitously by 20% to 40%, large amounts of fluid may be necessary. If hypotension persists after epinephrine, a normal saline bolus, and positioning, a continuous infusion of epinephrine should be started as previously described.

Other Therapy

The H_1-receptor antihistamines such as diphenhydramine (1 to 2 mg/kg intramuscularly or intravenously; maximum, 50 mg) are indicated in histamine-mediated allergic reactions. They work synergistically with the epinephrine therapy. Corticosteroids do not take effect during the initial resuscitative phase of anaphylaxis. In significant reactions, however, their early administration may block or reduce the late-phase reactions over the next several hours or days. They can be administered as methylprednisolone 1 to 2 mg/kg intravenously (maximum, 125 mg) or prednisone 1 to 2 mg/kg orally (maximum, 80 mg). Many authorities recommend H_2-blocking antihistamines such as cimetidine (5 mg/kg; maximum, 300 mg) or ranitidine (1 to 2 mg/kg; maximum, 50 mg) in addition to H_1-blocking antihistamines, particularly for more severe reactions.

Management of Limited Reactions

Most children with allergic reactions present with involvement limited to a diffuse pruritic rash, localized swelling, or benign involvement of the mucous membranes. Appropriate management of these children varies according to the specific presentation. Options include subcutaneous epinephrine (e.g., for evolving urticaria), antihistamines, and corticosteroids. Diphenhydramine (5 mg/kg per day divided

every 4 to 6 hours; maximum, 300 mg per day) and hydroxyzine (2 mg/kg per day divided every 4 to 6 hours; maximum, 200 mg per day) are the antihistamines most commonly prescribed for urticaria. In the case of cold urticaria, cyproheptadine (0.25 to 0.5 mg/kg per day divided every 12 hours; maximum, 32 mg per day) is the drug of choice, whereas hydroxyzine is preferred for cholinergic urticaria or most other chronic urticarias.

Disposition

Patients with severe reactions that involve upper airway obstruction or shock generally should be monitored for a minimum of 8 to 24 hours. Children with a history of asthma appear to be at increased risk of delayed and severe reactions and may require prolonged monitoring. Those with less severe manifestations can be discharged home on a course of antihistamines and, in selected cases, corticosteroids. As a rule, therapy initiated in the emergency department should be continued for a minimum of 48 hours. Follow-up with the child's primary care physician also is advised. All children with a history of significant anaphylaxis with an antigen that cannot be avoided totally (e.g., Hymenoptera venom or food) should be instructed to carry a preloaded syringe of epinephrine (EpiPen) to be used in emergencies.

SERUM SICKNESS

Clinical Findings

The reaction is characterized by fever, malaise, and a rash that is most commonly urticarial but also may appear as maculopapular or vasculitic. Other manifestations include arthralgias or arthritis, lymphadenopathy, angioedema, and nephritis. Less common problems include abdominal pain, carditis, anemia, and neuritis. Characteristically, the onset of symptoms occurs 7 to 14 days after the primary exposure. If there has been prior sensitization, however, reexposure can result in onset of a few days.

Examination of the skin may reveal a maculopapular eruption, urticaria, or the palpable purpura of a cutaneous vasculitis (Fig. 2.8). Painful angioedema is commonly present.

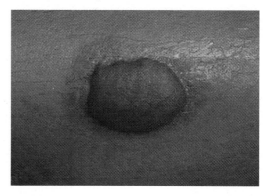

FIG. 2.8. Vasculitis. Hemorrhagic bulla in patient with vasculitis.

TABLE 2.5. *Possible laboratory evaluation of serum sickness[a]*

Blood tests
  Erythrocyte sedimentation rate
  Complete blood count with differential
  CH_{50}, C3, C4
  Blood, urea, nitrogen; creatinine
  Antinuclear antibody
  Rheumatoid factor
  Hepatic enzymes
  Hepatitis B screen
  Heterophil antibody
  Immune complex assay
Other ancillary tests
  Urinalysis
  Electrocardiogram
  Stool Hematest
  Computed tomography scan

[a] Laboratory evaluation should be tailored for each individual patient as noted in text.

Generalized lymphadenopathy often occurs. In more severe reactions, the joints show erythema, warmth, and effusion. Wheezes may be appreciated on auscultation of the lungs, and a pericardial friction rub may be audible if pericarditis is present. The liver and spleen often enlarge. Rarely, neurologic deficits occur secondary to a vasculitis of the central nervous system.

Table 2.5 provides a list of other studies that may be indicated for individual patients with immune complex–mediated disease. The erythrocyte sedimentation rate may be elevated. A complete blood count and differential may reveal leukopenia or leukocytosis. The C3, C4, and CH_{50} may decrease because of complement activation. Stool Hematest should be performed, and an echocardiogram should be considered for patients with abdominal pain or other symptoms involving the gastrointestinal tract. If carditis is suspected, a screening electrocardiogram should be performed. Severe headache or focal neurologic deficits are indications for a computed tomography scan.

Management

If possible, the offending antigen should be eliminated. Pharmacologic management usually involves one or more of the following: antihistamines, nonsteroidal antiinflammatory drugs (NSAIDs), and corticosteroids. Pruritus, rash, and angioedema can be managed with an antihistamine such as hydroxyzine (2 mg/kg per day divided every 6 to 8 hours; maximum, 200 mg per day). Although experience in the treatment of serum sickness is limited, use of the second-generation nonsedating antihistamines may also be considered (Table 2.6). Urticarial lesions and angioedema that evolve rapidly may respond acutely to subcutaneous epinephrine (1:1,000, 0.01 mL/kg subcutaneously; maximum, 0.30 mL) and/or longer acting Sus-Phrine (0.005 mL/kg subcutaneously; maximum, 0.15 mL). Mild joint involvement and/or fever often improve with use of an NSAID such as ibuprofen (30 to 50 mg/kg per day divided every 6 to 8 hours; maximum, 3.2 g per day). In more severe disease or after failure to respond to these measures, a burst of corti-

TABLE 2.6. *Emergency department management of allergic rhinitis*

Medication	Dose	Comments
Antihistamines		
First generation		
Chlorpheniramine maleate	0.35 mg/kg q 6–12 hr	Sedation, anticholinergic effects;
Brompheniramine maleate	depending on formulation	maximum; 24 mg/d
Second generation (nonsedating)		
Claritin (loratadine)	<30 kg 10 mg qd	≥3 yr
10-mg tablet or 10 mg/10 mL syrup		
Claritin-D		
12-hr (5 mg loratadine/120 mg pseudoephedrine)	1 tablet b.i.d.	≥12 yr
24-hr (10 mg loratadine/240 mg pseudoephedrine)	1 tablet qd	
Allegra (fexofenadine)		
60-mg capsules	1 capsule b.i.d.	≥12 yr
Zyrtec (cetirizine)		
5- or 10-mg tablets	2–6 yr: 5 mg/d	±sedating, FDA approved ≥2 yr
5 mg/5 mL syrup	6–12 yr: 5–10 mg/d	
Decongestants		
Oral		
Pseudoephedrine	4 mg/kg/d q 6–8 hr	
Topical		
Oxymetazoline	Age 2–5 yr: 0.025%; >6 yr: 0.05%; 2–3 drops each nostril b.i.d.	Limit use to >5 d to avoid rebound congestion

q, every; qd, every day; b.i.d., twice daily; FDA, U.S. Food and Drug Administration.

costeroids may be indicated. This involves the use of 1 to 2 mg/kg prednisone per day in divided doses for 7 to 10 days, followed by a taper for 3 to 4 weeks (maximum, 80 mg per day). In life-threatening serum sickness with significant circulating immune complexes, plasmapheresis may play a role, but this procedure has not been used extensively for treatment of this disease. Most children with serum sickness can be managed as outpatients with close follow-up by their primary care physicians. Children with more severe involvement may benefit from hospitalization.

ALLERGIC RHINITIS

Clinical Findings

The classic symptoms of allergic rhinitis include nasal congestion, paroxysmal sneezing, pruritus of the nose and eyes, and watery, profuse rhinorrhea. Other complaints may include noisy breathing, snoring, repeated throat clearing or cough, itching of the palate and throat, popping of the ears, and ocular complaints such as redness, itching, and tearing. The physical examination is variable but may reveal the gaping look of a mouth breather, dark discoloration of the infraorbital ridge caused by venous congestion "allergic shiners", and a transverse external nasal wrinkle secondary to chronic rubbing of the nose "allergic salute". Intranasal findings are variable. The mucosa often is edematous and may appear pale or violaceous. The nasal secretions may be clear, mucoid, or opaque.

Management

Recognizing that long-term therapy must be highly individualized, the emergency physician will generally limit interventions to those that safely provide rapid, symptomatic relief and then refer the child to the primary care physician for long-term therapy. In addition, topical corticosteroids, first-line therapy for chronic allergic rhinitis, may require as long as 2 weeks to achieve maximal relief. Rapid relief can generally be achieved by prescribing an antihistamine (Table 2.6). The first-line approach for patients who require long-term therapy is topical corticosteroids (Table 2.7) with or without a second-generation oral antihistamine. For completeness, other categories of topical treatment are also listed in Table 2.7. Children with significant ocular symptoms may also benefit from topical ophthalmic treatment (Table 2.8).

RHEUMATOLOGIC EMERGENCIES

Juvenile Rheumatoid Arthritis

A variety of demographic and clinical features may accompany the arthritis of JRA, so the condition has been divided into subtypes based on these factors and on the pattern of the

TABLE 2.7. *Topical treatment for allergic rhinitis*

Trade name	Generic name	Dose	Age (yr)
Corticosteroids			
Vancenase AQ (84 μg)	Beclomethasone (aqueous: 84 μg/spray)	1–2 sprays each nostril qd	≥.6
Vancenase AQ	Beclomethasone (aqueous: 42 μg/spray)	1–2 sprays each nostril b.i.d.	≥.6
Vancenase pocket inhaler	Beclomethasone (42 μg/puff)	1 spray each nostril t.i.d.	≥.6
Beconase	Beclomethasone (42 μg/spray)	1 spray each nostril t.i.d.	≥.6
Beconase AQ	Beclomethasone (aqueous: 42 μg/spray)	1–2 sprays each nostril b.i.d.	≥.6
Rhinocort	Budesonide (32 μg/actuation)	2 sprays each nostril b.i.d. or 2–4 sprays each nostril qd	≥.6
Flonase	Fluticasone (50 μg/spray)	1–2 sprays each nostril qd	≥.12
Nasacort	Triamcinolone (55 μg/puff)	2 sprays each nostril qd	≥.6
Nasacort AQ	Triamcinolone (55 μg/spray)	2 sprays each nostril qd	≥.12
Nasarel	Flunisolide	2 sprays each nostril b.i.d.	≥.6
Nasonex	Mometasonefuroate (50 μg/spray)	2 sprays each nostril qd	≥.12
Others			
Nasalcrom	Cromolyn (mast-cell stabilizer)	1 spray each nostril q 4–8 hr	≥.6
Astelin	Azelastine (137 μg/spray) (antihistamine)	2 sprays each nostril b.i.d.	≥.12

qd, every day; b.i.d., twice daily; t.i.d., three times daily.

TABLE 2.8. *Ophthalmic drops*

Trade name	Generic name	Category	Dose	Age (yr)
Naphcon-A	Naphazoline and pheniramine	Antihistamine-decongestant	1–2 drops q.i.d.	≥.6
Livostin	Levocabastine	Antihistamine	1–2 drops q.i.d.	≥.12
Alomide	Lodoxamide tromethamine	Mast-cell stabilizer	1–2 drops q.i.d.	≥.2
Patanol	Olopatadine	Mast-cell stabilizer and antihistamine	1–2 drops b.i.d.	≥.3
Acular	Ketorolac tromethamine	NSAID	1–2 drops q.i.d.	≥.12

q.i.d., four times daily; b.i.d., twice daily. NSAID, nonsteroidal antiinflammatory drug.

disease during the first 6 months after onset. Until better means of classifying and distinguishing these subtypes of JRA become available, what is likely to be several discrete conditions will continue to be grouped based on purely clinical features (Fig. 2.9, Table 2.9).

NSAIDs are now the mainstay of therapy for children with JRA (Table 2.10). For children who respond inadequately to NSAIDs, so-called disease-modifying antirheumatic drugs are generally added to the regimen. Several agents, including sulfasalazine, hydroxychloroquine, and methotrexate, are available.

Corticosteroids must be used judiciously in JRA because of the significant toxicity associated with their use. Systemic steroids are typically reserved for children with severe cardiac or pulmonary symptoms (Fig. 2.10), during brief flare-ups of severe arthritis, or while waiting for slower-acting agents to take effect. Topical steroids are also effective for localized manifestations of JRA. Intraarticular steroids may be used in patients with pauciarthritis or in children with polyarticular disease in whom selected joints require particularly aggressive management. Ocular steroids are the linchpin of therapy for iridocyclitis.

Patients with JRA may develope a multitude of complications that require timely diagnosis and appropriate therapy as outlined for many in Table 2.11.

Iridocyclitis (inflammation of the iris and ciliary body) (Fig. 2.11) occurs in approximately 10% to 20% of all children with JRA. Acute iridocyclitis is characterized by

TABLE 2.9. *Subgroups of juvenile rheumatoid arthritis*

Subgroup-positive	At onset % of JRA	Gender ratio	Age at onset	Joints affected	Serologic and genetic test	Extraarticular manifestations	Prognosis
Rheumatoid-polyarticular	15%	90% female	Late childhood	Any joints, especially hands, wrists	ANA 75%, RF 100%	Low-grade, fever, anemia, malaise, rheumatoid nodules	>50% severe arthritis
Rheumatoid-negative polyarticular	20%	70% female	Younger onset	Any joints	ANA 50%, RF negative	Low-grade fever, mild anemia malaise, growth retardation	20%–40% severe arthritis
Type I pauciarticular	45%	80% female	Early childhood	Few large joints (hips and sacroiliac joints spared)	ANA 50% RF negative	Few constitutional complaints, chronic iridocyclitis in 50%	Severe arthritis uncommon; 10%–20% ocular damage from iridocyclitis if untreated
Type II pauciarticular	5%	90% male	Late childhood	Few large joints (hip and sacroiliac involvement common)	ANA negative, RF negative, HLA-B27, 75%	Few constitutional complaints, acute iridocyclitis in 5%–10% during childhood	Clinically similar to spondyloarthritis
Systemic onset	20%	65% female	Any age	Any joints	ANA negative, RF negative	High fever, rash, organomegaly, polyserositis, leukocytosis, growth retardation	30% severe arthritis

ANA, antinuclear antibody; RF, rheumatoid factor; HLA-B27, histocompatibility antigen B27.
Modified from Schaller JG. In: Franklin EC, ed. *Clinical immunology update.* New York: Elsevier-North Holland, 1979.

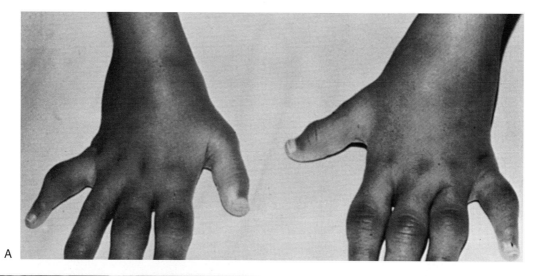

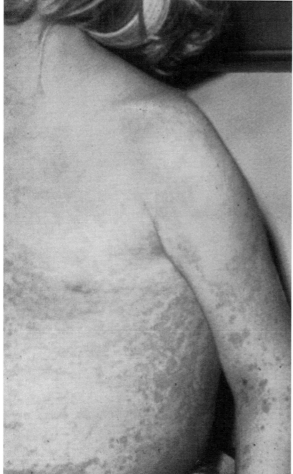

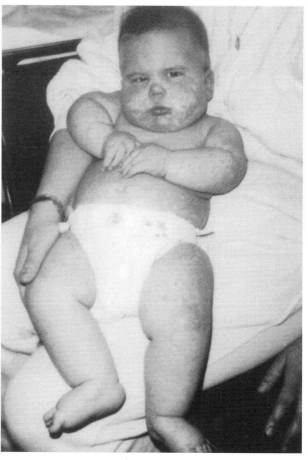

FIG. 2.9. Juvenile rheumatoid arthritis (JRA) subtype examples. **A:** Symmetric involvement of large and small joints of the hands in a child with polyarticular arthritis. **B:** Macular rash in a child with systemic type of JRA. **C:** The florid erythematous maculopapular rash of a child with systemic JRA. This rash appeared with fever (daily spike to 39.4°C or 103°F) and then faded. (Part C from Koopman W. *Arthritis and allied conditions: a textbook of rheumatology*, 14th ed. Philadelphia: Lippincott Williams & Wilkins, 2001:1280, with permission.)

CHAPTER 2: ALLERGIC/RHEUMATOLOGIC EMERGENCIES / 29

TABLE 2.10. *Nonsteroidal antiinflammatory drugs*

Drug	Dosing frequency	Dose range	Side effects
Ibuprofen (Motrin, Advil, Pediaprofen)	t.i.d.–q.i.d.	Antiinflammatory doses are 20–40 mg/kg/d	Gastric irritation, chemical hepatitis
Indomethacin	t.i.d.	Start at 0.5 mg/kg/d; increase to 2.5 mg/kg/d	Gastric irritation, headache, hematuria
Naproxen (Narosyn)	b.i.d.	10–20 mg/kg/d; maximal daily dose, 1,000 mg	Gastric irritation, behavioral changes, headache, rash
Tolmetin sodium (Tolectin)	t.i.d.–q.i.d.	Start at 15 mg/kg/d; increase to 30 mg/kg/d; maximal daily dose, 1,800 mg	Gastric irritation, headache, hematuria

t.i.d., three times daily; b.i.d., twice daily.

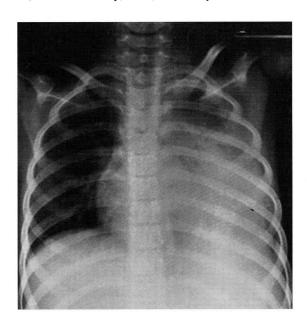

FIG. 2.10. Pericardial and pleural effusions in a child with systemic type of juvenile rheumatoid arthritis.

TABLE 2.11. *Complications in juvenile rheumatoid arthritis*

Complication	Symptoms and signs	Laboratory	Treatment[a]
Fever (>38.5°C)	Fatigue, malaise	CBC, U/A, ESR, appropriate cultures, chest radiograph	NSAID (prednisone 0.5–2 mg/kg/d)
Pericarditis	Fever, chest pain, dyspnea (possibly asymptomatic), friction rub, tachycardia, weak pulse, distended neck veins, distant heart sounds, hepatomegaly	Chest radiograph, ECG, echocardiogram, CBC, ESR, ANA, pericardiocentesis	NSAID (prednisone 2 mg/kg/d), pericardiocentesis as needed
Myocarditis	Tachycardia out of proportion to fever, arrhythmias	Chest radiograph, ECG, echocardiogram, CBC, ESR	Prednisone (2 mg/kg/d); diuretics
C-spine atlantoaxial subluxation	Neck stiffness, headache, torticollis, decreased range of movement, paresthesias	Lateral neck radiograph in flexion/extension, laminograms, CT scan	Cervical collar, surgical stabilization (rarely)
Pleural effusion	Dyspnea, fever, chest pain, decreased breath sounds	Chest radiograph, CBC, ANA, ESR, thoracentesis-cell count, Gram stain, protein, glucose, culture	NSAID (prednisone (2 mg/kg/d), oxygen, thoracentesis as needed
Cricoarytenoid arthritis	Hoarseness, inspiratory stridor, sore throat, ear pain, air hunger	Direct laryngoscopy	Prednisone (2 mg/kg/d), intubation as needed
Macrophage activation syndrome	Fever, lethargy, stupor, coma	DIC, hepatitis	Methyprednisolone (30 mg/kg intravenously), occasionally cyclosporine

[a] Treatment regimens assume that an infectious cause has been excluded.

CBC, complete blood count; U/A, urinalysis; ESR, erythrocyte sedimentation rate; NSAID, nonsteroidal antiinflammatory drug; ECG, electrocardiogram; ANA, antinuclear antibody; CT, computed tomography; DIC, disseminated intravascular coagulation.

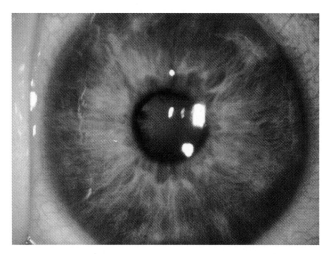

FIG. 2.11. Chronic changes in an eye with juvenile rheumatoid arthritis iritis: posterior synechiae (iris–lens adhesions at pupil margin); iris bombe (shallowing of the anterior chamber caused by blockage of aqueous flow from posterior chamber through pupil); secondary cataract. (From Hiles DA. Slide atlas of pediatric physical diagnosis. In: Zitelli BJ, Davis HW, eds. *Pediatric ophthalmology*. New York: Gower Medical, 1987:17.15, with permission.)

sudden onset of redness, tearing, pain, and photophobia, and urgent management is crucial. Consultation with an ophthalmologist is essential. The usual treatment includes topical corticosteroids and mydriatics.

In a patient known to have JRA who is taking antiinflammatory medication, acute swelling with pain and limitation of range of movement of a single joint raises a major management problem (Fig. 2.12). The differential diagnosis in this situation includes an acute flare-up of JRA versus infectious arthritis, and careful attention to physical examination and historical features are essential to avoid misdiagnosis.

If infection cannot be excluded with confidence, joint fluid must be aspirated, and the fluid sent for cell count, Gram stain, and culture. If there is any doubt about the diagnosis, it is best to obtain a blood culture and to initiate treatment for septic arthritis. For the acute swelling and pain in a single joint as a result of JRA, resting for 2 to 3 days and splinting the involved joint may be adequate. Local injection of the joint with a topical steroid preparation such as triamcinolone hexacetamide is sometimes indicated after infection has been excluded.

Almost all drugs used for the treatment of JRA have the potential for serious toxicity. If a child with JRA is being treated and develops a new symptom, drug toxicity must always be considered as one of the possible causes. Table 2.10 lists the common adverse reactions reported with NSAIDs.

Despite its favorable therapeutic profile, methotrexate is an antimetabolite with the potential to cause oral ulcers, nausea, and abdominal pain. Children must be monitored regularly for evidence of hepatic toxicity, and persistent elevation of hepatic transaminases identifies those at risk of

hepatic fibrosis or cirrhosis. Methotrexate may also cause lymphopenia, especially with prolonged use, or even pancytopenia caused by bone marrow suppression.

Sulfasalazine is a sulfa drug, and its most severe toxicity is typical of this class of medications. Headache and gastrointestinal upset, especially with preparations that are not enterically coated, are the most common side effects. Rarer, although more concerning, are bone marrow suppression, agranulocytosis, photosensitive eruptions, and hypersensitivity reactions, including Stevens–Johnson syndrome (Fig. 2.13).

Antimalarial agents such as hydroxychloroquine must be administered judiciously because they can cause irreversible ocular toxicity at high doses. Even at lower doses, children may develop rashes, gastric upset, or reversible visual disturbances secondary to altered accommodation. Finally, children with glucose-6-phosphate deficiency who receive hydroxychloroquine may develop hemolytic anemia, especially during intercurrent infections.

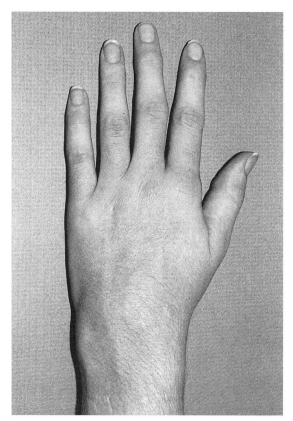

FIG. 2.12. Fusiform swelling and erythema about the proximal interphalangeal joints, most marked in the long finger. Swelling at the metacarpophalangeal joints has caused loss of definition of joint margins. The extensor carpi ulnaris tendon sheath (sixth dorsal compartment of the wrist) has synovial thickening and swelling. (From Koopman W. *Arthritis and allied conditions: a textbook of rheumatology*, 14th ed. Philadelphia: Lippincott Williams & Wilkins, 2001:1157, with permission.)

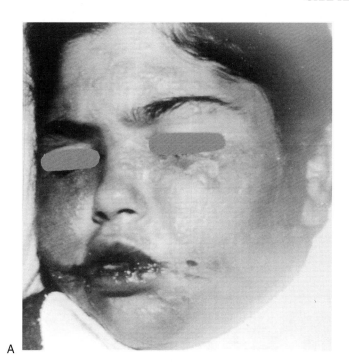

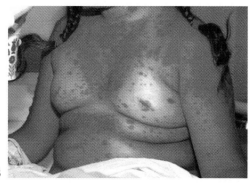

FIG. 2.13. Stevens–Johnson syndrome. **A:** Adolescent with Stevens–Johnson syndrome secondary to sulfonamides. Note the involvement of mucous membranes of the mouth. **B:** Same child. Note the distribution of lesions.

Systemic Lupus Erythematosus

The onset of systemic lupus erythematosus (SLE) may be insidious or acute. The initial presentation usually includes constitutional features such as fever, malaise, and weight loss, in addition to features of specific organ involvement such as rash (Fig. 2.14), pericarditis, arthritis, and seizures. Because virtually any part of the body may be affected, SLE may present with a bewildering variety of signs and symptoms.

Arthritis in SLE is usually symmetric, involving both large and small joints. Swollen joints may be painful but are usually not erythematous. Patients may lose function because of tendon involvement, but the erosive synovial proliferation seen in JRA is uncommon.

Cutaneous lesions are present in more than 85% of patients with SLE. The typical malar erythematous rash with butterfly distribution occurs in approximately half of pa-

tients at the time of diagnosis (Fig. 2.15A). Vasculitic skin lesions over the extensor surface of the forearm and on the fingertips are reported in approximately 20% of patients. These lesions are tender and may ulcerate. Nodules are less common. Mucosal lesions (macular and ulcerative) may involve the nose or mouth, particularly the palate, and are usually painless (Fig. 2.15B). Rarer types of mucocutaneous lesions in SLE include livedo reticularis, urticaria, erythema multiforme, and alopecia (Fig. 2.16).

Patients with mild disease (fever and/or arthritis) without nephritis generally receive one of the NSAIDs (Table 2.10). Severe systemic features usually require treatment with oral or IV corticosteroids, in divided doses three or four times daily in the most florid cases. As disease activity subsides, steroids may be carefully tapered; tapering too rapidly often results in a flare-up of the disease process.

Patients with life-threatening disease, particularly those with severe renal or central nervous system involvement, may require so-called pulse doses of corticosteroids (30 mg/kg IV methylprednisolone per day), plasmapheresis, or an immunosuppressive agent (especially azathioprine or cyclophosphamide). Symptomatic management may be necessary for the treatment of seizures, psychosis, or acute renal failure. Most patients also receive hydroxychloroquine, which has been shown to prolong disease-free remissions once signs and symptoms of active lupus are controlled. In any event, close follow-up is mandatory to detect clinical and serologic clues to exacerbations as rapidly as possible and to monitor drug toxicity. Finally, as with all chronic diseases, total management should include emotional support for patients and their families.

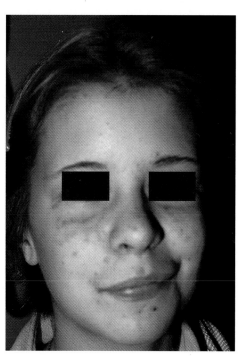

FIG. 2.14. Malar butterfly rash characteristic of systemic lupus erythematosus.

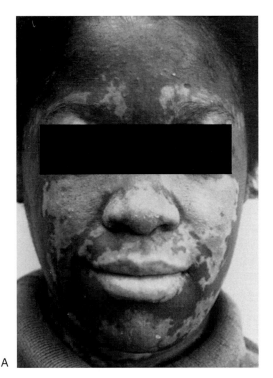

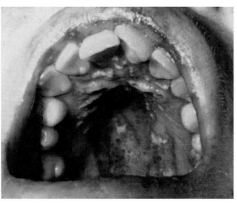

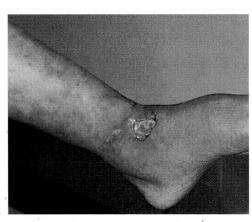

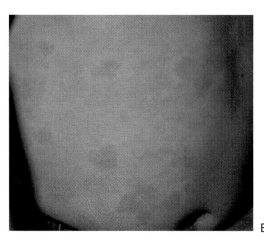

FIG. 2.15. Cutaneous lesions in systemic lupus erythematosus. **A:** Adolescent girl with discoid lesions in malar distribution. **B:** Mucosal lesions (macules and ulcers) of the palate in an adolescent girl with active systemic lupus erythematosus.

FIG. 2.16. Rarer types of mucocutaneous lesions in systemic lupus erythematosus (SLE). **A:** Livedo reticularis and ulceration of the leg in a patient with SLE and high-titer IgG anticardiolipin antibodies. **B:** Urticarial vasculitis in a patient with SLE. These urticaria-like lesions differ from true urticaria in that they produce pain and burning rather than itching, last longer than 24 hours, and heal with residual bruising, hyperpigmentation, or telangiectasia. The urticarial vasculitis lesions seen in patients with SLE are clinically indistinguishable from urticarial vasculitis lesions seen in patients without SLE. (From Wallace DJ, Hahn BH, Dubois EL. *Dubois' lupus erythematosus*, 5th ed. Philadelphia: Lippincott Williams & Wilkins, 605, with permission.)

TABLE 2.12. *Criteria for classification of systemic lupus erythematosus*

Criterion	Definition
Malar rash	Fixed erythema, flat or raised, over the malar eminences, tending to spare the nasolabial folds
Discoid rash	Erythematosus raised patches with adherent keratotic scaling and follicular plugging; atrophic scarring may occur in older lesions
Photosensitivity	Skin rash as a result of unusual reaction to sunlight, by patient history or physician observation
Oral ulcers	Oral or nasopharyngeal ulceration, usually painless, observed by a physician
Arthritis	Nonerosive arthritis involving two or more peripheral joints characterized by tenderness, swelling, or effusion
Serositis	Pleuritis if convincing history of pleuritic pain or rub heard by a physician or evidence of pleural effusion or pericarditis documented by electrocardiogram, rub, or evidence of pericardial effusion on echocardiography
Renal disorder	Persistent proteinuria >0.5 g/d or >3 if quantitation not performed or cellular casts, may be red cell, hemoglobin, granular, tubular, or mixed
Neurologic disorder	Seizures or psychosis in the absence of offending drugs or known metabolic derangements (uremia, ketoacidosis, or electrolyte imbalance)
Hematologic disorder	Hemolytic anemia with reticulocytosis or leukopenia (<4,000/mm^3 total on two or more occasions) or lymphopenia (<1,500/mm^3 on two or more occasions) or thrombocytopenia (<100,000/mm^3 in the absence of offending drugs)
Immunologic disorders	Positive antiphospholipid antibody or anti-DNA antibody to native DNA in abnormal titer or anti-Sm, presence of antibody to Sm nuclear antigen or false-positive serologic test for syphilis known to be positive for at least 6 mo and confirmed by *Treponema pallidum* immobilization or fluorescent treponemal antibody absorption test
Antinuclear antibody	An abnormal titer of antinuclear antibody by immunofluorescence or an equivalent assay at any time and in the absence of drugs known to be associated with drug-induced lupus syndrome

Management of Complications and Emergencies

Table 2.12 and Table 2.13 summarizes the myriad complications that plague patients with SLE, including clinical manifestations, laboratory findings, and initial treatment.

Juvenile Dermatomyositis, Scleroderma, and Polyarteritis Nodosa

The complications and treatment of dermatomyositis (Table 2.14), scleroderma (Table 2.15), and polyarteritis nodosa (Table 2.16) are summarized (Figs. 2.17 and 2.18).

Kawasaki Disease

Kawasaki disease is a clinical syndrome diagnosed based on fever and four of five signs of mucocutaneous inflammation (Table 2.17). These guidelines were established by Tomisaku Kawasaki in 1967 and remain the sine qua non for diagnosing Kawasaki disease. Nonetheless, as with all clinical criteria, these should be regarded as imperfect guidelines with less than 100% sensitivity and specificity. Children who do not meet criteria may indeed have Kawasaki disease, and some children with other conditions may nonetheless manifest five or six criteria of Kawasaki disease.

Fever is probably the most consistent manifestation of Kawasaki disease. A diagnosis of Kawasaki disease should be considered in all children with prolonged, unexplained fever, irritability, and laboratory signs of inflammation, especially in the presence of mucocutaneous inflammation. Conversely, the diagnosis must be suspect in the absence of fever (Fig. 11.69).

The remaining cardinal manifestations of Kawasaki disease vary considerably in frequency. As many as half of the children with Kawasaki disease do not have cervical lymphadenopathy, especially children younger than 2 years of age. When present, lymphadenopathy tends to involve the anterior cervical nodes overlying the sternocleidomastoid muscle. Diffuse lymphadenopathy, as well as other signs of reticuloendothelial involvement such as splenomegaly, should prompt a search for an alternative diagnosis.

Bilateral, nonexudative conjunctivitis is present in more than 90% of patients. A predominantly bulbar injection typically begins within days of the onset of fever, and eyes eventually develop a brilliant erythema, which spares the limbus. Children are also commonly photophobic, and 80% of patients have evidence of anterior uveitis during the first week of illness. Consequently, in ambiguous cases, slit-lamp examination may be helpful in confirming a diagnosis of Kawasaki disease.

Cracked, red lips and a strawberry tongue (Fig. 2.19A) are characteristic of the mucositis typically seen during the first week of Kawasaki disease. Discrete oral lesions, such as vesicles or ulcers and tonsillar exudate, suggest a viral or bacterial infection rather than Kawasaki disease. The cutaneous manifestations of Kawasaki disease are polymorphous. The rash typically begins as perineal erythema and desquamation (Fig. 2.19B), followed by macular, morbilliform, or targetoid lesions of the trunk and extremities. Vesicular or bullous lesions are rare. Changes in the extremities are generally the last clinical manifestation of Kawasaki disease to develop. Children demonstrate an indurated edema of the dorsum of their hands and feet, and a diffuse

TABLE 2.13. *Complications of systemic lupus erythematosus*

Complication	Symptoms and signs	Laboratory	Treatment[a]
Fever	Malaise	CBC, urinalysis, ESR, anti-DNA antibodies, CH_{50}, C3, cultures (blood, urine, CSF, stool, and appropriate secretions), chest radiograph, gallium scan	Prednisone (1–2 mg/kg/d)
Infection	Fever, headache, seizure, cough, sputum, skin lesions, arthritis, disease flare, weight loss	Same as above	Intravenous antibiotics (broad spectrum), reevaluate prednisone dose
Renal disease	Dehydration, fever, weight gain, hypertension, decreased urine output	Urinalysis, urine culture, 24-hr urine protein, serum creatinine, creatinine clearance, anti-DNA, CH_{50}, C3, C4, CBC, ESR, platelets, electrolytes, BUN	Prednisone pulse therapy (as needed), cytotoxic agents (azathioprine PO or cyclophosphamide PO or IV pulse), plasmapheresis
Hemolytic anemia	Fatigue, malaise, pallor, dyspnea, edema	CBC, Coombs, reticulocyte count, haptoglobin, peripheral smear, total bilirubin	Prednisone (2 mg/kg/d), transfusion, if acute emergency
Central nervous system	Seizures, coma, cranial nerve palsies, papilledema, hypertension	EEG, MRI, CT scan, CSF, opening pressure, cell count, Gram and special stains, cultures	ICU admission, prednisone (2 mg/kg/d) or pulse therapy, plasmapheresis, cytoxic agents
Pleural effusion	Fever, chest pain, dyspnea, decreased breath sounds, splinting	Chest radiograph, thoracentesis, cell count, Gram stain, protein, glucose, cultures, cytology	Thoracentesis, if indicated, oxygen, prednisone, cytotoxic agents
Peritonitis	Abdominal pain, fever, vomiting, diarrhea, tenderness, rigidity, hypoactive bowel sounds, melena	Radiograph (abdominal flat plate, cross-table, upright, and/or lateral decubitus), peritoneal aspiration, cell count, special stains, cultures, CBC, electrolytes, ESR, ANA, test for occult blood in gastric contents and stool, nuclear scan	Surgical consult, NPO, IV hydration, nasogastric tube, antacids, transfusion prednisone, interventional radiography (if available)
Pancreatitis	Same	Serum amylase, amylase clearance ratio	IV hydration, NPO, adjust steroid dose, hyperalimentation
Pericarditis	Fever, chest pain, distended neck veins, decreased heart sounds, hepatomegaly	Chest radiograph, ECG, two-dimensional echocardiogram, CBC, ESR, blood culture, ANA	NSAIDs (prednisone 2 mg/kg/d), pericardiocentesis as needed
Raynaud's phenomenon	Triple color change of fingers and/or toes, pain, swelling in digits	CBC, ESR, ANA, cryoglobulins, Doppler flow studies	Protection from cold, biofeedback, analgesia, prednisone, calcium channel blockers, sympathetic ganglion block
Ocular	Blurring or loss of vision headache	Funduscopic examination, CT scan	LP (caution), prednisone
Traverse myelitis	Paraplegia, paraparesis, pain, sensory level	CT, MRI, LP (once epidural abscess excluded), antiphospholipid antibody, lupus anticoagulant	Pulse dose methylprednisolone, cytotoxic agents, anticoagulation

[a] Treatment regimens (except for infectious category) assume that an infectious etiology has been excluded.

CBC, complete blood count; ESR, erythrocyte sedimentation rate; CSF, cerebrospinal fluid; BUN, blood urea nitrogen; PO, orally; IV, intravenous; EEG, encephalogram; MRI, magnetic resonance imaging; CT, computed tomography; ICU, intensive care unit; ANA, antinuclear antibody; NPO, nothing by mouth; ECG, electrocardiogram; NSAIDs, nonsteroidal antiinflammatory drugs; LP, lumbar puncture.

From Bohan A, Peter JB, Polymyositis and dermatomyositis. *N Engl Med* 1975;292:344, with permission.

TABLE 2.14. *Complications of juvenile dermatomyositis*

Clinical entity	Symptoms and signs	Investigations	Treatment
Respiratory failure	Air hunger, tachypnea, cyanosis, shallow respiration, alteration in mental status	Chest radiograph, arterial blood gas	Oxygen, mechanical ventilatory support, corticosteroids and immunosuppressives, plasmapheresis, antibiotics if evidence of aspiration pneumonia
Pneumothorax	Chest pain, breathlessness, tachypnea, cyanosis, diminished breath sounds, increased resonance to percussion	Chest radiograph	Chest tube
Velopalatine weakness	Pooling of secretions, drooling, nasal voice, aspiration pneumonia (recurrent)	Careful barium cineradiographic study, chest radiograph	Corticosteroids, nasogastric feedings, tracheostomy
Gastrointestinal hemorrhage	Abdominal pain, nausea, vomiting, guarding, diminished bowel sounds (may be masked by corticosteroids), hematemesis, melena, hematochezia	CBC (type and cross), abdominal radiograph (flat plate and upright), endoscopy, angiography, nuclear scan	NPO, NG tube, support of circulatory volume, antacids, corticosteroids, surgical consult, interventional radiography
Gastrointestinal perforation	May be silent (corticosteroids) or associated with abdominal pain, distention, vomiting	Abdominal radiographs (flat plate and upright)	NPO, NG tube, surgical consult
Calcinosis	Swelling resembling cellulitis around large joints, fever	CBC, radiograph, aspiration	Antibiotics if superinfection suspected
Carditis	Dyspnea, tachycardia, arrhythmias	Chest radiograph, ECG, echocardiogram	Digoxin, diuretics, antiarrhythmics, corticosteroids

CBC, complete blood count; NPO, nothing by mouth; NG, nasogastric; ECG, electrocardiogram.

TABLE 2.15. *Complications of systemic sclerosis*

Clinical entity	Symptoms and signs	Investigations	Treatments
Myocardial fibrosis	Exertional dyspnea, orthopnea, angina pectoris, distant heart sounds, gallop rhythm, arrhythmias	Chest radiograph, ECG, echocardiogram, gated nuclear ventricular scans	Digoxin, diuretics, antiarrhythmics
Pulmonary interstitial fibrosis	Cough, dyspnea, dry crackles, cor pulmonale	Chest radiograph, ECG, pulmonary function tests including CO diffusion, high-resolution CT, bronchoalveolar lavage, lung biopsy	Corticosteroids, oxygen, bronchodilators, treatment of right-sided heart failure
Pulmonary hypertension	Acute dyspnea, increased P2 and widely split S2	Chest radiograph, ECG, echocardiogram, right-sided heart catheterization, lung biopsy	Corticosteroids, calcium channel blockers, ACE inhibitors, direct PA installation of vasodilators
Scleroderma renal crisis	Severe headache, blurred vision, congestive heart failure, seizures, malignant hypertension, retinopathy	Electrolytes, BUN, creatinine, plasma renin activity	Captropril and other ACE inhibitors, minoxidil and other vasodilators, beta-blockers, diuretics, dialysis in refractory cases, nephrectomy
Impending gangrene	Pain, loss of sensation in distal digits, trophic changes	Cryoglobulins, Doppler flow studies	Topical vasolidators, sympathetic ganglionic blockade (digital, regional), prostaglandin E_1 infusion
Esophagitis	Retrosternal pain, pyrosis, melena	CBC, barium swallow, esophageal, pH probe and manometry	Antacids/cimetidine, surgical manipulation for chronic unremitting complaints

ECG, electrocardiogram; CO, carbon monoxide; CT, computed tomography; ACE, angiotensin-converting enzyme; PA, posteroanterior; BUN, blood urea nitrogen; CBC, complete blood count.

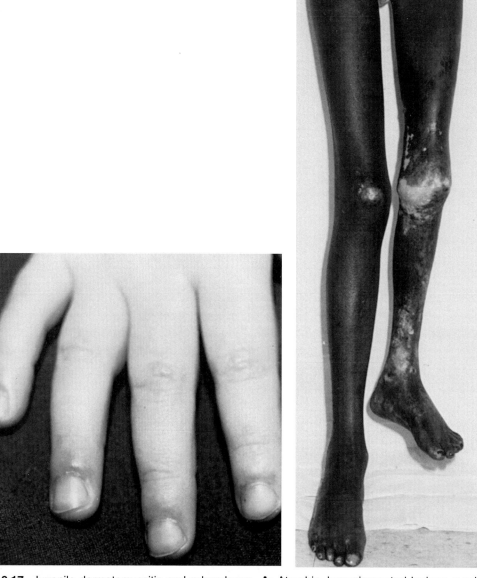

FIG. 2.17. Juvenile dermatomyositis and scleroderma. **A:** Atrophic, hypopigmented lesions overlying extensor surfaces of interphalangeal joints, with periungual erythema typical of juvenile dermatomyositis. **B:** Linear scleroderma involving left lower extremity in a 12-year-old girl.

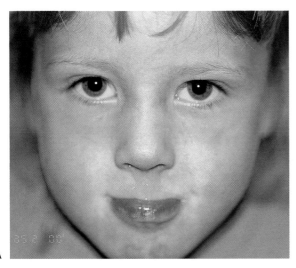 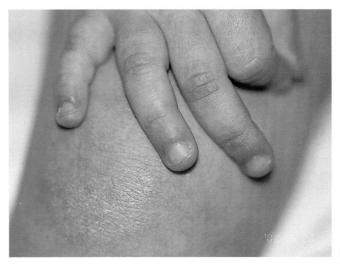

A B

FIG. 2.18. This patient with dermatomyositis has the characteristic facial **(A)** and extremity findings **(B)**.

TABLE 2.16. *Complications of polyarteritis nodosa*

Clinical entity	Symptoms and signs	Investigations	Treatment
Renal failure	Usually insidious; no symptoms until uremia sets in	Urinalysis (serial), BUN, creatinine, creatinine clearance, serum electrolytes	Fluidelectrolyte management, treatment of hypertension, peritoneal dialysis, hemodialysis
Renal infarction	Flank pain, high blood pressure	Urinalysis, BUN, creatinine, renal arteriogram	Management of renal failure as given above, hemodialysis
Renal artery aneurysm with hemorrhage	Severe, sudden flank pain; gross hematuria; shock; palpable abdominal mass	Serial hematocrit, renal arteriogram	Management of shock, surgical consult
Hypertension	Asymptomatic or headache, retinal changes, encephalopathy	Serial measurement of BP; BUN; creatinine; creatinine clearance; IVP or renal arteriogram	Diuretics, antihypertensive agents
Pericarditis	Chest pain, pericardial rub, pulsus paradoxus (if tamponade)	ECG, radiograph chest, echocardiogram, removal of fluid for analysis	Rest, steroids, removal of fluid (if tamponade). *Caution:* if tamponade is sudden, it may be caused by ruptured aneurysm with blood in pericardium
Myocardial infarction	Sudden chest pain, shock, arrythmia, dyspnea, congestive failure	ECG (continuous monitor), echocardiogram, thallium scan, coronary arteriography	Pain relief, oxygen, circulatory support, heparin, thrombolytic agents
Gastrointestinal hemorrhage	Abdominal pain, vomiting, melena, hematemesis or hematochezia; shock; tenderness and guarding of abdomen; bowel sounds absent	Plain radiograph of abdomen, peritoneal aspiration, endoscopy, celiac arteriogram	Treat shock, block bleeding vessel during angiography, surgical ligation
Gastrointestinal perforation	Sudden abdominal pain; shock; guarding, tenderness, and rigidity of abdomen; absent bowel sounds	Plain radiograph of abdomen (upright)	Treat shock, surgical repair
Aneurysm with rupture (intraabdominal)	Abdominal pain (chronic) with acute exacerbation, palpable mass, sudden onset of shock	Ultrasonography, celiac arteriogram	Treat shock, surgical repair
CNS lesions	Convulsions, gradual onset of loss of consciousness, hemiparesis	Exclude hypertensive encephalopathy, CT scan, MRI, carotid arteriography	Supportive care, control blood pressure, anticonvulsants, high-dose corticosteroids and/or immunosuppressives

BUN, blood urea nitrogen; BP, blood pressure; IVP, intravenous pyelogram; ECG, electrocardiogram; CNS, central nervous system; CT, computed tomography; MRI, magnetic resonance imaging.

erythema of their palms and soles. In addition, one-third of children develop arthritis. This is typically a small joint polyarthritis during the first week of illness, followed by a large joint pauciarthritis. During the convalescent phase of Kawasaki disease, sheetlike desquamation that begins in the periungual region of the hands and feet and linear nail creases (Beau lines) is characteristic (Fig. 2.19C).

Kawasaki disease is most commonly confused with exanthematous infections of childhood (Table 2.17).

No laboratory studies are included among the diagnostic criteria for Kawasaki disease, but some findings may support the diagnosis. Most characteristic is the systemic inflammation, with widespread elevation of acute-phase reactants (including C-reactive protein and erythrocyte sedimentation rate), leukocytosis, and a shift to left in the white blood cell count. By the second week of illness, platelet counts rise as well, reaching 1,000,000/mm^3 in the most severe cases.

Children with Kawasaki disease often present with a normocytic, normochromic anemia; hemoglobin concentrations more than 2 standard deviations below the mean for age are noted in approximately half of patients within the first 2 weeks of illness. Urinalysis commonly reveals white blood cells on microscopic examination; the cells are mononuclear and therefore are not detected by dipstick tests for leukocyte esterase. They also originate in the urethra, so they will be missed on urinalyses obtained by bladder tap or catheterization. Measurement of liver enzymes often reveals elevated transaminase levels or mild hyperbilirubinemia caused by intrahepatic congestion. In addition, a minority of children may develop obstructive jaundice from hydrops of the gall-

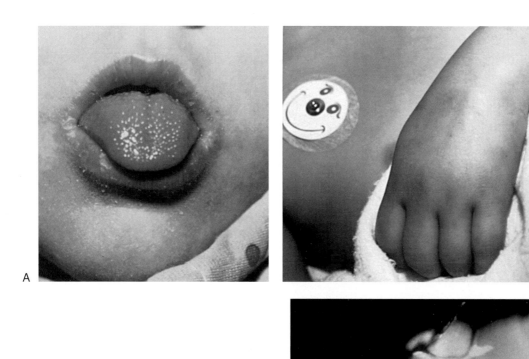

FIG. 2.19. Clinical findings in Kawasaki disease. **A:** Cracked, erythematous lips, and "strawberry" tongue in Kawasaki disease. **B:** Brawny edema of the dorsum of the hand and small joint polyarthritis in Kawasaki disease. **C:** Peeling of the skin on the thumbs in Kawasaki disease.

TABLE 2.17. *Differential diagnosis of Kawasaki disease*

	Kawasaki disease	Toxic shock syndrome	Streptococcal scarlet fever	Stevens–Johnson syndrome	Systematic juvenile rheumatoid arthritis
Age	<5 yr	>10 yr	2–8 yr	All ages	2–5 yr
Fever	≤12 days	<10 d	Variable	Prolonged	Prolonged
Eyes	Nonexudative conjunctivitis, limbal sparing, anterior uveitis	Conjunctivitis	Normal	Exudative conjunctivitis, keratitis	Normal
Oral mucosa	Erythema, "strawberry tongue"	Erythema	Pharyngitis, "strawberry tongue," circumoral pallor	Erythema, ulcerations, pseudomembrane formation	Normal
Extremities	Erythema of palms and soles, indurative edema, periungual desquamation	Peripheral edema	Fine flaking desquamation	Normal	Arthritis
Rash	Polymorphous; targetoid or purpuric in 20%	Erythroderma	Erythroderma, Pastia lines	Target lesions	Transient, salmon pink
Lymph nodes	Single anterior lymph node	Normal	Painful, diffuse cervical nodes	Normal	Diffuse
Other	Arthritis	Shock, coagulopathy, mental status changes	Positive throat culture	Arthralgia, associated herpes virus infection (30%–50%)	Pericarditis

Modified from Yanagihara R, Todd JK. Acute febrile mucocutaneous lymph node syndrome. *Am J Dis Child* 1980;134:603.

bladder. If sampled, other body fluids demonstrate inflammation as well: CSF typically displays a mononuclear pleocytosis (less than 100 cells/mm³) with normal glucose and protein concentrations, whereas arthrocentesis of involved joints demonstrates 50 to 300,000 white blood cells/mm³, primarily neutrophils.

Most characteristic of Kawasaki disease is inflammation of the coronary arteries. This progresses to ectasia or aneurysm formation in 15% to 25% of untreated children. Dilation of coronary arteries may be detected by echocardiography as early as 6 days after the appearance of fever and usually peaks 3 or 4 weeks after onset of illness. Cardiac catheterization need not be performed in patients with normal echocardiograms and electrocardiograms throughout the disease course because the likelihood of finding unsuspected lesions is negligible (Figs. 2.20 and 2.21).

IV immunoglobulin (IVIG) has truly revolutionized the care of children with Kawasaki disease; treatment within 10 days of onset significantly shortens disease duration and minimizes the incidence of complications. Overall, prompt diagnosis and appropriate therapy prevent aneurysm formation in approximately 95% of children and result in rapid symptomatic improvement in approximately 90%. Use of antiinflammatory medications, such as aspirin or NSAIDs, improves patient comfort and complements the disease-modifying effects of IVIG. Most recently, a single large infusion of IVIG (2 g/kg) administered over 8 to 12 hours has become the standard of care for Kawasaki disease.

Aspirin was the first medication to be used for treatment of Kawasaki disease, for both its antiinflammatory and antithrombotic effects. High-dose (more than 80 mg/kg per day) and lower dose regimens (30 mg/kg per day) are still used in conjunction with IVIG during the acute phase of the illness, despite the fact that aspirin has no known effect on the development of coronary artery aneurysms. Once fever resolves, patients are generally switched to antiplatelet doses of aspirin (3 to 5 mg/kg per day).

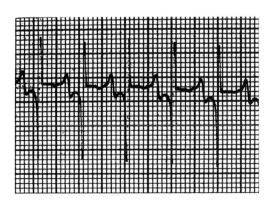

FIG. 2.20. Lead III from an electrocardiogram on a 15-month-old boy shows deep Q waves in Kawasaki disease.

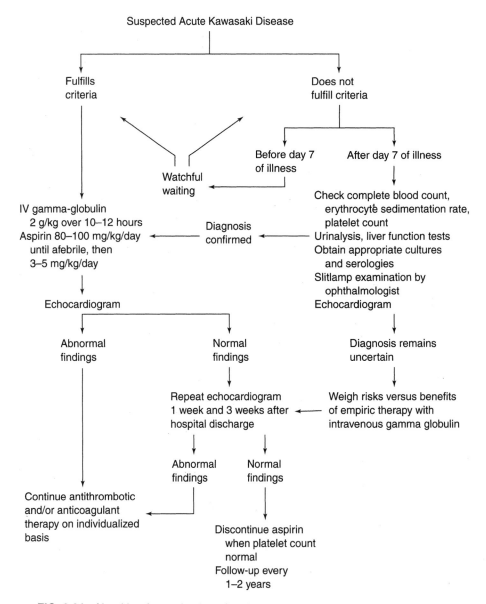

FIG. 2.21. Algorithm for evaluation of patients with suspected Kawasaki disease.

Complications of Kawasaki disease include myocardial infarction, congestive heart failure (CHF), vascular obstruction, and hyprups of gallbladder and arthritis.

Lyme Disease

Symptoms of *Borrelia burgdorferi* infection may be classified into three stages (Fig. 2.22A). Stage 1, or early infection, consists of a localized erythema migrans rash. This begins as a small, red, indurated papule at the site of the tick bite and then expands centrifugally for days or weeks. Lesions ultimately may reach an average diameter of 15 cm and may be accompanied by mild flulike symptoms, including fever, regional lymphadenopathy, and malaise (Fig. 2.22B, C, D).

Stage 2 of Lyme disease results from hematogenous dissemination of the spirochete. Integumental, musculoskeletal,

and central nervous systems are most commonly affected. Approximately half of patients develop secondary annular skin lesions similar to erythema migrans but smaller and without central puncta. Debilitating fatigue may accompany myalgias and migratory arthralgias, followed in somewhat more than 50% of patients by a large-joint oligoarthritis. Severe headache and meningismus, cranial neuritis (especially Bell palsy), and peripheral radiculoneuropathy may supervene. Finally, approximately 5% of patients demonstrate cardiac involvement, including conduction abnormalities or, more rarely, pancarditis. These symptoms generally resolve within weeks or months but may recur or persist.

Stage 3 disease is characterized by persistent infection and symptoms of prolonged latency. Acrodermatitis chronica atrophicans, a scleroderma-like skin rash, is seen most commonly in Europe. A potentially erosive chronic oligoarthritis may be seen months to years after the tick bite. Subtle neurologic findings, including peripheral neuropathies and organic brain syndromes, may become apparent long after other manifestations of spirochete infestation have resolved.

B. burgdorferi is extremely difficult to grow in culture, and spirochetes generally cannot be identified in infected tissues. A diagnosis of Lyme disease therefore is made based on characteristic clinical features accompanied by confirmatory serologic markers. Two caveats accompany serologic testing for Lyme disease. First, these tests are relatively difficult to perform, and standardization has been difficult to achieve. Many laboratories are plagued by both false-positive and false-negative results, so only experienced reference laboratories, preferably state or regional centers, should be used. Second, serologic tests for Lyme disease depend on the patient's antibody response. Titers may not be measurable until the second month after a tick bite in as many as 85% of cases, and they may be abrogated by early antibiotic therapy. Early Lyme disease is thus a clinical condition based on a typical erythema migrans rash, and serology should not be relied on to confirm the diagnosis.

In Lyme arthritis, synovial fluid analysis typically reveals elevated white blood cell counts ranging from 2,000 to 100,000 cells/mm^3. Polymorphonuclear leukocytes usually predominate, but Lyme disease is one of the few conditions in which a significant number of eosinophils may be identified in the synovial fluid. Total protein is elevated. Synovial biopsy reveals nonspecific synovial hypertrophy and mononuclear cell infiltration. In cases of neuroborreliosis, cerebrospinal fluid analysis may reveal a mononuclear pleocytosis ranging from 25 to 500 cells/mm^3. At times, how-

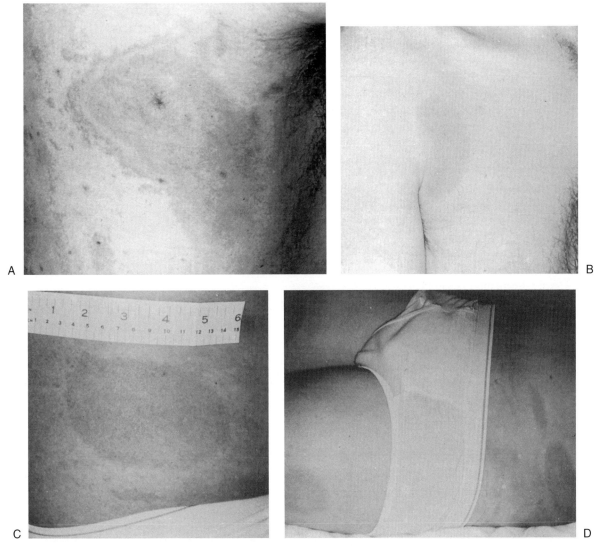

FIG. 2.22. Lyme disease. **A:** Primary erythema chronicum migrans lesion. Dermatologic manifestations of Lyme disease. **B:** Erythema migrans (EM). An early lesion is seen 4 days after detection. **C:** In a 10-day lesion of EM, the red outer ring has expanded, and central clearing is beginning. **D:** Eight days after onset of EM, similar secondary lesions have appeared, and several of their borders have merged. (From Koopman W. *Arthritis and allied conditions: a textbook of rheumatology*, 14th ed. Philadelphia: Lippincott Williams & Wilkins, 2001:2634, with permission.)

TABLE 2.18. *Treatment of Lyme disease*

Disease stage	Organ system	Treatment
Acute (stage 1)	General malaise, flulike symptoms; skin: erythema migrans	Oral regimens; 100 mg doxycycline b.i.d. for 14–21 d Children <9 yr: amoxicillin 25–50 mg/kg/d in 3 divided doses (maximum, 2 g/d) for 14–21 d
Chronic (stage 2)	Skin: multiple erythema migrans; neurologic: facial palsy; musculoskeletal: migratory arthralgias and arthritis	Oral regimen as for early disease, but for 21–28 d
Persistent (stage 3)	Skin: acrodermatitis chronica atrophicans; neurologic: meningitis, encephalitis; cardiac: heart block, myocarditis; musculoskeletal: chronic arthritis	Parenteral regimen: ceftriaxone 75–100 mg/kg/d IV or IM (maximum, 2 g/d) for 14–28 d or penicillin 300,000 U/kg/d IV divided in doses q 4 hr (maximum, 20 million U/d) for 14–28 d

b.i.d., twice daily; IV, intravenous; IM, intramuscularly. Modified from American Academy of Pediatrics. Lyme disease. In: Peter G, ed. *1997 red book: report of the Committee on Infectious Diseases,* 24th ed. Elk Grove Village, IL: American Academy of Pediatrics, 1997:332.

ever, cerebrospinal fluid may be entirely normal despite the presence of neurologic symptoms; even polymerase chain reaction testing might fail to reveal evidence of borrelial DNA. In such cases, magnetic resonance imaging of the brain might be useful, although other causes of the symptoms must also be considered. Suspected cardiac involvement may be confirmed by electrocardiography, which reveals varying degrees of atrioventricular block and nonspecific ST-T wave changes.

General Management

The cornerstone of treatment of Lyme disease is antibiotics. Oral antibiotic therapy is beneficial in early stages of the infection, whereas IV medications have a lower failure rate in chronic Lyme disease. Late manifestations of Lyme disease may represent a host autoimmune response rather than direct effects of the spirochete, but antibiotics may nonetheless be beneficial. Current treatment guidelines are shown in Table 2.18.

SUGGESTED READINGS

Albisetti M, Schaer G, Good M, et al. Diagnostic value of cerebrospinal fluid examination in children with peripheral facial palsy and suspected Lyme borreliosis. *Neurology* 1997;49:817.

American Academy of Pediatrics. Lyme disease. In: Peter G, ed. *1997 red book: report of the Committee on Infectious Diseases*, 24th ed. Elk Grove Village, IL: American Academy of Pediatrics, 1997.

Amirav I, Newhouse MT. Metered-dose inhaler accessory devices in acute asthma. *Arch Pediatr Adolesc Med* 1997;151:876–882.

Armstrong GP, Whalley GA, Doughty RN, et al. Left ventricular function in scleroderma. *Br J Rheum* 1996;35:983.

Asthma mortality and hospitalization among children and young adults—United States, 1980–1993. *MMWR Morb Mortal Wkly Rep* 1996;45; 350–353.

Athreya BH, Cassidy JT. Current status of the medical treatment of children with juvenile rheumatoid arthritis. *Rheum Dis Clin North Am* 1991;17:871.

Athreya BH. Vasculitis in children. *Pediatr Clin North Am* 1995;42:1239.

Atkinson TP, Kaliner MA. Anaphylaxis. *Med Clin North Am* 1992;76: 841–855.

Barnett PL, Caputo GZ, Baskin M, et al. Intravenous versus oral corticosteroids in the management of acute asthma in children. *Ann Emerg Med* 1997;29:212–217.

Barron KS. Kawasaki disease in children. *Curr Opin Rheumatol* 1998;10:29.

Bingham PM, Galetta SL, Athreya B, et al. Neurologic manifestations in children with Lyme disease. *Pediatrics* 1995;96:1053.

Bochner BS, Lichtenstein LM. Anaphylaxis. *N Engl J Med* 1991;324: 1785–1790.

Bray VJ, Singleton JD. Disseminated intravascular coagulation in Still's disease. *Semin Arthritis Rheum* 1994;24:222.

Carter ER, Webb, CR, Moffitt DR. Evaluation of Heliox in children hospitalized with acute severe asthma. A randomized crossover trial. *Chest* 1996;109:1256–1261.

Cassidy JT, Petty RE. Juvenile rheumatoid arthritis. In: *Textbook of pediatric rheumatology*, 3rd ed. Philadelphia: WB Saunders, 1995.

Ciarallo LM, Saver AH, Shannon MW. Intravenous magnesium therapy for moderate to severe pediatric asthma: results of a randomized placebo-controlled study. *J Pediatr* 1996;129:809–814.

DeNicola LK, Monem GF, Gayle MO, et al. Treatment of critical status asthmaticus in children. *Pediatr Clin North Am* 1994;41:1293–1324.

Dillon MJ, Ansell BM. Vasculitis in children and adolescents. *Rheum Dis Clin North Am* 1995;21:1115.

Dillon MJ. Rare vasculitic syndromes. *Ann Med* 1997;29:175.

Durongpisitkul K, Gurunaj VJ, Park JM, et al. The prevention of coronary artery aneurysm in Kawasaki disease: a meta-analysis on the efficacy of aspirin and immunoglobulin treatment. *Pediatrics* 1995;96:1057.

Fine LG. Systemic sclerosis: current pathogenic concepts and future prospects for targeted therapy. *Lancet* 1996;347:1453.

Fujita Y, Yamamori H, Hiyoshi K, et al. Systemic sclerosis in children: a national retrospective survey in Japan. *Acta Paediatr Jpn* 1997;39:263.

Fukushige J, Takahashi HN, Ueda Y, et al. Incidence and clinical features of incomplete Kawasaki disease. *Acta Paediatr* 1994;83:1057.

Fukushige J, Takahashi N, Ueda K, et al. Long-term outcome of coronary abnormalities in patients after Kawasaki disease. *Pediatr Cardiol* 1996;17:71.

Geelhoed GC, Landau LI, LeSouef PN. Oximetry and peak expiratory flow in assessment of acute childhood asthma. *J Pediatr* 1990;117:907–909.

Gershel JC, Goldman HS, Stein RE, et al. The usefulness of chest radiographs in first asthma attacks. *N Engl J Med* 1983;309:336–339.

Giannini EH, Calkwell GD. Drug treatment in children with juvenile rheumatoid arthritis. *Pediatr Clin North Am* 1995;42:1099.

Gonzalez-Lopez L, Gamez-Nava JI, Sanchez L, et al. Cardiac manifestations in dermato-polymyositis. *Clin Exp Rheum* 1996;14:373.

Haber PL. Clinical manifestations of scleroderma. *Pediatr Rev* 1995;16:49.

Harris JB, Weinberger MM, Nassif E, et al. Early intervention with short courses of prednisone to prevent progression of asthma in ambulatory patients incompletely responsive to bronchodilators. *J Pediatr* 1987;110: 627–633.

Heckbert SR, Stryker WS, Coltin KL, et al. Serum sickness in children after antibiotic exposure: estimates of occurrence and morbidity in a health maintenance organization population. *Am J Epidemiol* 1990;132:336–342.

Kaplan RF. Lyme encephalopathy: a neuropsychological perspective. *Semin Neurol* 1997;17:31.

Kato H, Sugimua T, Akagi T, et al. Long-term consequences of Kawasaki disease. A 10- to 21-year follow up study of 594 patients. *Circulation* 1996;94:1379.

Kearns GL, Wheeler JG, Childress SH, et al. Serum sickness-like reactions to cefaclor: role of hepatic metabolism and individual susceptibility. *J Pediatr* 1994;125:805–811.

Kerem E, Levison H, Schuh S, et al. Efficacy of albuterol administered by nebulizer versus spacer device in children with acute asthma. *J Pediatr* 1993;123:313–317.

Landwher LP, Boguniewicz M. Current prospectus on latex allergy. *J Pediatr* 1996;128:305–312.

Lemanske RF. A review of the current guidelines for allergic rhinitis and asthma. *J Allergy Clin Immunol* 1998;101:5392–5396.

Meltzer EO. Treatment options for the child with allergic rhinitis. *Clin Pediatr* 1998;37:1–10.

Mouy R, Stephan JL, Pillet P, et al. Efficacy of cyclosporine A in the treatment of macrophage activation syndrome in juvenile arthritis: report of five cases. *J Pediatr* 1996;129:750.

Nagi KS, Joshi R, Thakur RK. Cardiac manifestations of Lyme disease: a review. *Can J Cardiol* 1996;12:503.

Nakamura Y, Yanagawa H, Kato H, et al. Mortality rates for patients with a history of Kawasaki disease in Japan. Kawasaki disease follow-up group. *J Pediatr* 1996;128:75.

Newburger JW, Takahashi M, Beiser AS, et al. A single intravenous infusion of gamma globulin as compared with four infusions in the treatment of acute Kawasaki syndrome. *N Engl J Med* 1991;324:1633.

NHLBI. Highlights of the expert panel report 2: guidelines for the diagnosis and management of asthma. NIH publication no. 97-4051A, 1997.

Padeh S, Passwell JH. Intraarticular corticosteroid injection in the management of children with chronic arthritis. *Arthritis Rheum* 1998;41:1210.

Patel L, Radivan S, David TJ. Management of anaphylactic reactions to food. *Arch Dis Child* 1994;71:370–375.

Rachelefsky GS. Pharmacologic management of allergic rhinitis. *J Allergy Clin Immunol* 1998;101:5367–5369.

Rider LG, Miller FW. Classification and treatment of the juvenile idiopathic inflammatory myopathies. *Rheum Dis Clin North Am* 1997;23:619.

Rosenfeld EA, Corydon KE, Shulman ST. Kawasaki disease in infants less than one year of age. *J Pediatr* 1995;126:524.

Rowley AH. Controversies in Kawasaki syndrome. *Adv Pediatr Infect Dis* 1997;13:127.

Scarfone RJ, Fuchs SM, Nager AZ, et al. Controlled trial of oral prednisone in the emergency department treatment of children with acute asthma. *Pediatrics* 1993;92:513–518.

Scartone RJ, Loiselle JM, Wiley JR, et al. Nebulized dexamethasone versus oral prednisone in the emergency treatment of asthmatic children. *Ann Emerg Med* 1995;26:480–486.

Schaller JG. Juvenile rheumatoid arthritis. *Pediatr Rev* 1998;18:337.

Schuh S, Johnson DW, Callahan S, et al. Efficiency of frequent nebulized ipratropium bromide added to frequent high dose albuterol therapy in severe childhood asthma. *J Pediatr* 1995;126:639–645.

Schuh S, Parkin P, Rajan A, et al. High-versus low-dose, frequently administered, nebulized albuterol in children with severe, acute asthma. *Pediatrics* 1989;83:513–518.

Schuh S, Reider MJ, Canny G, et al. Nebulized albuterol in acute childhood asthma: comparison of two doses. *Pediatrics* 1990;86:509–513.

Shapiro ED. Lyme disease. *Pediatr Rev* 1998;19:147.

Silverman ED, Lang B. An overview of the treatment of childhood SLE [Editorial]. *Scand J Rheumatol* 1997;26:241.

Vancheeswaran R, Black CM, David J, et al. Childhood-onset scleroderma: is it different from adult-onset disease? *Arthritis Rheum* 1996;39:1041.

Wood RA. Anaphylaxis: causes and management. *Contemp Pediatr* 1996;13:89–96.

Wright DA, Newburger JW, Baker A, et al. Treatment of immune globulin-resistant Kawasaki disease with pulsed doses of corticosteroids. *J Pediatr* 1996;128:146.

Yell JA, Mbuagbaw J, Burge SM. Cutaneous manifestations of systemic lupus erythematosus. *Br J Dermatol* 1996;135:355.

Zeller V, Cohen P, Prieur AM, et al. Cyclosporin A therapy in refractory juvenile dermatomyositis. Experience and long-term follow-up of 6 cases. *J Rheumatol* 1996;23:1424.

CHAPTER 3

Bites and Stings

Editor: Stephen Ludwig

MARINE INVERTEBRATES

Phylum Coelenterata (Cnidaria)

Class Scyphozoa

In the category of marine invertebrates, the common purple jellyfish (*Pelagia noctiluca*) (Fig. 3.1) is only mildly toxic. Local skin irritation is the major clinical manifestation. Sea nettle (*Chrysaora quinquecirrha*) is a common jellyfish found along the Atlantic coast. The clinical manifestations are the same as those for purple jellyfish. Lion's mane (*Cyanea capillata*) is a highly toxic creature. Contact with the tentacles produces severe burning. Prolonged exposure causes muscle cramps and respiratory failure.

Treatment of hydrozoan and scyphozoan stings is based on the same general principles. It is directed at three objectives: relieving pain, alleviating effects of venom, and controlling shock. The most important step is to remove the tentacles. Inactivate the unexploded nematocysts by topical application of vinegar (3% acetic acid), a slurry of baking soda, or meat tenderizer (papain) for 30 minutes. The area should be washed with seawater or normal saline. Any adherent tentacles should be carefully removed with instruments or a gloved hand, and the wound area should be immobilized. General supportive measures for systemic reactions include oral antihistamines, oral corticosteroids, and codeine or meperidine for pain. Cardiac and respiratory support may be required. Muscle spasms have been treated with 0.1 mL/kg 10% solution of calcium gluconate given intravenously. Local dermatitis should be treated with a topical corticosteroid cream.

Class Anthozoa

The anemones found within United States tidal zones are only mildly toxic at worst. The clinical picture is one of a stinging sensation followed by wheal formation and itching. If the wound is untreated, an ulcer with an erythematous base may form within a few days. Cellulitis, lymphangitis, fever, and malaise commonly occur. Treatment consists of cleaning the wound and irrigation with copious amounts of saline. Removal of foreign particles must be accomplished, and debridement may be necessary. Broad-spectrum antibiotic therapy, particularly tetracycline, has been advocated but cannot be used in children younger than 8 years old. For children younger than 8 years, cephalexin or trimethoprim-sulfamethoxazole should be used.

Phylum Echinodermata

Phylum Echinodermata includes starfish, sea urchins, and sea cucumbers. Of the three classes, only the Echinoidea (sea urchins) have clinical relevance for American children. The spines may break off readily and can penetrate wet suits and sneakers. Clinically, penetration is accompanied by intense pain followed by redness, swelling, and aching. Complications include tattooing of the skin, secondary infection, and granuloma formation. In treatment, all spines should be removed as completely as possible. If spines break off in the wound, debridement should be performed with local anesthetic under aseptic conditions, but any spines not reachable will be absorbed in time. Soaking the wound in warm water may be helpful. Systemic antistaphylococcal antibiotics should be used if infection develops (Table 3.1).

MARINE VERTEBRATES

Stingrays

Because the barb is retropointed, the wound that it produces is a combination of puncture and laceration. The sting is followed immediately by pain, which spreads from the site of injury over the next 30 minutes and usually reaches its greatest intensity within 90 minutes. Pain and edema are most often localized to the area of injury; however, syncope, weakness, nausea, and anxiety are common complaints attributed to both the effects of the venom and the vagal response to the pain. Among other generalized symptoms are vomiting, diarrhea, sweating, and muscle fasciculations of the affected extremity. Generalized cramps, paresthesias, hypotension,

44

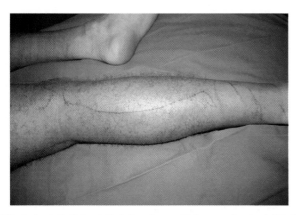

FIG. 3.1. Jellyfish. Jellyfish stings. Chironex fleckeri (Major Australian box jellyfish) sting on the leg at 24 hours demonstrating the cross-hatched whip-like lesion. [Image taken in Darwin, Northern Territory, Australia, 2000, by Geoff Isbister, MD. University of Newcastle, Newcastle Mater Hospital, Newcastle, Australia.]

arrhythmias, and death may occur. The wound often has a jagged edge that bleeds profusely, and the wound edges may be discolored. Discoloration may extend several centimeters from the wound within hours after injury and may subsequently necrose if untreated.

Treatment is aimed at (1) preventing complications evoked by the venom, (2) alleviating the pain, and (3) preventing secondary infection. On the patient's arrival in the emergency department, shock, if present, should be treated with intravenous fluids. An attempt should be made to remove any remnants of the integumentary sheath if it can be seen in the wound. The extremity should be placed in hot water [40° to 45°C (104° to 113°F)] for 30 to 90 minutes. After soaking, the wound should be reexplored. Pain relief may be

achieved with meperidine. Tetanus prophylaxis should always be considered, but antibiotics are reserved for wounds that become secondarily infected.

Sharks

Two types of bite wounds are described: tangential injury and a definitive bite. Tangential injury is caused by the slashing movement of the open mouth as the shark makes a close pass. Severe lacerations, incised wounds, and loss of tissue are seen. Definitive bite wounds vary according to the part of the body seized by the shark. Lacerations, loss of soft tissue, amputations, and comminuted fractures are recorded. Most injuries involve only one or two bites and are confined to the extremities. Hypovolemic shock is the immediate threat to life in shark attacks. Bleeding should be controlled. Tetanus toxoid and tetanus immunol globulin should be considered, and administering prophylactic antibiotics with a third-generation cephalosporin or trimethoprim-sulfamethoxazole is suggested.

Scorpaenidae

Severe pain at the site of the wound is the first and primary clinical sign for all species. The wound and surrounding area become ischemic and then cyanotic. Paresthesia and paralysis of the extremity may occur. Other clinical signs include nausea, vomiting, hypotension, tachypnea proceeding to apnea, and myocardial ischemia with electrocardiographic changes. Treatment involves irrigating the wound with sterile saline. The injured extremity is then immersed in very hot water (40° to 45°C [104° to 113°F]) for 30 to 60 minutes or until the agonizing pain is completely relieved. Meperidine hydrochloride may be required for pain. The patient should be monitored carefully for cardiotoxic effects

TABLE 3.1. *Treatment of marine envenomations: invertebrates*

Marine organism	Detoxification	Emergency department treatment
Hydroids	Irrigate with seawater (not fresh water); topical 5% acetic acid (vinegar); shave affected area	Topical corticosteroid cream for dermatitis
Fire coral	Same as for hydroids; topical 5% acetic acid	Topical corticosteroid cream for dermatitis
Portuguese man-of-war	Same as for hydroids; topical 5% acetic acid; use forceps or gloves to remove tentacles	Topical corticosteroid cream for dermatitis; All patients with systemic symptoms should be observed for 8 hr; severe systemic symptoms mandate hospitalization with supportive care
Sea nettles	Same as for hydroids; topical 5% acetic acid	Same as for Portuguese man-of-water
Box jellyfish	Same as for hydroids; topical 5% acetic acid; use forceps or gloves to remove tentacles	Give *Chironex* antivenom; supportive care for hypotension and respiratory depression
Anenomes	Same as hydroids; topical 5% acetic acid	Topical corticosteroid cream for dermatitis
Blue-ringed octopus	Pressure immobilization bandage	Supportive care for respiratory depression
Cone shell	Hot water [105°F (40.5°C)]; pressure immobilization bandage	Supportive care for hypotension and respiratory depression
Starfish	Irrigation with fresh water	Exploration and removal of any spines; Topical corticosteroid for dermatitis
Sea urchin	Hot water [105°F (40.5°C)]; removal of any spines or pedicellariae	Exploration and removal of any retained spines
Sea cucumber	Topical 5% acetic acid	Topical corticosteroid cream for dermatitis

Adapted from McGoldrick J, Marx JA. Marine envenomations. Part 2: invertebrates. *J Emerg Med* 1992;10:71–77.

and respiratory depression. Antivenin is available only for the stings of the stonefish of Australia.

Catfish

The spines inflict a puncture wound or laceration. The spines may become embedded in the flesh of the victim causing soft-tissue swelling, which may become infected or lead to a foreign body reaction. The venom produces a local inflammatory response of local intense pain, edema, hemorrhage, and tissue necrosis. Treatment (Fig. 3.2) involves irrigating the wound with sterile saline. The injured extremity is then immersed in hot water (40° to 45°C [104° to 113°F]) for 30 to 60 minutes or until the pain is relieved. Meperidine hy-

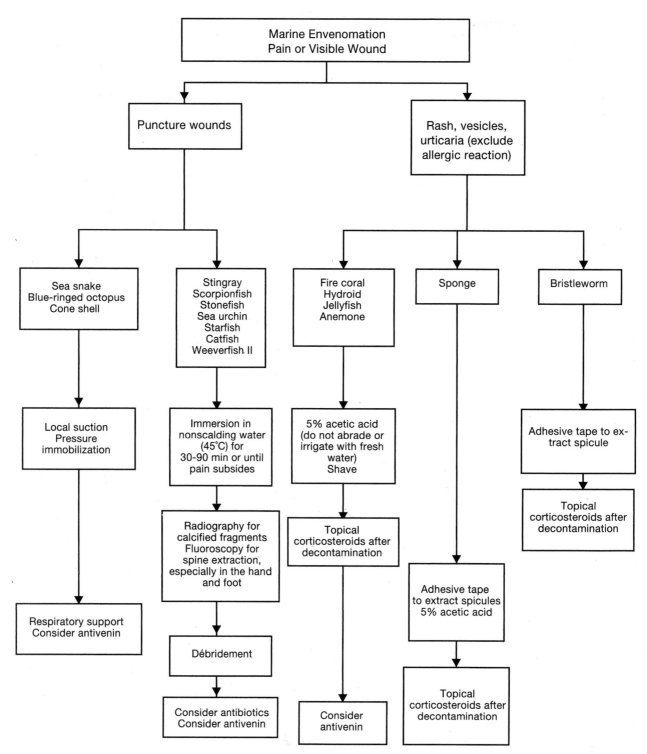

FIG. 3.2. Approach to emergency management of marine envenomation. (From Ellenhorn MJ, Schonwald SJ, Ordog G, et al., eds. *Ellenhorn's medical toxicology*, 2nd ed. Philadelphia: Lippincott Williams & Wilkins, 1996:1793, with permission.)

TABLE 3.2. *Treatment of marine envenomations: vertebrates*

Marine organism	Detoxification	Emergency department treatment
Stingray	Hot water [105°F (40.5°C)]	Irrigation with normal saline; exploration and debridement; observation for 3–4 hr to rule out systemic envenomation
Catfish	Hot water [105°F (40.5°C)]	
Weeverfish	Hot water [105°F (40.5°C)]	Same as outlined for stingray; intravenous calcium gluconate if pain persists
Scorpionfish (stonefish)	Hot water [105°F (40.5°C)]	Same as outlined for stingray; stonefish antivenom for severe systemic reactions
Sea snake	Limb immobilized in dependent position; pressure immobilization bandage	Give polyvalent sea snake antivenom for any evidence of envenomation; monitor respiratory and renal function and support as needed; if no signs of envenomation after 8 hr, patient can be discharged

Adapted from McGoldrick J, Marx JA. Marine envenomations; Part 1: vertebrates. *J Emerg Med* 1991;9:497–502.

drochloride may be required for analgesia. The wound should be explored to locate any retained spines. Systemic antibiotics to cover Gram-negative organisms are recommended (Table 3.2).

TERRESTRIAL INVERTEBRATES

Phylum Arthropoda

Scorpions

Common symptoms of scorpion stings include local pain, restlessness, hyperactivity, roving eye movements, and respiratory distress (Fig. 3.3). Other associated signs may include convulsions, drooling, wheezing, hyperthermia, cyanosis, and respiratory failure. The diagnosis may be difficult because a history of a sting may not be forthcoming. There is no laboratory test for confirmation of envenomation. Treatment modalities have been used in addition to general supportive care. Cryotherapy of the site of sting has been advocated to reduce swelling and local induration. Antivenin should be considered after general supportive care has been instituted only if the following symptoms persist: tachycar-

dia, hyperthermia, severe hypertension, and agitation. Antivenin that is not approved by the U.S. Food and Drug Administration is available through the Antivenom Production Laboratory at Arizona State University in Tempe, AZ. Sedative-anticonvulsants, in particular phenobarbital, have been used to treat persistent hyperactivity, convulsions, and/or agitation. Calcium gluconate has been given intravenously to reduce muscular contractions and associated pain, but benefit has not been proven.

Spiders

Loxoscelism (Bite of the Brown Recluse Spider)

The spectrum of reaction ranges from minor local reaction to severe necrotic arachnidism. The local reaction is characterized by mild to moderate pain 2 to 8 hours after the bite (Fig. 3.4). At the site of the bite, erythema develops with a central blister or pustule. Within 24 hours, subcutaneous discoloration appears and spreads over the next 3 to 4 days, reaching a size of 10 to 15 cm. At this time, the pustule drains, producing an ulcerated "crater." The local reaction varies with the amount of venom injected. Scar formation is rare if there

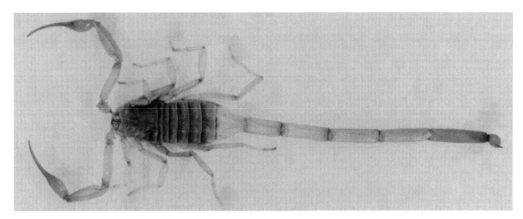

FIG. 3.3. Scorpion (*Centruroides exilicauda*).

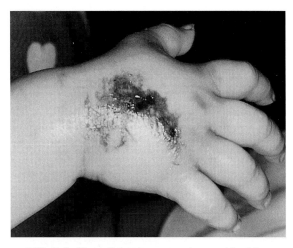

FIG. 3.4. Necrotizing brown recluse spider bite.

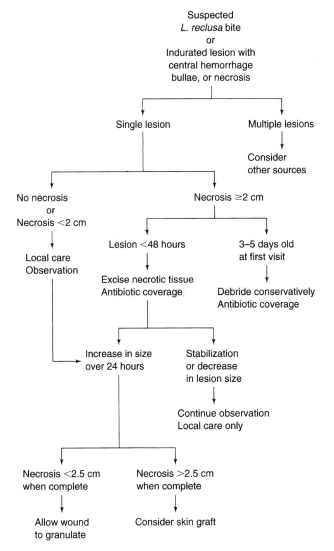

FIG. 3.5. Management of a suspected brown recluse spider bite.

is no clinical evidence of necrosis within 72 hours of the bite. Systemic reaction is most commonly noted in small children. Symptoms are noted 24 to 48 hours after the bite and include fever, chills, malaise, weakness, nausea, vomiting, joint pain, morbilliform eruption with petechiae, intravascular hemolysis, hematuria, and renal failure.

Because of the delay in initial diagnosis, treatment varies with the clinical stage of the bite. There is no specific serologic, biochemical, or histologic test to diagnose envenomation accurately. Table 3.3 lists the spiders found in the United States that are known to cause necrotic lesions. An algorithm for management of suspected bites is shown in Figure 3.5. Most victims will heal with supportive care. Dapsone should not be used in children because of methemoglobinemia. Antivenom is not yet commercially available. For systemic manifestations, vigorous supportive care is administered. Platelet count for evidence of hemolysis is needed as well as monitoring of hemoglobin, urine sediment, blood urea nitrogen, and creatinine for evidence of hemolysis and renal failure.

Latrodectism (Bite of the Black Widow Spider)

The reaction is generalized pain and rigidity of muscles 1 to 8 hours after the bite (Fig. 3.6). No local symptoms are associated with the bite itself. The pain is felt in the abdomen, flanks, thighs, and chest and is described as cramping. Nausea and vomiting are often reported in children.

Respiratory distress can occur. Chills, urinary retention, and priapism have been reported. There is a 4% to 5% mortality rate, with death resulting from cardiovascular collapse. The mortality rate in young children may be as high as 50%.

Because of the size, color, and distinctive markings of this spider, bites are seldom mistaken if the child is old enough

TABLE 3.3. *Spiders known to cause necrotic lesions*

Genus name	Common name	Geographic distribution
Argiope	Golden orb weaver	Throughout North America (individual species more restrictive)
Chiracanthium	Running spider	Throughout the United States
Loxoscelles	Brown recluse	Kansas and Missouri to Texas West to California
Lycosa	Wolf spider	Throughout the United States
Phidippus	Black jumping spider	Atlantic Coast to Rocky Mountains

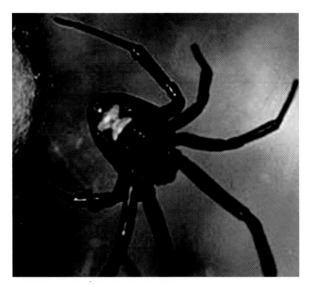

FIG. 3.6. A black widow spider. (From *http://www.nlm.nih.gov/medlineplus/ency/imagepage/1237.htm*, with permission.)

to describe the spider. A child who has severe pain and muscle rigidity after a spider bite should be considered a *Latrodectus* bite victim. A clinical grading scale was developed by Clark (Table 3.4). Treatment with *Latrodectus* antivenin (Lyovac; Merck, Sharp & Dohme) should be instituted as soon as a bite is confirmed in children who weigh less than 40 kg. Antivenin should be administered following instructions on the package insert and after skin testing to determine the risk of hypersensitivity to horse serum. Serum sickness is a possibility but uncommon, with a rate lower than those reported for other types of antivenom. Calcium gluconate (10% solution) is often given for control of leg and abdominal cramps. Muscle relaxants such as diazepam also have been advocated, but they are variably effective and the effects are short-lived. Analgesia may be achieved with morphine or meperidine.

Tarantulas and Others

Tarantulas, although fearsome in size and appearance, do not bite unless provoked. The venom is mild, and envenomation is not a problem. The wolf spider (*Lycosa* species) and the jumping spider (*Phidippus* species) also have been implicated in bites. Like the tarantula, they have a mild venom that

TABLE 3.4. *Grading scale for* Latrodectus *envenomation*

Grade	Symptoms
1	Asymptomatic, local pain at bite site, normal vital signs
2	Muscular pain, localized; diaphoresis, localized; normal vital signs
3	Muscular pain, generalized; abnormal vital signs; nausea, vomiting; headaches; diaphoresis

causes only local reactions. Bites from all three of these spiders should be treated with local wound care.

Tick Paralysis

After tick attachment, there is a latent period of 4 to 7 days followed by symptoms of restlessness, irritability, and ascending flaccid paralysis. Laboratory findings, including cerebrospinal fluid, are usually normal, but lymphocytic pleocytosis has been reported. Management is based on general supportive care and a diligent search for the tick. Ticks should be removed using blunt forceps or tweezers (Fig. 3.7). After the tick is removed, the paralysis is reversible without apparent sequelae.

Centipedes and Millipedes

Centipedes (class Myriapoda, order Chilopoda) are venomous, biting with jaws that act like stinging pincers. Bites can be extremely painful; however, the toxin is relatively innocuous, causing only local reaction. Treatment consists of injection of local anesthetic at the wound site and local wound care. American millipedes (order Diplopoda) are generally harmless.

Insects

Bees, Hornets, Yellow Jackets, and Wasps

Clinically, the stings of bees and wasps differ because the barbed stinger of the bee remains in the victim's skin, whereas the wasp may sting multiple times. The allergic reactions may be grouped by severity. Group I reactions consist of a local response at the site of the bite or sting (Figs. 2.5 and 3.8). Group II reactions include the mild systemic reactions typified by generalized pruritus and urticaria. Group III reactions consist of severe systemic reactions, including wheezing, angioneurotic edema, nausea, and vomiting.

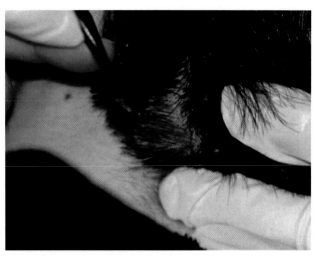

FIG. 3.7. A dog tick.

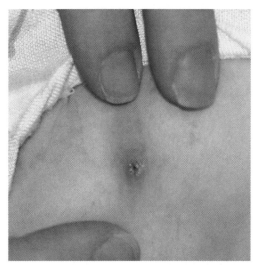

FIG. 3.8. An insect bite in a traveler, caused by a botfly infection.

Group IV reactions consist of life-threatening systemic reactions such as laryngoedema, hypotension, and shock. Anaphylactic reactions secondary to insect stings occur in 0.5% to 5% of the population.

Management

Because the barbed honeybee stinger with a venom sac is avulsed and often remains in the victim's skin, it must be removed if seen. Group I reactions can be treated with cold compresses at the site of sting. Group II reactions are treated with diphenhydramine hydrochloride for several days. Group III reactions are treated with 0.01 mL/kg epinephrine in a 1:1,000 solution injected subcutaneously followed by oral diphenhydramine. In addition H_2-blockers may provide additional benefit. Ranitidine or cimetidine can be used. These children should be observed in the hospital for 24 hours. Group IV reactions may require intubation if upper airway obstruction is present. Wheezing refractory to epinephrine should be treated with an aminophylline. Hypotension should be treated with a fluid bolus of saline or lactated Ringer solution. Intravenous epinephrine (1:10,000) should be considered if hypotension fails to respond to subcutaneous epinephrine and fluid bolus. Hydrocortisone may be given intravenously every 6 hours for 2 to 4 days.

Fire Ants

The clinical picture of a fire ant sting is one of immediate wheal and flare at the site. The local reaction varies from 1 to 2 mm to as much as 10 cm, depending on the amount of venom injected. Within 4 hours, a superficial vesicle appears. After 8 to 10 hours, the fluid in the vesicle changes from clear to cloudy (pustule) and becomes umbilicated. After 24 hours, it is surrounded by a painful erythematous area that persists for 3 to 10 days. Edema, induration, and

pruritus at the site occur in as many as 50% of patients. Occasionally, systemic reactions occur as with other Hymenoptera. Treatment of fire ant stings is symptomatic (Table 3.5).

TERRESTRIAL VERTEBRATES

Venomous Reptiles

Pit Vipers

Local pain after a *Crotalus* species envenomation is typically intense, and a sensation of burning occurs within a couple of minutes (Table 3.6). The pain is greater with ensuing edema and presumably increases with larger inocula of venom. Victims of a significant rattlesnake bite often complain within minutes of perioral numbness, extending to the scalp and periphery. This paresthesia may be accompanied by a metallic taste in the mouth. These patients also may have nausea, vomiting, weakness, chills, sweating, syncope, and other more ominous symptoms of systemic venom absorption. A copperhead or pygmy rattlesnake envenomation produces less localized symptoms, and systemic consequences are often minimal or nonexistent unless a small child, multiple bites, or a larger than average snake is involved. The water moccasin's effects are more variable. There is a relative lack of serious pain or swelling with the Mojave rattlesnake bite (Fig. 3.9), although, as in other *Crotalus* bites, the patient may complain of paresthesia in the affected extremity. Within several hours, these patients may develop neuromuscular symptoms such as diplopia, difficulty in swallowing, lethargy, nausea, and progressive weakness from the large portion of neurotoxin in this species.

The wound should be inspected for fang punctures, and if two are present, the distance between them should be noted. An interfang distance of less than 8 mm suggests a small snake; 8 to 12 mm, a medium snake; and more than 12 mm, a larger snake. Fang wounds by small snakes, such as the pygmy rattler, may be extremely subtle; in larger crotalid snakebites, the fang marks may be hidden within hemorrhagic blebs and edema. Occasionally, only one puncture or two scratches will be present, but both wounds may be potentially venomous. However, not all crotalid bites are envenomated; 10% to 20% of known rattlesnake strikes do not inject venom.

Pit viper envenomations are characterized by intense pain, erythema, and edema at the wound site within 5 to 10 minutes. There may be bloody serosanguinous fluid dripping from the fang punctures. Progressive swelling proportional to the inoculum of venom develops over the next 8 hours and may continue to some degree for an additional 24 hours. Rarely, the venom is deposited predominantly in a muscle compartment, resulting in a deceptively minimal amount of edema. The Mojave rattlesnake bite provides another example of a seemingly innocuous local wound in the setting of a potentially serious envenomation. In a severe diamondback rattlesnake bite, an entire extremity may be swollen within 1 hour.

TABLE 3.5. *Habits and effects of various arthropods*

Insect	Average length[a] (mm)	Usual location	Method of attack		Time of activity				Local reaction Onset		Local reaction Duration			Distribution of lesions			Residua
			Bite	Sting	Day	Night	Dusk	Dawn	Immediate	Delayed	Hr	D	Wk	Single	Scattered	Grouped	
Bumblebee	20–25	Flowers		X	X				X	X	X	X		X			None
Honeybee	10–15	Flowers		X	X				X	X	X	X		X			None
Mud dauber wasp	20–25	Orchards, garbage pails		X	X				X			X		X			None
Yellow jacket	10–15	Orchards, garbage pails		X	X				X			X		X			None
Hornet	20–30	Woods, flowers		X	X				X			X		X			None
Harvester ant	7–9	Vegetation, kitchen		X	X							X		X			None
Fire ant	6–7	Fields		X	X				X			X				X	Pigmented macules, occasionally nodules
Stable fly	6–7	Barns	X		X				X		X			X			None
Horsefly	10–20	Barns	X		X				X		X			X			None
Deerfly	7–9	Cattle	X		X				X		X			X	X		None
Blackfly	1–5	Woodlands, running water	X				X			X			X		X		Nodules, scars
Sand fly	1–4	Woodlands	X			X			X			X			X		Bluish spots
Biting midges	0.6–5	Marshlands	X					X	X		X				X		None
Chigger mite	0.2–1	Vegetation	X		X					X		X				X	Hyperpigmentation
Ticks	5–15	Vegetation	X								X	X		X	X		Granulomas
Brown recluse spider	10–15	Closets, attics	X						X		X	X		X			Scar
Tarantula	15–20	Vegetation	X											X			None
Black widow spider	10	Basements, outhouses							X		X	X		X			None
Scorpion	15–200	Stones and sand		X	X				X		X			X			None
Wheel bug	20+	Vegetation	X		X				X		X			X			None
Kissing bug	20+	Bedroom	X			X				X		X				X	

Adapted from Frazier VA. *Clin Symp (Ciba)* 1968;20:101.
[a] 10 mm = 3/8 in.

TABLE 3.6. *Poisonous snakes indigenous to the United States*

Family	Genus	Species	Common name
Crotalidae			Pit vipers
	Crotalus		Rattlesnakes
		C. adamanteus	Eastern diamondback
		C. atrox	Western diamondback
		C. horridus	Timber rattlesnake
		C. viridus	Western rattlesnake
		C. v. viridis	Prairie rattlesnake
		C. v. helleri	Southern Pacific rattlesnake
		C. v. oreganus	Northern Pacific rattlesnake
		C. v. abussus	Grand Canyon rattlesnake
		C. v. lutosus	Great Basin rattlesnake
		C. cerastes	Sidewinder
		C. ruber	Red diamond rattlesnake
		C. Mitchelli	Speckled rattlesnake
		C. lepidus	Rock rattlesnake
		C. tiaris	Tiger rattlesnake
		C. willardi	Ridge-nosed rattlesnake
		C. scutulatus	Mojave rattlesnake
		C. molossus	Black-tailed rattlesnake
		C. pricei	Twin-spotted rattlesnake
	Sistrurus		
		S. catenates	Massauga rattlesnake
		S. miliarius	Pygmy rattlesnake
	Agkistrodon		
		A. piscivorus	Water moccasin
		A. piscivorus	Copperhead
Elapidae		*Micruroides euryxanthus*	Sonoran (Arizona) coral snake
		Micrurus fulvius	Eastern coral snake

Local ecchymoses and vesicles usually appear within the first few hours, and hemorrhagic blebs are often present by 24 hours. Lymphadenitis and lymph node enlargement also may become apparent.

Without appropriate therapy (Fig. 3.10), these local manifestations progress to necrosis and may extend throughout the bitten extremity, effectively maiming the victim. Also, as in any animal wound, secondary infection is a risk; the snake's oral flora includes Gram-negative bacteria. Table 3.7 summarizes the local characteristics of pit viper bites.

The dramatic signs of crotalid envenomation are derived primarily from the victim's hypovolemic state, hemorrhagic tendencies, and neuromuscular dysfunction. These signs are outlined in Table 3.8), while Table 3.9 outlines the more notable physical signs.

Coral Snakes

Coral snakes leave unimpressive local signs but can neurologically cripple their prey (Fig. 3.11). The bite may have one or two punctures, at most 7 to 8 mm apart, as well as other small teeth marks. There is usually only mild pain and little, if any, swelling. Local wound and, eventually, extremity paresthesia and weakness may be reported. Over several hours, generalized malaise and nausea, fasciculations, and weakness develop insidiously. The patient may complain of diplopia and have difficulty talking or swallowing. Physical examination reveals bulbar dysfunction and generalized weakness. Respiratory failure may ensue.

One antivenin (antivenin crotalidae polyvalent, Wyeth Laboratories, Madison, NJ) is effective for the rattlesnake, water moccasin, and copperhead. For maximal venom binding, the antivenin should be given within 4 hours of the snake strike. Benefits of antivenin administration after 12 hours are questionable, and use is not indicated after 24 hours (an exception may be continued coagulopathy). The initial recommended dose varies with the severity of the envenomation. The amount of antivenin is not calculated on a weight basis;

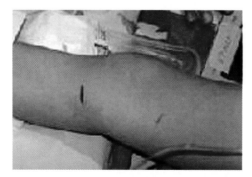

FIG. 3.9. The site of a snakebite in a severe Mojave rattlesnake envenomation. Note the minimal swelling and erythema. (From *http://emedicine.com/asp/image_search.asp? query=Snakebite*, with permission.)

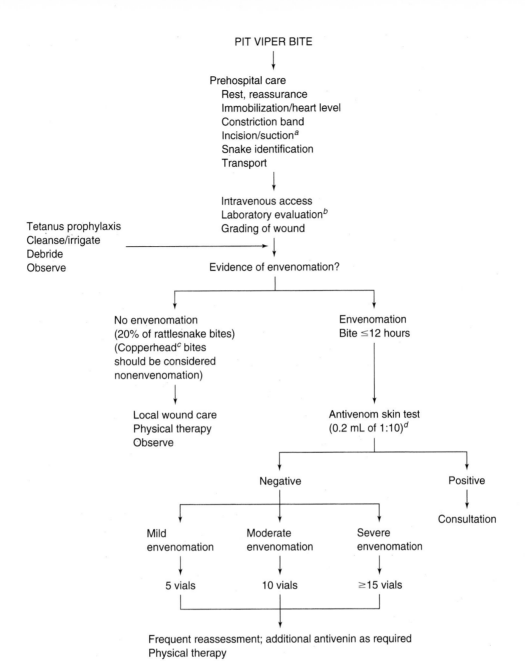

PIT VIPER BITE

Prehospital care
Rest, reassurance
Immobilization/heart level
Constriction band
Incision/suction[a]
Snake identification
Transport

Intravenous access
Laboratory evaluation[b]
Grading of wound

Tetanus prophylaxis
Cleanse/irrigate
Debride
Observe

Evidence of envenomation?

No envenomation
(20% of rattlesnake bites)
(Copperhead[c] bites
should be considered
nonenvenomation)

Envenomation
Bite ≤12 hours

Local wound care
Physical therapy
Observe

Antivenom skin test
(0.2 mL of 1:10)[d]

Negative

Positive

Consultation

Mild
envenomation

Moderate
envenomation

Severe
envenomation

5 vials

10 vials

≥15 vials

Frequent reassessment; additional antivenin as required
Physical therapy

FIG. 3.10. Management of a pit viper bite. **a:** Perform within 5 to 10 minutes of bite; continue suction for 30 to 60 minutes. **b:** Obtain a complete blood count, platelet count, prothrombin time, partial thromboplastin time, urinalysis, type and hold; in moderate or severe cases, add fibrinogen, arterial blood gases, electrolytes, blood urea nitrogen, and creatinine. **c:** Antivenin seldom needed except when large snakes and small children. **d:** Dilution of 1:100 if there is an allergy history; saline control; resuscitation medications at hand; antivenin seldom indicated if more than 12 to 24 hours since the bite.

TABLE 3.7. *Local signs of pit viper envenomation*

Pain
Edema
Erythema
Ecchymosis
Vesicles
Hemorrhagic blebs

TABLE 3.8. *Systemic signs of crotalid (pit viper) envenomation*

General
  Anxiety, diaphoresis, pallor, nonresponsiveness
Cardiovascular
  Tachycardia, decreased capillary perfusion, hypotension, shock
Pulmonary
  Pulmonary edema, respiratory failure
Renal
  Oliguria, hemoglobinuria, hematuria
Neuromuscular
  Fasciculations, weakness, paralysis, convulsions
Hematologic
  Bleeding diathesis

Table 3.9. *Grading of crotalid (pit viper) snakebites*

	Mild	Moderate	Severe
Local	Fang mark, intense pain, edema, erythema, ecchymosis, vesicles within 10–15 cm of bite	All local signs extend beyond wound site	Entire extremity involvement
Systemic	None, anxiety-related	Nausea/vomiting, weakness/fainting, perioral, scalp paresthesias, metallic taste, pallor, tachycardia, mild hypotension, fasciculations	As in moderate; hypotension, shock, bleeding, diathesis, respiratory distress
Laboratory	No abnormalities	Hemoconcentration, thrombocytopenia, hypofibrinogenemia	Significant anemia, prolonged clotting time, metabolic acidosis

children require more than adults as a rule. Doses in the higher range are used when snake or human variables associated with higher morbidity/mortality are present.

Wound care includes irrigation, cleansing, a loose dressing, and consideration of tetanus prophylaxis. The affected extremity should be maintained just below the level of the heart and in a position of function. Cotton padding between swollen digits is useful. Broad-spectrum prophylactic antibiotics are recommended by most authorities. Analgesics for pain may be offered if the cardiorespiratory status is not in question. Surgical excision of the wound, routine fasciotomy, and application of ice are contraindicated. Excision of the wound does not remove significant venom after 30 minutes, and cryotherapy has been associated with increased extremity necrosis and amputations. Fasciotomy should be reserved for the very rare case of a true compartmental syndrome. Necrosis is usually the result of the proteolytic enzymes or inappropriate therapy and is not caused by compartmental pressure. Superficial debridement will be required at 3 to 6 days; a wound care regimen suggested at this stage includes local oxygen, aluminum acetate (1:20 solution) soaks, and triple dye. Physical therapy is beneficial during the healing phase.

When coral snake wounds are present or the history or specimen is consistent with an eastern coral snakebite, antivenin for *Micrurus fulvius* (Wyeth) is administered before

development of further symptoms. This is also an equine serum and requires preliminary skin testing (see package insert). The initial recommended dose is three to five vials intravenously; an additional three to five vials may be given as needed for signs of venom toxicity. There is no antivenin available for the Arizona coral snake (*Micruroides euryxanthus*). Supportive care should provide a satisfactory outcome in these cases. Constriction bands, suction and drainage, and other local measures do not retard coral snake venom absorption and, hence, are not indicated (Table 3.10 and Fig. 3.12).

MAMMALIAN BITES

Clinical Manifestations

Mammalian bite wounds cause a spectrum of tissue injuries from trivial to life threatening. Scratches, abrasions, contusions, punctures, lacerations, and their complications are seen commonly in the emergency department. The complications usually involve secondary infections or damage to structures that underlie the bite. Dogs are the animals causing most bite wounds. The dog strikes the head and neck in 60% to 70% of victims 5 years old and younger and in 50% of those 10 years old and younger. These wounds most often involve the lips, nose, and cheek areas, and, on rare occasions, they penetrate the skull, with resulting depressed skull fractures and intracranial lesions; secondary infections complicate approximately 1% to 3% of such wounds (Figs. 3.13, 3.14, and 3.15). The uncommon life-threatening injuries occur almost exclusively in young children and include major vascular injury, visceral penetration, and chest trauma.

Cat bites are located in the infection-prone upper extremities in two-thirds of cases and usually are puncture wounds rather than lacerations or contusions. Infections that complicate these wounds result from the same organisms isolated in dog bites, but a higher incidence of *Pasteurella multocida* is found. *P. multocida* infections characteristically present within 12 to 24 hours of the injury and rapidly display erythema, significant swelling, and intense pain.

Cat scratches are most commonly located on the victim's upper extremities or periorbital region and are more likely to develop secondary bacterial infection than scratches from

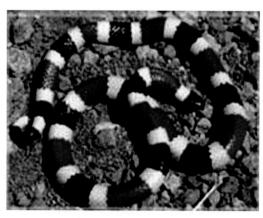

FIG. 3.11. Western coral snake.

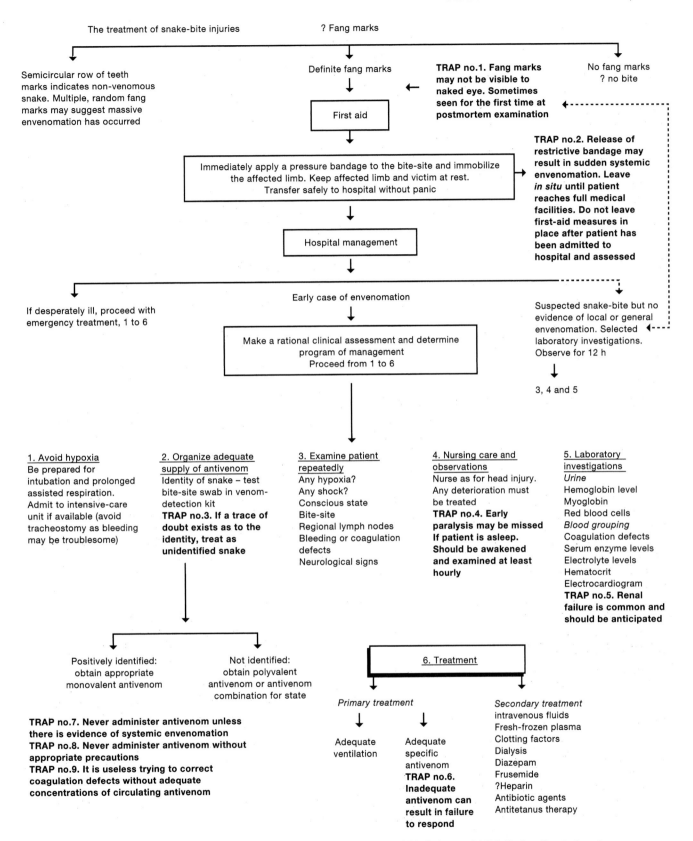

FIG. 3.12. Treatment of snake bite injuries. (From Ellenhorn MJ, Schonwald SJ, Ordog G, et al., eds. *Ellenhorn's medical toxicology*, 2nd ed. Philadelphia: Lippincott Williams & Wilkins, 1996:1750, with permission.)

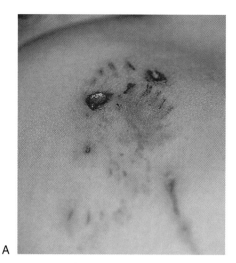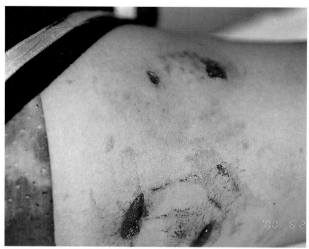

A   B

FIG. 3.13. This child was bitten multiple times by a dog in the back **(A)** and thigh **(B)**.

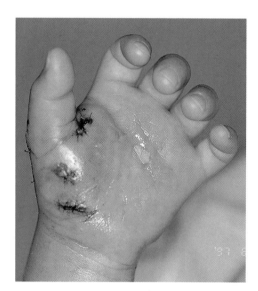

FIG. 3.14. An infected dog bite.

the other common domesticated species. Corneal abrasions also are occasionally associated with the periorbital wounds. Catscratch disease, an uncommon complication of these injuries, is characterized by a papule at the scratch site and subsequent regional lymphadenitis (see Fig. 11.67).

Human bites in older children and adolescents are most commonly incurred when a clenched fist strikes the teeth of an adversary. The wound typically overlies the metacarpalphalangeal joint, and on relaxation of the fist, the bacterial inoculum penetrates more deeply into the relatively avascular fascial layers. Hand infections, regardless of infection site, usually present with mild swelling over the dorsum of the hand 1 to 2 days after injury. Infected hand bites may be superficial and localized to the wound, but if there is pain with active or passive finger motion, a more serious deep compartmental infection or tendonitis should be suspected. Osteomyelitis occasionally occurs in hand infections. In younger children, human bites are more often on the face or

Table 3.10. *How not to treat a snakebite*

Although united medical professionals may not agree on every aspect of what to do for snakebite first aid, they are nearly unanimous in their views of what not to do. Among their recommendations are the following:

1. No ice or any other type of cooling on the bite. Research has shown this to be potentially harmful.
2. No tourniquets. This cuts blood flow completely and may result in the loss of the affected limb.
3. No electric shock. This method is under study and has yet to be proven effective. It could harm the victim.
4. No incisions in the wound. Such measures have not been proven useful and may cause further injury.

Adapted from Henkel J. *FDA Consumer* 1995;29:23–27.

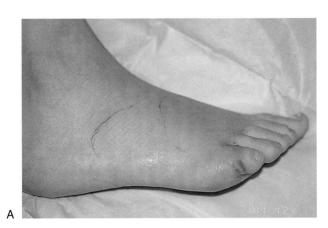
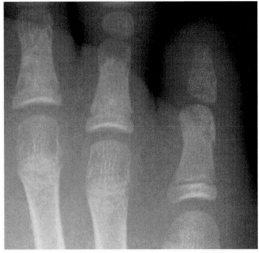

FIG. 3.15. This child sustained a dog bite to the foot, which was sutured at another institution. On follow-up, he had both cellulites **(A)** and a phalangeal fracture **(B)**, possibly complicated by osteomyelitis.

trunk than on the hands (Fig. 3.16). Often, a playmate inflicts the wound, but child abuse must always be considered. Some systemic diseases that may be spread by human bites are human immunodeficiency virus, hepatitis B, and syphilis.

Rodent bites have a relatively low incidence of secondary infection (10%) (Fig. 3.17). Ratbite fever is a rare disease that may present after a 1- to 3-week incubation period with chills, fever, malaise, headache, and a maculopapular or petechial rash. There are two forms: Haverhill fever (*Streptobacillus moniliformis*) and Sodoku (*Spirillum minus*), both of which are responsive to intravenous penicillin.

Another uncommon bacterium for which lagomorphs, particularly rabbits, are hosts is *Francisella tularensis*. Tularemia is usually spread to humans by rabbit bites, although contact

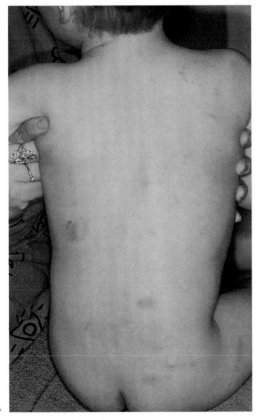
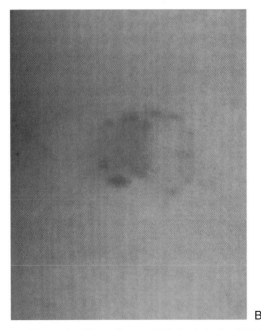

FIG. 3.16. A, B: A 3-year-old boy with human bites on his back. (From Reece RM, Ludwig S. *Child abuse: medical diagnosis and management*, 2nd ed. Philadelphia: Lippincott Williams & Wilkins, 2001:396, with permission.)

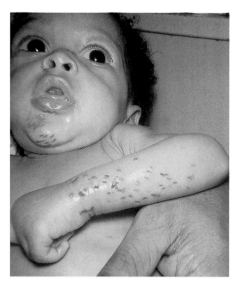

FIG. 3.17. Rat bites on an arm.

with or ingestion of contaminated animals or insect vectors is sufficient for transmission. Ulceroglandular tularemia is the most common form of the disease, and streptomycin is the agent of first choice in its treatment.

Serious infections from multiple bacteria, such as osteomyelitis, sepsis, endocarditis, and meningitis, have been reported as complications of mammalian bite wounds as well as the more esoteric diseases already mentioned. The risk of rabies or tetanus always must be considered in animal bites.

Management

Meticulous and prompt local care of the bite wound is the most important factor in satisfactory healing and prevention of infection. In more extensive wounds, local anesthesia is achieved before wound hygiene. Then, the skin surrounding the wound should be cleaned with a soft sponge and 1% povidone iodine solution can remove obvious contaminants. The wound itself should be forcefully irrigated with a minimum of 200 mL normal saline. A 19-gauge needle or catheter attached to a 30-mL syringe will supply sufficient pressure for wound decontamination and will decrease the infection rate by 20-fold. Stronger irrigant antiseptics e.g., povidone iodine scrub preparation, 20% hexachlorophene,

alcohols, hydrogen peroxide) may damage wound surfaces and delay healing. Soaking in various preparations has not proved helpful in reducing infections.

Extremities with extensive wounds should be immobilized in a position of function and kept elevated as much as possible. This is especially true of hand wounds, which should have bulky mitten dressings and be supported by an arm sling. All significant wounds should be rechecked in 24 to 48 hours.

SUGGESTED READINGS

Auerbach PS. Marine envenomation. *N Engl J Med* 1991;325:486–493.

Auerbach PS. *Wilderness medicine*, 4th ed. St. Louis: Mosby, 2001.

Brogan TV, Bratton SL, Dowd MD, et al. Severe dog bites in children. *Pediatrics* 1995;96:947–950.

Burgess JL, Dart RC, Egen NB, et al. Effects of constriction bands on rattlesnake venom absorption: a pharmacokinetic study. *Ann Emerg Med* 1992;21:1086–1093.

Clark RF, Wethern-Kestner S, Vance MV, et al. Clinical presentation and treatment of black widow spider envenomation: a review of 163 cases. *Ann Emerg Med* 1992;21:782–787.

Cruz NS, Alvarez RG. Rattlesnake bite complications in 19 children. *Pediatr Emerg Care* 1994;10:30–33.

Davidson TM, Schafer SF. Rattlesnake bites: guidelines for aggressive treatment. *Postgrad Med* 1994;96:107–114.

DeShazo RD, Butcher BT, Banks WA. Reactions to the stings of the imported fire ant. *N Engl J Med* 1990;323:462–466.

Dire DJ. Emergency management of dog and cat bite wounds. *Emerg Med Clin North Am* 1992;10:719–736.

Halstead BW, Vinci JM. Venomous fish stings. *Clin Dermatol* 1991;5:29–35.

Jerrard DA. ED management of insect stings. *Am J Emerg Med* 1996;14:429–433.

Koffman MB. Portuguese man-o'-war envenomation. *Pediatr Emerg Care* 1992;8:27–28.

Lindsey D, Christopher M, Hollenbach J, et al. Natural course of the human bite wound: incidence of infection and complications in 434 bites and 803 lacerations, in the same group of patients. *J Trauma* 1987;27:45–48.

Phillips S, Kohn M, Baker D, et al. Therapy of brown spider envenomation: a controlled trial of hyperbaric oxygen, dapsone and cyproheptadine. *Ann Emerg Med* 1995;25:363–368.

Rees R, Campbell D, Rieger E, et al. The diagnosis and treatment of brown recluse spider bites. *Ann Emerg Med* 1991;16:945–949.

Reeves JA, Allison EJ Jr, Goodman PE. Black widow spider bite in a child. *Am J Emerg Med* 1996;14:469–471.

Valentine MD, Lichtenstein LM. Anaphylaxis and stinging insect hypersensitivity. *JAMA* 1991;258:2881–2885.

Visscher PK, Veller RS, Camazine S. Removing bee stings. *Lancet* 1996;348:301–302.

Whitley RE. Conservative treatment of copperhead snakebites without antivenin. *J Trauma* 1996;41:219–221.

Woestman R, Perkin R, Van Stralen D. The black widow: is she deadly to children? *Pediatr Emerg Care* 1996;12:360–364.

Wright SW, Wrenn KD, Murray L, et al. Clinical presentation and outcome of brown recluse spider bite. *Ann Emerg Med* 1997;30:28–32.

CHAPTER 4

Cardiothoracic Emergencies

Editor: Marc N. Baskin

CARDIAC EMERGENCIES

Congestive Heart Failure

Congestive heart failure (CHF) is best described as a syndrome in which the heart cannot maintain a level of tissue perfusion adequate to meet metabolic needs. Although the primary cause of CHF in infants and children is congenital heart disease, a number of conditions can cause CHF in the presence of a normal cardiac structure.

Clinical Manifestations

The clinical manifestations of CHF are directly related to the compensatory mechanisms: (1) Cardiac enlargement usually is the result of ventricular dilation. The chest radiograph remains the most readily available method for assessing ventricular dilation. The other finding related to mechanical compensatory responses is ventricular hypertrophy, which is demonstrable on the electrocardiogram (ECG). (2) Tachycardia is a manifestation of catecholamine release that is part of the neurohumoral response to diminished cardiac output. (3) The protodiastolic gallop, or third heart sound (S_3), is a sign of decreased ventricular compliance and increased resistance to filling. (4) Tachypnea and often rales and wheezing are present. In older children, dyspnea with activity and orthopnea also may be present. (5) Feeding difficulties may be caused by the tachypnea. (6) Cool, moist extremities and pallor may be present as a result of peripheral vasoconstriction secondary to catecholamine release. (7) Pulmonary and peripheral fluid accumulation accompanies CHF, reflecting impaired cardiac emptying and impaired sodium and protein balance. Hepatomegaly and peripheral edema (Fig. 4.1) represent the clinical manifestations of this problem. Peripheral edema is an unusual finding in young infants.

Laboratory Findings

A chest radiograph may show an increased cardiothoracic ratio or evidence of pulmonary congestion such as Kerley B lines, thought to be caused by thickening of the interlobular septa (Fig. 4.2). Pleural effusions are common. The ECG is a nonspecific indicator of cardiac decompensation but may be helpful for establishing the cause of the CHF, such as cardiac arrhythmia, myocardial ischemia, or congenital heart disease (CHD). Echocardiography is helpful in evaluating the cardiac anatomy of a child with CHF. Ultrasonography can differentiate an enlarged cardiac silhouette secondary to ventricular chamber enlargement from pericardial fluid accumulation. Functional indices can be obtained as an objective measure of cardiac performance and response to therapy. Blood gas abnormalities may be present. Prolonged tissue hypoperfusion can result in metabolic acidosis, and the alveolar fluid accumulation may result in hypoxia. Prerenal azotemia may be present, and, in situations of suspected perfusion abnormalities or inflammatory myocardial diseases, cardiac enzymes (creatine phosphokinase or troponin) may be elevated.

Management

Initial medical therapy includes defining the cause, ensuring adequate ventilation, administering oxygen, initiating cardiorespiratory monitoring, achieving rhythm control, treating pulmonary edema (e.g., diuretics, morphine sulfate), and providing inotropic support (digitalis or catecholamines). Positive-pressure respiration by endotracheal intubation is indicated for respiratory decompensation ($PaCO_2 \geq 50$ mm Hg). Bicarbonate therapy sometimes is indicated to correct severe metabolic acidosis that arises from diminished tissue perfusion but only after adequate ventilation is ensured.

Newborn with Obstructed Systemic or Pulmonary Blood Flow

Clinical Manifestations/Management

Any newborn with sudden onset of either collapsed systemic circulation or intense cyanosis should be considered at risk of the presence of a ductus-dependent state. Typical conditions

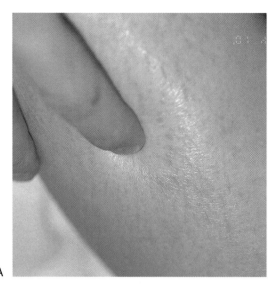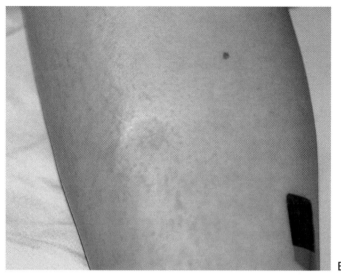

A   B

FIG. 4.1. This 12-year-old child presented with leg swelling and fatigue. Pressing the pretibial soft tissue for a few seconds **(A)** and then releasing it demonstrates the pitting edema **(B)**.

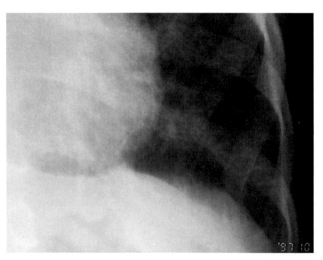

FIG. 4.2. This 8-year-old child presented with shortness of breath and puffy eyes. Her chest radiograph shows Kerley B lines, thin horizontal linear densities in the costophrenic angle area.

TABLE 4.1. *Duct-dependent cardiac lesions*

Ductus-dependent pulmonary blood flow
  Pulmonary atresia with intact ventricular septum
  Tricuspid atresia
  Critical pulmonary stenosis
Ductus-dependent systemic blood flow
  Coarctation of the aorta
  Aorta arch interruption
  Hypoplastic left heart syndrome (aortic atresia)

Adapted from Gewitz MH. Cardiac disease. In: Polin R, Yoder M, Burg F, eds. *Workbook in practical neonatology,* 2nd ed. Philadelphia: WB Saunders, 1993.

that are duct dependent are listed in Table 4.1. In these babies, closure of the ductus unmasks the underlying circulatory insufficiency resulting in the clinical picture of either severe hypoxemia, shock, or both. Prostaglandin E_1 is infused to keep the ductus open.

Cardiac Arrhythmias

Clinical Manifestations

Arrhythmias may come to the physician's attention in the following ways: (1) symptoms of CHF [e.g., poor feeding in a neonate (see previous section)], (2) symptoms related to decreased cerebral blood flow (e.g., syncope, dizziness, irritability, inappropriate behavior), (3) symptoms related to decreased coronary blood flow (anginal chest pain), (4) perception of a rhythm disturbance by the child (e.g., palpitations, skipped beats).

Management

Cardiac arrhythmias become emergencies when they produce hemodynamic alterations that result in a decreased cardial output or have the potential to do so. To treat cardiac arrhythmias effectively, one must be able to identify specific arrhythmias, recognize the signs and symptoms of cardiac decompensation, and understand which arrhythmias are likely to produce rapid cardiac decompensation. Table 4.2 represents an overview of the emergent management of arrhythmias. Table 4.3 illustrates ranges of rates accepted as normal.

Slow Heart Rates

Complete Heart Block

Complete (third-degree) atrioventricular (AV) heart block is the most common cause of significant bradycardia in infants

TABLE 4.2. *Emergent management of arrhythmias in children*

Arrhythmia	Initial treatment (IV)	Secondary treatment (IV)
Slow heart rate		
Complete heart block		
Congenital	Isoproterenol (I) infusion: 0.1–2.0 μg/kg/min Epinephrine(E): 0.1–0.5 μg/kg of 1:10,000 dilution Infusion: 0.1–2.0 μg/kg/min	Pacemaker
Acquired, nonsurgical	(I), (E)	Pacemaker
Postsurgical	(I), (E), pacemaker	None
Sick sinus syndrome	(I), (E) Atropine (At): 0.02–0.04 mg/kg (maximum, 1–2 mg)	Pacemaker
Fast heart rate		
Supraventricular tachycardia		
Critical	Adenosine (Ad): 100–400 μg/kg Cardioversion: 1–2 watt-sec/kg	Repeat cardioversion Digoxin: total digitalizing dose (TDD) for term infant-12 yr: 30–45 μ/kg IV over first 24 hours; first dose is $\frac{1}{2}$ of TDD; second dose $= \frac{1}{4}$ of TDD at 8–12 hrs; third dose $= \frac{1}{4}$ of TDD at 8–12 hours after second dose.
Noncritical	Adenosine	Digoxin, (Am), (Proc), Esmolol (Es) 500 μg/kg/min over 1 min followed by 50 μg/kg/min over 4 min; repeat in 5 min with 500 μg/kg/min over 1 min, 100 μg/kg/min over 4 min, Propranolol (Prop) 0.05–0.1 mg/kg over 5 min
Wolff–Parkinson–White syndrome	Adenosine	(Am), (Es), (Prop), (Proc)
Junctional tachycardia	Digoxin	(Am), (Proc)
Ventricular tachycardia		
Critical	Cardioversion 2–5 watt-sec/kg	Lidocaine 1 mg/kg and cardioversion 2–5 watt-sec/kg
Noncritical	Lidocaine 1 mg/kg	(Am), (Proc)
Ventricular fibrillation	Defibrillation: 2 J/kg, then	Lidocaine 1 mg/kg and defibrillation 4–10 watt-sec/kg
Irregular heart rate		
Premature ventricular contractions	Lidocaine 1 mg/kg	(Am), (Proc)
Second-degree heart block	Isoproterenol, epinephrine	Pacemaker

Many arrhythmias require treatment only when symptomatic.
Treatment of underlying disorders (e.g., electrolyte imbalance) and supportive therapy (e.g., airway management) are always the first priority.
Refer to the text for a more complete discussion.
IV, intravenous; IO, intraosseous; TDD, total digitalizing doses.

TABLE 4.3. *Normal heart rate ranges*

Age	Heart rate (beats per min)
Newborn	80–180
1 wk–3 mo	80–180
3 mo–2 yr	80–160
2–10 yr	65–130
10 yr–adult	55–90

and children. Complete heart block, which may be congenital or acquired, results from a complete failure of conduction from atria to ventricles (Fig. 4.3).

Congenital Heart Block

Congenital heart block may be idiopathic, associated with congenital heart defects, or associated with collagen disease in the mother. The infant with complete heart block who has severe CHF may require intubation for adequate ventilation and oxygenation. Infusion of isoproterenol or epinephrine may increase the heart rate slightly, allowing time for the placement of a temporary pacemaker.

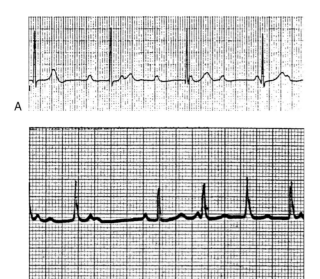

FIG. 4.3. Complete atrioventricular block. **A:** This 4-year-old child had an episode of syncope and was noted to have a heart rate of 45 beats per minute (bpm). The electrocardiogram shows no relationship between the P waves and QRS complexes. (Courtesy of Dr. Paul K. Woolf). **B:** This 16-year-old girl was asymptomatic but was noted to have an irregular heart rate. Her electrocardiogram showed no regular PR interval or relationship between the P wave and QRS complex. Her ventricular rate is approximately 110 beats per minute (bpm), and her atrial rate approximately 95 bpm.

An older child with congenital complete heart block occasionally presents with dizziness, syncope, exercise limitation, or fatigue rather than symptoms associated with CHF.

Acquired Heart Block

Acquired heart block may be idiopathic, occur after cardiac surgery, or may be associated with congenital heart defects, infectious diseases such as myocarditis (viral or Lyme), inflammatory processes (lupus, rheumatic fever), Kawasaki disease, muscle diseases, cardiac tumors, or cardiac sclerosis. The emergency treatment of congenital or acquired nonsurgical heart block is similar. Pharmacologic therapy (Table 4.2) plays a role if adequate ventilation, oxygenation, and treatment of acidosis do not produce a normalization of the blood pressure and peripheral perfusion.

Sinus Bradycardia

Sinus bradycardia is a heart rate that is below the normal range for age (Table 4.3). An ECG is necessary to rule out second-degree or complete heart block; P waves with a normal PR interval must precede each QRS complex in sinus bradycardia. It often occurs in the athletic child or in the adolescent as a normal variant, especially during sleep. Other causes of sinus bradycardia are anorexia-induced weight loss, hypothyroidism, increased intracranial pressure, and drugs such as propranolol or digoxin. Therapy of the under-

lying disorder is indicated, but in symptomatic patients, atropine may be useful as a temporizing measure (Table 4.2).

Sick Sinus Syndrome

Sick sinus syndrome is a condition in which sinus node function is depressed and may present with syncope and a sinus

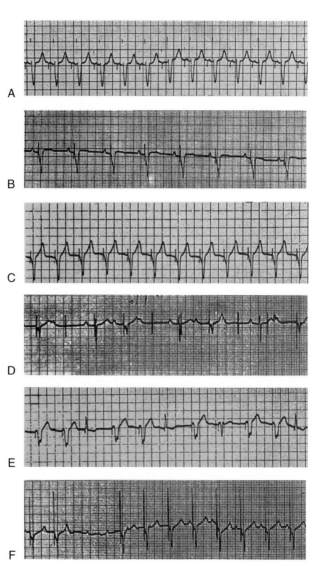

FIG. 4.4. A: An electrocardiogram shows a pacemaker that paces the atrium and after 150 milliseconds paces the ventricle. Note the pacemaker stimulus artifact before the P wave and QRS complex. **B:** An electrocardiogram shows a pacemaker that senses the atrium and paces the ventricle after a 150-millisecond delay. Note that pacemaker stimulus artifact only precedes the QRS complex. **C:** An electrocardiogram shows ventricular pacing at 100 beats per minute (bpm) with normal capture. Note the pacemaker stimulus artifact preceding the QRS. **D:** An electrocardiogram shows ventricular pacing at 85 bpm with intermittent failure of capture. Note that several pacemaker stimulus artifacts are not followed by a QRS complex, indicating failure of capture. **E:** An electrocardiogram shows ventricular pacing at 90 bpm, with normal sensing of the patient's intrinsic rhythm. **F:** An electrocardiogram shows ventricular pacing at 100 bpm, with inappropriate sensing and failure to stimulate the heart secondary to a wire fracture.

bradycardia often in association with episodes of tachycardia. This rhythm may be seen in children who have undergone cardiac surgery, may be in association with myocarditis, or may be idiopathic.

Pacemakers

When a pacemaker malfunction is suspected, a chest radiograph should be obtained to look for wire fractures or lead displacement. An ECG lead that shows the largest possible pacemaker stimulus artifact should be chosen (Fig. 4.4). A cardiology consultation should be obtained for any patient with evidence of pacemaker malfunction.

Fast Heart Rates

Supraventricular Tachycardia

Clinical Manifestations

The clinical findings in the patient with supraventricular tachycardia (SVT) depend on the duration of the arrhythmia and the presence or absence of an underlying heart defect or myocardial dysfunction. In the patient with no congenital heart defect or myocardial dysfunction, CHF usually appears only after 24 hours of a rapid rate. The infant with SVT may present with only a fast rate, have varying degrees of CHF (poor feeding, irritability, respiratory distress), or appear to be in shock or septic. The child older than 5 or 6 years of age will usually complain of chest pain, dyspnea, or a rapid heartbeat.

Diagnosis

The ECG is usually characteristic (Fig. 4.5). The rate in infants ranges from 220 to 320 beats per minute (bpm). Older children have rates ranging from 150 to 250 bpm.

Management

The main principle of treatment of any cardiac arrhythmia is that the type of therapy is determined by the urgency of the situation (Table 4.2)

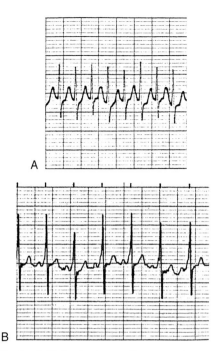

FIG. 4.6. A: Initial electrocardiogram demonstrates a supraventricular tachycardia at a rate of 290 beats per minute. Note the rapid, unvarying rate and narrow QRS complex. P waves may be different from the usual sinus P wave or may be obscured by the ST segment. **B:** After pacing has slowed the rhythm, the P wave, short PR interval, and initial slurring of the QRS complex (the "delta wave") can be seen, suggesting Wolff–Parkinson–White syndrome.

When the SVT is caused by reentry using the AV node (AV nodal reentry) or AV reentry using a bypass tract, any intervention that interrupts the relationship of conduction and refractoriness in the AV node can interrupt the tachycardia. The methods used most often are those that slow AV nodal conduction.

In the emergency department, the cardiologist may use esophageal overdrive pacing to terminate SVT. A small bipolar electrode catheter is passed via the nasogastric route and positioned in the esophagus behind the left atrium. As with intracardiac methods, esophageal rapid atrial pacing at

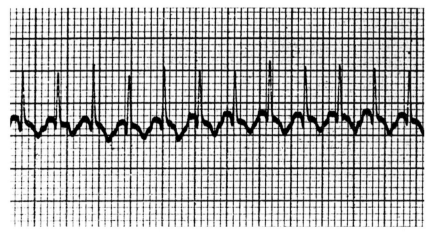

FIG. 4.5. An electrocardiogram shows a rapid, unvarying rate of 290 beats per minute and a narrow QRS complex. P waves may be different from the usual sinus P wave or may be obscured by the ST segment.

a rate faster than the SVT can capture the atrium and interrupt a reentrant circuit, ending the SVT (Fig. 4.6).

Patients with Wolff–Parkinson–White syndrome, a congenital conduction anomaly due to the presence of a bypass tract, only show their ECG abnormalities between episodes of tachycardia. Wolff–Parkinson–White syndrome is a preexcitation syndrome resulting from the conduction through an anomalous path (the Kent bundle) between the atrium and the ventricle. The part of the ventricle attached to the anomalous pathway is depolarized prematurely, slowly producing the short PR and the slurred upstroke of the QRS (the delta wave). A premature systole transmitted through the AV node is conducted in a retrograde manner back up the anomalous tract to the atrium. This action can initiate the tachycardia because the bypass tract has a shorter refractory period than the AV node.

As soon as the patient converts from SVT, an ECG in sinus rhythm should be obtained. This allows diagnosis of the Wolff–Parkinson–White syndrome or other abnormalities that might direct long-term therapy.

Sometimes patients may appear to have SVT, only to have the underlying arrhythmia e.g. atrial flutter recognized when the rate is slowed temporarily with adenosine or other interventions (Fig. 4.7).

Atrial Flutter and Atrial Fibrillation

Atrial flutter and fibrillation occur uncommonly in children. Atrial flutter consists of rapid, regular atrial excitation at rates of 280 to 480 bpm. The ventricular response depends on AV nodal conduction that may allow 1:1, 2:1, 3:1, or 4:1 conduction. The typical ECG reveals saw-toothed flutter waves (Fig. 4.8). Atrial flutter is most commonly seen in children with CHD, especially postoperatively after Mustard repair of D-transposition of the great arteries or Fontan repair, but it also can occur idiopathically or congenitally.

Children with atrial fibrillation or flutter raise the same

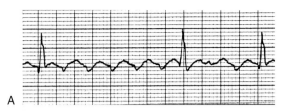

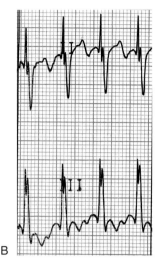

FIG. 4.8. Atrial flutter. **A:** In this electrocardiogram, the sawtooth baseline representing atrial flutter with a varying ventricular response of 6:1 to 3:1 is easy to see. **B:** All leads need to be carefully examined. On this electrocardiogram, the flutter waves are difficult to see in lead II but are more obvious in lead III.

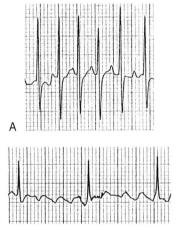

FIG. 4.7. This 18-month-old child had a fever of 103°F (39.4 °C) and a heart rate "too fast to count." **A:** The electrocardiogram initially shows a narrow complex tachycardia of 290 beats per minute. **B:** After adenosine administration, the rate slows temporarily and a sawtooth baseline suggestive of atrial flutter is seen.

therapeutic problems as those with SVT. If cardiac compromise does not necessitate immediate cardioversion, the initial treatment is digoxin. Adenosine increases the AV block and therefore may help diagnostically (Fig. 4.7), but it usually will not correct the atrial flutter or fibrillation to sinus rhythm. For the child who is stable and has a normal blood pressure and adequate perfusion, the physician should allow 24 hours for a response to digoxin before adding a second drug such as procainamide.

Automatic Atrial or Junctional Tachycardia

Automatic atrial or junctional tachycardias may be difficult to control and often are associated with inflammatory states such as myocarditis.

Ventricular Tachycardia

Ventricular tachycardia (VT) is defined as three or more consecutive premature ventricular contractions (PVCs) (Fig. 4.9). The heart rate usually is 150 to 200 bpm, and the contractions may be hemodynamically inefficient and resulting in syncope and death. The cause may be electrolyte imbalance, metabolic disturbances, cardiac tumors, drugs, cardiac catheterization or surgery, CHD, cardiomyopathies, acquired heart disease, right ventricular dysplasia, prolonged QT syndrome, or idiopathic. VT is being seen more commonly in

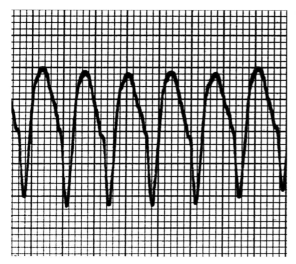

FIG. 4.9. Ventricular tachycardia. There is a wide QRS complex with a rate of approximately 250 beats per minute and a sinusoid pattern.

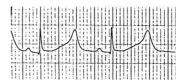

FIG. 4.11. Prolonged QTc syndrome. This 1-year-old child presented after her first short generalized tonic-clonic seizure. She had a medical history of congenital deafness. The electrocardiogram shows a rate of 71, a QT of 0.53 seconds, and a prolonged QTc of 0.57 seconds. (Courtesy of Dr. Mary Chris Bailey.)

children who can be divided into three groups: (1) patients with identifiable noncardiac causes (electrolyte imbalance, toxins, drug overdoses, or drug toxicity), (2) patients with no known underlying heart disease and no extracardiac disturbances (may have small Purkinje cell tumors or foci in the right ventricular outflow tract or left ventricle septum), and (3) patients with either congenital or acquired heart disease.

In children with identifiable extracardiac abnormalities, the underlying disturbance is treated. Children with no known cardiac or extracardiac causes for VT require treatment if they have a sustained, rapid arrhythmia. The urgency of treatment depends on the clinical status. Those with Purkinje cell tumors or ectopic foci may be amenable to catheter radiofrequency ablation or surgical ablation in selected cases (Fig. 4.10).

The congenital long QT syndrome is a special case (Fig. 4.11). Patients with prolonged QT syndromes may present with seizures, syncope, or sudden death. Congenital prolonged QT syndromes include the Jervell and Lange–Nielson syndrome associated with deafness and the Romano–Ward syndrome in families with normal hearing. Sudden death occurs in many patients who are not treated. The sudden death

is secondary to ventricular tachyarrhythmias (torsade de pointes) of the type that often degenerates to ventricular fibrillation. Acquired prolonged QT intervals can be caused by hypocalcemia, myocarditis, increased intracranial pressure, and medications (e.g., procainamide, phenothiazines, some antihistamines, tricyclic antidepressants). Any patient who presents with VT, especially of the polymorphic or torsade de pointes type, should have corrected QT intervals determined in sinus rhythm.

Emergent treatment of these patients includes lidocaine and synchronized DC cardioversion when needed. If the VT is polymorphic, nonsynchronized cardioversion or defibrillation is indicated. Intravenous propranolol, phenytoin, and magnesium have been used in these patients. The class I agents that prolong the QT interval in normal patients should be avoided in patients with these long QT intervals.

Ventricular Fibrillation

Ventricular fibrillation consists of chaotic irregular ventricular contractions with cessation of circulation. These patients are treated according to Advanced Cardiac Life Support guidelines.

Irregular Heart Rates

Premature Depolarizations

Clinical Manifestations

PVCs are seen as premature, wide, bizarrely shaped QRS complexes. Generally, the T wave is opposite in direction to the main deflection of the QRS. A compensatory pause usually follows the premature beat. Children who present with PVCs are often asymptomatic. If the PVC is appreciated, the child may complain of a skipped beat, pounding in the chest, difficulty breathing, or chest pain. If the PVCs are frequent and/or associated with heart disease (congenital or acquired), the child may note dizziness or a rapid heartbeat.

Management

PVCs that require treatment are those likely to cause hemodynamic compromise. This generally is seen in the context

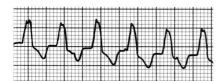

FIG. 4.10. Ventricular tachycardia. This 9-year-old boy, seen because of a 1-week history of malaise and fatigue, was noted to have a rapid pulse and appeared ill. His electrocardiogram shows a wide complex tachycardia at a rate of 155 beats per minute (lead I). His tachycardia only resolved after surgical excision of the tachycardia focus.

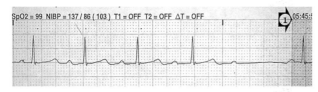

FIG. 4.12. Second-degree atrioventricular block, Mobitz type I (Wenckebach phenomenon). This 12-year-old child presented after fainting at home. The electrocardiogram shows a progressively prolonged PR interval and eventual dropped beat.

of frequent PVCs in a patient with abnormal cardiac function. Symptoms of dizziness or chest pain may accompany PVCs in these patients. Such patients may be found to have myocarditis, cardiomyopathy, or a congenital heart defect (preoperative or postoperative) and abnormal underlying cardiac function. Their treatment may include lidocaine, procainamide, or amiodarone (Table 4.2).

Isolated multiform or coupled PVCs or nonsustained VT ($\geq$150 bpm) in an asymptomatic patient with a normal heart may not require treatment, but this decision must be individualized after consultation with a cardiologist. Rarely is emergency treatment of this type of patient required. It sometimes is helpful to observe the patient's response to activity. If the PVCs abate completely with sinus tachycardia (140 to 150 bpm), they are likely to be benign in terms of clinical significance and need for therapy, although this is not universally true.

Isolated PVCs in an asymptomatic patient in the presence of a structurally and functionally normal heart do not require treatment. Continuous 24-hour ambulatory monitoring should be performed to rule out the presence of undetected VT or complex ventricular arrhythmias.

Premature atrial contractions generally do not require treatment. Patients with frequent premature atrial contractions or PVCs should be evaluated appropriately to rule out myocarditis. Continuous 24-hour ambulatory monitoring should be performed to rule out the occurrence of SVT.

First- and Second-degree Heart Block

First-degree heart block reflects slowed conduction from the sinus node to the ventricle and is manifested by a prolonged PR interval. It is seen with digoxin and other antiarrhythmic drugs, atrial septal defects, and inflammatory diseases such as rheumatic, viral, or Lyme myocarditis. Second-degree heart block results in the failure of some impulses to traverse the AV node. Second-degree heart block, Mobitz type I (Wenckebach phenomenon) is a result of progressive slowing of AV conduction (Fig. 4.12). In Mobitz type II, there is either normal AV conduction or the conduction is completely blocked. The ventricular rate depends on the degree of AV block. Children with first- and second-degree heart block rarely are symptomatic and do not require therapy unless the associated heart rate is low enough to decrease the cardiac output. In this instance, the management is the same as that outlined for complete heart block.

Electrocardiographic Abnormalities Associated with Electrolyte Abnormalities

Any patient with significant arrhythmias should be evaluated for an electrolyte disturbance. The ECG changes may be characteristic and lead to suspicion of a specific electrolyte abnormality. Normal ECG intervals (PR, QRS, QTc) are listed in Table 4.4.

Hyperkalemia

Hyperkalemia is a true life-threatening emergency, often seen in patients with end-stage renal failure. ECG abnormalities and management are discussed in Chapter 17 (Renal and Electrolyte Emergencies).

Hypokalemia

Serum potassium concentrations less than 2.7 mEq/L generally produce typical ECG changes in ventricular repolarization. These changes include U waves and ST segment depression. The QTc interval lengthens and the T wave flattens

TABLE 4.4. *PR interval and QRS duration related to rate and age (and upper limits of normal)*

Rate	0–6 mo	1–6 mo	6 mo–1 yr	1–3 yr	3–8 yr	8–12 yr	12–16 yr	Adult
PR								
<60						0.16 (0.18)	0.16 (0.19)	0.17 (0.2)
60–80					0.15 (0.17)	0.15 (0.17)	0.15 (0.18)	0.16 (0.2)
80–100	0.10 (0.12)				0.14 (0.16)	0.15 (0.16)	0.15 (0.17)	0.15 (0.2)
100–120	0.10 (0.12)			(0.15)	0.13 (0.16)	0.14 (0.15)	0.15 (0.16)	0.15 (0.1)
120–140	0.10 (0.11)	0.11 (0.14)	0.11 (0.14)	0.12 (0.14)	0.13 (0.15)	0.14 (0.15)		0.15 (0.1)
140–160	0.09 (0.11)	0.10 (0.13)	0.11 (0.13)	0.11 (0.14)	0.12 (0.14)			(0.17)
160–180	0.10 (0.11)	0.10 (0.12)	0.10 (0.12)	0.10 (0.12)				
>180	0.09	0.09 (0.11)	0.10 (0.11)					
QRS (sec)	0.05 (0.065)	0.05 (0.07)	0.05 (0.06)	0.06 (0.07)	0.07 (0.08)	0.07 (0.09)	0.07 (0.10)	0.08 (0.10)
QTc = QT/$\sqrt{R-R}$		Average normal, <0.450 msec.						

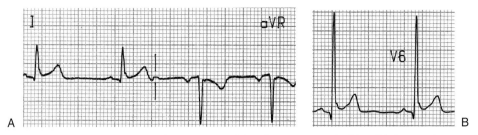

FIG. 4.13 A,B: Early repolarization. This 19-year-old patient presented with mild chest pain associated with coughing. The ST segments are elevated in all the leads with upright T waves and depressed in the leads with negative T waves. Note lead I compared with lead aVR.

with progressive hypokalemia. The PR interval may be prolonged, and intraventricular conduction may be delayed with widening of the QRS complex.

Hypocalcemia

Hypocalcemia prolongs the ST segment causing QTc interval prolongation. Abnormal rhythms, although uncommon, have been reported and include SVT, heart block, and torsade de pointes VT.

Hypercalcemia

Hypercalcemia, with levels higher than 12 mg/dL, shortens the ST segment, causing a shortened QTc interval and normal or prominent U waves. Severe hypercalcemia causes PR interval prolongation, QRS prolongation, and, occasionally, second- and third-degree heart block.

Normal Variants

Early repolarization is often seen in healthy adolescents (Fig. 4.13). In mild pericarditis, the ST segments may also be elevated, especially in the leads representing the left ventricle.

Pericardial Disease

Clinical Manifestations

Respiratory difficulty and chest pain are common with pericardial inflammation. The child with significant pericardial effusion may show clinical signs similar to those of patients with CHF such as tachycardia, tachypnea, and cool extremities.

The cardiac auscultatory findings directly relate to the degree of pericardial fluid accumulation. A friction rub, the scratching, harsh sound heard throughout the cardiac cycle, is commonly heard. The heart sounds usually are distant and muffled.

Pericardial disease can be caused by infections (bacterial, viral, tuberculous, or others), trauma (e.g., chest wall injury, postpericardiotomy syndrome), noninfectious inflammation (e.g., acute rheumatic fever, systemic lupus erythematosus, uremia, drugs), leukemia, or tumors.

Laboratory Findings

The ECG shows diminished precordial voltage in most instances of significant pericardial fluid accumulation (Fig. 4.14). Diffuse T-wave inversions and elevations in the ST segments are common. The heart size is increased on the

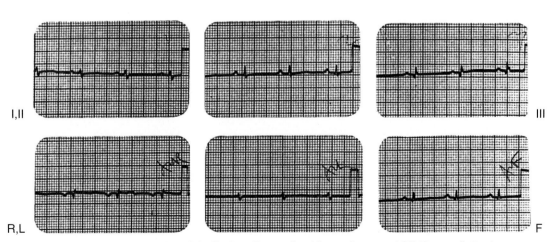

FIG. 4.14. Electrocardiogram in pericardial effusion. Generalized low-voltage and ST-T wave flattening are present.

chest radiograph with pericardial effusion but can be entirely normal if the effusion is small. Echocardiography is the diagnostic procedure of choice for determining the presence of intrapericardial fluid.

Management

For pericarditis without evidence of pericardial effusion, symptomatic therapy for pain should be prescribed, and bed rest in the hospital is advisable. The patient should be followed closely for the development of complications such as myocarditis, pericardial effusion, and cardiac tamponade.

For pericardial effusion, diagnostic pericardiocentesis often is required. Antibiotic therapy alone is not adequate for treatment of purulent pericarditis, and usually an open drainage procedure is indicated. Initial antibiotic therapy should include antimicrobials to cover *Staphylococcus aureus* and *Haemophilus influenzae* (e.g., oxacillin, cefotaxime).

Infective Endocarditis

Although the most common setting for this problem is the child with preexisting CHD, a minority of cases develop in children with no history of cardiac abnormality.

Clinical Manifestations

In the context of CHD, some conditions should prompt an evaluation for endocarditis. These include (1) a protracted febrile course in a presumed viral syndrome, (2) the development of a new neurologic deficit, (3) the onset of hematuria, and (4) signs of systemic or cutaneous embolization.

The classic findings of fever, a change in the cardiac examination, splenomegaly, and evidence of emboli often are present in severe cases. Embolic phenomena may be noted by examining the fundus for Roth spots (retinal hemorrhages), the palms and soles for Janeway lesions (painless hemorrhages), and the fingers and toes for Osler nodes (red painful lesions on the pads), and performing a urinalysis to evaluate for hematuria.

Management

Treatment of infective endocarditis should be started as soon as appropriate blood cultures are obtained. For empiric therapy, many experts recommend the combination of an aminoglycoside, such as gentamicin with either oxacillin or ampicillin.

Hypoxemic Attacks

Clinical Findings

Children with cyanotic CHD in which pulmonary blood flow is reduced, such as tetralogy of Fallot, may experience episodes of intense hypoxemia and hyperpnea. The child may be crying, lethargic, or even unconscious. During a spell, there may be an absence or lessening of a previously heard heart murmur because pulmonary blood flow through the stenotic right ventricular outflow tract is reduced. Laboratory investigations, such as arterial blood gas analysis, ordinarily should be avoided in the initial evaluation. Monitoring with transcutaneous oxygen saturation meters may be helpful.

Management

Knee–chest positioning, oxygen, and administration of morphine are the standard initial therapeutic measures, and these usually result in prompt abatement of the attack.

Acute Rheumatic Fever

Clinical Manifestations

The presence of two major or one major and two minor Jones criteria (Table 4.5) usually establishes the diagnosis. Polyarthritis is the most commonly found major criterion. In contrast to other forms of collagen disease, joint involvement in rheumatic fever usually is migratory and multiple and tends to localize to the larger joints. The minor criteria defined by Jones are nonspecific indices of inflammatory disease and, often, are sources of overdiagnosis of acute rheumatic fever.

It must be emphasized that the modified Jones criteria include evidence of recent streptococcal infection in the history. The antistreptolysin O test is a commonly used, single serologic test and is well standardized.

TABLE 4.5. *Rheumatic fever manifestations*

Major
    Carditis
    Arthritis
    Subcutaneous nodules
    Erythema marginatum
    Chorea
Minor
    Clinical findings
    Arthralgia
    Fever
    Laboratory findings
    Elevated acute phase reactants
    Erythrocyte sedimentation rate
    C-reactive protein
    Prolonged PR interval
    Supporting evidence of antecedent group A streptococcal infections
    Positive throat culture of rapid streptococcal antibody titer
    Elevated or rising streptococcal antibody titer

Adapted from Jones TD. The diagnosis of rheumatic fever. *JAMA* 1944;126:481, as modified in Guidelines for the diagnosis of rheumatic fever. *JAMA* 1992;268:2069.

Management

Acute rheumatic fever requires admission to the hospital and long-term management. Principles of management include (1) treatment of the active streptococcal infection, (2) rest, (3) antiinflammatory agents, and (4) treatment of chorea. All patients with acute rheumatic fever should receive a course of penicillin to eradicate any streptococci. Intramuscular benzathine penicillin is preferable. Occasionally, the child with acute rheumatic fever may present with significant cardiac compromise that involves CHF associated with a large degree of valvar regurgitation or cardiac tamponade due to a pericardial effusion.

NONTRAUMATIC THORACIC EMERGENCIES

Airway Compromise

Obstructive emergencies relating to the oropharynx, larynx, and proximal trachea are discussed in Chapters 11 and 24. Compromise of the more distal tracheobronchial tree may be caused by lesions in the lumen, the wall, or outside the wall of the bronchus. Examples of intraluminal obstruction include tumor (e.g., carcinoid tumor), foreign body, aspiration, hemoptysis or a mucous plug. Obstructions by lesions in the wall of the bronchus include collapse from tracheomalacia and stenosis after tracheostomy. Extrinsic lesions make patients symptomatic by producing impingement on a bronchus by some adjacent structure such as inflamed lymph nodes or mediastinal tumors.

Airway Obstruction

Tracheal Obstruction

Tracheal obstruction may be produced by lesions within the lumen of the trachea, in the wall of the trachea, or extrinsic to the tube. Intrinsic obstruction most commonly occurs in children because of an aspirated foreign body. Intrinsic obstruction may also occur because of a subglottic stenosis after tracheostomy. A hemangioma may also occur but is rare. Tracheomalacia is characterized by a floppy trachea that collapses during expiration. Laryngomalacia, or tracheomalacia outside the thoracic inlet, may produce obstruction during inspiration. Extrinsic compression may occur both from mass lesions and as a result of anomalous arteries.

Clinical Findings

Occasional episodes of respiratory infection that are thought to result from croup or bronchitis may be the only symptom. Stridor, wheezing, or coughing occurs in patients with more significant obstruction, and there may be a history of multiple hospitalizations for croup or bronchitis. Severe tracheal compromise usually is manifested by stridor at rest.

Evaluation/Management

Radiographic evaluation of the stable patient should begin with posteroanterior and lateral chest radiographs, ideally obtained at full inspiration and again at full expiration. Computed tomography to evaluate mass lesions or bronchoscopy to evaluate obstructive lesions may be indicated.

Intubation of the airway to within a short distance of the carina supports most patients with lesions extrinsic to the trachea or in the tracheal wall with a critical obstruction. Lesions within the lumen will likely require endoscopic management in an operating theater.

Vascular Rings

Vascular rings are developmental anomalies of the aorta and great vessels. They may produce obstruction of the esophagus, trachea, or both. The level of obstruction is usually at the trachea, but compression of a bronchus by the ductus arteriosus or by a pulmonary artery sling may produce compression more distally.

Clinical Findings

Vascular rings should be suspected in infants with stridor, dysphagia, failure to thrive associated with difficult feeding, or recurrent pneumonia. Chest radiographs may be supplemented by a variety of diagnostic tests; angiography, echocardiography, magnetic resonance imaging, and digital subtraction angiography are needed in some combination to define the anatomy.

Management

Surgical treatment is usually indicated to relieve the obstruction. This is accomplished by dividing the vascular ring and preserving the blood supply to the aortic branches.

Bronchial Lesions

Right Middle Lobe Syndrome

The right middle lobe is anatomically predisposed to compression of its bronchus by the lymph nodes in its vicinity, which tend to encircle it. Because the right middle and lower lobes are favored sites for aspirated material, recurrent inflammation caused by pneumonia leads to adenopathy.

Clinical Presentation

Recurrent episodes of pneumonia and associated atelectasis in the right middle (and often lower) lobes occur in these patients and are not responsive antibiotic treatment. The mechanical compression of the bronchus leads to a sequestered infection, which may require resection of the right middle or right middle and lower lobes.

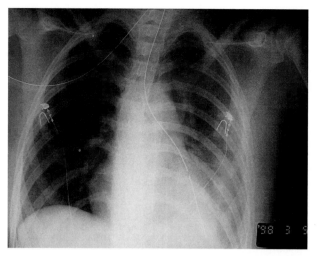

FIG. 4.15. This adolescent had a nasogastric tube placed after a polydrug ingestion. Charcoal was administered, and the patient's respiratory status deteriorated. The chest radiograph shows the nasogastric tube in the left lower lung and alveolar opacification.

Iatrogenic

Nasogastric tubes may occasionally be malpositioned in the tracheobronchial tree. Medications may then be administered into the distal airways or the nasogastric tube may perforate the bronchus. Patients with a depressed mental status or cough reflex are at especially high risk (Fig. 4.15).

Clinical Findings

The development of persistent cough, gag, or abnormal voice suggests malposition into the tracheobronchial tree. If the gastric contents cannot be aspirated, radiographic confirmation may be necessary.

Management

The nasogastric tube should be removed immediately and therapy with ventilatory support, if needed, pulmonary toilet, and antibiotics provided.

Esophagus-related Causes of Airway Difficulties

Tracheoesophageal Fistula

Tracheoesophageal fistula occurs in children both as a congenital lesion and as an acquired problem after suppuration of mediastinal nodes. A congenital fistula is accompanied by atresia of the esophagus in more than 85% of patients. However, in approximately 3% of all patients with a tracheoesophageal fistula, the connection between the tracheal tube and the esophagus creates the shape of the letter H without accompanying esophageal atresia. It is this H-type fistula that is most likely to be seen in the emergency department.

Clinical Findings

These fistulae are notoriously difficult to diagnose. Children generally develop recurrent pulmonary infections for which no source is evident. The characteristic history of choking or gagging when swallowing that accompanies esophageal atresia with tracheoesophageal fistula may not be present.

Management

Contrast esophagram may identify the lesion. Most of these fistulae are small in diameter (much less than 1 cm) and short (less than 1 cm), making radiographic identification difficult.

Gastroesophageal Reflux

Introduction/Pathophysiology

Common causes of repetitive soilage of the tracheobronchial tree include primary aspiration of oropharyngeal secretions, often in children with impaired swallowing mechanisms, and gastroesophageal reflux (GER). GER is universal in babies and is usually outgrown. In the neurologically impaired patient, however, GER may require medical or surgical treatment.

Clinical Presentation

GER presents with symptoms of spitting up or vomiting after eating. Aspiration may lead to presentation with recurrent pneumonia or with an acute life-threatening event in which laryngospasm or bronchospasm precipitated by aspiration of gastric contents produces profound hypoxia and even respiratory or cardiac arrest.

Evaluation/Management

If the diagnosis is evident clinically and the child responds to medical management, no further evaluation may be needed. Recalcitrant GER may be an indication for an upper gastrointestinal contrast study to establish that there is no esophageal web or anatomic obstruction to gastric emptying such as a duodenal web or annular pancreas.

GER is managed by a three-tiered approach. Initially, elevating the head of the bed, thickening the feeds, and decreasing the volume of individual feeds are useful to allow gravity and mechanical effects to help. Medical management includes efforts to decrease gastric acidity using H_2-receptor antagonists such as ranitidine or proton pump–inhibiting drugs or to improve the gastric motility using prokinetic medications such as metoclopramide. Indication for surgery is the failure of nonoperative management or occurrence of a complication that cannot be tolerated such as esophageal stricture or repeated acute life-threatening events without other evident cause. At present, the favored surgical treatment in North America is fundoplication: wrapping the

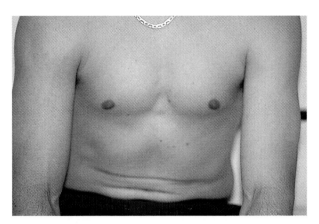

FIG. 4.16. Thoracic outlet syndrome. This 20-year-old pitcher developed "burning" pain, swelling, and erythema of the right arm. His right arm has distended veins. Computed tomography confirmed right subclavian vein thrombosis.

fundus of the stomach either partially or completely (the Nissen operation) around the esophagus just above the gastroesophageal junction.

Thoracic Outlet Obstruction

Thoracic outlet syndrome is a collection of symptoms caused by obstruction of the thoracic neurovascular bundle. This bundle includes the subclavian vessels and brachial plexus.

Clinical Findings

Patients usually present with swelling of the upper chest or extremity and paresthesias or weakness of the arm. If the ob-

struction is mainly venous, the patient may have color changes, venous dilation, and diffuse pain.

Management

Once the diagnosis is suspected, a chest radiograph to rule out a cervical rib should be obtained. Doppler flow ultrasonography, computed tomography (CT), or magnetic resonance angiography can evaluate the great vessels for obstruction (Fig. 4.16). Therapy for deep venous thrombosis is often initiated with alteplase, a thrombolytic agent, and enoxaparin, an anticoagulant.

Pleural Disease

Pneumothorax

Seemingly spontaneous episodes of pneumothorax may occur in children or adolescents. For example, a patient with one or more emphysematous blebs on the surface of the lung may develop spontaneous rupture. In patients with cystic fibrosis, spontaneous pneumothorax is the second most common pulmonary complication of this condition. Patients with Marfan syndrome also have a high incidence of spontaneous pneumothorax (Fig. 4.17).

A tension pneumothorax can cause rapid decompensation of the patient resulting from air accumulating in the hemithorax with each inspiration via a one-way valve effect. The air continues to accumulate in the pleural cavity with inspiration but cannot be extruded on expiration, resulting in total collapse of the lung and hypoxemia. In addition, the accumulating air causes shifting of the mediastinum, impeding the venous return from below the diaphragm and resulting in circulatory failure.

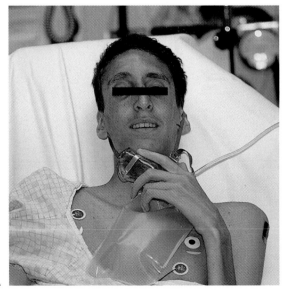
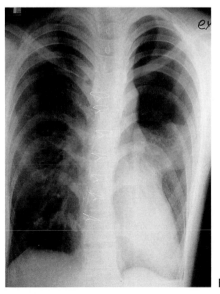

FIG. 4.17. Spontaneous pneumothorax. **A:** This tall, thin, 16-year-old patient with long, slender fingers developed sudden onset of dyspnea and chest pain at rest. **B:** The chest radiograph shows a large left pneumothorax. (Courtesy of Dr. Mark Waltzman.)

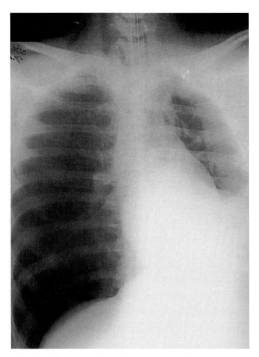

FIG. 4.18. A right-sided tension pneumothorax displaces the heart to the left.

Clinical Findings

The symptoms and signs of pneumothorax depend on the size of the pneumothorax and how rapidly it occurred. A patient with spontaneous rupture of an emphysematous bleb may complain of sudden acute pain on the involved side of the chest followed by tachypnea, pain at the tip of the ipsilateral shoulder, and a sense of shortness of breath.

A patient with a larger pneumothorax may have acute pain, dyspnea, agitation, tachypnea, tachycardia, diminished breath sounds, and increased resonance on the involved side. A radiograph can confirm the diagnosis (Fig. 4.18).

Management

If the patient's condition is not severe, an immediate upright posteroanterior and lateral chest radiographs should be taken. If the pneumothorax is less than 15% and the patient asymptomatic, observation in the hospital and administration of 100% oxygen are all that are necessary.

Lung Lesions

Bronchogenic Cyst

Bronchogenic cysts are thought to result from aberrant budding from the primitive foregut or tracheobronchial tree.

Clinical Presentation

Centrally located cysts may present with symptoms caused by compression of an airway. Wheezing, coughing, fever, and recurrent pneumonia may result in such children. In contrast, patients with peripherally located cysts develop respiratory symptoms only 50% of the time.

Management

Detection of bronchogenic cysts usually occurs radiographically. A chest radiograph often suggests the process, but a CT scan is usually indicated to clarify the anatomy. Plain film findings include a homogeneous, water-density mass without sharply defined borders (Fig. 4.19).

Treatment of bronchogenic cysts is by surgical resection. Asymptomatic cysts should be removed to establish the diagnosis and to prevent the complications of secondary bronchial communication. Carcinoma and fibrosarcomas have been reported to arise in benign-appearing bronchogenic cysts.

Congenital Cystic Disease of the Lung

Congenital Cystic Adenomatoid Malformation and Sequestration

A congenital cystic adenomatoid malformation is the result of an excessive overgrowth of bronchioles and an increase

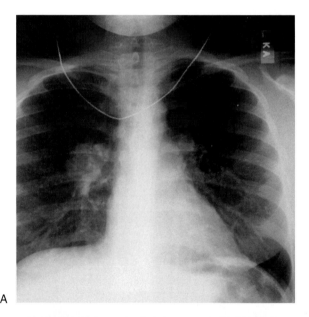

A

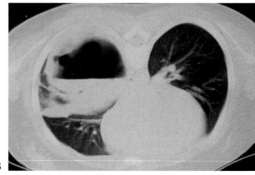

B

FIG. 4.19. A. Plain film of patient with bronchogenic cyst arising off the right mainstem bronchus. **B.** Computed tomography scan of sinular lesion reveals large fluid-filled cyst compressing adjacent lung tissue.

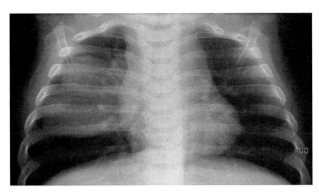

FIG. 4.20. Cystic adenomatoid malformation. This 5-month-old infant had fever, cough, and wheezing for 2 weeks. His radiograph shows a lobular consolidation of the superior segment of the right lower lobe. Computed tomography confirmed the diagnosis of cystic adenomatoid malformation.

in terminal respiratory structures and mucous cells lining the cyst walls. Pulmonary sequestrations arise from an accessory bronchopulmonary bud of the foregut. Histologically, they are portions of pulmonary tissue; however, they are not connected with bronchi or vessels to the rest of the lung (and hence the pulmonary tissue is sequestered).

Clinical Findings Recurrent respiratory infections often lead to a chest radiograph, which confirms the condition. Clinical findings may be identical to those of lobar pneumonia (Fig. 4.20).

Management Chest radiographs in the posteroanterior, lateral, and bilateral decubitus positions should be obtained to evaluate any areas with air–fluid levels. After control of superimposed infection, the lesion should be resected to prevent recurrent infection. A CT scan will help to define the anatomy and exclude other conditions, such as a diaphragmatic hernia, postpneumonic pneumatoceles, or esophageal duplication.

Congenital Lobar Emphysema

Congenital lobar emphysema is caused by overexpansion of the air spaces of a segment or lobe of the lung. There is no significant parenchymal destruction. This entity accounts for approximately half of all congenital lung malformations.

Clinical Findings Infants with congenital lobar emphysema are often normal in appearance at birth but develop tachypnea, coughing, wheezing, and/or cyanosis within a few days. The onset of symptoms may be more gradual, but 80% of patients are symptomatic by 6 months of age, usually presenting with wheezing. Chest radiographs show striking radiolucency in the involved (usually upper) lobe. The diaphragm is usually flattened on the affected side. It can be difficult to tell whether pulmonary markings are present at all in the involved lobe, and pneumothorax may be suspected (Fig. 4.21). The compressed normal lung may be erroneously thought to be atelectatic with the emphysematous lobe compensatory.

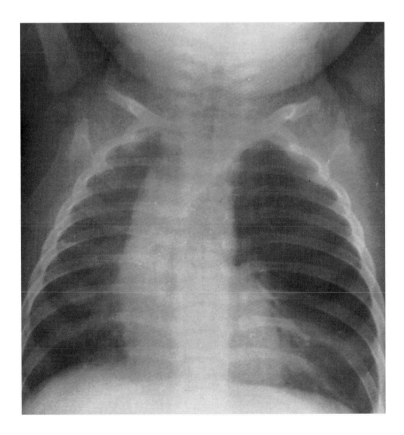

FIG. 4.21. Congenital lobal emphysema of the left upper lobe in a 3-month-old baby girl who presented with decreased breath sounds and rales in this area. Note the secondary compression atelectasis of the left lower lobe.

Management Patients with life-threatening pulmonary insufficiency from compression of normal pulmonary tissue should be treated. Lobectomy is curative if the cause of the obstruction is also relieved.

Congenital Pulmonary Arteriovenous Fistula or Malformation

A congenital pulmonary arteriovenous fistula, a congenitally occurring communication between a major pulmonary artery and a vein within the lung, is usually an aneurysmal sac. Direct right-to-left shunting leads to hypoxemia.

Clinical Findings

The initial presentation of this disorder is frequently either wheezing or persistent pneumonia. Clubbing may suggest chronic hypoxemia. Examination of the chest may demonstrate a palpable thrill or murmurs. Telangiectasias or hemangiomas of the skin and mucous membranes may be observed. Evaluation of the family may also reveal the presence of hereditary hemorrhagic telangiectasis (Osler–Weber–Rendu disease), which is present in more than half the patients with congenital pulmonary arteriovenous fistulae (Fig. 4.22).

Management

Chest films may demonstrate the aneurysmal areas as rounded or lobulated discrete lesions in the parenchyma. CT, magnetic resonance imaging, or arteriography may be necessary. Resection of the fistula, often involving a lobectomy, is indicated if the lesion is localized.

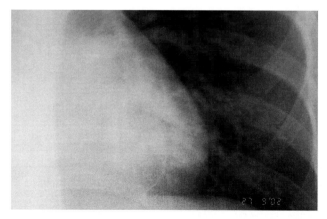

FIG. 4.22. This 12-year-old girl had been treated for recurrent left lower lobe pneumonia and hypoxemia. Her mother had buccal hemangiomas and Osler–Weber–Rendu disease. The chest radiograph shows the persistent retrocardiac density confirmed by computed tomography as an arteriovenous malformation.

Mediastinal Tumors

The mediastinum is commonly divided into anterior, superior, middle, and posterior compartments. Neurogenic tumors are the most common cause of mediastinal masses, with lymphomas and germ cell tumors being second and third in frequency. Thymic enlargement may mimic an anterior mediastinal mass.

Clinical Presentation

Mediastinal masses usually present with respiratory symptoms secondary to airway obstruction or erosion. As a result, patients may present with coughing, wheezing, recurrent respiratory infections, bronchitis, atelectasis, hemoptysis, chest pain, or sudden death. Dysphagia and hematemesis may occur with compression of the esophagus. Superior vena cava syndrome is a rare complication, usually in association with a rapidly growing tumor. If the recurrent laryngeal nerve is compressed as a result of the mass, hoarseness and inspiratory stridor may result. Spinal cord compression syndrome and vertebral erosion can be seen with a posterior mediastinal tumor.

Management

Children with tumors of the anterior or superior mediastinum should be admitted to a hospital to undergo urgent evaluation. CT scan of the chest is usually needed to supplement plain radiographs and assess the likelihood of tracheal compression.

Airway compression by large mediastinal masses is often significant. If a general anesthetic is administered, the thoracic trachea may be occluded by a tumor because the anesthetic eliminates the negative intrathoracic pressure caused by expansion of the chest wall. This situation can be difficult to manage; passage of a rigid bronchoscope may be necessary to stent the trachea open to allow gas exchange.

Diaphragmatic Problems

Congenital Diaphragmatic Hernia

A congenital diaphragmatic hernia is the presence of intestinal viscera in the chest through an opening in the diaphragm not caused by trauma. Approximately 90% occur on the left, usually through the foramen of Bochdalek, which is at the back of the thoracic cavity. Herniation may rarely occur through the foramen of Morgagni, which lies just posterior to the sternum. Traumatic diaphragmatic rupture may occur through any portion of the diaphragm and may present in a delayed time frame.

Pathophysiology

Most babies with a congenital diaphragmatic hernia become symptomatic as newborns, when profound respiratory compromise leads to diagnosis. Mechanical compression, pulmonary hypertension, surfactant deficiency, and a vicious cycle of hypoxia, acidosis, and intrapulmonary shunting lead to the death of approximately half of newborns with this diagnosis. A congenital diaphragmatic hernia may be also identified after the neonatal period. Pulmonary hypoplasia and hypertension may not occur in the older infant. These patients may be presented with features of bowel obstruction and visceral ischemia or the abnormality may only be noted on a radiograph obtained due to a mild respiratory infection.

Clinical Presentation

When found in older babies and children, identification usually is by a chest radiograph obtained for nonspecific symptoms such as fever, cough, chest or abdominal pain, and vomiting. The presence of loops of intestine on the chest radiograph may be confirmed by passing a nasogastric tube, which will often end up with its tip in the thorax. The chest radiograph may suggest pneumonia with pneumatocele formation; in fact, these pneumatoceles may be loops of bowel (Fig. 4.23). A gastrointestinal contrast study or chest and abdominal CT scan may clarify confusing findings.

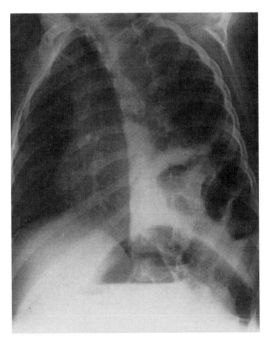

FIG. 4.23. A 4-year-old boy was admitted with a 1-day history of recurrent severe upper abdominal colicky pain with dyspnea and decreased breath sounds in the left base. A posteroanterior chest radiograph demonstrates multiple bowel loops in the lower left chest, indicative of a congenital diaphragmatic hernia.

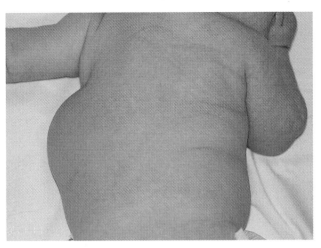

FIG. 4.24. The mother of this 7-week-old infant noted a left chest mass. The child was behaving and feeding normally. The mass was soft and nontender. A lymphatic malformation was diagnosed by chest magnetic resonance imaging.

Management

Surgical repair is indicated to prevent incarceration of the bowel even in asymptomatic patients.

Chest Wall Tumors

Tumors of the chest wall occurring in childhood are likely to be malignant. Benign tumors may arise from the ribs (e.g., aneurysmal bone cysts, chondromas, osteochondromas) or subcutaneous tissue (e.g., lymphatic malformations) (Fig. 4.24).

Clinical Findings

Benign tumors of the chest wall are usually asymptomatic until trauma or fracture brings them to light. Malignancy is signaled by a rapid increase in size, pain, tenderness, or local inflammation. The site of the lesion may give a clue. A Ewing tumor typically involves the lateral aspects of the ribs. Chondrosarcoma typically involves the costal cartilage between the sternum and distal rib end. The sternum is a favored site of anaplastic sarcomas. Chest radiographs may show pleural effusion, a mass adjacent to the pleura, or bone erosion of the ribs (Fig. 4.25).

Management

Radiographic evaluation of these areas should include a CT scan of the pertinent area and bone scans of the entire body for metastases. Multiple-modality, coordinated treatment is usually required involving surgery, chemotherapy, and radiotherapy.

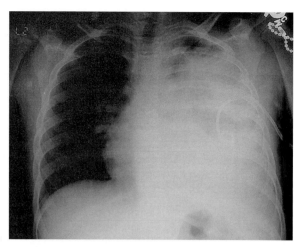 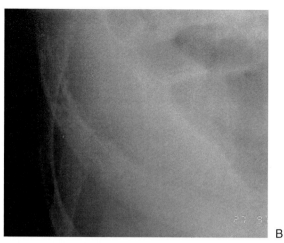

FIG. 4.25. Ewing sarcoma. This 9-year-old boy had fever and cough for 5 days. **A:** The chest radiograph shows a large left pleural effusion. **B:** A close-up of his left 10th rib shows bone erosion owing to an Ewing sarcoma.

SUGGESTED READINGS

General

Fish F, Benson DW Jr. Disorders of cardiac rhythm and conduction. In: Emmanouilides GC, Allen HD, Riemenschneider TA, et al., eds. *Moss and Adams heart disease in infants, children, and adolescents*, 5th ed. Baltimore: Williams & Wilkins, 1995:1555.

Gewitz MH, ed. *Primary pediatric cardiology*. Armonk, NY: Futura, 1995.

Talner NS. Heart failure. In: Emmanouilides GC, Allen HD, Riemenschneider TA, et al., eds. *Moss and Adams heart disease in infants, children, and adolescents*, 5th ed. Baltimore: Williams & Wilkins, 1995.

Vetter VL. What every pediatrician needs to know about arrhythmias in children who have had cardiac surgery. *Pediatr Ann* 1991;20:378–385.

Vincent GM, Timothy KW, Leppert M, et al. The spectrum of symptoms and QT intervals in carriers of the gene for the long QT syndrome. *N Engl J Med* 1992;327:846–852.

Thoracic Emergencies

Bailey PV, Tracy T Jr, Connors RH, et al. Congenital bronchopulmonary malformations. Diagnostic and therapeutic considerations. *J Thorac Cardiovasc Surg* 1990;99:597–603.

Lazar RH, Younis RT, Bassila MN. Bronchogenic cysts: a cause of stridor in the neonate. *Am J Otolaryngol* 1991;12:117–121.

Livingston GL, Holinger LD, Luck SR. Right middle lobe syndrome in children. *Int J Pediatr Otorhinolaryngol* 1987;13:11–23.

Risher, WH, Arensman RM, Ochsner JL. Congenital bronchoesophageal fistula. *Ann Thorac Surg* 1990;49:500–505.

CHAPTER 5

Dental Emergencies

Editor: Marc N. Baskin

NATAL TOOTH

Natal (present at birth) or neonatal teeth may cause excessive maternal pain during breast-feeding. The teeth are usually mandibular and occur in approximately 1:2,000 births (Fig. 5.1). The tooth may lacerate the infant's tongue, and there is a small risk of aspiration when the tooth disengages. Decisions about extractions should be made in consultation with a pediatric dentist.

EXFOLIATING TEETH

Occasionally, exfoliating teeth cause dental pain and anxiety. A careful examination can rule out a dental infection as the cause of the exfoliation (see Dentoalveolar Abscess section) (Fig. 5.2).

ERUPTION CYSTS OR HEMATOMAS

As new teeth erupt, a swelling over the alveolar ridge may be noted. These are eruption cysts (Fig. 5.3). When the cysts fill with blood, they are called eruption hematomas (Fig. 5.4). Treatment is unnecessary because the new tooth will soon emerge.

BABY BOTTLE CARIES

Decay due to children sleeping with their bottles is seen in children of all social and economic strata but is more common in medically underserved areas. These children need referral to a pediatric dentist (Fig. 5.5).

POSTEXTRACTION COMPLICATIONS

Hemorrhage

It is expected that any extraction site may ooze for 8 to 12 hours and perhaps longer for a permanent site. Treatment may include the following.

1. Apply pressure using folded gauze sponges placed over the socket with biting pressure applied for 30 minutes.

2. Close the socket with sutures: Administer local anesthesia (2% Xylocaine with 1:100,000 epinephrine infiltration) and approximate the extraction site with the appropriate sutures. Alternatively, the socket may be packed with Gelfoam.

3. A possible home remedy before going to the emergency department is to apply a tea bag that has been dipped in hot water, allowed to cool, and then placed over the socket with pressure; the tannic acid in the tea bag may initiate coagulation.

Alveolar Osteitis

Alveolar osteitis, or dry socket, is a painful postoperative condition produced by a disintegration of the clot in the tooth socket. Under local anesthesia, the socket may be debrided and then packed with 0.25 in. iodoform gauze or paste (bismuth, iodoform). Oral analgesic medication should also be prescribed with antibiotics.

ORAL INFECTIONS

Dentoalveolar Abscess

In a dentoalveolar abscess, the causative factors are usually decay or trauma. Suppuration is usually confined to the bone around the tooth. If the infection is long-standing, it can perforate the thin buccal bony plate adjacent to the root of the involved tooth and spread into the surrounding soft tissues. If it does not drain intraorally, the infection can spread rapidly through the fascial planes of the face or neck.

The following are clinical manifestations of a dentoalveolar abscess in a child: (1) pain, (2) fever, (3) gingival swelling (Fig. 5.6), (4) fistulous tracts to the gingiva (Fig. 5.7), and (5) facial erythema and swelling (Fig. 5.8). The treatment of choice for a localized dentoalveolar abscess is local in its focus (e.g., drainage, moist heat). In cases of facial cellulitis caused by an acute dentoalveolar abscess (Fig. 5.9), the antibiotic of choice is penicillin (or erythromycin, if there is a known allergy to penicillin). The initial

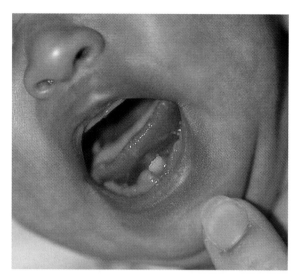

FIG. 5.1. A natal tooth. This 16-day-old neonate was seen due to difficulty feeding.

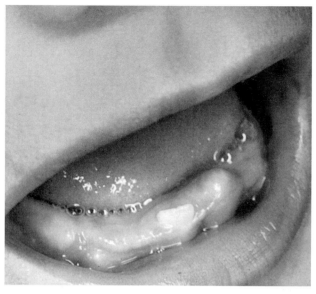

FIG. 5.3. An eruption cyst associated with an erupting primary central incisor is shown.

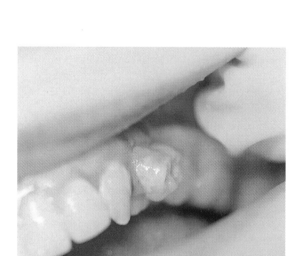

FIG. 5.2. An exfoliating tooth. This 13-year-old child presented with tooth pain. The permanent tooth can be seen behind the exfoliating molar. The gingival margin shows no signs of infection.

dose for children who weigh more than 60 lb (27 kg) is 1 g orally followed by 500 mg every 6 hours until the patient can be seen by a dentist. For children who weigh less than 60 lb (27 kg), the initial penicillin dose is 500 mg followed by 250 mg every 6 hours. As with infection elsewhere in the body, basic surgical principles must be used: establish drainage and remove the cause. An abscessed primary tooth must be vigorously treated because such infections can affect the developing, unerupted permanent tooth bud. Facial cellulitis can have severe systemic consequences, including cavernous sinus thrombosis, airway obstruction, brain abscess, and septicemia.

Pericoronitis

Pericoronitis is a localized infection surrounding an erupting tooth. It is usually associated with erupting molars in the

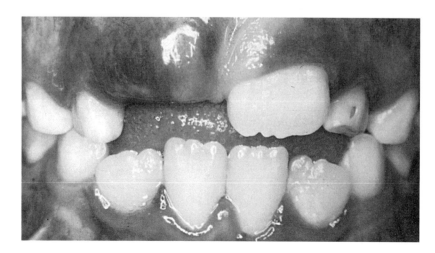

FIG. 5.4. An erupting hematoma over an erupting maxillary permanent central incisor.

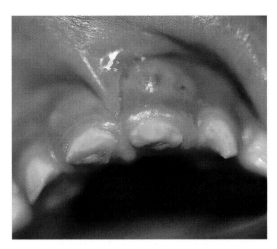

FIG. 5.5. Baby bottle caries. This 3-year-old boy was brought to the emergency department for mouth pain. His eroded incisors are due to baby bottle caries. In addition, the gingival swelling above the incisor is caused by a dentoalveolar abscess. This infection is discussed in the section on oral infections.

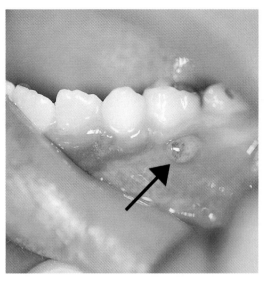

FIG. 5.6. This 8-year-old girl had fever, dental pain, and a "bump" for 2 days. The bump (arrow) is localized gingival swelling and was caused by her dentoalveolar abscess.

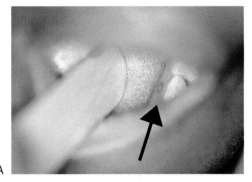

A

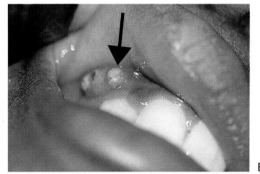

B

FIG. 5.7. This fistula may be suggested by a small, red papule (arrow) **(A)** or a large fluctuant swelling (arrow) **(B)**.

FIG. 5.8. Swelling can be extensive and mimic periorbital cellulitis **(A)**, especially if the abscess is associated with the maxillary cuspids and bicuspids, or more subtle, as in this patient with an early abscess of a mandibular tooth **(B)**.

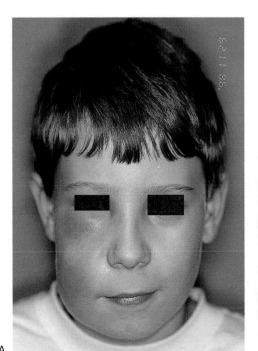

A

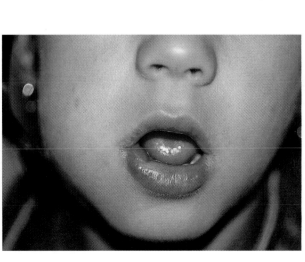

B

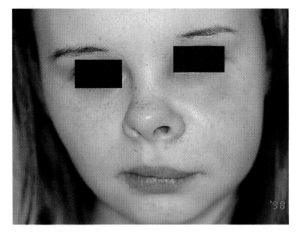

FIG. 5.9. This child had a painful swollen cheek and infraorbital cellulitis caused by a dentoalveolar abscess. (Courtesy of Dr. Debra Weiner.)

adolescent patient, although a mild form may be associated with the eruption of the first permanent molar at age 6 years (Table 5.1). Symptoms usually include pain distal to the last erupted tooth in the dental arch, along with erythema and edema localized to the gingiva in the retromolar area. Lymphadenopathy, trismus, and dysphagia may accompany these symptoms. Fever is an occasional finding.

Emergency treatment includes local curettage, oral rinses, heat, and scrupulous oral hygiene. Penicillin may be necessary (for dose, see Dentoalveolar Abscess section) when there are systemic symptoms.

Primary Herpetic Gingivostomatitis or Herpes Simplex Virus Type 1

This is discussed in Chapter 11 (Infectious Disease Emergencies).

Acute Necrotizing Ulcerative Gingivitis (Vincent's Disease or Trench Mouth)

Acute necrotizing ulcerative gingivitis (Vincent's disease or trench mouth) is characterized by increases in the fusiform

TABLE 5.1. *Eruption schedule for specific teeth*

	Age at eruption (mo)		Age at shedding (yr)	
	Lower	Upper	Lower	Upper
Primary teeth				
Central incisor	6	7.5	6	7.5
Lateral incisor	7	9	7	8
Cuspid	16	18	9.5	11.5
First molar	12	14	10	10.5
Second molar	20	24	11	10.5
Incisors	Range, 2 mo			
Molars	Range, 4 mo		Range, 6 mo	

	Age (yr)	
	Lower	Upper
Permanent teeth[a]		
Central incisors	6–7	7–8
Lateral incisors	7–8	8–9
Cuspids	9–10	11–12
First bicuspids	10–12	10–11
Second bicuspids	11–12	10–12
First molars	6–7	6–7
Second molars	11–13	12–13
Third molars	17–21	17–21

[a] The lower teeth erupt before the corresponding upper teeth. The teeth usually erupt earlier in girls than in boys.

Modified from Massler M, Schour I. *Atlas of the mouth and adjacent parts in health and disease.* The Bureau of Public Relations Council on Dental Health, American Dental Association, 1946.

bacillus and *Borrelia vincentii*, a spirochete that usually coexists in a symbiotic relationship with other oral flora. Adolescents complain of soreness and point-tenderness at the gingiva and often tell the physician that they feel as if they "cannot remove a piece of food" that feels painfully stuck between their teeth. They may also complain of a metallic taste in their mouth and of bleeding gums. On examination, the breath has an obvious fetid odor. The gingivae are hyperemic, and the usually triangular gingiva between the teeth is missing or "punched out" (Fig. 5.10). Intense pain is produced with probing, and a gray, necrotic pseudomembrane may cover some areas of gingiva.

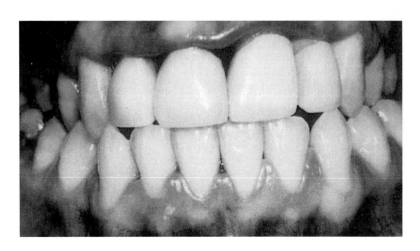

FIG. 5.10. A child with typical "punched out" gingiva, pathognomonic for acute necrotizing ulcerative gingivitis. (Courtesy of Dr. Mark Snyder.)

The adolescent should be advised to maintain better oral hygiene and to use frequent hydrogen peroxide mouth rinses. Diluted 1:1 with warm water, the hydrogen peroxide is vigorously swished and forced between the teeth as often as possible throughout the acute phase. Because of the rapidity of tissue destruction and sensitivity of the organisms as well as the risk of secondary infection, penicillin should be prescribed for the first week. When the acute phase is over, the patient should be sent to the dentist for a thorough debridement of the area.

HEMATOLOGIC PATHOLOGY PRESENTING AS DENTAL EMERGENCIES

Occasionally leukemia or thrombocytopenia may cause complaints referred to the oral cavity. If the patient's dental complaints seem atypical, a comprehensive history and physical examination should be done to assess for other systemic illness (Fig. 5.11).

ORAL AND PERIORAL PATHOLOGY PRESENTING AS DENTAL EMERGENCIES

Neoplasms

Orofacial neoplasms in children are rare but may be frightening to the patient and family. Common benign and malignant neoplasms may result in emergency visits and, therefore, are included.

The oral papilloma is a benign epithelial neoplasm that is an exophytic elevation of the surface epithelium with small, fingerlike projections from its surface. These lesions, which rarely become malignant, occur on the tongue and (in

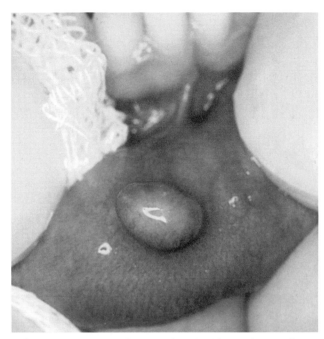

FIG. 5.12. A mucocele associated with a minor salivary gland of the lower lip.

decreasing order of frequency) palate, buccal mucosa, gingiva, and lip. If spontaneous involution does not occur, the usual treatment is surgical removal.

The fibroma is a common smooth-surfaced lesion with a sessile base. Its consistency varies from soft to firm, and its size ranges from a few millimeters to a centimeter or more in diameter. It may become whitened secondary to the overlying hyperkeratosis caused by trauma. Fibromas occur during the first and second decades of life and are usually found on the palate, tongue, cheek, and lip. Surgical removal is sometimes indicated, and recurrence is rare if the source of the irritation is removed.

The mucocele appears as a soft, raised, fluid-filled, and well-delineated nodule, most commonly on the lower lip. Superficial lesions appear translucent and are bluish, whereas deep-seated lesions have a normal color (Fig. 5.12). A mucocele in the floor of the mouth is termed a ranula (see Chapter 15, Ophthalmic and Otolaryngologic Emergencies) and is seen as a dome-shaped, fluid-filled lesion. Mucoceles are thought to result from the severance or obstruction of a salivary gland duct, with pooling of mucin in the lamina propria. Complete excision of the mucocele or marsupialization of the ranula is indicated.

Traumatic injuries are discussed in Chapter 24 (Trauma: Head and Neck).

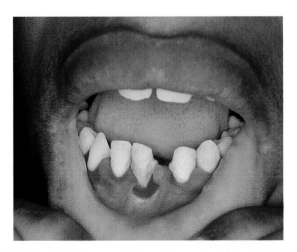

FIG. 5.11. This 14-year-old boy with mouth pain was referred for a dental consultation due to a dental abscess. He had mild jaundice and generalized gingivitis with gingival hemorrhage. His complete blood count was consistent with hemolytic anemia and thrombocytopenia. His final diagnosis was Evans syndrome, a chronic immune hemolytic anemia with immune-mediated thrombocytopenia.

SUGGESTED READINGS

Kaban L. *Pediatric oral and maxillofacial surgery.* Philadelphia: WB Saunders, 1990.
Shusterman S. Pediatric dental update. *Pediatr Rev* 1994;15:311–318.

CHAPTER 6

Dermatology

Editor: Gary R. Fleisher

ATOPIC DERMATITIS

Clinical Manifestations

During infancy, exudative lesions appear most often on the cheeks and extensor surfaces. At times, the process becomes generalized. Near the age of 2 years, the more characteristic flexural involvement occurs (Fig. 6.1). Other findings of atopic dermatitis are (1) hypopigmentation of varying size, especially prominent on the cheeks (pityriasis alba); (2) patchy or diffuse, fine papules (follicular accentuation); (3) scaling on the scalp with or without hair loss; and (4) hyperlinear palms and soles, which may show desquamation. Involvement of the feet in such a manner often leads to the misdiagnosis of tinea pedis, which occurs less often in the pediatric population before adolescence. During adolescence, the distribution remains the same; however, a greater incidence of involvement of the face, neck, posterior auricular areas, and hands and feet occurs. The major physical findings of chronicity, hyperpigmentation, and lichenification are often present. Other possible features are listed in (Table 6.1). Many immune and metabolic disorders are also associated with a rash that is similar in appearance to atopic dermatitis (Table 6.2). Colonization and infection with *Staphylococcus aureus* or *Streptococcus pyogenes* is common among atopic children and may account for flare-ups or failure to respond to therapy. The usual cause for what is termed Kaposi varicelliform eruption, characterized by groups of umbilicated vesicles or areas of increased crusting and ulceration, is herpes simplex virus (eczema herpeticum) infection (Fig. 6.2).

Management

The four main objectives in the treatment of uncomplicated atopic dermatitis are (1) reduction of pruritus, (2) reduction of inflammation, (3) protection of the skin from unknown irritants, and (4) removal of known irritants (Table 6.3). Reduction of pruritus can be accomplished in numerous ways. Most important of these methods are limitation of bathing (at times, to only once per week) and the use of a mild soap (e.g., Dove). Lubrication of the skin with a moisturizing cream ameliorates dryness, which may be a factor in producing pruritus. Antihistamines can be helpful, although during infancy, the necessity for soporific doses results in their being less useful therapeutically. A newer preparation includes topical doxepin and oral cetirizine. Control of inflammation is accomplished with the use of topical steroids. Appropriate antibiotics are important in the treatment of secondary bacterial infections; 40 mg/kg erythromycin per day or 50 mg/kg dicloxacillin per day provides suitable coverage. Eczema herpeticum that is localized can be treated orally with acyclovir at a dose of 40 mg/kg per 24 hours in four to five divided doses for 10 days. With severe infection, especially in young infants, more aggressive therapy is indicated with a daily dose of 700 mg/m^2 per 24 hours of acyclovir, given in a 1-hour intravenous infusion every 8 hours.

SEBORRHEIC DERMATITIS

Clinical Manifestations

The two common locations of skin involvement during infancy are the scalp (cradle cap) (Fig. 6.3) and diaper area. Most commonly, yellow, greasy scales are found over the anterior fontanel. Occasionally, the scaling spreads to the forehead, eyebrows, nose, ears, and neck. The intertriginous and flexural areas may also become involved. This reaction is especially seen in the diaper area. The child is not irritable, and pruritus is not present. From infancy to adolescence, scaling of the scalp usually indicates causes other than seborrheic dermatitis (atopic dermatitis or tinea capitis). In fact, true seborrheic dandruff does not appear until puberty, when excessive production of sebum occurs. Seborrheic dermatitis of the scalp during the adolescent period is similar in nature to the condition in adults. Scaling in the scalp appears, and the seborrheic areas are variably involved. Erythema and scaling occur between the eyebrows, on the eyelid margins, and in the nasolabial creases, sideburns, beards, mustache, posterior auricular areas, and aural canals.

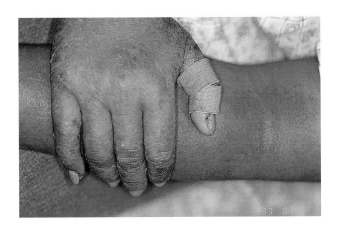

FIG. 6.1. Atopic dermatitis. The typical findings of atopic dermatitis include eczematous eruptions and lichenification or thickening of the skin, particularly in the antecubital and popliteal fossae.

TABLE 6.1. Diagnostic features of atopic dermatitis

Major
  Typical morphology and distribution
  Pruritus
  Chronically relapsing course
  Personal or family history of atopic disease
Additional features
  Xerosis
  Hyperlinear palms and soles
  Follicular accentuation
  Pityriasis alba
  Scaling of the scalp
  Ichthyosis
  Tendency toward nonspecific hand and foot dermatitis (pseudotinea pedis)
  Tendency toward repeated cutaneous infections
  White dermographism
  Elevated serum immunoglobulin E
Minor
  Cataracts
  Keratoconus
  Dennie–Morgan (infraorbital) fold

TABLE 6.2. Immune and metabolic disorders causing rash that resembles atopic dermatitis

Metabolic disorders	Immunologic disorders
Phenylketonuria	Ataxia-telangiectasia
Acrodermatitis enteropathica	Letterer–Siwe disease
	Wiskott–Aldrich syndrome
Histidinemia	X-linked agammaglobulinemia
Gluten-sensitive enteropathy	Hyperimmunoglobulin E syndrome
	Selective immunoglobulin A deficiency
Hartnup syndrome	
Hurler syndrome	Severe combined immunodeficiency

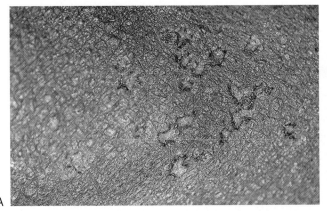
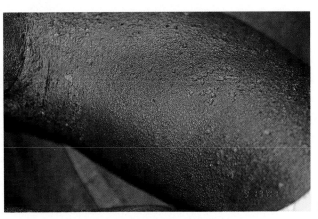

A   B

FIG. 6.2. Eczema herpeticum. Ulcers and excoriations, as in these two cases [patient 1 **(A, B)**, patient 2 **(C)**], usually characterize the eruption, although vesicles may be seen at times **(D)**. *(continued)*

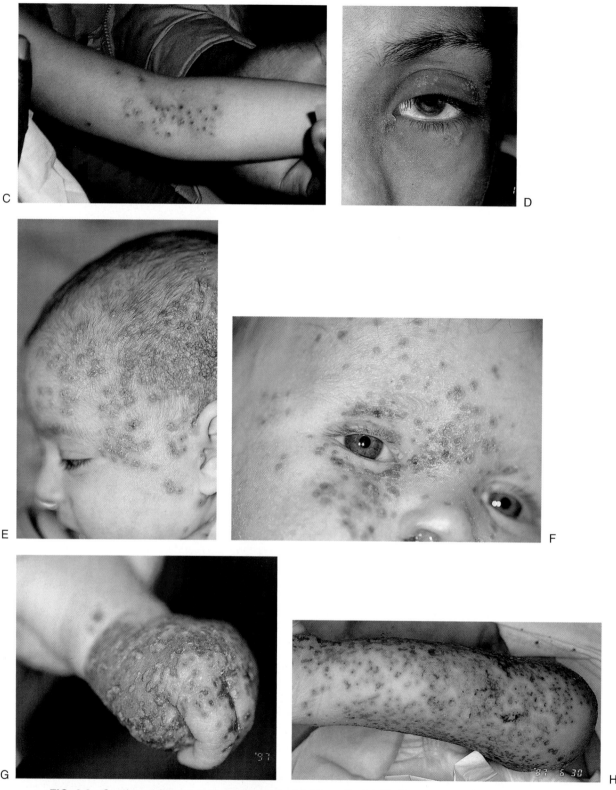

FIG. 6.2. *Continued.* More severe cases [patient 3 **(E)**, patient 4 **(F, G)**, patient 5 **(H)**], with generalized eruptions, require intravenous therapy with acyclovir.

TABLE 6.3. *Acute treatment of atopic dermatitis*

Reduction of pruritus
  Mild soaps
  Infrequent washing skin care
  Skin lubrication
  Topical steroids (high potency)
  Systemic steroids (rarely necessary)
  Antihistamines (children >4 yr)
Reduction of inflammation
  Skin care
  Topical steroids (high potency)
  Systemic steroids (rarely necessary)
Control of infection
  Penicillinase-resistant antibiotics

Management

Seborrheic dermatitis of the scalp responds readily to antiseborrheic shampoos (i.e., selenium sulfide) and topical steroids such as fluocinolone acetonide or betamethasone valerate. Secondary infection with bacteria can be treated with appropriate antibiotics. If *Candida albicans* secondarily invades the lesions, topical clotrimazole cream, applied twice daily, is useful.

ALLERGIC CONTACT DERMATITIS

Clinical Manifestations

The acute onset of linear or geometric areas of erythema, edema, eczematization, and papulovesiculation usually indicates the presence of allergic contact dermatitis (Fig. 6.4). Because skin involvement is limited to areas of contact, the distribution, pattern, and shape of the dermatitis provide important clues for the clinician (Table 6.4). Therefore, a round lesion on the back of the wrist would incriminate a wristwatch; a linear pattern encircling the waist points to the rubber in the waistband of a garment; linear lesions on exposed portions of the body indicate brushing against the leaves of a poison ivy plant; and extensive involvement of exposed areas of skin suggests an airborne allergen, as with ragweed or vaporized oil transmitted in the smoke of burning poison ivy. The most common causes of contact dermatitis, in order of frequency, are rhus (poison ivy, oak, sumac), nickel, and rubber compounds.

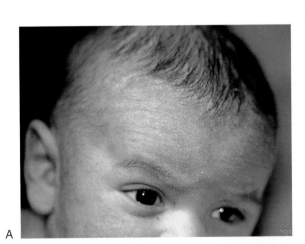
A

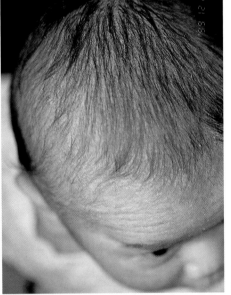
B

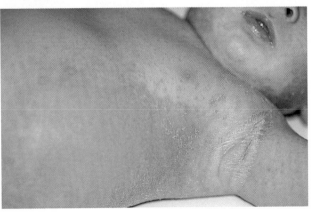
C

FIG. 6.3. Seborrhea typically manifests with an oily, scaly rash involving the face **(A)** and scalp **(B)** (cradle cap). More extensive involvement may be seen as in this second infant, with disease of both the head and the trunk **(C)**.

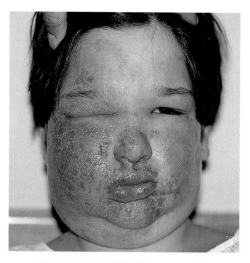

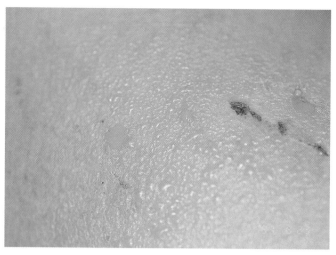

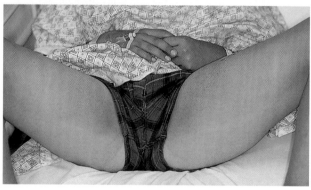

FIG. 6.4. Contact dermatitis may be quite localized as in this patient with facial involvement **(A)** or more diffuse, as in this child with a rash on the extremities **(B, C)**.

Management

Rhus

Avoiding exposure is the best prophylaxis. After the oil has been removed, spread does not occur, even from vesicular fluid. Antipruritic lotions such as calamine are useful. Topical steroids are minimally effective, and topical antihis-

tamines and anesthetics should be avoided because they can be sensitizers. Oral antihistamines can be helpful. With generalized reactions, 1 to 2 mg/kg oral prednisone once daily for 1 week then tapered over the next week is advisable.

Nickel Contact Dermatitis

Treatment consists of removing the offending object, avoiding further contact with nickel-containing jewelry, and applying topical steroids to the affected areas of skin.

Shoe Contact Dermatitis

Control is achieved by avoiding shoes when possible, treating secondary infection with appropriate antibiotics, and using topical steroids. Oral antihistamines are helpful for reducing pruritus. An id reaction consisting of huge bullae on the hands and feet can occur.

DIAPER DERMATITIS

Clinical Manifestations

Occlusion Dermatitis

Occlusion dermatitis arises from two causes (Fig. 6.5). The first, friction, occurs mainly on those portions of the diaper

TABLE 6.4. *Regional predilection of various substances that cause contact dermatitis*

Head and neck
 Scalp: hair dye, hair spray, shampoo
 Ear canal: neomycin
 Forehead: hat band
 Eyelids: nail polish, volatile gases, false eyelash cement, mascara, eye shadow/cosmetics
 Perioral: dentrifices, bubble gum, chewing gum
 Ears: earrings, perfume
Trunk
 Axilla: deodorant, clothing dye
 Breasts: metal, elastic in bra
Arms
 Wrist: cosmetic jewelry (nickel), leather (*p*-phenylenediamine, chrome)
Abdomen
 Waistline: rubber dermatitis from elastic in pants, jockstrap (lower)
Lower extremities
 Feet: shoe dermatitis

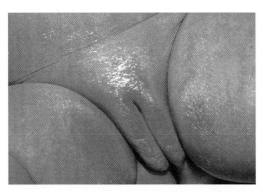

FIG. 6.5. This infant has a typical occlusion diaper dermatitis. Another common cause of diaper dermatitis is monilia, which usually manifests with satellite lesions and is more prominent in the skin folds.

area where contact with the diaper is greatest (inner thighs, lower abdomen, and prominent surfaces of the genitalia and buttocks). The rash waxes and wanes and often has a shiny, glazed surface appearance. Occasionally, papules are associated with the rash. The second component, trapped moisture, causes the erythema and maceration that occurs in the intertriginous parts of the diaper area (inguinal, genital, intergluteal, and folds of the thighs).

Atopic Dermatitis

The appearance of the rash in the diaper area is not different from occlusion dermatitis. It is however, more chronic and difficult to treat. Examination may disclose lesions on other body surfaces (e.g., cheeks, antecubital and popliteal spaces) typical of atopic involvement.

Seborrheic Dermatitis

Generally, the rash has an erythematous, salmon-colored base that is covered with yellow, greasy scaling. Similar involvement of other seborrheic locations such as the scalp, postauricular area, or flexures helps to establish the diagnosis.

Moniliasis

The skin in the diaper area has clusters of erythematous papules and pustules that go on to coalesce into an intensely red, confluent rash with sharp borders. Beyond these borders are satellite papules and pustules. At times, the infant has concomitant oral thrush.

Mixed or Not Diagnosable Rash

Mixtures of the above categories of diaper dermatitis are often found on infants. A diagnosis is often difficult to make. Secondary invasion with *C. albicans* is common, as men-

tioned. The potential for secondary bacterial infection exists. If blistering occurs, *S. aureus* infection should be considered.

Management

Treatment is determined by the cause of the dermatitis. In general, proper skin care, which includes decreased frequency of washing, use of mild soaps, and keeping the diaper off as much as possible, will help to resolve diaper dermatitis from any cause. With occlusive dermatitis, avoidance of tightly fitting diapers, plastic-covered paper diapers, and rubber pants is important. When atopic dermatitis is present, 1% hydrocortisone cream no more than twice daily for a short period is recommended. Hydrocortisone (1%) is also effective for seborrheic diaper dermatitis and can be used intermittently. With monilial diaper dermatitis, the use of preparations such as econazole twice daily is effective. If thrush is also present, 200,000 U (2 mL) oral nystatin four times daily for 7 days is advisable. Patients with id reactions, as described before, require oral nystatin, econazole on the diaper and intertriginous areas, and 1% hydrocortisone applied to the plaques. Secondarily infected dermatitis, such as bullous impetigo, should be treated with the appropriate systemic antibiotics. Whether traditional diaper creams and ointments are effective is still unproved.

DRUG REACTIONS IN THE SKIN

Clinical Manifestations

Urticaria

Urticaria (Fig. 6.6) constitutes the most common expression of drug sensitivity. Usually, reactions occur within 1 week of drug exposure. When an individual is on multiple agents and has a reaction, the clinician should suspect those agents that were most recently introduced or those medications that are known to be commonly associated with drug reactions (Table 6.5).

Maculopapular Eruptions Similar to Those of a Viral Exanthem

Maculopapular eruptions are the second most common of all drug-induced rashes and may be caused by many different agents. These eruptions are symmetric and consist of erythematous macules and papules with areas of confluence. Variable involvement of the palms, soles, and mucous membranes as well as purpura may occur. The presence and severity of pruritus are variable. Ampicillin is a medication often associated with this type of skin reaction, particularly in patients with infectious mononucleosis.

Erythema Multiforme

Erythema multiforme (Fig. 6.7) is an acute and often recurrent inflammatory syndrome, often secondary to drugs

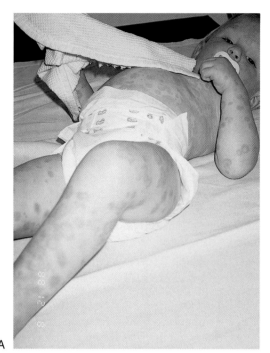 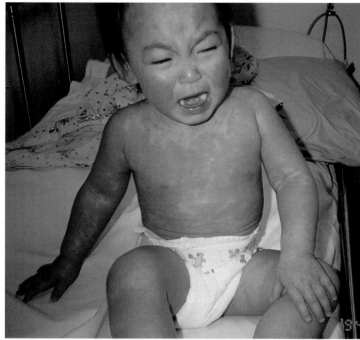

A   B

FIG. 6.6. (A, B) Urticaria lesions are erythematous and irregular. Urticaria may be a manifestation of a more generalized anaphylaxis, but when the pathology is limited to the skin, the patients appear otherwise well.

(e.g., penicillins, sulfonamides, hydantoins, barbiturates) or infections. Recent observations suggest that some cases of idiopathic erythema multiforme cases may be caused by herpes simplex virus. The skin findings include macules, papules, vesicles, and pathognomonic target or iris lesions that tend to be more or less symmetrically distributed. Bullous lesions may also be present. In the more severe cases, constitutional symptoms occur; when mucous membranes are involved, the term Stevens–Johnson syndrome is used. Erythema multiforme consists of two lesion types: macular-urticarial and vesicular-bullous. There is a predilection for the backs of the hands, palms, soles, and extensor surfaces

of the limbs. The lesions may begin at these sites and then spread diffusely or may begin in a generalized manner. In 25% of the patients, the mucous membranes are involved and, in fact, can be the sole site of involvement. The usual sites of mucous membrane involvement are the lips, buccal mucosa, palate, conjunctivae, urethra, and vagina. With severe involvement, the pharyngeal, tracheobronchial, and esophageal mucous membranes are also affected. Less common sites are the anal and nasal mucosa. Lesions may continue to erupt in crops for as long as 2 to 3 weeks. Death occurs in 3% to 15% of patients.

Vasculitis

The classic lesions of vasculitis are palpable purpura (Fig. 6.8). Although these lesions are characteristic, vasculitis may be manifest by erythematous macules, papules, urticaria, and hemorrhagic vesicles and bullae. The diagnosis can be confirmed by a skin biopsy.

Erythema Nodosum

The lesions of erythema nodosum (Fig. 6.9) appear as deep, tender, erythematous nodules or plaques of the extensor surfaces of the extremities. They are thought to be hypersensitivity phenomena secondary to infections (e.g., streptococcal pharyngitis, tuberculosis, coccidioidomycosis, histoplasmosis), inflammatory bowel disease, sarcoidosis,

TABLE 6.5. *Drugs most commonly associated with allergic skin reactions*

Trimethoprim–sulfamethoxazole
Ampicillin
Semisynthetic penicillins (carbenicillin, cloxacillin, dicloxacillin, methicillin, nafcillin, oxacillin)
Sulfisoxazole
Penicillin G
Gentamicin
Cephalosporins
Dipyrone
Nitrazepam
Barbiturates
Nitrofurantoin
Glutethimide
Indomethacin

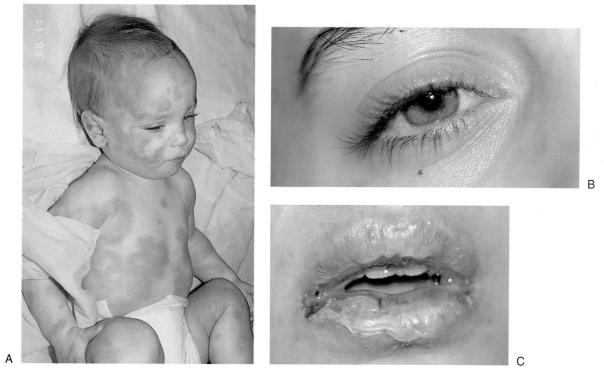

FIG. 6.7. Erythema multiforme. Target lesions **(A)**, which consist of a red ring around a clear area (sometimes with a central bull's eye), characterize erythema multiforme. In severe cases **(B, C)** or with involvement of the mucous membranes (Stevens–Johnson syndrome), vesicles may appear.

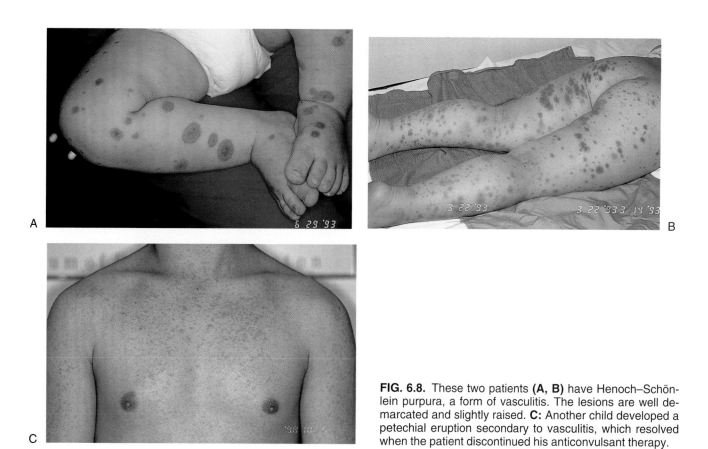

FIG. 6.8. These two patients **(A, B)** have Henoch–Schön-lein purpura, a form of vasculitis. The lesions are well de-marcated and slightly raised. **C:** Another child developed a petechial eruption secondary to vasculitis, which resolved when the patient discontinued his anticonvulsant therapy.

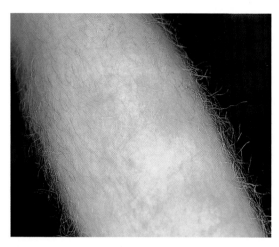

FIG. 6.9. Erythema nodosum. This teenager has the typical erythematous and nodular lesions of erythema nodosum along his anterior tibia. Palpation accentuates appreciation of the nodularity and elicits tenderness. Evaluation of this boy was positive only for streptococcal pharyngitis.

malignancies, and, occasionally, drugs, including oral contraceptives.

Toxic Epidermal Necrolysis

Drug-induced toxic epidermal necrolysis must be differentiated from an illness caused by a circulating staphylococcal exotoxin (Fig. 6.10). If a child who has toxic epidermal necrolysis has been taking drugs long term or shortly before the onset of the rash, is older than 6 years of age, or has a mixed rash (i.e., areas with the appearance of erythema multiforme as well as toxic epidermal necrolysis), a biopsy must be performed to distinguish between the two disorders. With drug-induced toxic epidermal necrolysis, dermal-epidermal separation is visible on histologic examination. If epidermolytic toxin has been released by staphylococci, epidermal cleavage occurs in the granular layer. With extensive exfoliation of skin, fluid and electrolyte disturbances may occur, and the potential for bacterial sepsis is present.

Management

Vital to the management of any suspected drug reaction is the identification and removal of the offending drug. Pruritus can be controlled with oral antihistamines, and open lesions are responsive to compressing with Burow solution and topical silver sulfadiazine. When extensive exfoliation occurs, attention to fluid and electrolyte balance and secondary infection is essential. Any patient with mucous membrane involvement should have an ophthalmologic examination to rule out the presence of corneal lesions. Hospitalization should be considered in any patient who has severe involvement of the skin, is toxic, or has extensive exfoliation. The literature suggests that steroid therapy of Stevens–Johnson syndrome and

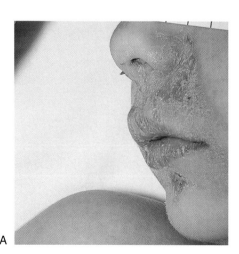

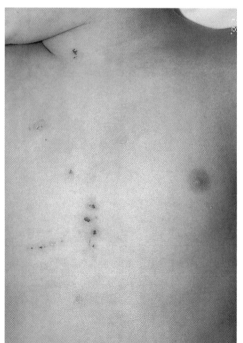

A   B

FIG. 6.10. Staphylococcal scalded skin syndrome. **A:** The thin, yellow crusting around the mouth and nares of this boy characterizes this syndrome, which is most often secondary to impetigo in the perioral and nasal regions. **B:** In addition, desquamation secondary to circulating toxin produced by the organism appears on the chest. Toxic epidermal necrolysis may be virtually identical to these truncal lesions but does not cause crusting on the face.

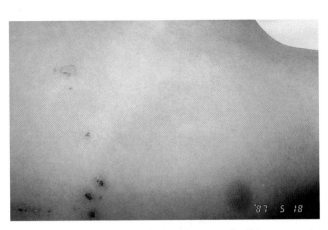

FIG. 6.11. Nikolsky sign. The application of mild pressure to this child's chest by the examiner with his thumb has left a clear thumbprint visible. The upper layer of the skin, even in areas that appear visually normal, may be partially disrupted by the toxin and easily induced to cleave from its base by mechanical pressure.

drug-induced toxic epidermal necrolysis is of no value, will prolong hospital stays, and may in fact be harmful. If denudation progresses to greater than 25% of body surface area, the child should be considered for transfer to a burn unit.

Staphylococcal Scalded Skin Syndrome

Clinical Manifestations

The illness begins with malaise, fever, and irritability. The irritability is often caused by significant tenderness of the skin when touched. A "sunburn" erythema follows, which first begins and is most intense around the neck, the intertriginous areas, and periorificially (especially the eyes and mouth) (Fig. 6.10). The erythema spreads to varying portions of the skin surface, and the child may be very toxic. With mild involvement of the skin, superficial desquamation (flaking) then follows, similar to the reaction that occurs after ordinary sunburn. With severe involvement, large sheets of skin shear away, leaving a denuded, oozing surface similar to the reaction that occurs after a burn. The skin can often be rubbed off (Nikolsky sign) (Fig. 6.11). Vesicles, pustules, and bullae can also occur during the exfoliative phase. Often, a purulent discharge emits from the eyes, but no conjunctival injection is present. Mucous membranes are not involved. Most children do well, and clearing of the skin occurs in 12 to 14 days, leaving no residua. Causes other than *S. aureus* or drugs may produce a similar clinical picture.

Management

Most of the time, staphylococcal scalded skin syndrome is a self-limited disorder. Antibiotics probably ameliorate the course of the disease, but steroids have no beneficial effects. Neonates and children younger than 1 year of age should be

admitted to the hospital and started on intravenous anti-staphylococcal antibiotics (e.g., cefazolin, oxacillin) after blood cultures are obtained. In addition, any older child who is toxic or who has severe skin involvement with significant denudation should be admitted.

BITES AND INFESTATIONS

Mosquitoes and Fleas

Mosquito bites are generally limited to the warm months of the year. Conversely, fleabites, which predominate from spring to fall, can also occur during the winter months as a result of cats and dogs living indoors. The distribution of lesions is a valuable clue in making the diagnosis of mosquito or fleabites. Insect bites generally involve the exposed surfaces of the head, face (Fig. 2.5A), and extremities. The lesions are usually urticarial wheals that occur in groups or along a line on which the insect was crawling. On occasion, both mosquito bites and fleabites can cause blistering lesions. These lesions are not caused by secondary infection but rather by a violent immune response to the bite. Certainly, excoriation with resulting secondary infection with *S. aureus* or group A streptococci can complicate a simple bite. A recurrent papular eruption called papular urticaria can occur in young children who become sensitized to insect bites. Although the lesions tend to occur on exposed parts of the body, with sensitization they may appear at sites distant from the primary bite. Unfortunately, no specific treatment exists for insect bites.

Tick Bites

Tick bites (Fig. 6.12) may cause local reactions. For removal of ticks, the only safe method is to use a blunt curved forceps, tweezers, or fingers protected by rubber gloves. The tick is grasped close to the skin surface and pulled upward with a steady even force. The tick must not be squeezed, crushed, or punctured. If mouth parts are left in the skin, they should be removed.

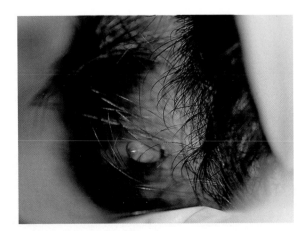

FIG. 6.12. Tick bite. Typical appearance of an engorged tick.

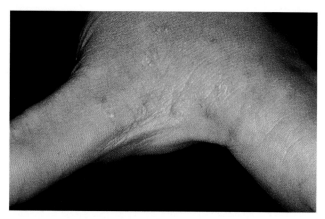

FIG. 6.13. Scabies typically involves the web spaces between the fingers and/or the toes.

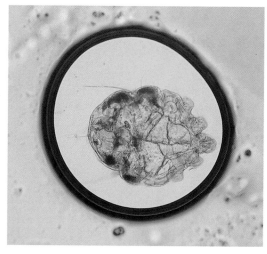

FIG. 6.15. Microscopy of a skin scraping often demonstrates the presence of mites in patients with scabies.

Scabies Infestation

The cardinal symptom of any infestation with scabies is pruritus. Infants and many children excoriate themselves to the point of bleeding. Two clues should be considered when attempting to make this diagnosis: (1) distribution (concentration on the hands, feet, and folds of the body, especially the finger webs) (Fig. 6.13) and (2) involvement of other family members. In contrast to adults, infants may develop blisters and exhibit lesions on the head and face (Fig. 6.14). The diagnosis is made by scraping involved skin and looking for mites under the 10× microscope objective (Fig. 6.15).

Treatment is with 5% permethrin cream (Elimite), applied from head to toe and left on for 8 to 12 hours. The preparation is then washed off with soap and water. Its safety for use in pregnant females has not been proven. All family members and close contacts should be treated.

Louse Infestation

Three forms of lice infest humans: (1) the head louse, (2) the body louse, and (3) the pubic (Fig. 6.16) or crab louse. The

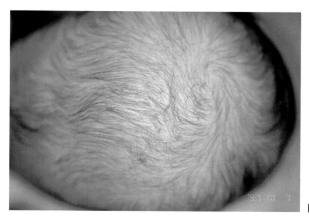

A

B

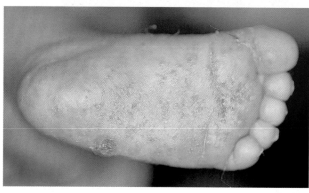

C

FIG. 6.14. The rash of scabies may be more diffuse in infants, spreading to the trunk **(A)** and scalp **(B)** in addition to the extremities **(C)**.

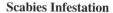

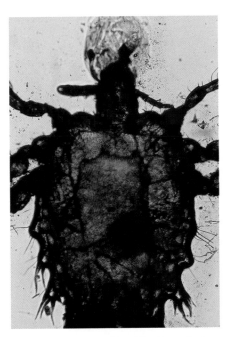

FIG. 6.16. Louse infestation. Identification of a louse, as pictured here under 10× magnification, or nits supports the diagnosis of an infestation.

major louse infestation in children involves the scalp and causes pruritus. The female attaches her eggs to the hair shaft. The egg then hatches, leaving behind numerous nits that resemble dandruff. Secondary infection can occur from vigorous scratching. Body lice generally reside in the seams of clothing and lay their eggs there. They go to the body to feed, particularly the interscapular, shoulder, and waist areas. Red pruritic puncta that become papular and wheal-like then occur. Pubic lice occur in the genital area, lower abdomen, axillae, and eyelashes. Transmission is usually venereal. Blue macules (maculae caeruleae) that are 3 to 15 mm in diameter can be seen on the thighs, abdomen, or thorax of

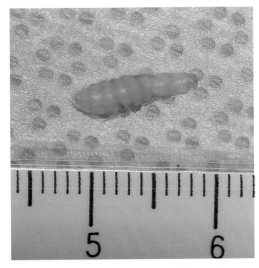

FIG. 6.17. Botfly bite. The bite of a botfly produces a large, red papule from which larvae extrude.

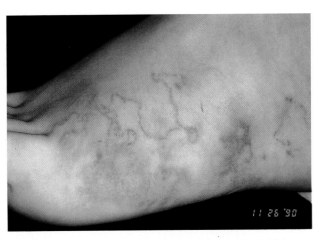

FIG. 6.18. Cutaneous larval migrans. The larvae of this parasite penetrate the skin and migrate subcutaneously, causing serpiginous lesions. Invasion generally occurs through the sole of the foot when children walk on contaminated sand or soil without shoes. Treatment is with thiabendazole.

infested persons. These macules are secondary to bites. Because the body louse resides in clothing, therapy consists mainly of disinfecting the clothing with steam under pressure. Pediculosis capitis and pubic infestations are most effectively treated with 1% permethrin creme rinse (Nix). Any nits are removed with a fine-toothed comb. The safest treatment for lice in the eyelashes is the application of white petrolatum twice daily for 7 days.

Bites in Travelers

Children returning after travel to tropical areas are susceptible to a variety of common and unusual bites and infestations. Both mosquito and fly bites are common, with secondary impetigo a frequent complication. The botfly causes a characteristic eruption, in which larva can be seen to emerge from the center (Figs. 6.17 and 3.8). Because they are likely to go without shoes more often than adults, children are particularly predisposed to cutaneous larval migrans, an infestation that involves larvae in the ground gaining access to the skin through direct contact (Fig. 6.18).

SUPERFICIAL FUNGAL INFECTIONS OF THE SKIN

Tinea Corporis

Tinea corporis is characterized by one or more sharply circumscribed scaly patches (Fig. 6.19). The center of the circular patch generally clears as the leading edge spreads out. The leading edge may be composed of papules, vesicles, or pustules. The lesions are most commonly confused with nummular eczema. These lesions do not fluoresce under a Wood light. Treatment with topical antifungal agents such as clotrimazole, miconazole, or econazole produces clearing in 7 to 10 days. Therapy should be continued for 2 weeks. If improvement

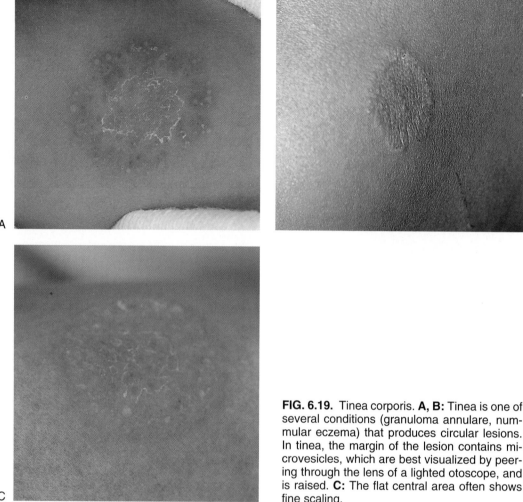

FIG. 6.19. Tinea corporis. **A, B:** Tinea is one of several conditions (granuloma annulare, nummular eczema) that produces circular lesions. In tinea, the margin of the lesion contains microvesicles, which are best visualized by peering through the lens of a lighted otoscope, and is raised. **C:** The flat central area often shows fine scaling.

does not occur, treatment with 15 mg/kg oral griseofulvin in two divided doses per day will usually resolve the problem.

Tinea Capitis

The *Microsporum* species generally causes round patches of scaling alopecia. Illumination of a lesion with a Wood lamp gives a blue-green fluorescence. Kerion formation can occur as a swollen, boggy abscess (Fig. 6.20). The *Trichophyton* species usually causes scattered alopecia, not always oval or rounded; the alopecia is irregular in outline with indistinct margins. Normal hairs grow within the patches of alopecia and may break off at the surface, leaving a black dot appearance. Diffuse scaling may simulate dandruff, and although minimal hair loss is present, it is not perceived. Wood light examination of the lesion does not produce fluorescence. The clinician should consider the presence of tinea capitis when a nonresponsive seborrheic or atopic dermatitis of the scalp is present, black dots are seen, or increased scaling follows the use of topical steroids. Culture on fungal media may be necessary to confirm the diagnosis.

Treatment of tinea capitis consists of 15 to 20 mg/kg oral griseofulvin daily in two divided doses with a glass of milk for 6 weeks. Adjunctive therapy includes the use of 2.5% selenium sulfide shampoo twice weekly. If a kerion is present, the swelling (allergic reaction to the fungus) can be controlled by a combination of oral prednisone and griseofulvin.

Tinea Versicolor

Tinea versicolor refers to a superficial infection of the skin caused by *Pityrosporum orbiculare*, which produces color changes of the skin, hypopigmentation, hyperpigmentation, and redness (Fig. 6.21). Wood light examination usually shows yellowish brown fluorescence. Because moisture promotes growth of the organism, exacerbations occur in warm weather or in athletes who sweat excessively. A potassium hydroxide preparation shows large clusters of spores and short, stubby hyphae, often called meatballs and spaghetti. Treatment consists of lathering the entire body with selenium sulfide shampoo (2.5% concentration) after wetting the skin surface in a shower. The lather is left on for 20 minutes

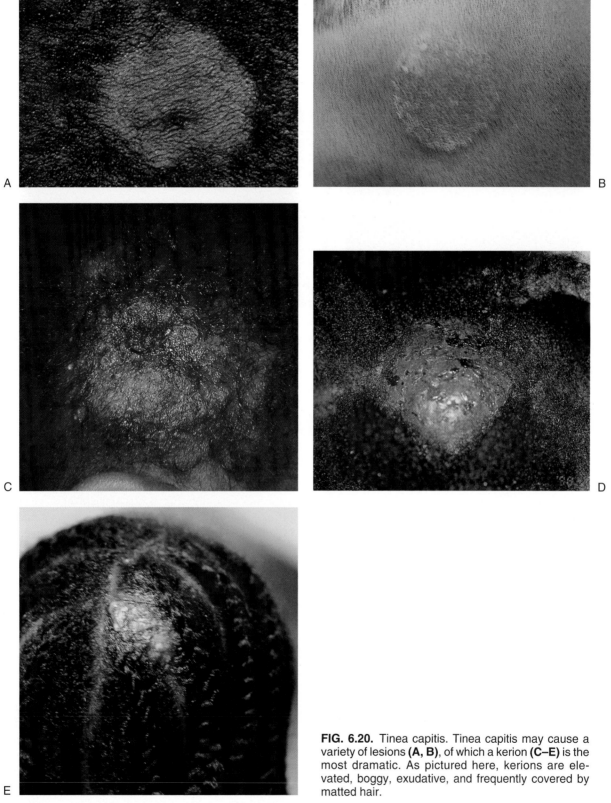

FIG. 6.20. Tinea capitis. Tinea capitis may cause a variety of lesions **(A, B)**, of which a kerion **(C–E)** is the most dramatic. As pictured here, kerions are elevated, boggy, exudative, and frequently covered by matted hair.

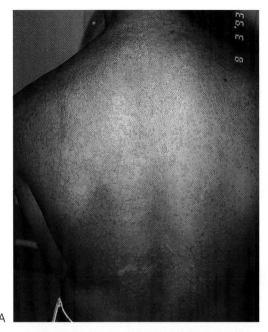
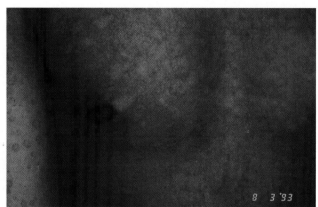

FIG. 6.21. A, B: Tinea versicolor. Tinea versicolor occurs most often in the summer, as tanning of the skin accentuates the hypopigmented lesions that are characteristic of this condition. As in this adolescent, the eruption typically involves the trunk.

and is then showered off. This procedure is carried out multiple times during the first week, with decreasing frequency over the ensuing weeks. Maintenance therapy is advisable because of the high incidence of recurrence. Localized areas of involvement can be treated with topical antifungal agents (e.g., econazole, ketoconazole topically). Adolescents can be treated with 400 mg oral ketoconazole initially and then 200 mg at monthly intervals during the warm summer months or during a sports season when the child sweats frequently.

URTICARIA

Urticaria can be localized or generalized (Fig. 6.6). At times, the lesions are huge with serpiginous borders. Indi-

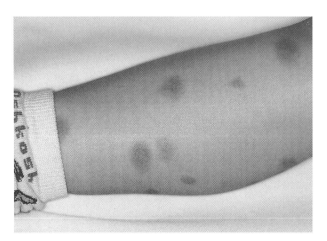

FIG. 6.22. Urticaria pigmentosa. Urticaria pigmentosa is a genetic condition. The lesions in this condition are brown macules that form urticaria in response to rubbing or pressure.

vidual wheals rarely last more than 12 to 24 hours. Most commonly, the lesions appear in one area for 20 minutes to 3 hours, disappear, and then reappear in another location. The total duration of an episode is usually 24 to 48 hours; however, the course can last 3 to 6 weeks. Some children are susceptible to recurrent urticaria, caused by either an underlying allergic diathesis or urticaria pigmentosa, a cutaneous condition (Fig. 6.22). Acute relief can be accomplished with 0.01 mL/kg subcutaneous epinephrine (1:1,000) and 1 mg/kg intramuscular diphenhydramine. Oral antihistamines are useful for maintenance therapy for transient urticaria.

PITYRIASIS ROSEA

Pityriasis rosea can occur in all age groups but is seen predominantly after 10 years of age and only rarely in children younger than 5 years of age. In 80% of children, a large, oval, solitary lesion known as the herald patch appears on the trunk before the eruption of subsequent lesions. Individual lesions are oval and slightly raised, pink to brown, with peripheral scaling (Fig. 6.23). Because the lesions follow the cleavage lines of the skin, the backs of patients have a "Christmas tree" appearance. Generally, the face, scalp, and distal extremities are spared. On occasion, an inverse distribution occurs (lesions on the face and extremities with truncal sparing). The rash is pruritic early in the course but then becomes asymptomatic. It lasts 4 to 8 weeks. When pityriasis rosea appears in adolescence, it must be differentiated from secondary syphilis. Clinical clues are helpful, but serologic testing is necessary. Antihistamines and topical emollients can help the pruritus.

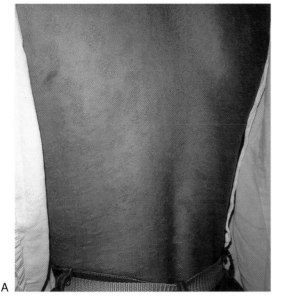

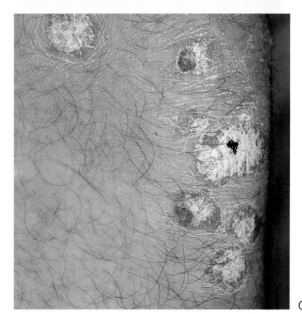

FIG. 6.23. Pityriasis rosea. **A:** Pityriasis rosea causes a papulosquamous eruption that frequently involves the thorax and assumes a characteristic "Christmas tree" appearance. **B:** The individual lesions are elongated maculopapules with a rough surface. They follow the skin lines, which leads to the branching pattern of the chest. **C:** Psoriasis, another papulosquamous eruption more often appears on the extensor surface and has a silvery scale.

ERYTHEMA NODOSUM

Erythema nodosum (Figs. 2.6B and 6.9) seems to be a hypersensitivity reaction to infection (streptococci, tuberculosis, coccidioidomycosis, histoplasmosis), inflammatory bowel disease, sarcoidosis, and drugs. The entity occurs predominantly in adolescents during the spring and fall. Females are affected more often than males. Ibuprofen helps with lesions, which are painful.

WARTS (VERRUCAE)

The common wart resembles a tiny cauliflower. The shape of the wart varies with its location on the skin. It may be long and slender (filiform) on the face and neck or flat (ver-

ruca plana) on the face, arms, and knees. When located on the soles, they are called plantar warts, and when in the anogenital area, they are referred to as condyloma acuminata (Fig. 6.24). Because most warts disappear spontaneously with time, procedures that are least traumatic for the child should be attempted first (Table 6.6). The simple, nontraumatic method of airtight occlusion with plain adhesive tape for 1 month has been shown to be successful on many occasions. Topical application of salicylic acid in flexible collodion (Duofilm) (Table 6.7) is good for home use, as are some of the over-the-counter preparations (e.g., Compound W). When simple methods are unsuccessful, touching the warts with liquid nitrogen for 20 to 30 seconds or surgical removal can be attempted. Plantar warts can be treated with 40% salicylic acid plaster. Anogenital warts are treated with 20% podophyllin.

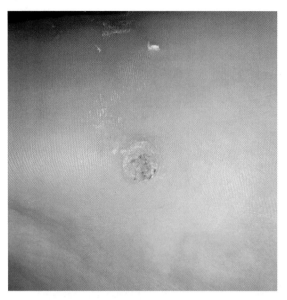

FIG. 6.24. Plantar wart. As opposed to warts on other surfaces, those on the sole of the foot are flat.

MOLLUSCUM CONTAGIOSUM

Clinical Manifestations

These lesions, produced by the common poxvirus, consist of papules with white centers (Fig. 6.25). They occur at any age during childhood. Most cases of molluscum resolve in 6 to 9 months, but some may persist for more than 3 years. Spread is by autoinoculation. Lesions can be single or numerous and favor intertriginous areas such as the groin. They are usually 2 to 5 mm in diameter, but several can coalesce and form a lesion 1.5 cm in diameter. They may become inflamed, which sometimes heralds spontaneous disappearance. At times, an eczematous reaction occurs around some lesions, and they can become secondarily infected.

Management

Treatment should be gentle. Removal of the white core will cure the lesion. This treatment can be performed by applying eutectic mixture of local anesthetic cream under occlusion to the lesion 1 to 2 hours before treatment. This procedure will anesthetize the area and allow the physician to prick the skin open over the core with a 26-gauge needle and squeeze the core out with a comedone extractor. Multiple light touches with liquid nitrogen can also be effective. With widespread lesions, nonpainful procedures are preferable. Application of 0.1% retinoic acid one to two times daily may induce enough inflammation to hasten the host's immune response or cause extrusion of the central core.

Table 6.6. *Management of warts*

Decrease irritation; cover with tape (1–2 mo)
Over-the-counter preparations such as Compound W (1 mo)
Salicylic in collodion (Duofilm) (1 mo)
Refer to dermatologist

Table 6.7. *Use of Duofilm*

1. Soak wart for 5 min.
2. Dry.
3. Surround with petroleum jelly.
4. Apply Duofilm (let dry for few minutes).
5. Cover with tape.
6. Repeat twice daily.
7. Pare dead skin.

MISCELLANEOUS LESIONS

Parents occasionally bring their children to the emergency department for evaluation of a chronic lesion, particularly when a sudden change occurs. Pyogenic granuloma represents a specific example of this situation because minor trauma may produce sudden hemorrhage that is difficult to control (Fig. 6.26).

Additionally, the physician should pay attention to cutaneous findings, even those of long standing because they may offer clues to the diagnosis of an underlying disease of importance, whether or not related to the acute presentation. Patients with neurofibromatosis (Fig. 6.27) may develop seizures acutely and are at risk of malignancy over the years.

FACTITIOUS DERMATITIS

Children may present with a factitious dermatitis, either self-inflicted or a result of Munchausen syndrome by proxy. Whenever the characteristics of a rash do not fit with any known disease pattern or the morphology is highly geometric, the physician should suspect nonaccidental trauma (Figs. 6.28 and 6.29).

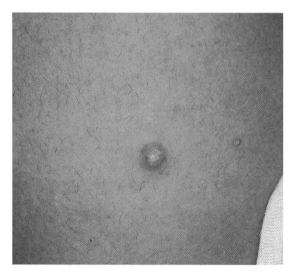

FIG. 6.25. Molluscum contagiosum. Molluscum contagiosum usually results in an isolated lesion or a localized grouping of four or five papules. Close inspection reveals a central core ("pearl") in the macules, which varies from 2 to 3 mm to 1 cm in diameter.

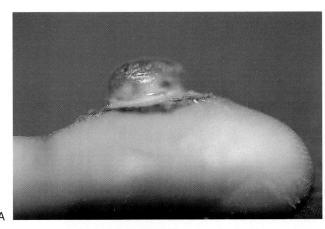
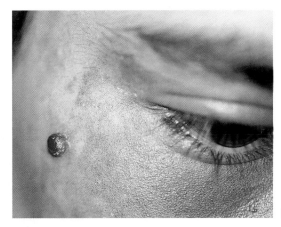

FIG. 6.26. These patients demonstrate the characteristic findings of pyogenic granuloma, one having a lesion on the finger **(A)** and the other on the face **(B)**. The lesions are raised, but not pedunculated, and have a fleshy, friable appearance.

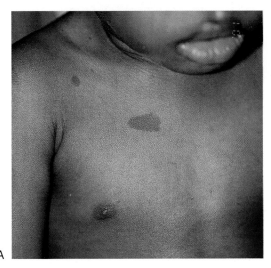
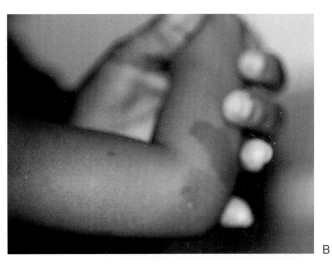

FIG. 6.27. A, B: This boy has the characteristic large café-au-lait lesions of neurofibromatosis.

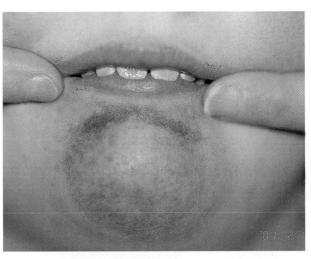
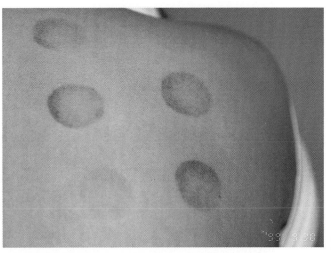

FIG. 6.28. A: This boy produced a rash on his chin, by applying a suction cup from a toy dart. The lesion is geometric in appearance and in an area accessible to the patient. **B:** In contrast, the parents of this child used "cupping" as a folk remedy to treat a fever, and the marks appear on the back, an area that could not be reached by the patient.

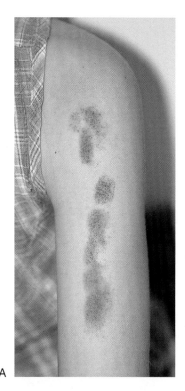

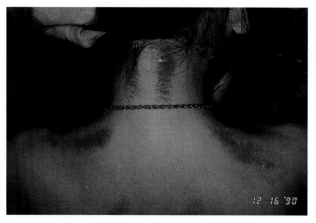

FIG. 6.29. This 11-year-old girl complained of the sudden appearance of a linear lesion on her left arm **(A)**. After a thorough evaluation, she confessed to self-injurious behavior. **B:** In contrast, the parents of this child rubbed the back of her neck with a hot coin, as part of a traditional "remedy" for the relief of throat pain.

FIG. 6.30. Alopecia areata is an idiopathic disorder causing noncicatricial hair loss. The lesions may be localized **(A)**, patchy **(B)**, diffuse **(C)**, or occasionally universal.

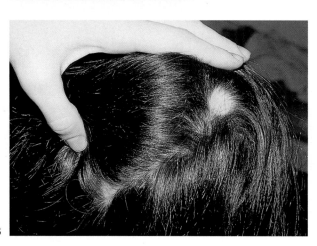

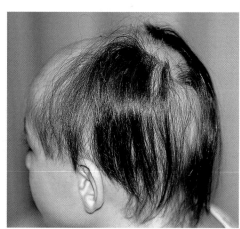

ALOPECIA

Alopecia radically alters the appearance of a child and may lead parents to seek urgent medical attention as soon as the disorder is noticed. Diseases causing alopecia are characterized as cicatricial (the underlying skin is abnormal) or noncicatricial. Tinea capitis (Fig. 6.20) represents the most common cause of cicatricial hair loss. Baldness with normal skin may be secondary in children to traction on the hair from braiding, hair pulling by the child, or alopecia areata (Fig. 6.30).

SUGGESTED READINGS

Berg RW, Buckingham KW, Stewart RL. Etiologic factors in diaper dermatitis: the role of urine. *Pediatr Dermatol* 1986;3:102–106.

Ghosh S, Kanwar AJ, Kaur A. Urticaria in children. *Pediatr Dermatol* 1993;10:107–110.

Goodyear HM, Wilson P, Cropper L, et al. Rapid diagnosis of cutaneous herpes simplex infections using specific monoclonal antibodies. *Clin Exp Dermatol* 1994;19:294–297.

Gupta AK, Sauder DN, Shear NH. Antifungal agents: an overview. Part I. *J Am Acad Dermatol* 1994;30:677–700.

Gupta AK, Sauder DN, Shear NH. Antifungal agents: an overview. Part II. *J Am Acad Dermatol* 1994;30: 911–936.

Honig PJ, Caputo GL, Leyden JJ, et al. Treatment of kerions. *Pediatr Dermatol* 1994;11:69–71.

Needham GR. Evaluation of five popular methods for tick removal. *Pediatrics* 1985;75:997–1002.

Paller AS. Scabies in infants and small children. *Semin Dermatol* 1993;12:3–8.

Rothe MJ, Grant-Kels JM. Atopic dermatitis: an update. *J Am Acad Dermatol* 1996;35:1–16.

Weston WL, Lane AT. *Color textbook of pediatric dermatology*, 2nd ed. St. Louis: Mosby, 1996.

CHAPTER 7

Endocrinologic Emergencies

Editor: Stephen Ludwig

Major clinical features, recommended investigations, and treatments of pediatric endocrinologic emergencies are summarized in Table 7.1.

DIABETIC KETOACIDOSIS

In cases of new-onset diabetes, the child usually has a history of polyuria and polydipsia for a few days or weeks before the acute decompensation. Significant weight loss often occurs despite a vigorous appetite. In children known to have diabetes, the prodrome may be less than 24 hours and precipitated by an intercurrent illness, inappropriate sick-day management, or omission of insulin doses. Patients may complain of nausea, vomiting, and abdominal pain, and the parents may have noticed increasing listlessness. On physical examination, particular attention should be paid to the degree of dehydration, including skin turgor and dryness of mucous membranes. In severe cases, the child may exhibit signs of shock, including a thready pulse, cold extremities, and hypotension. The smell of ketones on the breath and the presence of deep sighing (Kussmaul) respirations reflect the ketoacidosis. The patient's consciousness level, which may range from full alertness to deep coma, should be noted. The child may have exquisite abdominal tenderness with guarding and rigidity, which can mimic an acute abdomen. The ears, throat, chest, and urine should be examined because infection is often a precipitating factor.

Typical laboratory findings include a serum glucose level greater than 200 mg/dL (usually 400 to 800 mg/dL), the presence of glucose and ketones in the urine, acidosis [venous pH <7.3 and bicarbonate (HCO) <15 mEq/L], high or normal plasma potassium level, and a slightly elevated blood urea nitrogen level. Occasionally, diabetic ketoacidosis (DKA) can occur with normoglycemia when persistent vomiting and decreased intake of carbohydrates are accompanied by continued administration of insulin. The serum sodium is usually low or in the low-normal range. Leukocytosis may be noted but does not necessarily signify an underlying infection.

Management

This section primarily focuses on the child who is significantly dehydrated, acidotic, and unable to take oral fluids because of vomiting or altered level of consciousness. Many cases of mild DKA can be managed with rehydration, either orally or intravenously, and with supplemental insulin either at home or in the emergency department. For the severely dehydrated child, initial treatment is directed toward rapid expansion of intravascular volume and correction of the acidosis because these conditions are life threatening. Subsequent treatment is directed at the normalization of all biochemical parameters by the use of insulin. Medical intervention carries significant risks of hypokalemia and cerebral edema (Tables 7.2 and 7.3).

Fluid and Electrolyte Replacement

In the first hour, isotonic (0.9%) saline should be infused intravenously at 20 mL/kg per hour to establish an adequate vascular volume and to improve tissue perfusion. This procedure may need to be repeated if the pulse rate and capillary refill rate do not decrease. After adequate intravascular volume is established, the fluid deficit can be replaced over the next 24 to 48 hours, depending on the degree of hyperosmolality; however, when the child is able to drink, rehydration may occur enterally. It can be assumed that the fluid deficit is 10% of the body weight in children with DKA. Dehydration may actually be greater than that estimated based on clinical appearance because of the hyperosmolar state.

Alkali

The use of $NaHCO$ for correction of acidosis remains controversial because of the potential for paradoxical acidosis of the central nervous system (CNS) and resultant cerebral depression. Most children will correct their acidosis during rehydration and initiation of insulin therapy without recourse to alkali. HCO therapy is generally reserved for children

TABLE 7.1. *Summary of clinical features, investigations, and initial treatment of pediatric endocrinologic emergencies*

Condition	Major clinical features	Urgent investigations	Initial treatment
Diabetic ketoacidosis	Polyuria, polydipsia, dehydration, ketotic breath, hyperpnea, nausea, vomiting, abdominal pain, coma	Blood glucose, pH	20 mL/kg 0.9% saline in first hour IV; 0.1 u/kg/hr insulin infusion; later, may need KCl 20–30 mEq/L ½ KPhos; 20–30 mEq/L
Hypoglycemia	Older child: hunger, sweatiness, dizziness, convulsions, coma; neonate: apnea, hypotonia, hypothermia, irritability, tremor, convulsions	Blood glucose, serum for growth hormone, cortisol, insulin; first voided urine for organic acids and toxic screen	1–2 mL/kg 25% dextrose IV bolus or 5–10 mg/kg/min 10% dextrose IV infusion, 0.5–1 mg glucagon, IM stat (if hyperinsulinism)
Congenital adrenal hyperplasia	Ambiguous genitalia in females; poor feeding, weight loss, irritability, vomiting, dehydration	Plasma sodium, potassium, glucose, 17-hydroxyprogesterone; karyotype and pelvic ultrasonography	20 mL/kg 0.9% saline in first hour IV; 0.5–1 mg deoxycorticosterone acetate IM stat; 25 mg hydrocortisone IV stat
Adrenal insufficiency	Nausea, vomiting, abdominal pain, weakness, malaise, hypotension, dehydration, hyperpigmentation	Plasma sodium, potassium, glucose, cortisol, and ACTH (for retrospective confirmation of diagnosis)	100 mg hydrocortisone IV stat; 20 mL/kg 10% dextrose in 0.9% saline in first hour
Hypercalcemia (hyperparathyroidism)	Headache, irritability, anorexia, constipation, polyuria, polydipsia, dehydration, band keratopathy	Plasma calcium, phosphate	0.9% saline at 2–3 times maintenance rate; 1 mg/kg furosemide
Hypocalcemia (hypoparathyroidism)	Cramps, carpopedal spasms, paresthesias, lethargy, apathy, convulsions	Plasma calcium, phosphate, alkaline phosphatase	0.6% mg/kg 10% calcium gluconate (or 5 mg Ca/kg) IV over 15 min
Diabetes insipidus	Polyuria, polydipsia, dehydration, irritability, fever, drowsiness, coma	Paired plasma and urine osmolality and sodium	Central: 1.5 times maintenance rate; DDAVP 0.4 μg/kg nasally; Nephrogenic: 5% dextrose at 1.5 times maintenance
Syndrome of inappropriate antidiuretic hormone secretion	Anorexia, headache, nausea, vomiting, irritability, seizures, coma	Paired plasma and urine osmolality and sodium	Seizures: 1–3 mL/kg 3% saline; 1 mg/kg V furosemide IV stat, otherwise, fluid restriction
Thyroid storm	Goiter, exophthalmos, high fever, tachycardia, congestive cardiac failure, delirium, stupor	Serum T$_4$ or free T$_4$, TSH	10 μg/kg propranolol IV over 15 min; 15 drops/d Lugol iodine PO; 2–3 mg/kg propylthiouracil t.i.d. PO; tepid sponging
Neonatal thyrotoxicosis	Goiter, failure to gain weight, irritability, tachycardia, congestive cardiac failure	Serum T$_4$ or free T$_4$, TSH	1 mg/kg propranolol t.i.d. PO; potassium iodide 2 drops/d PO; 2–3 mg/kg propylthiouracil t.i.d. PO
Congenital hypothyroidism	Asymptomatic; hypothermia, hypoactivity, poor feeding, constipation, prolonged jaundice, large posterior fontanelle	Serum T$_4$, TSH	37.5 μg l-thyroxine PO if weight >3 kg, 25 μg if <3 kg
Hypopituitarism	See features listed for adrenal insufficiency and hypoglycemia		

ACTH, adrenocorticotropic hormone; TSH, thyroid-stimulating hormone.
IV, intravenous/intravenously; IM, intramuscularly; DDAVP, 1-deamino-8-D-arginine vasopressin; t.i.d., three times daily; PO, orally.

TABLE 7.2. *Principles of management of diabetic ketoacidosis*

Life-threatening complications immediate (within the first hours after admission)
  Cardiovascular collapse
  Profound metabolic acidosis
Short-term (within 8–24 hr after start of therapy)
  Hypokalemia
  Cerebral edema
Areas of management decisions
  Fluids
    Treat hypovolemia with extracellular fluid expander. Use normal saline (154 mEq/L) and infuse 20 mL/kg in the first hour. (Avoid hypotonic solutions initially because they are inefficient volume expanders and may contribute to cerebral edema.) Continue infusion at this rate until the blood pressure is normal. After first 1–2 hr, start half-normal saline. Total fluid administration in first 24 hr = maintenance % fluid deficit (10% body weight). If calculated serum osmolality is >320 mOsm/L, replace fluid deficit over 36–48 hr.
  Alkali
    Consider administering $NaHCO_3$ if blood pH $\leq$7.10. Usual dose, 2 mEq/kg $NaHCO_3$ infused over 1–2 hr. Then recheck pH, Pco_2, and HCO_3. (Avoid bolus infusion of HCO_3 because this may acutely lower serum potassium.)
  Potassium
    Start potassium therapy after the patient urinates (usually 1–2 hr after start of fluid therapy). Potassium replacement should be 40 mEq/L as a combination of potassium chloride and potassium phosphate. If the patient is hypokalemic (<4 mEq/L), a higher concentration of potassium (60 mEq/L) may be necessary. Administer high concentrations of potassium only with electrocardiographic monitoring.
  Insulin
    Low-dose insulin is safe and effective. May be given as either a continuous intravenous infusion (0.1 U/kg/hr) or an intramuscular injection (0.25 U/kg initially, followed by 0.1 U/kg/hr).
  Glucose
    Add 5% glucose to solutions when serum glucose is approximately 300 mg/dL. This may be given as 5% dextrose in half-normal saline solution.
Monitoring
  Clinical monitoring
    Blood pressure, pulse, respirations, neurologic status, and fluid intake and output.
  Laboratory monitoring
    Obtain initial glucose, electrolytes, blood gases, and blood urea nitrogen. Measure blood glucose every hour initially as guide to insulin dose. Repeat electrolytes and pH measurements as necessary. Use flow sheet.

with an initial arterial pH of less than 7.1 and for those who are unable to compensate for their acidosis by hyperventilation. The adequacy of compensation can be evaluated if the Pco_2 and serum HCO are known. If the Pco_2 is more than (1.5 HCO) + 8, respiratory effort is inadequate for the degree of acidosis, and HCO is required. The amount of HCO needed may be calculated using the formula: amount of HCO (mEq) = base deficit (mEq/L) body weight (kg) 0.6 (distribution factor for HCO). Half of this amount is given intravenously over 2 hours. Biochemical studies are then repeated; the need for continued HCO is reevaluated, and if necessary, a new dose of HCO is calculated and administered. Alternatively, 1 to 2 mEq/kg may be given intravenously every hour until the pH is more than 7.25 and the HCO is more than 15 mEq/L.

Insulin

Regular insulin is used for the treatment of ketoacidosis. Insulin should be started at the same time as initial fluid expansion to correct the acidosis and may be either infused intravenously or injected intramuscularly at hourly intervals. Subcutaneous injections of insulin should be avoided because of the uncertainties of absorption in a dehydrated pa-

tient. The starting dose of insulin for continuous infusion is 0.1 U/kg per hour, which is normally infused by a regulated pump. The rate of insulin infusion should be adjusted to sustain a decrease in the blood glucose of approximately 100 mg/dL per hour. It is unnecessary to give an initial bolus of insulin. The dose for the hourly intramuscular injection is 0.25 U/kg as a priming dose followed by 0.1 U/kg per hour. When the blood sugar is less than 300 mg/dL, glucose should be added to the intravenous fluids. As long as the child remains acidotic, insulin infusion should never be stopped; instead, the amount of glucose in the intravenous infusion should be increased and the insulin infusion adjusted to maintain the blood sugar between 100 and 200 mg/dL. When the child is able to eat and is no longer significantly acidotic, intravenous infusion of insulin can be discontinued.

MILD KETOACIDOSIS

Some children with new-onset diabetes may also have hyperglycemia without ketoacidosis or with only mild acidosis. Generally, these patients are hospitalized for at least 12 to 24 hours to allow time to educate the family and stabilize the insulin dose. These children require rehydration similar to patients with known diabetes and mild ketoacidosis. Insulin

TABLE 7.3. *Guide to treatment of severe diabetic ketoacidosis*

Calculated osmolality	Time (hr)[b]	Type of fluid	Approximate hourly Infusion amount by age (and body weight)[a]				Potassium replacement	Bicarbonate replacement	Insulin infusion rate (μ/kg/hr)
			1 (10 g)	5 (18 kg)	10 (30 kg)	15 (50 kg)			
Not relevant	Initial hour[b]	0.9% saline	200	360 mL	600 mL	1,000 mL	None	Consider if pH <7.1 or inadequate respiratory compensation	0.1
<320 mOsm/L	1–8[c,d]	0.45% saline	105	170	260	400	If K% >4 mEq/L, 20 mEq/L KCl %	If acidosis does not begin to resolve within the first 8-hr period, suspect either inadequate hydration, insulin, or underlying illness (e.g., pneumonia)	0.1, adjust to maintain rate decrease of glucose to ~100 mg/dL/hr
>320 mOsm/L[e]	1–16	0.45% saline[f]	75	120	160	250	20 mEq/L K phosphate if K% <4 mEq/L		
<320 mOsm/L	9–24	0.45% saline	75	120	160	250	30 mEq/L KCl %		
>320 mOsm/L	16–48	0.45% saline	60	90	110	170	30 mEq/L K phosphate		

[a] Suggested rate does not include ongoing fluid losses secondary to osmotic diuresis. Urine output in excess of 5 mL/kg/hr should be replaced milliliter for milliliter.

[b] If the child is severely volume depleted, an additional bolus of normal saline (20 mL/kg) may be required. The adequacy of the initial bolus can be evaluated by improving capillary refill and by declining pulse rate.

[c] Rates are based on 10% dehydration and replacement of the deficit in the first 8 hours along with maintenance fluids. Some clinicians now simply distribute the deficit replacement over the entire 23-hour period. The initial bolus of fluids to establish vascular sufficiency is not included in these calculations.

[d] Glucose will need to be added to the infusion when glucose is less than 300 mg/dL. Because the rate of decrease in glucose is predictable, the appropriate fluid can be ordered well in advance of this time to avoid the possibility of hypoglycemia.

[e] Rates are based on 10% dehydration and replacement of the deficit in the first 16 hours along with maintenance fluids. The initial bolus of fluids to establish vascular sufficiency is not included in these calculations.

[f] More concentrated saline may be required to prevent excessively rapid decrease in osmolality.

therapy can be initiated subcutaneously at a total daily dose of 0.25 to 0.5 U/kg per day for the prepubertal child and 0.5 to 0.75 U/kg per day for the adolescent. Two-thirds of the total daily dose is administered in the morning, and one-third before dinner; two-thirds of the morning dose and one-half of the evening dose should be as an intermediate-duration insulin (NPH, lente insulin).

Children with known diabetes often develop mild ketoacidosis during the course of intercurrent illness, especially gastroenteritis, or secondary to omission of insulin doses. Even the mildly dehydrated (5%) child with slight acidosis who presents to the emergency department benefits from a fluid bolus (20 mL/kg of normal saline); furthermore, this bolus will be given while awaiting laboratory test results. When the laboratory results are available, the physician must decide whether to hospitalize the child, continue treatment in the emergency department, or send the child home. For purposes of definition, mild DKA is defined as a pH of more than 7.3, HCO of more than 15 mEq/L, and a calculated osmolality of less than 320 mOsm/L. Children who are significantly acidotic or hyperosmolar should be hospitalized and managed as outlined in the earlier section of this chapter.

HYPOGLYCEMIA

A differential diagnosis of hypoglycemia, as it may present in the emergency department, is provided in Table 7.4. The acutely ill child warrants a glucose determination if the level of consciousness is altered because hypoglycemia may accompany an illness that interferes with oral intake. Historical evidence may aid in establishing the cause of hypoglycemia.

TABLE 7.4. *Causes of childhood hypoglycemia*

Decreased availability of glucose
  Decreased intake (fasting, malnutrition, illness)
  Decreased absorption (acute, diarrhea)
  Inadequate glycogen reserves
  Defects in enzyme of glycogen synthetic pathway
  Ineffective glycogenolysis (defects in enzymes of glycogenolytic pathways)
  Inability to mobilize glycogen, glucagon deficiency
  Ineffective gluconeogenesis (defects in enzymes of gluconeogenic pathway)
  Increased use of glucose hyperinsulinism
  Islet cell adenoma or hyperplasia, nesidioblastosis, ingestion of oral hypoglycemic agents, insulin therapy
  Large tumor (Wilms tumor)
Diminished availability of alternative fuels
  Decreased or absent fat stores
  Inability to oxidize fats (enzymatic defects in acid oxidation)
Unknown or complex mechanisms
  Sepsis/shock
  Reye syndrome
  Salicylate ingestion
  Ethanol ingestion
  Adrenal insufficiency
  Hypothyroidism
  Hypopituitarism

The possibility of ingestion should be considered because ethanol, propranolol, and oral hypoglycemic agents are in common use. The clinical findings of hypoglycemia reflect both the decreased availability of glucose to the CNS and the adrenergic stimulation caused by a decreasing or low blood sugar level. Adrenergic symptoms and signs include palpitations, anxiety, tremulousness, hunger, and sweating. Irritability, headache, fatigue, confusion, seizure, and unconsciousness are neuroglycopenic symptoms. Any combination of these symptoms should lead to a consideration of hypoglycemia. Any child presenting with a seizure or unconsciousness should have a serum glucose determination (Fig. 7.1).

Management

If hypoglycemia is suspected, blood should be collected, if possible, before treatment. An extra tube (3 mL, red top) should be obtained and refrigerated until the laboratory glucose screen result is known. Rapid screening should be performed using a portable glucose monitor while awaiting definitive laboratory results. Therapy should be instituted if this screen is suggestive of hypoglycemia. If the laboratory glucose screen confirms that the blood glucose was less than 50 mg/dL, the reserved serum can be used for chemical (β-hydroxybutyrate, acetoacetate, free fatty acids, carnitine), toxicologic, and hormonal (insulin, growth hormone, cortisol) studies and may provide the correct diagnosis without extensive additional testing. The first voided urine after the hypoglycemic episode should be saved for toxicologic and organic acid evaluation.

The preferred treatment of hypoglycemia is 0.25 g dextrose/kg body weight (2.5 mL/kg of 10% dextrose/kg, 1.0 mL/kg of 25% dextrose/kg) rapidly. The serum glucose level should then be maintained by an infusion of dextrose at a rate of 6 to 8 mg/kg per minute. Generally, this goal can be accomplished by providing 10% dextrose at 1.5 times maintenance rates. Glucagon (1 mg intramuscularly) may be used to treat hypoglycemia that is known to be caused by hyperinsulinism but is not indicated as part of the routine therapy of hypoglycemia.

ACUTE ADRENAL INSUFFICIENCY

The historical information suggestive of adrenal insufficiency depends on the cause. Children with a primary adrenal defect are more likely to have had a gradual onset of symptoms, such as general malaise, anorexia, fatigue, and weight loss. Salt craving and postural hypotension may also have been noted. A child with secondary adrenal insufficiency is more likely to have a history of neurosurgical procedures, head trauma, CNS pathology, or chronic disease necessitating the prolonged use of glucocorticoids. Findings on physical examination are more likely to be characteristic of the precipitating illness or trauma rather than specifically suggestive of adrenal insufficiency (Fig. 7.2). Although a lack of

FIG. 7.1. Hypoglycemia. **A:** A 25-month-old child with untreated type Ia glycogen storage disease with failure to thrive (length and weight less than the third percentile), a markedly protuberant abdomen with hepatomegaly, and eruptive xanthomas (serum triglycerides 12,300 mg/dL) on the arms and legs. **B:** Same child at 7.5 years of age after nearly 3 years of continuous glucose therapy (frequent feeds supplemented with oral glucose at 2- to 3-hour intervals during the day and overnight intragastric glucose infusion via a gastrostomy). Growth is normal (height and weight more than the 50th percentile); the liver size has decreased, the abdomen is less protuberant, and the serum triglyceride concentration is reduced to within the normal range. (From Becker KL, Bilezikian JP, Brenner WJ, et al. *Principles and practice of endocrinology and metabolism*, 3rd ed. Philadelphia: Lippincott Williams & Wilkins, 2001:1495, with permission.)

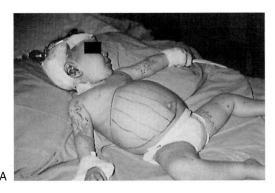

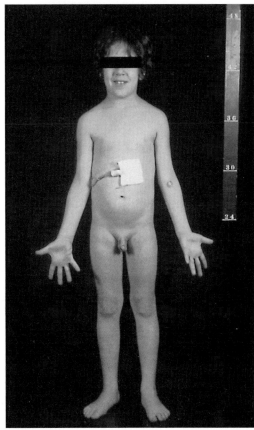

A

B

glucocorticoid and aldosterone can be associated with hypotension and dehydration, a better clue to the possibility of adrenal insufficiency is inappropriately rapid decompensation in the face of metabolic stress. Hyperpigmentation may be present in primary adrenal insufficiency, especially of long duration. Biochemical evidence suggestive of adrenal insufficiency includes hyponatremia, hyperkalemia, hypoglycemia, and hemoconcentration. Mild metabolic acidosis and hypercalcemia may be present. The definitive diagnosis depends on the demonstration of an inappropriately low level of cortisol in the serum.

Management

Treatment of adrenal crisis is based on rapid volume expansion and the administration of glucocorticoids. Immediate management consists of 50 to 100 mg hydrocortisone intravenously. Subsequent management is 50 mg/m^2 hydrocortisone per 24

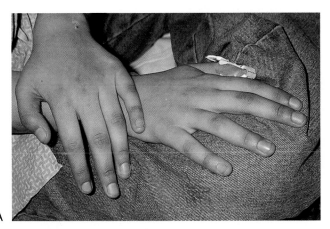

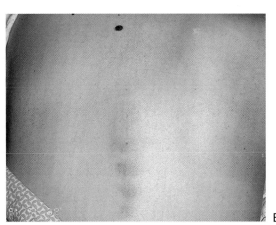

A

B

FIG. 7.2. Addison disease. This teenager was referred to the emergency department with a diagnosis of anorexia nervosa. Patient has hyperpigmentation over the joints of his hands **(A)** and the spine **(B)**.

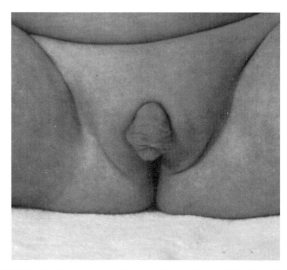

FIG. 7.3. External genitalia of a 2-month-old infant girl with 21-hydroxylase deficiency. (From Becker KL, Bilezikian JP, Brenner WJ, et al. *Principles and practice of endocrinology and metabolism*, 3rd ed. Philadelphia: Lippincott Williams & Wilkins, 2001:744, with permission.)

hours given continuously intravenously or 7.5 mg/m² methylprednisolone (Solu-Medrol) per 24 hours divided and administered every 8 hours intravenously. Volume expansion is accomplished with 20 mL/kg normal saline in the first hour, followed by fluids appropriate for maintenance and replacement. Additional Na⁺ may be needed in primary adrenal insufficiency because of ongoing urinary Na⁺ losses. These fluids should contain 10% dextrose and should not contain potassium until the serum potassium is within the normal range. Mineralocorticoid therapy is rarely important in the acute phase, if fluid therapy is adequate; however, patients with primary adrenal insufficiency may need replacement with a mineralocorticoid for long-term management.

CONGENITAL ADRENAL HYPERPLASIA

Initial evidence of congenital adrenal hyperplasia (CAH) may be acquired at birth with the discovery of ambiguous genitalia (Fig. 7.3), between 2 to 5 weeks of age when the baby presents with an acute salt-losing crisis, or during childhood with the onset of precocious puberty. The subsequent discussion deals primarily with the recognition and management of the acute salt-losing crisis, which is life threatening. Salt wasting is present soon after birth, but acute crisis usually does not occur until the second week of life. The appearance of symptoms can be insidious, with a history of poor feeding, lack of weight gain, lethargy, irritability, and vomiting. The nonspecificity of symptoms may lead to consideration of diagnoses far removed from CAH and delay initiation of treatment.

In severe cases, there may be shock and metabolic acidosis. The genitalia should be examined carefully because the degree of ambiguity of the genitalia varies considerably.

Virilized females may have an enlarged clitoris and fusion of the labial folds (Fig. 7.4). An undervirilized male may have a small phallus and/or hypospadias (Fig. 7.5). The presence of gonads in the inguinal canals or labioscrotal fold is suggestive of a male karyotype. Hyperpigmentation of the labioscrotal folds and nipples is occasionally present in the neonatal period; however, it is rarely prominent enough to alert the examiner to the possibility of CAH.

In the emergency department, the most urgent investigations are plasma electrolytes and blood glucose. The combination of hyperkalemia and hyponatremia is often the first clue to the diagnosis of CAH, especially in males. The plasma potassium is elevated, but in the presence of vomiting and diarrhea, the rise may be blunted. Levels between 6 and 12 mEq/L are commonly encountered, often without any clinical cardiac dysfunction or electrocardiographic changes. The plasma HCO level is usually low, reflecting the metabolic acidosis that results from the retention of hydrogen ions in exchange for sodium loss.

Management

If the child is dehydrated, fluid replacement is urgent. Volume expansion should be effected by the rapid infusion of 20 mL/kg normal saline in the first hour or more rapidly, if needed. Because the dehydration in salt-losing CAH represents urinary losses of isosmotic fluid, replacement should consist of normal saline (0.9%). The volume to be replaced should constitute the child's daily requirements and the estimated fluid loss. Principal management of the mineralocorticoid deficit is by the provision of sodium. In addition, hydrocortisone has some mineralocorticoid effect, particularly at high doses. For long-term management, the child will require mineralocorticoid replacement (0.1 mg fludrocortisone per day). Most infants also require oral Na⁺ supplements for the first several months of life. Hydrocortisone (25 mg) should be given in an intravenous bolus, followed by 50 mg/m² hydrocortisone per 24 hours as a constant infusion. Alternatively, 25 mg cortisone acetate intramuscularly immediately, followed by 25 mg every 24 hours, may be used.

Infants with CAH tolerate hyperkalemia far better than do other children and adults, with potassium levels as high as 12 mEq/L reported without clinical signs. Volume restoration with normal saline is the major and, usually, only measure needed to lower the potassium. In the presence of arrhythmias, intravenous 10% calcium gluconate can be given for its membrane-stabilizing properties.

PHEOCHROMOCYTOMA

The most common symptoms are headache, palpitations, and excessive or inappropriate sweating. The headache, characteristically, is pounding and may be severe. The palpitations may be accompanied by tachycardia. Almost all patients will have one of these three symptoms, and most will have at

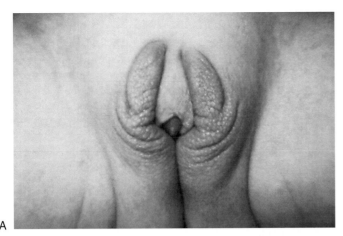

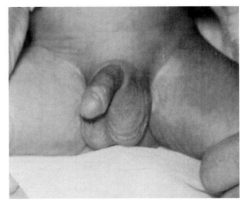

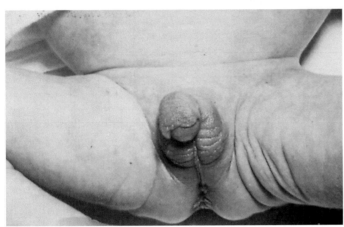

FIG. 7.4. Congenital adrenal hyperplasia in three newborns, all with 21-hydroxylase deficiency. The female newborns depicted in **A** and **B** have different degrees of ambiguity of the external genitalia. **A:** Clitoromegaly with labial enlargement. **B:** Severe clitoral hypertrophy and nearly complete labial fusion. Note the scrotal appearance of the labia. **C:** Male infant with precocious development of the external genitalia and rapid somatic growth. (From Becker KL, Bilezikian JP, Brenner WJ, et al. *Principles and practice of endocrinology and metabolism*, 3rd ed. Philadelphia: Lippincott Williams & Wilkins, 2001:808, with permission.)

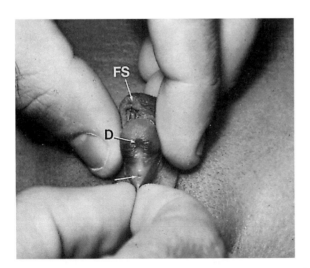

FIG. 7.5. Hypospadias. Glanular hypospadias demonstrated by pulling ventral penile tissue outward; the hypospadiac meatus becomes more apparent. *Arrow* points to the hypospadias. (From Becker KL, Bilezikian JP, Brenner WJ, et al. *Principles and practice of endocrinology and metabolism*, 3rd ed. Philadelphia: Lippincott Williams & Wilkins, 2001:911, with permission.)

least two. Other symptoms may include nervousness, tremor, fatigue, chest or abdominal pains, and flushing. The most useful screening tool for pheochromocytoma is the blood pressure cuff because most pheochromocytomas are associated with hypertension. Because this hypertension may be continuous or paroxysmal, frequent and repeated blood pressure determinations may be necessary. Hypertension is most likely to be found when the patient is symptomatic. A hypertensive patient who is asymptomatic is unlikely to have a pheochromocytoma.

The diagnosis of a pheochromocytoma should also be considered in patients with malignant hypertension, in those who fail to respond or respond inappropriately to antihypertensive medications, and in those who develop hypertension during the induction of anesthesia or during surgery. The incidence of pheochromocytomas is increased among patients with neurofibromatosis (Fig. 7.6) and with the multiple endocrine neoplasia syndromes types II and III. Documentation of excess catecholamine in either the urine or serum confirms the diagnosis of a pheochromocytoma. The most readily available and widely used test for this purpose is the measurement of urinary catecholamines or their metabolites (3-methoxy-4-hydroxymandelic acid and total metanephrines) in a 24-hour urine collection (Fig. 7.7).

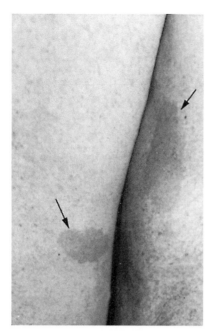

FIG. 7.6. Neurofibromatosis. Discrete, hyperpigmented macules (*arrows*), referred to as café-au-lait spots, are visible on the backs of the legs of a patient with neurofibromatosis. (From Becker KL, Bilezikian JP, Brenner WJ, et al. *Principles and practice of endocrinology and metabolism*, 3rd ed. Philadelphia: Lippincott Williams & Wilkins, 2001:1999, with permission.)

Management

The focus of emergency department management should be on controlling hypertension and hypertensive crisis that may occur before the surgical procedure. α-Adrenergic blocking agents are useful in controlling hypertension and minimizing blood pressure fluctuations during the surgical procedure. Preferred drugs for controlling hypertension are phenoxybenzamine (Dibenzyline) and prazosin (Minipress). Dosing schedules and quantity must be tailored to the individual for adequate control of hypertension. Hypertensive crisis may be appropriately managed with 1 mg intravenous phentolamine mesylate intravenously for children and 5 mg for adolescents or 0.5 to 8.0 μg/kg sodium nitroprusside per minute.

DIABETES INSIPIDUS

Either a deficiency of antidiuretic hormone secretion from the hypothalamus and posterior pituitary gland or renal unresponsiveness to antidiuretic hormone can cause this disease (Table 7.5). Urine excretion is increased in both volume and frequency in the child with diabetes insipidus (DI). This condition may manifest as enuresis in the younger child. If the thirst mechanism is intact and fluids are accessible, the child can compensate for the water loss by drinking more. A history may be elicited of the child's awakening in the middle of the night to drink. If fluids are not available or if fluid intake is interrupted because of a viral illness, dehydration rapidly ensues.

Physical examination may be normal, or signs of dehydration, such as dryness of mucous membranes, decreased

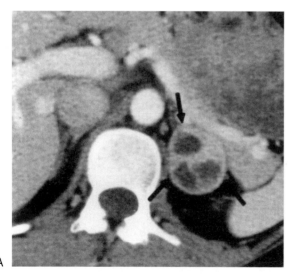

A

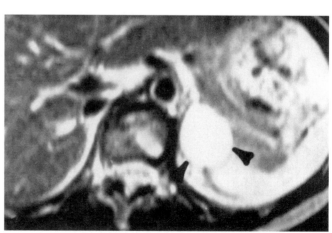

B

FIG. 7.7. Pheochromocytoma. **A:** This contrast-enhanced computed tomography scan shows a 3-cm pheochromocytoma in the left adrenal gland that contains focal areas of necrosis (*arrows*). **B:** T2-weighted magnetic resonance imaging (MRI) shows very high signal intensity (*arrowheads*), typical for a pheochromocytoma. This characteristic high signal intensity on a T2-weighted MRI scan makes it the preferred localization technique for ectopic pheochromocytomas. (From Becker KL, Bilezikian JP, Brenner WJ, et al. *Principles and practice of endocrinology and metabolism*, 3rd ed. Philadelphia: Lippincott Williams & Wilkins, 2001:840, with permission.)

TABLE 7.5. *Causes of diabetes insipidus in children*

Antidiuretic hormone deficiency
Head injury
Meningitis
Idiopathic
Suprasellar tumors and their treatment by surgery and/or
  radiotherapy
Craniopharyngioma
Optic nerve glioma
Dysgeminoma
Septooptic dysplasia
Association with midline cleft palate
Familial (dominant or sex-linked recessive)
Wolfram syndrome (diabetes insipidus, diabetes mellitus,
  optic atrophy, deafness)
Histiocytosis X (Hand–Schüller–Christian disease)
Nephrogenic diabetes insipidus (sex-linked recessive)
Renal disease
Polycystic kidneys
Hydronephrosis
Chronic pyelonephritis
Hypercalcemia
Hypokalemia
Toxins
Demeclocycline
Lithium
Sickle cell disease
Idiopathic

skin turgor, sunken eyes, and, in an infant, a depressed anterior fontanel, may be present. Because of the hyperosmolarity, the degree of dehydration may be underestimated on physical examination. Hypothalamic or pituitary lesions (Fig. 7.8) can lead to other endocrine abnormalities such as secondary hypothyroidism and growth failure. A craniopharyngioma or optic nerve glioma may affect the visual fields or cause increased intracranial pressure, which is indicated by papilledema (Fig. 7.9).

DI is diagnosed by demonstrating that the kidneys fail to concentrate urine when fluid intake is restricted. This condition can be difficult to prove in children. Nonetheless, an adequate working diagnosis is usually obtained by finding an elevated serum osmolality (normal, <290 mOsm/L) and an elevated serum (Na) (normal, <145 mmol/L) in the presence of dilute urine (normal osmolality, >150 mOsm/L). Blood glucose and serum creatinine levels are normal. The definitive diagnosis is made by a formal water deprivation test.

Management

In most cases, a diagnosis of DI is not known at the time of presentation; therefore, the acute management is directed toward correction of the dehydration and the hyperosmolar state. The treatment of DI is similar to that described for hypernatremic dehydration with the notable addition that the fluid required for the replacement of urinary fluid losses will be far greater. In fact, the high urinary output, despite significant dehydration, often provides the first and most convincing evidence of DI. If the child is hypotensive or if the serum Na$^+$ is greater than 160 mmol/L, initial volume expansion is necessary, using 20 mL/kg normal saline during the first hour or more rapidly, if needed. Once an adequate intravascular volume has been achieved, further fluid replacement is accomplished slowly because overly rapid volume correction can cause cerebral edema, seizures, and death.

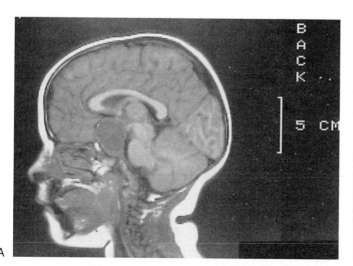
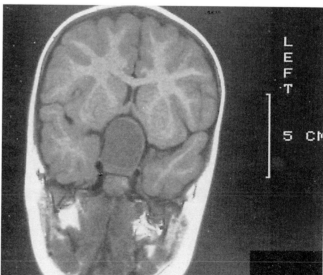

A
B

FIG. 7.8. Craniopharyngioma. Computed tomography scans of the brain of a 3-year-old girl with a craniopharyngioma. **A:** Sagittal view shows a large suprasellar mass. **B:** Coronal view shows compression of the pituitary gland and a large suprasellar mass. (From Becker KL, Bilezikian JP, Brenner WJ, et al. *Principles and practice of endocrinology and metabolism*, 3rd ed. Philadelphia: Lippincott Williams & Wilkins, 2001:196, with permission.)

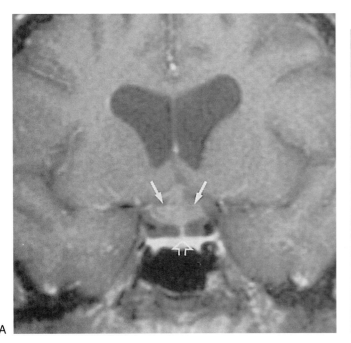
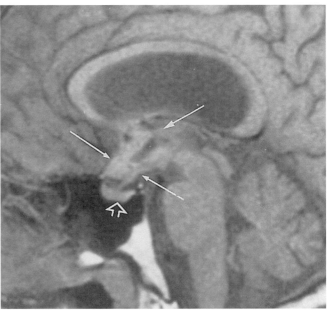

A

B

FIG. 7.9. Hypothalamic and optic pathway glioma. This young man presented with vision problems. He had a history of neurofibromatosis type 1. **A:** Coronal contrast-enhanced T1-weighted magnetic resonance image. The optic chiasm and hypothalamus (*solid white arrows*) are thickened and globular in configuration. The anterior third ventricular recess is not well seen. The pituitary stalk and pituitary gland (*open white arrow*) are normal in configuration. **B:** Sagittal noncontrast-enhanced T1-weighted magnetic resonance image. An irregular mass fills the anterior third ventricle, optic chiasm, and hypothalamic area (*long, thin white arrows*). A segment of the lesion may be cystic and appears as low signal regions. The pituitary gland infundibulum is normal (*open white arrow*). (From Becker KL, Bilezikian JP, Brenner WJ, et al. *Principles and practice of endocrinology and metabolism*, 3rd ed. Philadelphia: Lippincott Williams & Wilkins, 2001:228, with permission.)

SYNDROME OF INAPPROPRIATE ANTIDIURETIC HORMONE SECRETION

Most patients with syndrome of inappropriate antidiuretic hormone secretion (SIADH) (Table 7.6) are asymptomatic until the plasma sodium decreases to below 120 mmol/L. Symptoms associated with hyponatremia range from anorexia, headache, nausea, vomiting, irritability, disorientation, and weakness to seizures and coma, leading ultimately to death. Absence of edema and dehydration are significant clinical findings. Laboratory investigations for diagnostic purposes must include concomitant serum and urine samples (Table 7.7). Hyponatremia, hypoosmolality (serum), and low blood urea nitrogen will be present. In contrast, the urinary osmolality and sodium are inappropriately elevated for the hypotonicity of the serum. The underlying cause of the syndrome should be investigated according to the physician's' clinical judgment. In the presence of hyperglycemia, hyperlipidemia, or hyperproteinemia, the serum sodium may be falsely low. Renal salt wasting, secondary to adrenal insufficiency, should be accompanied by hyperkalemia and dehydration. The urine osmolality in water intoxication states is usually low compared with that found in SIADH.

Management

Patients with a persistent seizure attributable to severe hyponatremia and those who are lethargic or comatose need urgent treatment. Hypertonic (3%) saline is the preferred treatment. Infusing small amounts of 3% saline in the range of 3 mL/kg every 10 to 20 minutes until symptoms remit is probably the safest course of treatment. A single dose of 1 mg/kg furosemide can also be administered intravenously. Close monitoring of fluid balance, plasma and urinary sodium, potassium, and osmolality is essential. Intravenous phenytoin inhibits antidiuretic hormone release and may be helpful in the patient with seizures secondary to CNS causes of SIADH. The underlying cause of SIADH, such as meningitis, should be treated when possible; successful treatment is usually accompanied by remission of inappropriate antidiuresis.

HYPERPARATHYROIDISM

Hyperparathyroidism has two common presentations in children. The first presentation is the critically ill infant (Fig. 7.10) who is found to have severe hypercalcemia during the course of diagnostic investigations. The second presentation

TABLE 7.6. *Some causes of syndrome of inappropriate antidiuretic hormone secretion in children*

Disorders of the central nervous system
Infection (meningitis, encephalitis)
Trauma, postneurosurgery
Hypoxic insults, especially in the perinatal period
Brain tumor
Intraventricular hemorrhage
Guillain–Barré syndrome
Psychosis
Intrathoracic disorders
Infection (tuberculosis, pneumonia, empyema)
Positive-pressure ventilation
Asthma
Cystic fibrosis
Pneumothorax
Patent ductus arteriosus
Ligation
Miscellaneous pain (e.g., after abdominal surgery)
Severe hypothyroidism
Congenital deficiency
Tumors (e.g., neuroblastoma)
Idiopathic deficiency
Drug-induced
Increased antidiuretic hormone secretion
Vincristine
Cyclophosphamide
Carbamazepine
Adenine arabinoside
Phenothiazines
Morphine
Potentiation of antidiuretic hormone effect
Acetaminophen
Indomethacin

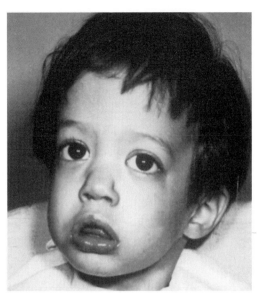

FIG. 7.10. Hypercalcemia. Idiopathic hypercalcemia (Williams syndrome) in a 3-year-old boy. Note the typical broad forehead, depressed bridge of the nose, anteverted nares, long philtrum (the vertical median groove extending from beneath the nose to the upper lip), and the large ears. The cheeks are full and dependent, and there is mandibular hypoplasia. (From Becker KL, Bilezikian JP, Brenner WJ, et al. *Principles and practice of endocrinology and metabolism*, 3rd ed. Philadelphia: Lippincott Williams & Wilkins, 2001:689, with permission.)

is a child in the early to mid teens with nonspecific symptoms including nausea, constipation, unexplained weight loss, personality changes, and headaches. Diffuse bone pain or renal colic may be reported, although these symptoms are less common in children than in adults. The physical findings of hypercalcemia are hypotonia, weakness, and listlessness. Rarely, a palpable mass is located in the parathyroid region. Radiographic findings consistent with hyperparathyroidism include evidence of demineralization and bone resorption (Figs. 7.11 and 7.12).

Hypercalcemia is usually present but may be subtle or intermittent in mild cases. The serum inorganic phosphate level is usually low but may be normal, especially in patients

with decreased renal function. Mild hyperchloremic acidosis may be present. Alkaline phosphate level and urinary hydroxyproline excretion may be elevated secondary to increased osteoclast activity.

Management

Acute management of hyperparathyroidism is essentially the same as management of hypercalcemia. The specific management of hyperparathyroidism depends on the level of calcium and on the presence of signs and symptoms. In the asymptomatic patient with a serum calcium of less than 12 mg/dL, careful follow-up with close attention to both bone mass and renal function is recommended. If the child is persistently hypercalcemic, parathyroid surgery is the preferred treatment.

HYPOPARATHYROIDISM

The predominant historical features and clinical manifestations of hypoparathyroidism are the same as those of hypocalcemia. The particular symptoms and signs found depends on the age at onset of the disease, the chronicity of the disease, and the presence of other autoimmune or syndromic phenomena. Papilledema without hemorrhage may be seen during the initial examination and tends to resolve within several days after the initiation of therapy (Fig. 7.13A).

TABLE 7.7. *Criteria for diagnosis of syndrome of inappropriate antidiuretic hormone secretion*

Hyponatremia, reduced serum osmolality
Urine osmolality that is inappropriately elevated (a urine osmolality <100 mOsm/kg usually excludes the diagnosis)
Urinary sodium concentration that is excessive compared with the degree of hyponatremia (usually >18 mEq/L)
Normal renal, adrenal, and thyroid function
Absence of volume depletion

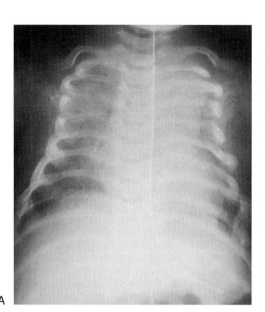
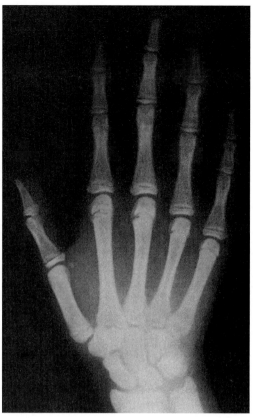

A

B

FIG. 7.11. Hyperparathyroidism. **A:** Primary hyperparathyroidism in a 3-day-old newborn girl. Chest radiograph shows profound demineralization of the skeleton with loss of a well-defined cortical margin. Cystic changes in rib and subperiosteal bone resorption in the humerus are seen. **B:** Secondary hyperparathyroidism in a 12-year-old girl with chronic pyelonephritis. There is moderate subperiosteal erosion on the radial side of the middle phalanges; note a lacy appearance of the periosteum and small-tuft erosion. Subperiosteal bone resorption is the most significant radiographic finding in hyperparathyroidism; subperiosteal bone resorption and tuft erosion are seen in both primary and secondary hyperparathyroidism.

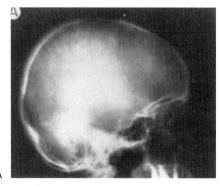
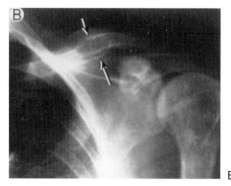

A

B

FIG. 7.12. Radiographic representations of osteitis fibrosa cystica in primary hyperparathyroidism. **A:** Salt-and-pepper erosions of the skull. **B:** Cystic bone disease in the clavicle (*arrows*).

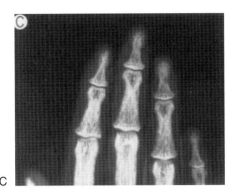
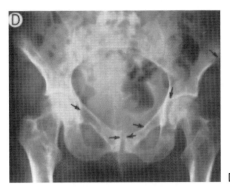

FIG. 7.12. *Continued.* **C:** Subperiosteal bone resorption of the digits. **D:** Cortical erosions (*arrows*). (From Becker KL, Bilezikian JP, Brenner WJ, et al. *Principles and practice of endocrinology and metabolism*, 3rd ed. Philadelphia: Lippincott Williams & Wilkins, 2001:565, with permission.)

Lenticular cataracts (Fig. 17.13B) are common in hypoparathyroidism and are associated with long-standing hypocalcemia of any cause. Psychiatric and neurologic disorders occur in association with hypoparathyroidism. Subnormal intelligence occurs in approximately 20% of children with the idiopathic form of hypoparathyroidism, and the severity correlates closely with the period of untreated hypocalcemia. Dry, scaly skin is a common finding, as is patchy alopecia. Psoriasis or mucocutaneous candidiasis may be found on occasion. Unusually brittle fingernails and hair are often found. Hypoplasia of tooth enamel may be seen if hypoparathyroidism was present at the time of dental development. Intestinal malabsorption and steatorrhea have been reported in association with hypoparathyroidism.

Management

Acute management of hypoparathyroidism is essentially the same as management of hypocalcemia. Long-term management consists of treatment with vitamin D, usually with one of its more active analogues [1,25-(OH)$_2$D$_3$]. Supplemental oral calcium is usually necessary.

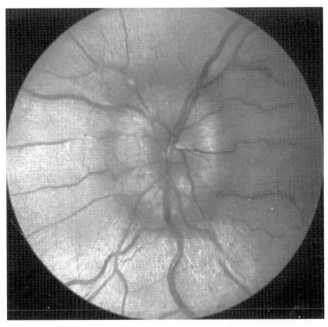
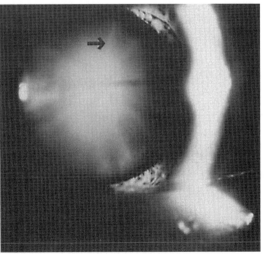

FIG. 7.13. Hypoparathyroidism signs and symptoms. **A:** Patient with papilledema; there is swelling of the optic disk as a result of increased intracranial pressure. Note the loss of the central cup. **B:** Cortical spoking cataract. Note the spokes of lens opacification (*arrows*) radiating from the center of the lens cortex. (From Becker KL, Bilezikian JP, Brenner WJ, et al. *Principles and practice of endocrinology and metabolism*, 3rd ed. Philadelphia: Lippincott Williams & Wilkins, 2001:1969, 1972, with permission.)

RICKETS

Children with rickets may come to medical attention because of specific physical abnormalities (bowed legs), limb pain and swelling, seizures, failure to thrive (renal tubular acidosis), biochemical abnormalities (hypocalcemia), or radiographic findings (broadened, frayed metaphysis) (Figs. 7.14 and 7.15). Thorough social and dietary histories are helpful in delineating the probable cause and in sparing the patient an extensive and expensive evaluation. A family history may be useful in identifying the 21-hydroxylase deficiency or renal phosphate wasting.

The clinical findings in rickets may vary considerably depending on the underlying disorder, the duration of the problem, and the child's age. Most features are related to skeletal deformity, skeletal pain, slippage of epiphyses, bony fractures, and growth disturbances (Fig. 7.16). Muscular weakness, hypotonia, and lethargy are often noted. Failure of calcification affects those parts of the skeleton that are growing most rapidly or that are under stress. For example, the skull grows rapidly in the perinatal period; therefore, craniotabes is a manifestation of congenital rickets. Conversely, the upper limbs and rib cage grow rapidly during the first year of life, and abnormalities at these sites are more common at this

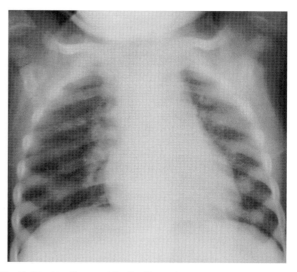

FIG. 7.15. Radiographic findings in rickets of the chest. Rickets in an 11-month-old boy breast-fed since birth. Chest radiograph shows demineralization of the skeleton with cupping of the distal end of ribs and humerus.

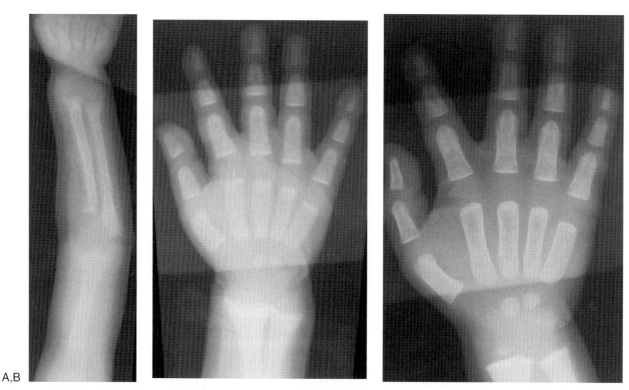

A,B   C

FIG. 7.14. Radiographic findings in rickets of the upper extremity. **A:** Rickets in an 11-month-old boy breast-fed since birth. Radiograph of the upper extremity shows profound demineralization of the skeleton, with frayed, irregular cupping of the end of the metaphysis and poorly defined cortex. Note the retardation of skeletal maturation. **B:** Same patient with some healing 4 weeks after supplemental vitamin D. Severe rachitic changes are noticeable. Periosteal cloaking of both the metacarpals and radius and ulna is evidence of healing. **C:** Complete healing of the rickets after 8 months of treatment. Note the reappearance of the provisional zone of calcification.

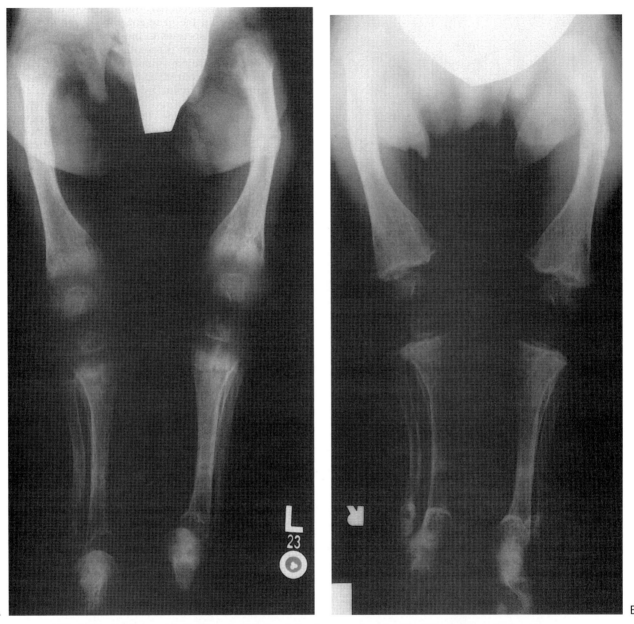

A

B

FIG. 7.16. Radiographic findings in rickets of the lower extremity. Rachitic changes in the lower extremities of a 2.5-year-old girl with hereditary resistance to vitamin D. **A:** At presentation, severely deformed epiphyses, demineralization, and bilateral fractures of the femora and tibiae are evident. **B:** After 4 months of therapy with high-dose calcitrol, dramatic remodeling of the metaphyseal edges has occurred. (From Becker KL, Bilezikian JP, Brenner WJ, et al. *Principles and practice of endocrinology and metabolism*, 3rd ed. Philadelphia: Lippincott Williams & Wilkins, 2001:692, with permission.)

age (e.g., rachitic rosary, flaring of the wrist) (Fig. 7.17). Bowing of the legs is unlikely to be noted until the child is ambulatory (Fig. 7.18). Dental eruption may be delayed, and enamel defects are common (Fig. 7.19).

Radiography is the optimal way to confirm the clinical diagnosis because the radiographic features reflect the histopathology (Fig. 7.20). Characteristic findings include widening and irregularity of the epiphyseal plates, cupped metaphyses, fractures, and bowing of the weight-bearing

limbs. The clinical laboratory is often helpful in correctly identifying the cause of rickets. Frank hypocalcemia (<7 mg/dL) is unusual in rickets. Calcium levels in the 7- to 9-mg/dL range are common and warrant careful attention because the initiation of vitamin D treatment increases bony deposition of calcium and may lead to a decrease in serum calcium. Phosphate levels are often low. An amino aciduria is often present and may lead to some confusion of simple vitamin D deficiency with Fanconi syndrome. Alkaline

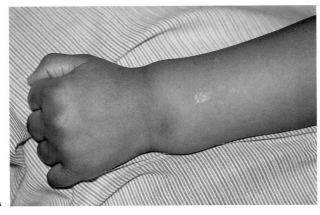

A

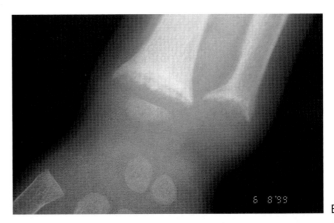

B

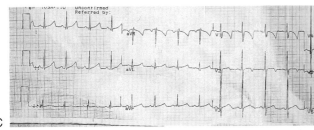

C

FIG. 7.17. This infant shows the characteristic widening of the wrist **(A)** caused by flaring at the end of the radius and ulna. **(B)** His electrocardiogram demonstrates prolongation of the QT interval, secondary to hypocalcemia **(C)**.

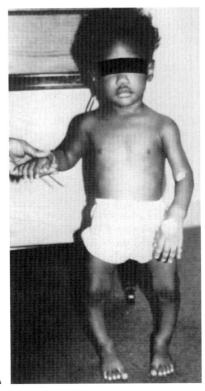

A

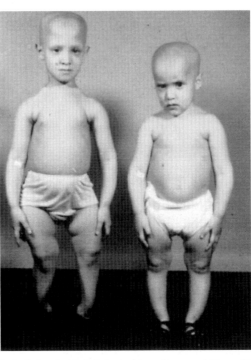

B

FIG. 7.18. Bowing of the legs. **A:** Nutritional rickets (vitamin D deficiency) in a 3-year-old boy. Note the severe bowing of the lower extremities and the wider wrists and ankles. **B:** Two siblings with vitamin D–dependent rickets type II and alopecia. (From Becker KL, Bilezikian JP, Brenner WJ, et al. *Principles and practice of endocrinology and metabolism*, 3rd ed. Philadelphia: Lippincott Williams & Wilkins, 2001:539, 690, with permission.)

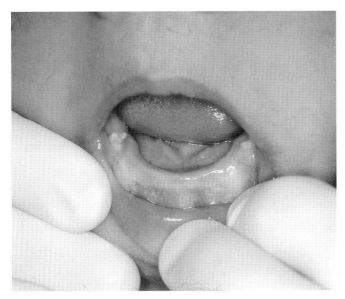

FIG. 7.19. The limited eruption of teeth (oligodontia), as shown here, is characteristic of some kindreds with hereditary resistance to vitamin D. (From Becker KL, Bilezikian JP, Brenner WJ, et al. *Principles and practice of endocrinology and metabolism*, 3rd ed. Philadelphia: Lippincott Williams & Wilkins, 2001:693, with permission.)

phosphatase levels are significantly increased, reflecting extremely active bony metabolism.

Management

Treatment depends on the nature of the underlying disease. The response to treatment may be helpful in differentiating

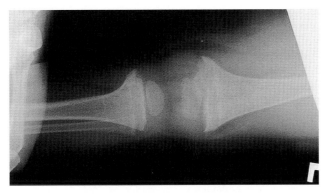

FIG. 7.20. Rickets, osteopenia.

simple dietary vitamin D deficiency from more complex causes of rickets. In the absence of chronic disease, dietary rickets may be adequately treated with daily doses of 1,000 to 2,000 IU of vitamin D until healing occurs. If the initial serum calcium is borderline low or low, supplemental calcium should be initiated 48 hours before the institution of vitamin D, especially in the young child. Otherwise, the institution of vitamin D may cause a further decrease in serum calcium and elicit frank hypocalcemia. Children with symptomatic hypocalcemia or an initial serum calcium of less than 7 mg/dL on presentation warrant hospitalization and frequent calcium determinations.

SUGGESTED READINGS

General

August GP. Treatment of adrenocortical insufficiency. *Pediatr Rev* 1997; 18:59–62.

Buonocore CM, Robinson AG. The diagnosis and management of diabetes insipidus during medical emergencies. *Endocrinol Metab Clin North Am* 1993;22:411–413.

Butkiewicz EK, Liebson CL, Obrien PC, et al. Insulin therapy for diabetic ketoacidosis: bolus injection versus continuous insulin infusion. *Diabetes Care* 1995;18:1187–1190.

Caty MG, Coran AG, Geagen M, et al. Current diagnosis and treatment of pheochromocytoma in children. *Arch Surg* 1990;125:978–981.

Cutler GG Jr, Laue L. Congenital adrenal hyperplasia due to 21-hydroxylase deficiency. *N Engl J Med* 1990;323:1906–1913.

Ein SH, Pullerits J, Crighton R, et al. Pediatric pheochromocytoma: a 36-year review. *Pediatr Surg Int* 1997;12:595–598.

Finberg L. Why do patients with diabetic ketoacidosis have cerebral swelling, and why does treatment sometimes make it worse? *Arch Pediatr Adolesc Med* 1996;150:785–786.

Foley TP Jr. Thyrotoxicosis in childhood. *Pediatr Ann* 1992;21:43–49.

Ganong CA, Kappy MS. Cerebral salt wasting in children: the need for recognition and treatment. *Am J Dis Child* 1993;147:167–169.

Jacobson AD, Hauser ST, Willett J, et al. Consequences of irregular versus continuous follow-up in children and adolescents with insulin dependent diabetes mellitus. *J Pediatr* 1997;131:727–733.

Kappy MS, Ganong CA. Cerebral salt wasting in children: the role of atrial natriuretic factor. *Adv Pediatr* 1996;43:271–308.

Klekamp J, Churchwell KB. Diabetic ketoacidosis in children: initial clinical assessment and treatment. *Pediatr Ann* 1996;25:387–393.

Lawson ML, Miller SF, Ellis G, et al. Primary hyperparathyroidism in a paediatric hospital. *Q J Med* 1996;89:921–932.

Lindsey R, Bolte RG. The use of insulin bolus in low-dose insulin infusion for pediatric diabetic ketoacidosis. *Pediatr Emerg Care* 1989;5:77–79.

Newfield RS, New MI. 21-hydroxylase deficiency. *Ann N Y Acad Sci* 1997;816:219–229.

Pang S. Congenital adrenal hyperplasia. *Endocrinol Metab Clin North Am* 1997;26:853–891.

Pheochromocytoma

Rosenbloom AL, Hamas R. Diabetic ketoacidosis (DKA): treatment guidelines. *Clin Pediatr* 1996;35:261–266.

CHAPTER 8

Gastrointestinal Emergencies

Editor: Stephen Ludwig

GASTROINTESTINAL BLEEDING

Upper Gastrointestinal Bleeding

Background

Upper gastrointestinal (GI) bleeding is generally regarded as originating proximal to the Treitz ligament. Hematemesis or bloody gastric aspirates from a nasogastric tube may originate from the mouth, nasopharynx, esophagus, stomach, biliary tree, or duodenum (Fig. 8.1). The most common causes of upper GI bleeding in children are mucosal lesions, including esophagitis (Fig. 8.2), gastritis (Fig. 8.3), Mallory–Weiss tear, peptic ulcer disease, and duodenitis. Less common but important causes include bleeding esophageal varices and vascular lesions. Endoscopy, when performed by a well-trained physician, is the most sensitive and specific diagnostic procedure for determining the cause and site of upper GI bleeding. A specific diagnosis should be pursued in patients who have (1) active bleeding documented by nasogastric lavage; (2) evidence of severe hemorrhage (hemodynamic instability or equilibrated hemoglobin level less than 10 g/dL); (3) conditions that affect healing or clotting, such as a catabolic state or serious chronic disease; (4) a history of unexplained gross or occult bleeding or unexplained iron deficiency anemia; or (5) a history of chronic dyspepsia (vomiting, abdominal pain, nausea, oral regurgitation, heartburn, dysphagia) (Fig. 8.4).

General Principles of Nasogastric Lavage

Most patients can be effectively lavaged with a nasogastric sump tube (12 French in small children, 14 to 16 French in older children). Verification of the location of the tube in the stomach by injection of air and auscultation over the stomach is essential. Return volumes should approximate input volumes, and discrepancies should be recorded. If aspiration meets with significant resistance, the physician should either reposition the tube, reposition the patient, or increase the amount of solution introduced (Fig. 8.5).

Blood-flecked gastric aspirate or coffee-ground material indicates a low rate of bleeding (Fig. 8.1). In contrast, bright red blood, especially if it does not clear with repeated lavage for 5 to 10 minutes, suggests a significant or ongoing hemorrhage. No benefit is derived from continuous lavage longer than 10 minutes if return is not clearing.

Nonspecific Mucosal Lesions

GI bleeding may be a complication of all acute and chronic nonspecific upper GI mucosal lesions (esophagitis, gastritis, Mallory–Weiss tears, and duodenitis). Regardless of the cause, upper GI bleeding usually stops spontaneously, often by the time the patient arrives in the emergency department (ED). Esophagitis caused by gastroesophageal reflux is being diagnosed more often with improved pediatric fiberoptic endoscopes. Increasing use of endoscopic biopsy has documented esophagitis in 60% of patients with clinically significant gastroesophageal reflux. Exposure to aspirin and nonsteroidal antiinflammatory drugs (e.g., ibuprofen, naproxen) has also been associated with gastritis and mucosal ulceration.

Management

For patients who have significant bleeding and for whom nasogastric lavage was initiated, if gastric contents clear after initial saline lavage and immediate endoscopy is not planned, gastric irrigation is performed every 15 minutes for 1 hour, then every hour for 2 to 3 hours.

For patients with significant symptoms or blood loss, H_2-antagonists may be given initially by the intravenous route, switching to the oral route when the nasogastric tube is removed. Either ranitidine or cimetidine is appropriate.

In general, all patients with a history suggestive of significant upper GI bleeding should be admitted to the hospital for observation. Unremitting or recurrent mucosal bleeding requires either therapeutic endoscopy, therapeutic angiography, or surgery. In the hands of a qualified endoscopist, therapeutic endoscopy using either a heater probe or multipolar electrocoagulation is the treatment of choice.

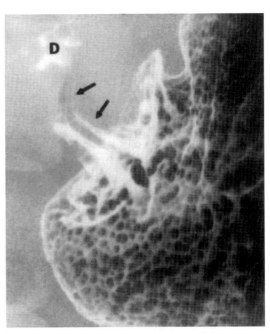

FIG. 8.3. Gastritis. Note the diffuse mucosal nodularity throughout the stomach. In addition, note spasm of the antrum (*arrows*) and duodenal bulb (*D*). (From Swischuk LE. *Emergency imaging of the acutely ill or injured child*, 4th ed. Philadelphia: Lippincott Williams & Wilkins, 2000:218, with permission.)

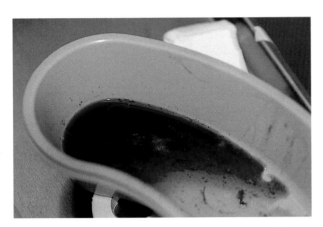

FIG. 8.1. Hematemesis from a child with gastritis.

FIG. 8.2. Esophagitis. **A:** Herpes. Note the fine nodularity and mucosal fold thickening (*arrows*) in the upper esophagus. (From Swischuk LE. *Emergency imaging of the acutely ill or injured child*, 4th ed. Philadelphia: Lippincott Williams & Wilkins, 2000:219, with permission.) **B:** Esophageal stricture. Lateral barium esophagram shows narrowing of mid-esophagus in an infant with gastroesophageal reflux.

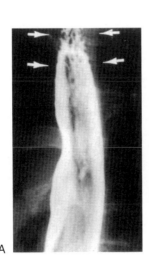

A

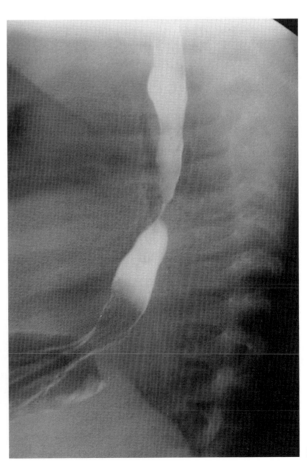

B

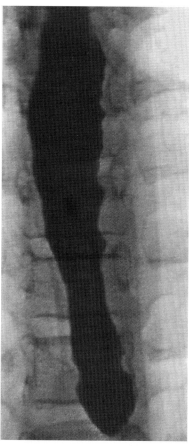

FIG. 8.4. Dysphagia. Upper gastrointestinal series of a 14-year-old girl presenting with dysphagia. The series demonstrates a significantly dilated upper esophagus, with a functional spasmodic obstruction of the lower esophagus, characteristic of achalasia.

Esophageal Varices

Portal hypertension and esophageal varices (Fig. 8.6) may result from either extrahepatic presinusoidal obstruction (50% to 65% of cases in children) or from hepatic parenchymal disorders. Extrahepatic obstruction (e.g., portal or splenic vein obstruction) is associated with omphalitis, dehydration, sepsis, and umbilical vein catheterization. Hepatic parenchymal disease may result from biliary cirrhosis associated with biliary atresia (Fig. 8.7), cystic fibrosis, hepatitis, α_1-antitrypsin deficiency, or congenital hepatic fibrosis. Patients with both types of portal hypertension are susceptible to GI hemorrhage from bleeding esophageal varices and congestive or hemorrhagic gastritis. After development of portal hypertension, the onset of esophageal varices can be variable, from a few months to many years (Fig. 8.8).

Patients with portal hypertension may have occult bleeding, but more commonly, the bleeding is brisk, and patients will have melena and/or hematemesis. The possibility of bleeding esophageal varices should be considered in any patient with a history of jaundice (beyond the newborn period), hepatitis, blood transfusion, chronic right-sided heart failure, pulmonary hypertension, omphalitis, umbilical vein catheterization, or one of the hepatic parenchymal diseases previously noted. Accordingly, the physical examination may reveal stigmata of the underlying disease leading to portal hypertension, including jaundice, ascites, rectal hemorrhoids, and hepatosplenomegaly.

Management

The initial management of suspected variceal hemorrhage is identical to that of massive upper GI bleeding from any source. Overexpansion of the intravascular volume should be avoided because it contributes to rebleeding. Coagulation abnormalities should be managed aggressively with intravenous vitamin K, fresh frozen plasma, and platelets. Bleeding varices may be the initial sign of sepsis in patients who have cirrhosis; therefore, any patient who has fever should be started on broad-spectrum antibiotics, such as ampicillin and gentamicin, pending results of blood cultures.

Suspicion of variceal bleeding is not a contraindication to pass a nasogastric tube. If bleeding ceases during the initial gastric lavage, the tube should be managed as previously described.

Gastroesophageal balloon tamponade is a high-risk procedure. It should be considered only for endoscopically proven gastric or esophageal varices. Indications of these varices include massive, life-threatening hemorrhage or continued

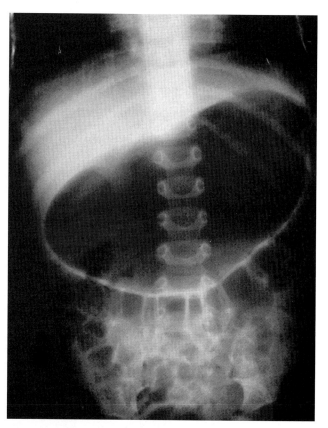

FIG. 8.5. Radiograph of a patient with gastric distention. The patient's respiratory distress resolved after a nasogastric tube was inserted.

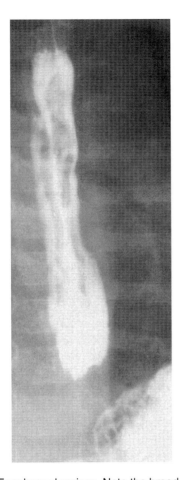

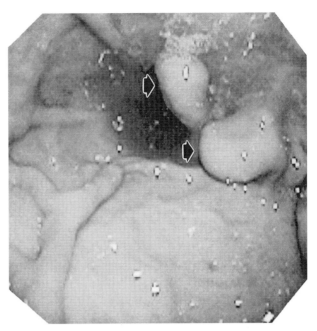

FIG. 8.8. Gastric varices. Two large, blood-filled varices in the gastric cardia (*arrows*).

FIG. 8.6. Esophageal varices. Note the broad, tortuous radiolucent bands running throughout the length of the esophagus. These are characteristic of esophageal varices. (From Swischuk LE. *Imaging of the Newborn, Infant and Young Child*, 4th ed. Philadelphia: Lippincott Williams & Wilkins, 1997:376, with permission.)

bleeding despite 2 to 6 hours of intravenous vasopressin. A Sengstaken–Blakemore or Linton tube may be used. The Sengstaken–Blakemore tube has both gastric and esophageal balloon tubes, whereas the Linton tube has a single lavage gastric balloon. Gastroesophageal tamponade is reported to arrest bleeding initially in 50% to 80% of cases. However, the reported incidence of major complications from the use of the Sengstaken–Blakemore tube ranges from 9% to 35%. Death directly attributed to the use of the tube has been reported in 5% to 20% of patients in whom the tube was used.

Endoscopic sclerotherapy should be performed on an elective basis within 6 to 24 hours after active bleeding has

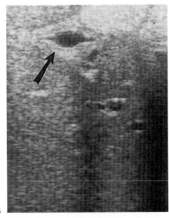

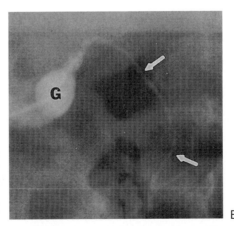

FIG. 8.7. Extrahepatic biliary atresia: various configurations. **A:** The gallbladder (*arrow*) is very small in this patient. **B:** Operative cholangiogram demonstrates the small gallbladder (*G*) and the thin common bile duct (*arrows*). No intrahepatic radicals are demonstrated. (From Swischuk LE. *Imaging of the Newborn, Infant and Young Child*, 4th ed. Philadelphia: Lippincott Williams & Wilkins, 1997:489, with permission.)

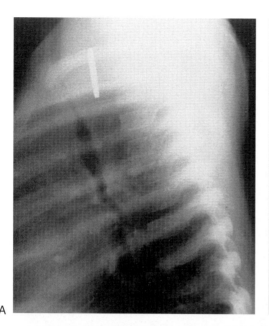

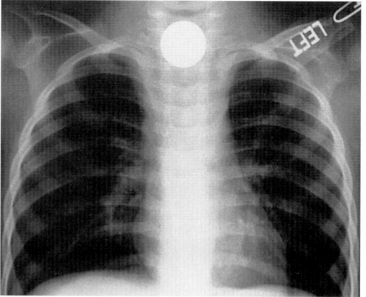

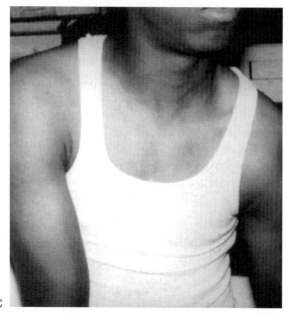

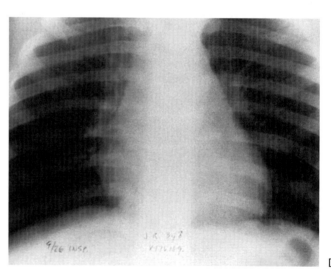

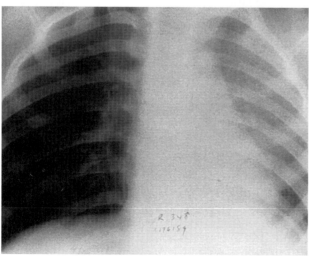

FIG. 8.9. Chest radiographs of swallowed foreign bodies. **A, B:** A two-view chest radiograph demonstrates impacted esophageal coin located at the thoracic inlet. **C:** A two-view chest radiograph demonstrates aspirated radiopaque foreign body (an earring) located in the left bronchus. **D, E:** Inspiratory and expiratory chest radiographs demonstrate air trapping in the right lung during expiration, indicating the likelihood of a right-sided foreign body. A peanut was removed at bronchoscopy.

been controlled by pharmacologic therapy or balloon tamponade. Recent reports have noted success with endoscopic variceal ligation using an elastic band ligature device in children. Randomized studies of endoscopic variceal sclerotherapy versus endoscopic variceal ligation in adults have demonstrated that endoscopic variceal ligation has a lower complication rate, less recurrent bleeding, and better variceal eradication than endoscopic variceal sclerotherapy.

Miscellaneous Causes of Upper Gastrointestinal Bleeding

In the first few days of life or in breast-fed infants, swallowed maternal blood may be the cause of hematemesis or melena in an infant who otherwise appears healthy. Performing a guaiac test on expressed breast milk may suggest the diagnosis. An Apt–Downey test should be performed on a sample of emesis or nasogastric aspirate to definitively diagnose the condition. Blood from the aspirate is placed on filter paper and mixed with 1% NaOH. Adult hemoglobin will be reduced to form a rusty brown or yellow color. Fetal hemoglobin is resistant to denaturation and will retain a bright pink or red color.

Dieulafoy erosion is an unusual cause of GI bleeding in which massive hemorrhage occurs from a pinpoint nonulcerated arterial lesion, usually high in the fundus of the stomach. The bleeding results from an unusually large submucosal artery that travels a tortuous course through the submucosa and may erode through a mucosal defect. Its characteristic presentation is one of recurrent, massive hematemesis, usually without any prodromal symptoms. Management is similar to that for any patient with a significant GI hemorrhage. Diagnosis can be made by endoscopy, during which the Dieulafoy erosion can usually be located.

Finally, swallowed foreign bodies can cause significant trauma and GI bleeding. Most swallowed foreign bodies, even those with sharp edges, will pass spontaneously and require no specific therapy (Fig. 8.9). However, on occasion, a sharp foreign body may be the cause of GI bleeding. Removal by endoscopy is indicated if significant bleeding occurs (Fig. 8.10).

Lower Gastrointestinal Bleeding

Rectal bleeding is a relatively uncommon but worrisome complaint in the ambulatory or ED setting. The cause of lower GI bleeding varies with age. Among infants younger than 6 months of age, the most common diagnoses are milk-protein sensitivity (allergic colitis), anorectal fissures, and infectious gastroenteritis. Children 1 to 5 years of age are most likely to have infectious gastroenteritis, intussusception (Fig. 8.11), Meckel diverticulum (Fig. 8.12), colonic polyps, and anorectal fissures. Older children typically have infectious gastroenteritis, inflammatory bowel disease (IBD), and hemorrhoids/rectal varices. The pathophysiology, clinical manifestations, and specific management indicated for the most common conditions causing lower GI bleeding in children are discussed in the following sections.

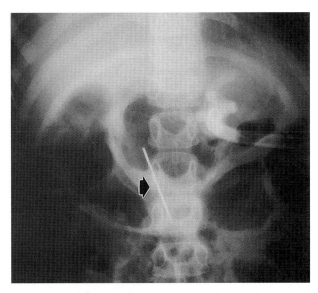

FIG. 8.10. Gastric foreign body and gastrointestinal bleeding. This 6-year-old developmentally delayed patient ingested a large straight pin (*arrow*) that caused bleeding of the gastric antrum. An opaque gastrostomy tube is also radiographically present.

Anorectal Fissures and Hemorrhoids

Anal fissures are the most common proctologic disorder during infancy and childhood. Most occur in infants younger than 1 year of age. Anal fissure may result from diarrhea, which causes perineal irritation, but it is more commonly associated with constipation. The fissure usually starts when passage of a hard stool tears the sensitive squamous lining of the anal canal. Subsequent bowel movements are associated with pain and/or bleeding. Bright red blood is seen coating the stool. The infant begins to withhold stool, leading to increasing constipation and a vicious cycle of hard stools, bleeding, and pain. An anal fissure can be seen by spreading the perineal skin to evert the anal canal. Simply spreading the buttocks to view the anal opening is not sufficient. Treatment consists of local skin care combined with stool softeners. Malt extract (Maltsupex 1 to 3 tablespoons per day) or mineral oil (1 to 3 tablespoons per day) can be given to soften the stool. Local care involves sitz baths four times daily, a perianal cleansing lotion (Balneol) after bowel movements, and an emollient protective ointment (Balmex) after each bowel movement.

All patients with perianal excoriation, multiple anal fissures, a recurrent anal fissure, or a fissure resistant to conservative management should have perianal cultures for β-hemolytic streptococcus. If this organism is recovered, the patient should receive a 10-day course of oral penicillin.

Polyps

There are two major types of polyps that may be diagnosed in infancy or childhood: hamartomatous and adenomatous.

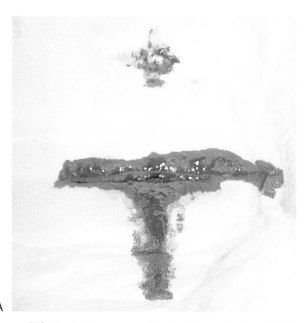

A

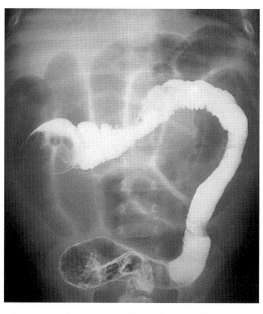

B

FIG. 8.11. Intussusception. **A:** Currant jelly stool characteristic of intussusception. **B:** Ileocolic intussusception. Barium enema shows the intussusception as the filing defect within the hepatic flexure surrounded by spiral mucosal folds. Significant distended small bowel represents distal small bowel obstruction.

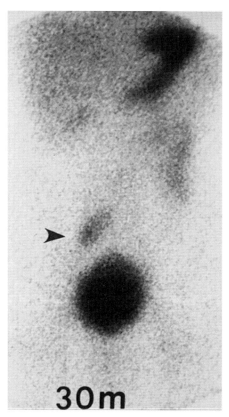

FIG. 8.12. Meckel diverticulum. Anterior image at 30 minutes shows an oval focal accumulation of technetium-99m–pertechnetate in the right lower quadrant of the abdomen (*arrowhead*).

Hamartomatous polyps are generally benign and are the usual type of polyp found in juvenile polyps, juvenile polyposis coli, and Peutz–Jeghers syndrome. Adenomatous polyps are potentially premalignant and are found in a number of syndromes, including familial adenomatous polyposis and Gardner syndrome.

Juvenile polyps are the most common of the polyp syndromes in children, found in 15% of patients in one series who had colonoscopy for rectal bleeding (Fig. 8.13). More than one polyp may be found in more than 50% of cases of juvenile polyps. Most (75%) of the polyps are rectosigmoid or in the descending colon, 15% are found in the transverse colon, and 10% in the ascending colon. Autoamputation of juvenile polyps, especially in the rectum, occurs spontaneously in most cases. In juvenile polyposis coli, multiple juvenile polyps are found throughout the colon. Peutz–Jeghers syndrome is the association of mucocutaneous pigmented lesions and hamartomatous polyps. It has autosomal dominant inheritance with a high degree of penetrance. The macular, melanin-containing pigmented lesions characteristically occur on the buccal mucosa, lips, face, arms, palms and soles, and perianal region. The polyps are typically located in the small intestine but can be found throughout the GI tract.

Familial adenomatous polyposis is an autosomal dominant inherited syndrome consisting of multiple adenomatous polyps that are generally confined to the colon but that can be found throughout the GI tract (Fig. 8.14).

A 6% incidence of malignant transformation of these lesions is present by 15 years of age, prompting recommendations for total proctocolectomy by age 18. Gardner syndrome

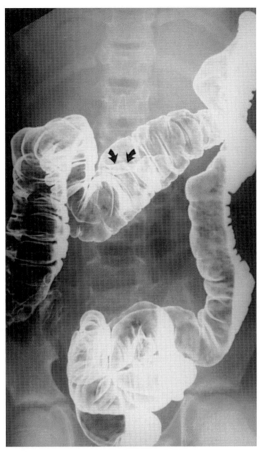

FIG. 8.13. Juvenile polyps. Double air-contrast barium enema shows a single polyp with a long stalk in transverse colon (*arrow*).

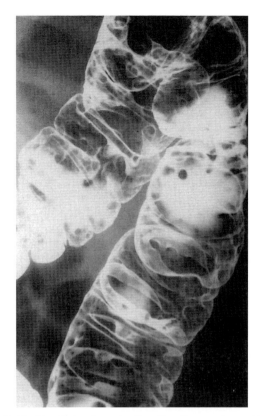

FIG. 8.14. Familial polyposis. Small uniform polyps virtually carpet the colon. This patient had familial adenomatous polyposis. (From Swischuk LE. *Imaging of the Newborn, Infant and Young Child*, 4th ed. Philadelphia: Lippincott Williams & Wilkins, 1997:486, with permission.)

is an autosomal dominant inherited syndrome consisting of hereditary adenomatous polyps of the small and large intestine and soft-tissue and bony tumors. The tumors are often epidermoid cysts (Fig. 8.15), fibromas, or osteomas of the skull and mandible and are often the initial manifestation of the disease.

The most common presentation of juvenile polyps is painless rectal bleeding, often with blood streaking the outside of the stools. The peak incidence for presentation is between 4 and 5 years of age. Prolapse of the polyp through the rectum may occur. The polyp may also form the lead point of an intussusception. All patients with rectal bleeding should have a careful rectal examination because 30% to 40% of polyps are palpable by rectal examination.

Polyps may be part of various inherited syndromes; therefore, a complete physical examination should be performed on any patient with rectal bleeding. A careful search for pigmented lesions or soft-tissue and bony tumors may aid in the diagnosis of inherited polyposis syndromes as previously described.

Management

The initial ED management of patients who have suspected polyps is aimed at assessing the amount of blood loss and

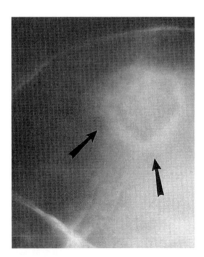

FIG. 8.15. Epidermoid cyst. Large epidermoid cyst with moderate sclerosis (*arrows*). This epidermoid cyst was located predominantly in the external table. (From Swischuk LE, John SD. *Differential Diagnosis in Pediatric Radiology*, 2nd ed. Philadelphia: Lippincott Williams & Wilkins, 2001:381, with permission.)

arranging the appropriate diagnostic study. Blood loss is rarely life threatening, but significant losses may be noted from chronic intermittent bleeding. All patients should have a complete blood count (CBC) performed, and if the history of blood loss is significant, a type and cross-match may also be indicated.

Dietary Protein Sensitivity Syndromes (Allergic Colitis)

Dietary proteins are capable of inducing significant bowel injury and may be the cause of several different types of enterocolitis presenting throughout childhood. Each condition, by definition, is induced by a dietary protein and resolves completely after the protein is eliminated from the diet. Immunologic responses may vary from classic allergic mast cell activation to immune complex formation. The development of proctocolitis in response to cow's milk protein exposure was among the first to be described. Subsequently, a similar condition has been described in response to soybean-based formula and among exclusively breast-fed infants, presumably in response to maternal dietary protein intake.

The typical presentation of milk-protein sensitivity colitis is that of acute onset of blood-streaked, mucoid diarrheal stools in an otherwise well-appearing infant younger than 6 months of age. Mean age at onset among 35 infants in one series was 4.3 + 4.1 weeks. It is unusual to present within the first week of life. Blood loss is typically limited, infants do not appear acutely dehydrated and are afebrile, and weight gain has typically been within normal limits since birth. The differential diagnosis includes anal fissures and infectious enterocolitis. External anal fissures can be ruled out by careful physical examination. Appropriate viral and bacterial cultures of stool may be indicated to rule out infectious causes.

Management

These patients are rarely hemodynamically unstable or seriously ill; therefore, initial ED management is focused on making a presumptive diagnosis based on initial laboratory testing, initiation of appropriate dietary therapy, and arranging adequate follow-up with the patient's primary care physician or a pediatric gastroenterologist. Initial laboratory testing should consist of a CBC with white blood cell differential, assessing the hemoglobin as well as assessing for leukocytosis and eosinophilia (Fig. 8.16). Patients with histologically proven milk-protein sensitivity colitis have higher mean peripheral eosinophil counts compared with age-appropriate normal values. However, in the individual patient, a higher than normal eosinophil count is actually an insensitive marker (10% sensitivity) for histologically proven colitis. In addition, a serum albumin level should be obtained because hypoalbuminemia has been demonstrated to have a sensitivity of approximately 80% for histologic colitis. Examination of stool for blood, fecal leukocytes, and routine bacterial culture should be performed on all infants. Infants who have milk-protein sensitivity colitis will charac-

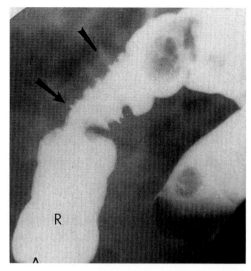

FIG. 8.16. Segmental colitis: cow's milk allergy. Note area of intense spasm (*arrows*) above the rectum (*R*). This patient presented with bleeding per rectum. The sigmoidoscope could not be passed through the area of spasm. (From Swischuk LE. *Imaging of the newborn, infant and young child*, 4th ed. Philadelphia: Lippincott Williams & Wilkins, 1997:482, with permission.)

teristically have leukocytes seen on fecal smear, although eosinophils may not be present in the stool.

Treatment consists of elimination of the offending protein from the infant's diet. The diagnosis is typically confirmed by the rapid resolution of symptoms within 72 hours of the dietary change. Infants receiving cow's milk–based or soy protein formulas should be changed to a formula containing casein hydrolysate as the protein source.

Infectious Enterocolitis

Infectious causes of GI bleeding are predominantly a result of bacterial pathogens, including *Campylobacter*, pathogenic *Escherichia coli*, *Salmonella*, and *Shigella*. Less commonly, infection with *Giardia* or rotavirus is associated with heme-positive stools.

Pseudomembranous colitis is a form of inflammatory colitis characterized by the pathologic presence of pseudomembranes consisting of mucin, fibrin, necrotic cells, and polymorphonuclear leukocytes. The entity develops as a result of colonic colonization and toxin production by the gram-positive obligate anaerobe *Clostridium difficile*, in most cases after normal bowel microflora have been altered by antibiotic therapy. All classes of antibiotics have been associated with pseudomembranous colitis. Patients usually present with profuse diarrhea, tenesmus, and crampy abdominal pain, usually beginning during the first week of antibiotic therapy.

Miscellaneous Causes of Lower Gastrointestinal Bleeding

Henoch-Schönlein purpura (HSP) is a systemic vasculitis that may cause edema and hemorrhage in the intestinal wall.

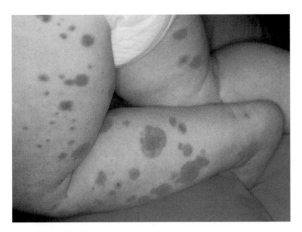

FIG. 8.17. Henoch–Schönlein purpura rash.

Peak age at onset is between 3 and 7 years and the male/female ratio is 2:1. The presentation consists of the onset of a purpuric rash, typically confined to the buttocks and lower extremities, followed by arthralgias, angioedema, and diffuse abdominal pain (Fig. 8.17). GI symptoms may precede the usual cutaneous symptoms and include abdominal pain (60% to 70%), occult bleeding (50%), gross bleeding (30%), massive hemorrhage (5% to 10%), and intussusception (3%). In a recent series, thickening of the duodenal wall was noted by ultrasonography in 82% of children who had HSP, with multiple hemorrhagic duodenal erosions noted by endoscopy in two patients. All children with suspected HSP and GI symptoms should have a stool guaiac test performed as well as a urinalysis to monitor for the onset of renal involvement (nephritis). Children with HSP limited to involvement of the skin and joints can often be managed as outpatients. However, severe abdominal pain or GI hemorrhage are indications for admission.

Hemolytic uremic syndrome is a disorder characterized by the triad of acute microangiopathic hemolytic anemia, thrombocytopenia, and oliguric renal failure. The disease is heralded by a prodrome of intestinal symptoms ranging from diarrhea (in 100% of patients) to hemorrhagic colitis (80%). Fever (20% to 30%), vomiting (75% to 80%), and abdominal pain (60%) are also commonly seen. Acute infectious gastroenteritis or colitis secondary to infection with *E. coli* O157:H7 is now considered the most important initial causative event in both sporadic and epidemic cases of hemolytic uremic syndrome.

All children with hemolytic uremic syndrome require admission to the hospital. Laboratory studies should be obtained, including a CBC, platelet count, prothrombin time (PT), partial thromboplastin time, electrolytes, blood urea nitrogen, and creatinine. Intravenous access needs to be secured immediately for the correction of dehydration and the administration of blood products. As with HSP, the GI manifestations of hemolytic uremic syndrome resolve, usually without sequelae or the need for antibiotic treatment of the initial intestinal infection.

GI vascular malformations, including hemangiomas, angiodysplasia, and arteriovenous malformations, are rare causes of GI bleeding in children and are often seen as part of congenital syndromes. GI hemangiomas may be part of the Klippel–Trenaunay–Weber syndrome (Fig. 8.18), which consists of a capillary or large vessel hemangioma on an extremity with hypertrophy of that limb. Diffuse visceral hemangiomatosis is rare, often fatal, and always associated with cutaneous vascular lesions. GI hemangiomatosis should be suspected in any child with unexplained anemia and a syndrome of cutaneous hemangiomata.

Intestinal arteriovenous malformations are rare in the pediatric age group, may occur both as solitary and multiple arteriovenous malformations, and are typically part of a congenital syndrome (e.g., Osler–Weber–Rendu disease). Many GI vascular malformations, particularly cavernous hemangiomas and arteriovenous malformations, can be detected using computed tomography scans with intravenous contrast. Intestinal angiography or tagged red blood cell scans

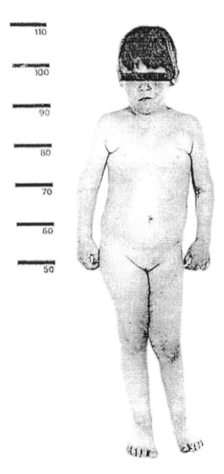

FIG. 8.18. A patient with Klippel–Trenaunay syndrome shows hemangiomas of the skin and hemihypertrophy of the right limb. (From Schmitt B, Posselt HG, Waag KL, et al. Severe hemorrhage from intestinal hemangiomatosis in Klippel-Trenaunay syndrome: pitfalls in diagnosis and management. *J Pediatr Gastroenterol Nutr* 1986;5:156, with permission.)

are often used to identify the source of bleeding during an acute hemorrhage. ED management of patients with GI bleeding from vascular malformations is the same as for any patient with potentially significant blood loss. After initial stabilization, referral to an appropriate subspecialist for diagnosis and definitive treatment is warranted.

Inflammatory Bowel Disease

Clinical Manifestations

Clinical manifestations of IBD can be varied and related to either GI inflammation or the development of either GI tract or extraintestinal complications. Severe abdominal pain is among the most common complaints prompting an ED visit by the patient with IBD. Abdominal pain and diarrhea with or without occult blood are the most common symptoms at presentation. The pain is often colicky and in Crohn disease may localize to the right lower quadrant or periumbilical area, prompting a consideration of acute appendicitis in the differential diagnosis. The abdominal examination may elicit guarding and rebound tenderness. Frank rectal bleeding occurs in fewer than 25% of all cases but is more common in ulcerative colitis. Perianal disease, including fissures, skin tags, fistulae, and abscesses, occurs in 15% of children with Crohn disease. Perianal disease may precede the appearance of the intestinal manifestations of Crohn disease by several years (Fig. 8.19).

A low-grade fever and mild leukocytosis commonly occur. Approximately 10% of children with ulcerative colitis (Fig. 8.20) and a lower percentage of those with Crohn disease present with a fulminant onset of fever, abdominal cramps, and severe diarrhea with blood, mucus, and pus in the stools. A fulminant episode may also occur in the patient

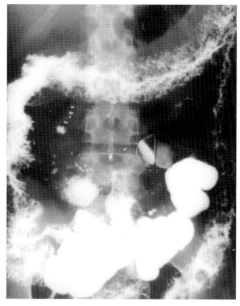

FIG. 8.20. Colitis: ultrasonographic findings. Barium enema in the same patient. Severe ulcerative colitis: the mucosa appears granular, nodular, and edematous and is actively bleeding. (From Swischuk LE. *Emergency Imaging of the Acutely Ill or Injured Child*, 4th ed. Philadelphia: Lippincott Williams & Wilkins, 2000:215, with permission.)

who has a known disease. There may be associated anemia and dehydration. IBD occasionally causes massive lower GI bleeding. Rarely, Crohn disease causes complete intestinal obstruction (Fig. 8.21). The patient always gives a history of antecedent abdominal pain, diarrhea, and weight loss. The presence of abdominal distention, accompanied by diminished or absent bowel sounds, should raise the suspicion of

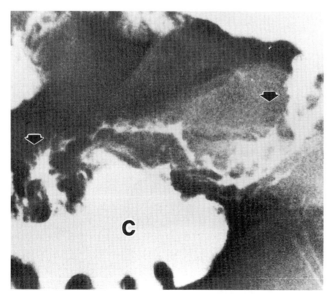

FIG. 8.19. Crohn disease of the terminal ileum demonstrated by severe narrowing of the terminal ileum (*area between the two arrows*). *C*, cecum.

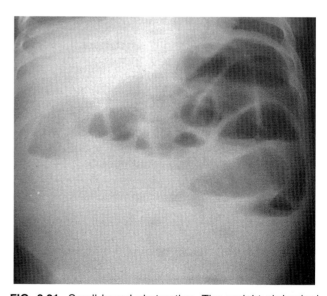

FIG. 8.21. Small bowel obstruction. The upright abdominal radiograph shows numerous dilated loops in the small bowel with differential fluid levels in one loop indicating mechanical bowel obstruction.

actual or impending perforation, even in the absence of severe pain. Perforation may occur after even minor abdominal trauma and must be ruled out when patients with known IBD complain of abdominal pain after trauma (Fig. 8.22).

Toxic megacolon usually involves the transverse colon (Fig. 8.23). The pathophysiology is believed to be an extension of the inflammatory process through all layers of the bowel wall with resulting microperforation, localized ileus, and loss of colonic tone. The result is imminent major perforation, peritonitis, and overwhelming sepsis. Antecedent

barium enema, opiates, or anticholinergics may all precipitate toxic megacolon. The differential diagnosis of acute fulminant colitis includes acute bacterial enteritis, amebic dysentery, ischemic bowel disease, and radiation colitis.

Management

The initial ED management of IBD is determined primarily by whether the patient is known to have been previously diagnosed with ulcerative colitis or Crohn disease and by an

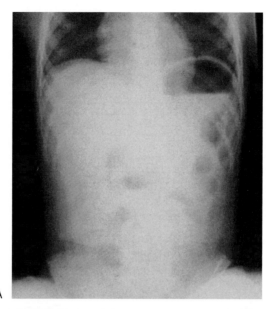

A

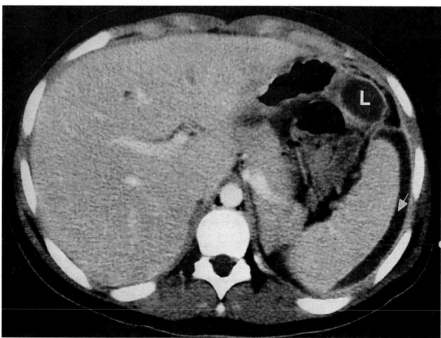

B

FIG. 8.22. Perforation. **A:** Perforated viscus. **B, C:** Perforated appendicitis. Appendiceal perforation with peritoneal spread producing lesser sac (*L*), perisplenic (*arrow*), interloop (*open arrows*), and pelvic (not shown) abscesses, seen on computed tomography as areas of fluid density with enhancing margins. (From Balistreri WF, Vonderhoof JA. *Pediatric gastroenterology and nutrition.* Philadelphia: JB Lippincott, 1990:252, with permission.) *(Continued on next page.)*

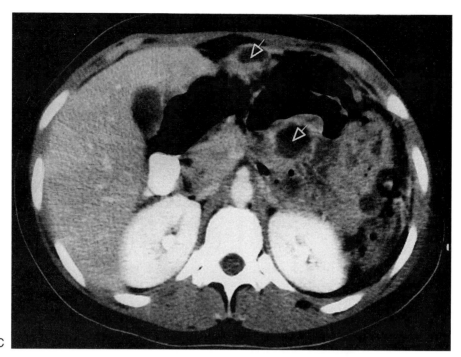

C

FIG. 8.22. *Continued.*

assessment of the severity of GI symptoms and systemic toxicity. Several clinical classification systems are used, but in general, mild disease is associated with fewer than six stools per day and an absence of systemic signs such as fever and severe anemia. Moderate disease is characterized by more than six stools per day, fever [higher than 38°C (100.4°F)], hypoalbuminemia (serum protein less than 3.2 g/dL), and anemia (hemoglobin concentration less than 10 g/dL). Severe

disease is indicated by more than eight stools per day, marked abdominal cramping and tenderness, high fever, significant anemia (hemoglobin concentration less than 8 g/dL), leukocytosis (white blood cell count greater than 15,000/mm^3), and, occasionally, toxic megacolon.

The goal of initial management of patients with moderately severe disease is supportive, and intravenous hydration with crystalloid solutions is often necessary to correct acute

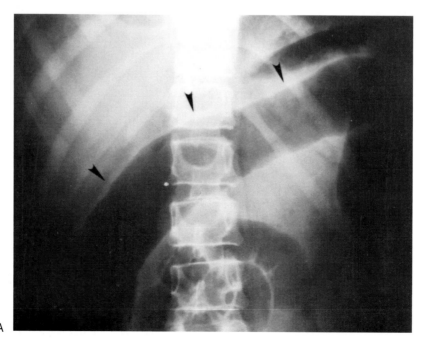

A

FIG. 8.23. Toxic megacolon. **A:** Note dilated but smooth transverse colon with no haustral markings (*arrows*).

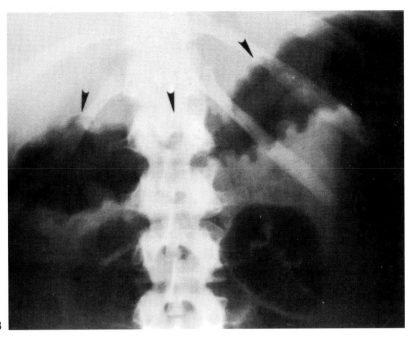

FIG. 8.23. *Continued.* **B:** Another patient with a dilated colon, but in this case note the nodular projections into the lumen of the dilated colon (*arrows*). The findings represent thickening, edema, and pseudopolyp formation of the colon. (From Swischuk LE. *Emergency imaging of the acutely ill or injured child*, 4th ed. Philadelphia: Lippincott Williams & Wilkins, 2000:216, with permission.)

dehydration. Normal saline may be given as a 20 mL/kg bolus infusion and repeated as necessary to achieve hemodynamic stability. An infusion of a dextrose-containing electrolyte solution may then be initiated based on the initial serum electrolytes. When severe abdominal pain occurs in a patient who is not known to have IBD, surgical consultation is indicated if diagnoses such as acute appendicitis or bowel obstruction are possibilities. Hospitalization of patients with moderately severe disease is often indicated to initiate or modify specific therapy such as systemic corticosteroids or immunosuppressive agents such as azathioprine or 6-mercaptopurine. In addition, improved nutritional intake, either via enteral or parenteral means, is often necessary.

Peptic Ulcer Disease

Symptoms of peptic ulcer disease vary with the patient's age. Nonspecific signs and symptoms predominate among infants and preschool-age children, with boys and girls affected equally. The older the child, the more specific (and similar to adult patterns of presentation) the signs and symptoms become (Fig. 8.24). Among teenagers with peptic ulcer disease, a male predominance is seen, with boys outnumbering girls nearly 4:1. Infants with peptic ulcer disease (usually secondary to some other condition) may present with either nonspecific feeding difficulties and vomiting or more fulminantly with upper GI bleeding or perforation. Preschool-age children often complain of poorly localized abdominal pain, vomiting, or GI hemorrhage and either manifest as hematemesis or melena. Older children and adolescents present

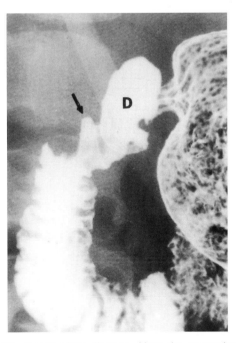

FIG. 8.24. Peptic ulcer disease. Note the postapical ulcer crate (*arrow*). There are edematous folds radiating from its base and marked spasm of the postapical portion of the duodenum. *D*, duodenal bulb. (From Swischuk LE. *Emergency imaging of the acutely ill or injured child*, 4th ed. Philadelphia: Lippincott Williams & Wilkins, 2000:218, with permission.)

almost invariably with abdominal pain, which is described as waxing and waning, sharp or gnawing, and localized to the epigastrium. It may awaken the child at night or in the early hours of the morning. The presence of nocturnal pain may assist in distinguishing recurrent abdominal pain as a result of peptic ulcer disease from functional abdominal pain, which rarely occurs at night. A careful history of the pain and a family history of peptic ulcer disease will often suggest the diagnosis of peptic ulcer disease in the older child. History should also be obtained regarding the presence of predisposing factors such as smoking or regular use of nonsteroidal antiinflammatory drugs.

Gastritis, distal esophagitis, giardiasis, and pancreatitis may all cause epigastric pain and tenderness. Biliary tract disease and an ureteropelvic junction obstruction may cause right upper quadrant tenderness. Children who have IBD, HSP, or diabetes mellitus may also present with abdominal pain, tenderness, or GI bleeding.

Flexible fiberoptic esophagogastroduodenoscopy with mucosal biopsy is the most accurate method of diagnosing peptic ulcer disease in children. In most tertiary care referral centers, this procedure can be performed safely even on infants. It is typically not performed in the presence of active hemorrhage, although some centers are gathering experience with the use of therapeutic endoscopy to control significant bleeding. When performed, biopsy specimens should routinely be obtained from any area of endoscopic abnormality and from the distal esophagus, antrum, and second part of the duodenum. No clear guidelines exist to indicate which pediatric patients should undergo endoscopy for evaluation of peptic ulcer disease. Suggested guidelines include any child with chronic abdominal pain (longer than 3 months) associated with any of the following signs and symptoms: (1) hematemesis, (2) a history of peptic ulcer disease in a first-degree relative, (3) nocturnal pain, (4) pain occurring within 1 hour of eating or relieved by eating, (5) recurrent vomiting, (6) weight loss, or (7) abdominal tenderness localized to the epigastrium (particularly in older children). In addition, endoscopy should be strongly considered in any patient presenting acutely with significant upper GI bleeding.

All patients for whom an obvious cause of secondary gastric or duodenal ulceration (e.g., stress, sepsis, burns) does not exist should undergo diagnostic evaluation for the presence of *Helicobacter pylori* infection. *H. pylori* infection can be confirmed in a variety of ways in patients with primary peptic ulcer disease. Histologic examination of biopsy specimens obtained during endoscopy should routinely be performed because *H. pylori* is readily seen using a variety of staining techniques. Various commercially available assays take advantage of the urease activity of the organism for diagnostic purposes. A biopsy specimen is mixed with the assay, which typically contains urea and an indicator dye that changes color when the urea is converted to ammonia by the organism. The urease activity can also be detected through the use of breath tests in which radiolabeled (^{13}C or ^{14}C) urea is ingested by the patient. Degradation of the urea by *H. py-*

lori results in the release of the radiolabeled carbon, which can be detected in the expired air. Finally, enzyme-linked immunosorbent assays are available for the detection of immunoglobulin G antibodies to *H. pylori* in serum.

Management

The focus of ED management of patients with suspected peptic ulcer disease is on the detection and stabilization of life-threatening complications such as perforation and major GI hemorrhage and on ruling out other potential serious or life-threatening conditions that may require urgent intervention. Depending on the suspected amount of blood loss, all patients with GI bleeding should have a CBC and blood type and screen obtained. If vomiting has been prominent, electrolytes, blood urea nitrogen, creatinine, serum amylase, and lipase levels should be obtained.

Several approaches are available for treatment of peptic ulcer disease in children. Therapies can be categorized as those that neutralize acid and block acid secretion, are cytoprotective, or are antiinfective.

Acute Biliary Tract Disease

The pain of biliary colic is acute in onset, often follows a meal, and is usually localized to the epigastrium or right upper quadrant. Some children may localize the pain to the periumbilical area. Characteristically, the pain increases to a plateau of intensity over 5 to 20 minutes, typically after meals, and persists for a variable duration, usually less than 4 hours (although less than 1 hour in 50% of patients). In contrast to the colicky pain of intestinal or ureteral origin, biliary colic does not worsen in relatively short cyclic paroxysms or bursts but instead is characterized by its sustained, intense quality. Unlike pancreatitis, the patient tends to move about restlessly and the pain is not improved by changes in position. In addition, referred pain is common, particularly to the dorsal lumbar back near the tip of the right scapula. Nausea and vomiting are commonly associated with biliary colic but are not severe and protracted as seen with pancreatitis. Mild jaundice occurs in 25% of patients, but the serum bilirubin rarely exceeds 4 mg/dL. An attack of acute cholecystitis begins with biliary colic (Fig. 8.25), which increases progressively in severity or duration. Pain lasting longer than 4 hours suggests cholecystitis. As the inflammation worsens, the pain changes character, becoming more generalized in the upper abdomen and increased by deep respiration and jarring motions. The temperature is usually mildly elevated, ranging from 37.5° to 38.5°C (99.5° to 101.3°F).

In contrast, acute cholangitis should be suspected in the patient who has right upper quadrant abdominal pain, shaking chills, and spiking fever [temperature higher than 39°C (102.2°F)] with jaundice (Charcot triad). These patients usually have a history of abdominal surgery. The danger of this disorder is that overwhelming sepsis can develop rapidly. Listlessness and shock are characteristic of advanced or

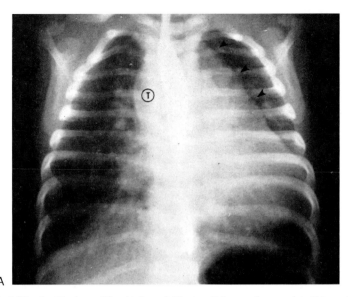
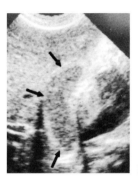

FIG. 8.25. A: Cholecystitis. Note calcified gallstones (*arrows*) in this patient with sickle cell disease. **B:** Acute cholecystitis. Another patient with acalculous cholecystitis demonstrates a distended gallbladder full of sludge (*arrows*). (From Swischuk LE. *Emergency imaging of the acutely ill or injured child*, 4th ed. Philadelphia: Lippincott Williams & Wilkins, 2000:207, with permission.)

severe cholangitis and usually reflect gram-negative septicemia. Cholangitis can evolve rapidly before development of significant jaundice. Clinically apparent jaundice may be absent even in postsurgical biliary atresia patients. Hydrops of the gallbladder is associated with a palpable right upper quadrant mass and pain (Fig. 8.26). Fever and jaundice generally do not occur.

In addition to scleral icterus, nonspecific physical findings that suggest gallbladder disease include right upper quadrant guarding, Murphy sign (production of pain by deep inspiration or cough when the physician's fingers are depressing the abdomen below the right costal margin in the midclavicular line and abrupt cessation of inspiration because of pain), and production of pain or tenderness by a light blow applied with the ulnar surface of the hand to the subcostal area. In approximately one-third of patients with cholecystitis, the gallbladder is palpable as a sausage-shaped mass lateral to the midclavicular line. A rigid abdomen or rebound tenderness suggests local perforation or gangrene of the gallbladder.

Laboratory tests are typically nonspecific. A CBC and blood smear may show evidence of hemolysis. The white blood cell count averages 12,000 to 15,000/mm^3 with a

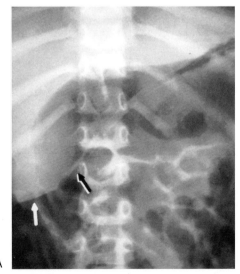
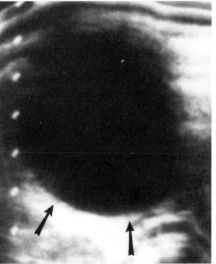

FIG. 8.26. Acute hydrops of the gallbladder. **A:** Note the large, distended gallbladder (*arrows*). **B:** Ultrasonographic study demonstrates a hydropic gallbladder in another patient (*arrows*). (From Swischuk LE. *Emergency imaging of the acutely ill or injured child*, 4th ed. Philadelphia: Lippincott Williams & Wilkins, 2000:206, with permission.)

neutrophilic leukocytosis. White blood cell counts greater than 15,000/mm^3 suggest cholangitis. The serum bilirubin may be elevated but rarely exceeds 4 mg/dL. Higher values are more compatible with either complete common duct obstruction or cholangitis. Serum transaminases, alanine aminotransferase and aspartate aminotransferase, and alkaline phosphatase may be mildly elevated but are often normal. Marked elevation of transaminases may occur with acute, complete common duct obstruction. Serum amylase may be mildly elevated without other evidence of pancreatitis. Abdominal flat and upright radiographs may show right upper quadrant calcification of gallstones, particularly in patients with hemolytic anemia (pigment stones), or a right upper quadrant mass. Abdominal radiographs are particularly important to rule out perforation. The erythrocyte sedimentation rate is often elevated in children with cholangitis, and organisms may be recovered by blood culture.

Abdominal ultrasonography is the most commonly used test to confirm gallbladder disease. This test is noninvasive and easily performed and provides information on the surrounding organs such as the liver, pancreas, and kidneys. Ultrasonography can determine the presence of most gallstones, dilated bile ducts, a thickened gallbladder wall or hydropic gallbladder, sludge, and hepatic abscesses. Other radiographic tests, such as cholecystograph or radionuclide testing, are not typically used in the emergency setting.

Management

All patients with suspected acute biliary tract disease and acute symptoms should be admitted to the hospital. The exception is patients with biliary colic that has resolved spontaneously, in which case an urgent outpatient evaluation by ultrasonography can be pursued. Conditions associated with acalculous cholecystitis should be evaluated and treated if identified. General ED management includes discontinuation of oral intake, support with intravenous fluids, and surgical consultation. Cholecystitis and cholangitis associated with gallstones are general indications for surgery. The patient should receive nothing by mouth and given intravenous fluids, pain medication, and antibiotics if cholangitis is considered. Antibiotic coverage should include gram-negative organisms and enterococci.

Acute Pancreatitis

Epigastric abdominal pain is the most consistent symptom of pancreatitis and may vary from tolerable distress to severe incapacitating pain. Symptoms may be chronic and insidious, but they typically progress rapidly, building to a crescendo over several hours. The pain is usually localized to the epigastrium and may radiate to the back (left or right scapula) or the right or left upper quadrants. The pain is usually described as knifelike and boring in quality and is aggravated when the patient lies supine. Classically, the pain of pancreatitis is constant, as opposed to colicky pain, which

waxes and wanes. Nausea and vomiting are the most common associated symptoms. Vomiting may be severe and protracted. Low-grade fever [below 38.5°C (101.3°F)] is present in 50% to 60% of cases. In cases of severe necrotic pancreatitis, patients may complain of dizziness. Mental aberrations are common in necrotic pancreatitis; patients may act overtly psychotic or present in coma.

Early in the course of the disease, there may be a discrepancy between the severity of the patient's subjective pain and the objective physical findings. During the examination, patients are usually quiet and prefer to sit or lie on their side with knees flexed. The abdomen may be distended but is usually not rigid. There may be mild to moderate voluntary guarding in the epigastrium. A palpable epigastric mass suggests pseudocyst. Ascites is rare. Bowel sounds may be decreased or absent. Associated physical findings may include signs of parotitis, mild hepatosplenomegaly, epigastric mass, pleural effusions (Fig. 8.27), and mild icterus. Although rare, rebound tenderness or a rigid abdomen are poor prognostic signs if present. A bluish discoloration around the umbilicus (Cullen sign) or flanks (Grey Turner sign) is also a poor prognostic indicator and evidence of hemorrhagic pancreatitis. Signs of overt hemodynamic instability are rarely evident at initial presentation. It is particularly important to evaluate patients for clinical signs of hypocalcemia (Trousseau and Chvostek signs).

The clinical diagnosis is often tentative because the same constellation of symptoms (abdominal pain, vomiting, and low-grade fever) and signs (abdominal tenderness and guarding) may be mimicked by several other conditions, including penetrating peptic ulcer, gastritis, esophagitis, biliary colic, acute cholecystitis, intestinal obstruction, and appendicitis.

Radiographically, abdominal ultrasonography (Fig. 8.28) provides a noninvasive, direct view of the pancreas and is probably the most useful test in diagnosing pancreatitis. Ultrasonography can assess pancreatic size, contour, and the presence of calcifications and pseudocyst formation. Ultrasonography should be considered in all cases of suspected pancreatitis. Abdominal computed tomography and endoscopic retrograde cholangiopancreatography are being used more often to assess the severity of pancreatitis and pseudocyst formation and to determine possible causes of pancreatitis. However, endoscopic retrograde cholangiopancreatography should not be performed in the acute phase or in patients with acute pseudocyst formation or pancreatic abscess formation but should be reserved for patients with chronic, recurrent pancreatitis. Rarely, endoscopic retrograde cholangiopancreatography may be indicated in acute pancreatitis if an obstructing gallstone is present in the common bile duct.

Management

All patients with evidence of pancreatitis or suspected pancreatitis should be admitted to the hospital. Treatment,

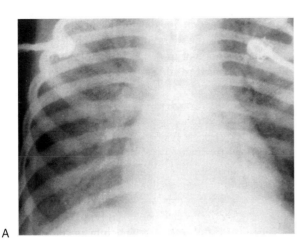
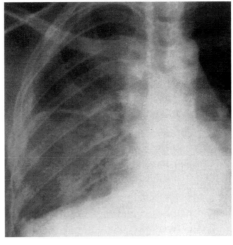

A   B

FIG. 8.27. Pancreatitis with chest findings. **A:** Note the bilateral interstitial pulmonary edema causing haziness of the lungs in this patient with acute pancreatitis. **B:** Another patient with a semiopacified right hemithorax caused by a pleural effusion secondary to pancreatitis. Pulmonary edema of the right lung also probably is present. (From Swischuk LE. *Emergency imaging of the acutely ill or injured child*, 4th ed. Philadelphia: Lippincott Williams & Wilkins, 2000:205, with permission.)

however, should begin in the ED. The goals of medical treatment include suppression of pancreatic secretion and relief of pain. Morbidity and mortality in pancreatitis are directly related to complications that may already be present at the time of initial presentation. Therefore, aggressive early maintenance of intravascular volume and treatment of hypocalcemia, respiratory distress, and suspected infection are mandatory.

Fulminant Liver Failure

Many patients do not exhibit serious clinical features of acute liver failure. Typically, pediatric patients who develop acute liver failure were previously healthy and had no prior medical problems. Patients may initially complain of fatigue, nausea, vomiting, and diffuse abdominal pain. Occasionally, right upper quadrant pain may be severe. Commonly, a history of a prodromal viral illness can be elicited. The presence of jaundice usually initiates the first visit to the physician. As liver failure progresses, patients become more jaundiced and lethargic and begin to develop tremors. In a short time, they become confused or somnolent and may begin to have problems with easy bruising or bleeding.

The onset of encephalopathy occurs in conjunction with the severity and progression of liver failure. Encephalopathy is graded on a scale from I to IV. Grade I is manifested by a coherent individual who shows mild or episodic drowsiness, poor concentration, and impaired intellect. In grade II, the patient continues to be coherent and conversant but becomes disoriented and fatigued. Agitation and aggressive behavior

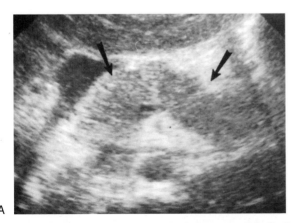
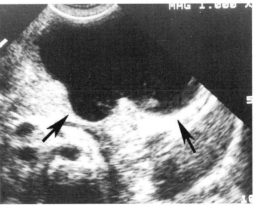

A   B

FIG. 8.28. Acute pancreatitis: ultrasonographic findings. **A:** Note the enlarged and slightly hypoechoic pancreas (*arrows*). **B:** Pseudocyst: ultrasonographic findings. Note the anechoic, lobulated pancreatic pseudocyst (*arrows*). (From Swischuk LE. *Emergency radiology of the acutely ill or injured child*, 4th ed. Philadelphia: Lippincott Williams & Wilkins, 2000:203–204, with permission.)

in conjunction with extreme drowsiness are manifested in grade III encephalopathy. Unresponsive patients who respond only to painful stimuli and who have evidence of cerebral edema are labeled as having grade IV encephalopathy. The clinical features of increased intracranial pressure include systemic hypertension, decerebrate posturing, hyperventilation, abnormal pupillary responses, and impairment of brainstem reflexes. Cerebral edema is associated with increased mortality and requires aggressive supportive management. Finally, bleeding esophageal and gastric varices as well as ascites may rapidly develop secondary to increased portal hypertension.

Because it may be difficult to diagnose patients clinically, biochemical evidence may be collected that provides evidence of liver failure. The liver plays an important role in hemostasis because the liver synthesizes a number of coagulation factors. An uncorrectable coagulopathy is usually the first laboratory manifestation of liver failure. Other factors may have a shorter half-life, but the PT is the most commonly used marker of the severity of liver disease. A prolonged PT despite intravenous supplementation of vitamin K should alert the physician to impending liver failure. Other laboratory markers suggestive of liver failure include evidence of increasing cholestasis manifested by an increasing serum bilirubin, hypoalbuminemia, and hypoglycemia.

It is also important to monitor serum transaminases. Decreasing transaminase levels usually indicate resolving liver disease, whereas a decrease in transaminases in association with increasing jaundice and coagulopathy indicates hepatocyte death rather than hepatocyte repair. Monitoring for hypoglycemia is extremely important because the liver is the primary organ for gluconeogenesis. Serum fibrinogen is usually decreased in patients with liver failure. In cases in which the patient has splenomegaly, thrombocytopenia and leukocytopenia may be present (Fig. 8.29).

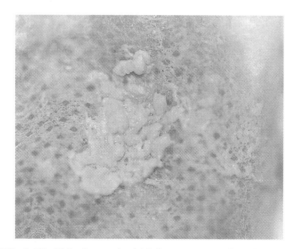

FIG. 8.29. This 3-month-old infant presented to the emergency department with jaundice and lethargy. Laboratory studies revealed the following: total bilirubin, 8.9 mg/dL; directed bilirubin, 6.9 mg/dL; aspartate aminotransferase, 199 IU/L; alanine aminotransferase, 160 IU/L. In the emergency department, he passed an acholic stool.

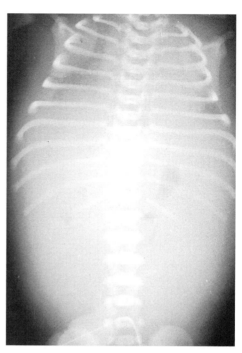

FIG. 8.30. Ascites. Massive ascites in a young infant produce marked distention and opacity of the abdomen, obliteration of the inferior liver edge, and obliteration of all retroperitoneal structures. In the right upper quadrant, a slight difference in density between the medially displaced liver and the adjacent ascitic fluid can be seen. (From Swischuk LE. *Emergency imaging of the acutely ill or injured child*, 4th ed. Philadelphia: Lippincott Williams & Wilkins, 2000:166, with permission.)

Hypoglycemia almost always accompanies acute liver failure and may complicate the signs of encephalopathy. Portal hypertension may cause bleeding from esophageal varices or ascites (Fig. 8.30). Hepatorenal syndrome occurs in approximately 75% of patients who reach grade IV encephalopathy. The cause of hepatorenal syndrome is unclear; however, the result is oliguria in the presence of near normal intravascular pressures. Metabolic acidosis occurs in approximately 30% of patients who have liver failure, and the risk of sepsis is increased secondary to the patient's compromised immune function.

Management

All patients suspected of having liver failure should undergo a complete physical examination, including a thorough neurologic evaluation. Laboratory testing should include serum glucose, transaminases, total and direct bilirubin, albumin, PT, γ-glutamyl transpeptidase, CBC with differential, electrolytes, blood culture, and fibrinogen. Patients with hypoglycemia should be given intravenous fluids with 10% dextrose and should undergo frequent blood glucose monitoring (every 1 hour) until their blood sugar stabilizes. Metabolic acidosis should be corrected; however, correction of hyponatremia should be gradual in patients with ascites.

Patients who have a coagulopathy should be given intravenous vitamin K. A repeat PT should be performed 6 to 8 hours after administration.

Acute Viral Hepatitis

Most childhood cases of acute hepatitis produce minimal symptoms, are anicteric, and, unless suspected by palpation of tender hepatomegaly, are usually confused with a GI flu-like illness. Clinical hepatitis classically consists of a 5- to 7-day prodrome of variable constitutional symptoms (low-grade fever, anorexia, nausea, vomiting, malaise, fatigue, and epigastric or right upper quadrant abdominal pain), followed by acute onset of scleral icterus, jaundice, and passage of dark urine. Pruritus and diarrhea are rare. Physical examination after the onset of jaundice may reveal tender hepatomegaly. Mild splenomegaly is present in 25% to 50% of patients. Patients with hepatitis B virus (HBV) may also present with extrahepatic signs and symptoms, such as arthralgia, arthritis, or papular acrodermatitis (on face, buttocks, and extensor surfaces of arms and legs). When the rash is associated with lymphadenopathy and fever, it is called Gianotti–Crosti syndrome. Onset of the icteric phase of acute hepatitis most commonly is temporarily associated with improvement in the constitutional symptoms. In as many as 15% of cases, severe fatigue, anorexia, nausea, and vomiting persist. The icteric period usually lasts 1 to 4 weeks. Occasionally, the jaundice is prolonged for 4 to 6 weeks with increasing pruritus at 2 to 3 weeks.

Several infectious agents may mimic a viral hepatitis–like illness. The most common are Epstein–Barr virus (infectious mononucleosis) and cytomegalovirus. Both agents rarely produce clinical jaundice, and a high fever and diffuse adenopathy are more characteristic. Less common agents include herpes, adenovirus, coxsackievirus, reovirus, echovirus, rubella, arbovirus, leptospirosis, toxoplasmosis, and tuberculosis.

Management

No specific treatment is available for acute viral hepatitis. Most patients can be managed at home. No restrictions in diet or ambulation are necessary. The traditional recommendations of a low-fat, high-carbohydrate diet and bed rest are now recognized to have no effect on the symptoms or duration of the disease. Parents should be told that anorexia and fatigue are common symptoms. Small, frequent feedings may be helpful. Drugs should be strictly avoided. The key for both the patient and other household contacts is personal hygiene. Infants and children should avoid contact with the patient even after they have received immunoprophylaxis. In hepatitis A virus (HAV), shedding of the virus may occur for as long as 2 weeks after the onset of jaundice. Patients should be kept at home during this time. After this, they may return to school. Indications for hospitalization of a patient who has acute hepatitis include the following: (1) dehydration secondary to anorexia and vomiting, (2) bilirubin level greater than 20 mg/dL, (3) abnormal PT, (4) white blood cell count greater than 25,000/mm^3, and (5) level of transaminases greater than 3,000 U/L.

Postexposure Prophylaxis

Hepatitis A Virus

The mean incubation period for HAV infection is approximately 4 weeks (range, 15 to 45 days). Conventional immune serum globulin (0.02 mL/kg intramuscularly) confers passive protection against clinical HAV infection if given during the incubation period up until 6 days before the onset of symptoms. Individuals exposed during the late incubation period or early acute phase of illness should also be promptly immunized. Seventy-five percent of this group will develop detectable levels of anti-HAV immunoglobulin M, suggesting passive-active immunity. Postexposure immunoprophylaxis is suggested for (1) household and close personal contacts, (2) institutionalized contacts, and (3) contacts within a day care facility. Grade-school classroom contacts of an isolated case and routine play contacts do not require immune serum globulin. However, a second case within a class is indication for immunoprophylaxis for the rest of the class. An alternative method for determining who should receive immune serum globulin is to test high-risk contacts for anti-HAV immunoglobulin G.

Hepatitis B Virus

Prophylactic treatment to prevent infection after exposure to HBV should be considered in the following situations seen in the ED: (1) sexual exposure to the HBV surface antigen–positive patient, (2) inadvertent percutaneous or permucosal exposure to HBV surface antigen–positive blood, and (3) household exposure of an infant younger than 12 months of age to a primary caregiver who has acute HBV. Before treatment in the first two situations, testing for susceptibility is recommended if it does not delay treatment beyond 14 days after exposure. Testing for anti-HBV core antibody is the most efficient prescreening procedure. All susceptible persons should receive a single dose of HBV immunoglobulin (0.06 mL/kg) intramuscularly and HBV vaccine in recommended doses.

SUGGESTED READINGS

Aideyan UO, Smith WL. Inflammatory bowel disease in children. *Radiol Clin North Am* 1996;34:885–902.

Bharucha AE, Gostout CJ, Balm RK. Clinical and endoscopic risk factors in the Mallory-Weiss syndrome. *Am J Gastroenterol* 1997;92:805–808.

Bode G, Rothenbacher D, Brenner H, et al. *Helicobacter pylori* and abdominal symptoms: a population-based study among preschool children in southern Germany. *Pediatrics* 1998;101:634–637.

Bourke B, Jones N, Sherman P. *Helicobacter pylori* infection and peptic ulcer disease in children. *Pediatr Infect Dis J* 1996;15:1–13.

Bujanover Y, Reif S, Yahav J. *Helicobacter pylori* and peptic disease in the pediatric patient. *Pediatr Clin North Am* 1996;43:213–234.

Chong SK, Lou Q, Asnicar MA, et al. *Helicobacter pylori* infection in recurrent abdominal pain in childhood: comparison of diagnostic tests and therapy. *Pediatrics* 1995;96:211–215.

Gore RM, Ghahremani GG. Radiologic investigation of acute inflammatory and infectious bowel disease. *Gastroenterol Clin North Am* 1995;24: 353–384.

Grand RJ, Ramakrishna J, Calenda KA. Inflammatory bowel disease in the pediatric patient. *Gastroenterol Clin North Am* 1995;24:613–632.

Harris JM, DiPalma JA. Clinical significance of Mallory-Weiss tears. *Am J Gastroenterol* 1993;88:2056–2058.

Hirsch BZ. Breast milk-induced allergic colitis. *J Pediatr Gastroenterol Nutr* 1995;20:480.

Kato S, Ebina K, Ozawa A, et al. Antibiotic-associated hemorrhagic colitis without *Clostridium difficile* toxin in children. *J Pediatr* 1995;126: 1008–1010.

Katz PO, Salas L. Less frequent causes of upper gastrointestinal bleeding. *Gastroenterol Clin North Am* 1993;22:875–889.

Kelso JM, Sampson HA. Food protein-induced enterocolitis to casein hydrolysate formulas. *J Allergy Clin Immunol* 1993;92:909–910.

Kirsh BM, Lam N, Layden TJ, et al. Diagnosis and management of fulminant hepatic failure. *Compr Ther* 1995;21:166–171.

Latt TT, Nicholl R, Domizio P, et al. Rectal bleeding and polyps. *Arch Dis Child* 1993;69:144–147.

Levine JB, Lukawski-Trubish D. Extraintestinal considerations in inflammatory bowel disease. *Gastroenterol Clin North Am* 1995;24:633–646.

Lidofsky SD. Fulminant hepatic failure. *Crit Care Clin* 1995;11:415–430.

Macarthur C, Saunders N, Feldman W. *Helicobacter pylori*, gastroduodenal disease, and recurrent abdominal pain in children. *JAMA* 1995;273: 729–734.

Machida HM, Catto Smith AG, Hall DG, et al. Allergic colitis in infancy: clinical and pathologic aspects. *J Pediatr Gastroenterol Nutr* 1994;19:22–26.

Mahony MJ, Wyatt JI, Littlewood JM. Management and response to treatment of *Helicobacter pylori* gastritis. *Arch Dis Child* 1992;67:940–943.

Manoop SB, Rostami G, Gopalswamy N. Hepatobiliary complications of inflammatory bowel disease. *Am Fam Physician* 1995;52:1440–1444.

Mezoff AG, Balistreri WF. Peptic ulcer disease in children. *Pediatr Rev* 1995;16:257–265.

Odze RD, Wershil BK, Leichtner AM, et al. Allergic colitis in infants. *J Pediatr* 1995;126:163–170.

O'Hara SM. Acute gastrointestinal bleeding. *Radiol Clin North Am* 1997; 35:879–895.

Sherlock S, Dusheiko G. Hepatitis C virus updated. *Gut* 1991;32:965–967.

Sherman PM. Peptic ulcer disease in children: diagnosis, treatment and the implication of *Helicobacter pylori*. *Gastroenterol Clin North Am* 1994;23:707–725.

Teach SJ, Fleisher GR. Rectal bleeding in the pediatric emergency department. *Ann Emerg Med* 1994;23:1252–1258.

Thompson EC, Brown MF, Bowen EC, et al. Causes of gastrointestinal hemorrhage in neonates and children. *South Med J* 1996;89:370–374.

Vinton NE. Gastrointestinal bleeding in infancy and childhood. *Gastroenterol Clin North Am* 1994;23:93–122.

Wolf DC, Giannela RA. Antibiotic therapy for bacterial enterocolitis: a comprehensive review. *Am J Gastroenterol* 1993;88:1667–1683.

CHAPTER 9

Genitourinary Emergencies

Editor: Gary R. Fleisher

PENILE PROBLEMS

Phimosis and Paraphimosis

Phimosis exists when tightness of the distal foreskin precludes its being withdrawn to expose the glans. Although inflammation of the foreskin from severe chronic ammoniacal rash or infection may lead to scarring and a true phimosis, this is uncommon in children. More often, normal penile adhesions are confused with phimosis (Fig. 9.1A). In the uncircumcised male, if the foreskin is retracted behind the glans and left in that position, venous congestion and edema of the foreskin result, making it difficult to reduce the foreskin to a normal position. This condition of a swollen, retracted foreskin is called paraphimosis (Fig. 9.1B). The application of ice and steady local manual compression usually reduces the edema and permits manual reduction of the paraphimosis. Injecting local anesthetic to block the dorsal nerve of the penis at the base of the shaft will reduce the discomfort experienced by the child during compression of the edematous foreskin. After a portion of the edema has been reduced, pressure on the glans (like turning a sock inside out) usually permits reduction of the foreskin back to its normal position. If manual reduction fails, a surgical division of the foreskin to permit reduction is indicated. That usually may be accomplished with sedation and local anesthetic.

Balanoposthitis

Balanoposthitis is an infection of the foreskin that may extend onto the glans. It is a form of cellulitis and has its origin in a break in the penile skin, commonly associated with ammoniacal dermatitis (Fig. 9.2). It may be the result of local trauma or may, in the older boy, be associated with poor penile hygiene. Scarring after the inflammatory reaction may lead to true phimosis. The acute infection is dealt with adequately by warm soaks and the administration of an appropriate antibiotic, usually 50 to 100 mg/kg ampicillin every 24 hours in four doses.

Penile Swelling

Although most penile swelling is painful and the result of either infection, as discussed previously, or trauma, to be described later, occasionally a child has isolated penile edema that is either nontender or minimally tender. This may result from an insect bite, with local edema secondary to histamine release. A history of a bite or the finding of a small punctate lesion may give the clue to diagnosis. Painless penile edema may be present with a generalized allergic reaction or as part of the manifestation of a general edematous state secondary to renal, cardiac, or hepatic problems. Here, the diagnosis is suggested by evidence of dysfunction in these organ systems on general examination. It is also important to remember that penile swelling may be caused by a strangulation injury.

Priapism

Prolonged, painful penile erection unaccompanied by sexual stimulation is called priapism. In the pediatric age group, this entity may be caused by trauma or leukemic infiltration, but it is most often seen in African-American males with sickle cell disease. Pain results from ischemia. Although recommendations for treating priapism have ranged from ice or hot packs, estrogens, and spinal anesthesia to radiation therapy, the best treatment for priapism associated with sickle cell disease now appears to be hydration and irrigation of the corporal bodies with saline in combination with vasoactive substances.

Strangulation

The penis may be encircled by a constricting ring formed by hair, fiber, or thread, just as occurs with digits. Many times the cause of the problem is not immediately evident because local edema may hide the ring of hair. After the source of the problem has been identified, therapy requires the division of the hair and the release of the constriction. This may require a general anesthetic.

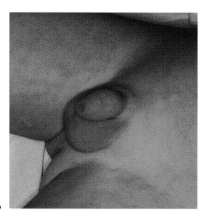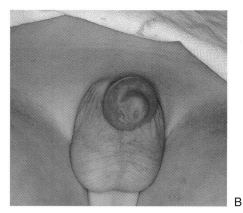

A   B

FIG. 9.1. The parents of this boy with physiologic phimosis **(A)** retracted his foreskin, causing a paraphimosis **(B)**.

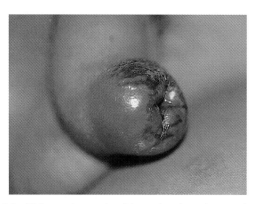

FIG. 9.2. This uncircumcised boy developed a moderately severe case of balanoposthitis.

SCROTAL PROBLEMS

Painless Swelling

Hydrocele

A hydrocele is an accumulation of fluid within the tunica vaginalis that surrounds the testis (Fig. 9.3). Hydroceles present at birth are physiologic and reabsorb. Those appearing later in childhood, particularly if they increase and decrease in size, usually accompany an inguinal hernia. Acute onset of a hydrocele suggests infection, torsion, trauma, or tumor.

Hernia

A hernia occurs when the processus vaginalis fails to obliterate before birth and is 10 times more common in males than females. Infants and children usually present with a painless inguinal bulge (Fig. 9.4), often appearing during straining or crying. If the prolapsing tissue, usually a loop of intestine, becomes entrapped, incarceration has occurred. Persistent incarceration leads to strangulation. The examiner should attempt to reduce an incarcerated inguinal hernia by

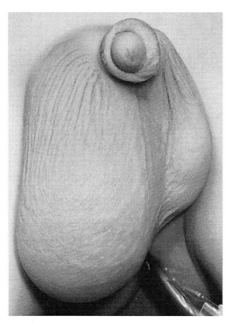

FIG. 9.3. Hydrocele. Increasing and decreasing size indicates a communicating hydrocele with a patent processus vaginalis, requiring surgical correction.

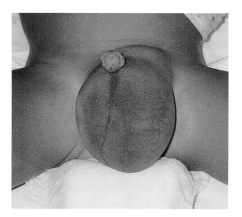

FIG. 9.4. This infant has a large left inguinal hernia, seen as a bulge in the inguinal canal and a swelling of the left hemiscrotum.

using the thumb and index finger of one hand to compress the inguinal ring area, while the other hand gently "milks" fluid and gas out of the entrapped bowel back into the abdominal cavity. All children with an inguinal hernia require surgical repair, which may need to be done emergently if reduction of an incarceration is unsuccessful.

Varicocele

Varicoceles are abnormal dilations of the cremasteric and pampiniform venous plexuses surrounding the spermatic cord (Fig. 9.5). They generally present as an asymptomatic scrotal swelling about the time of puberty and are rare in the prepubertal boy. Almost all are of congenital origin and affect the left testis. If the varicocele does not disappear when the child lies down, it suggests a varicocele secondary to obstruction of the left renal vein, and renal and bladder ultrasonography is appropriate. Varicoceles are rarely symptomatic; a heavy or tugging sensation is occasionally reported.

Painful Swelling

Torsion of the Testis and the Appendix Testis

Torsion of the testis (Fig. 9.6) typically affects prepubertal boys and causes sudden, severe scrotal pain, often with radiation to the abdomen, and associated nausea and vomiting. The scrotum is usually swollen (Fig. 9.7), and palpation reveals an enlarged, tender, high riding testis. The cremasteric

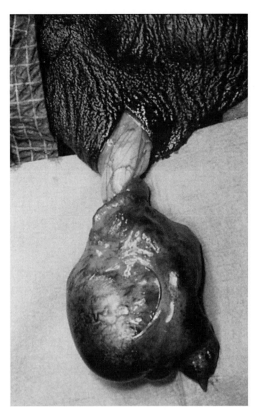

FIG. 9.6. Torsion of testis. Surgically exposed testis shows torsion of cord structures. Testis was infarcted and was removed.

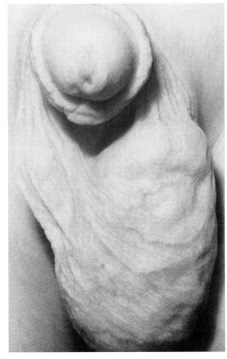

FIG. 9.5. Varicocele: abnormal dilation of cremasteric and pampiniform venous plexuses surrounding the spermatic cord, giving scrotum the appearance of a bag of worms.

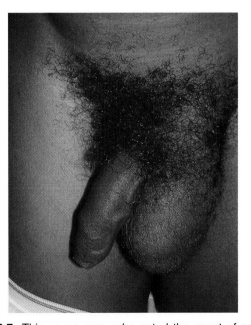

FIG. 9.7. This young man, who noted the onset of severe scrotal pain and a swollen right hemiscrotum, was diagnosed with a testicular torsion.

reflex disappears in nearly 100% of patients, but its presence does not absolutely rule out this diagnosis. In most cases, an imaging study, particularly Doppler ultrasonography, is required for confirmation and to exclude other conditions. Less commonly, radionuclide scanning may be used (Fig. 9.8). Management consists of prompt surgical reduction.

Torsion of the Appendix Testis

Torsion of the appendix testis also affects primarily prepubertal boys and causes the acute onset of scrotal gain, only occasionally with nausea and vomiting. Initially, palpation reveals a normal-sized testis with focal tenderness, but diffuse swelling and tenderness ensue over time. Rarely, a blue dot may be seen on the scrotal wall, overlying the torsed appendix. Confident differentiation from torsion of the testis, usually accomplished only with imaging, allows discharge home with analgesic agents.

Epididymitis/Orchitis

Epididymoorchitis occurs predominantly in postpubertal males and causes a gradual onset of swelling and pain. On palpation, the examiner may note swelling and tenderness confined to the epididymis, but the testis itself becomes inflamed and enlarges over time. White blood cells often appear in the urine. Imaging, either with Doppler ultrasonography or radionuclide scanning (Fig. 9.9), is required to differentiate epididymitis and/or orchitis from torsion of the testis in prepubertal patients; however, clinical findings suffice in most cases for diagnosis after puberty. Treatment of epididymitis includes analgesic agents, sitz baths, elevation of the scrotum, and antibiotics, such as 40 mg/kg trimethoprim-sulfamethoxazole per day. Isolated orchitis, such as that due to mumps in the prepubertal male, is viral in origin and requires only symptomatic therapy.

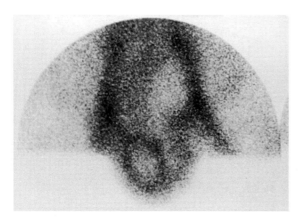

FIG. 9.8. Torsion of testis (several days old). Testicular scan (technetium-99m) shows central photopenic area surrounded by photon dense area reflecting inflammatory reaction around necrotic testis.

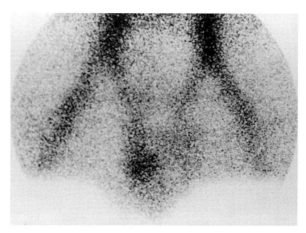

FIG. 9.9. Epididymitis. Testicular scan (technetium-99m). Diffuse photon dense area in scrotum reflects uptake of radionuclide into inflamed epididymis.

CONGENITAL VAGINAL OBSTRUCTION

Clinical Manifestations

Infancy

Although vaginal obstruction should properly be identified during the initial examination of the newborn female, infants with hydrocolpos often go unrecognized until days or weeks later when they develop the three hallmarks of this condition: (1) a lower abdominal mass, (2) difficulty with urination, and (3) a visible bulging membrane at the introitus. Inspection of the perineum should immediately indicate the proper diagnosis.

Adolescence

The girl with congenital vaginal obstruction who escapes notice during infancy will not come to attention until late in puberty when she presents with either primary amenorrhea or lower abdominal pain. She will have had satisfactory pubertal development until her menarche apparently fails to occur. Accumulating menstrual blood will then eventually produce vague lower abdominal pain that is not necessarily cyclic. As the hematocolpos grows, it will finally interfere with comfortable micturition, producing symptoms of urgency, frequency, or dysuria. The history of amenorrhea and the finding of a lower abdominal mass (Fig. 9.10) may lead the physician to suspect a tumor or even pregnancy, but the characteristic appearance of the introitus covered by a bluish bulging membrane is diagnostic of hematocolpos with imperforate hymen (Fig. 9.11). Rarely, the blood-filled vagina may rupture causing a labial hematoma (Fig. 9.12). Patients with a high transverse vaginal septum will not be as easily diagnosed because the introitus will appear normal. However, palpation of the vagina will promptly show that it is obstructed and that the cervix cannot be felt.

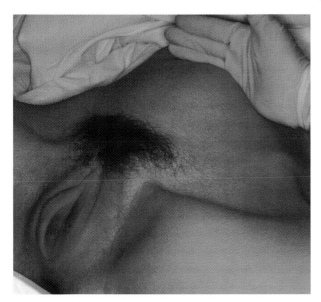

FIG. 9.10. Palpation of the abdomen in this 14-year-old girl revealed a distended uterus, rising to the level of the umbilicus.

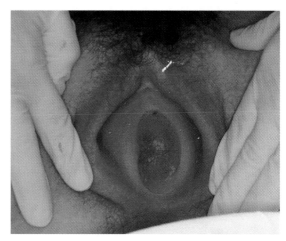

FIG. 9.11. On inspection of the same young girl as in Figure 9.10, an imperforate hymen is seen.

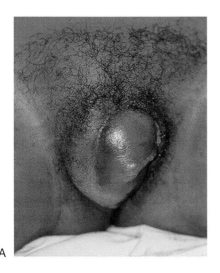

A

FIG. 9.12. This 15-year-old girl presented with a labial hematoma **(A)** secondary to an imperforate hymen and rupture of her obstructed vagina, which was filled with blood. **B, C:** Computed tomography scans show the vagina and uterus distended by blood.

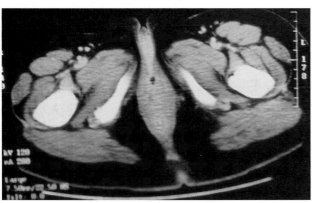

B

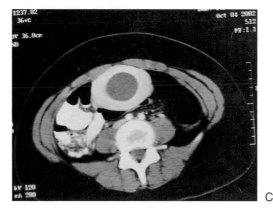

C

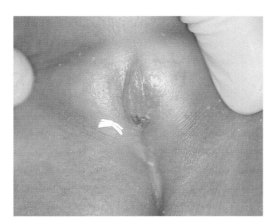

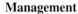

FIG. 9.13. This infant developed a fever. When a physician attempted to obtain a urine specimen by catheterization, she noticed the labial adhesions.

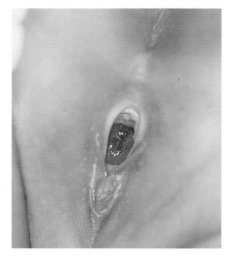

FIG. 9.14. This young girl developed urethral prolapse, manifesting with the characteristic donut sign.

Management

Patients with congenital vaginal obstruction need surgical treatment. Surgery should be scheduled promptly for adolescents but can be performed electively for asymptomatic infants and children.

Labial Adhesions

The parent who notices a daughter's labial adhesion at home usually brings her to the emergency department with a chief complaint that the child's vagina is closing up. Alternatively, a physician may detect the adhesions during the child's routine physical examination or when attempting catheterization of the bladder as part of an evaluation for fever. When the labia majora are gently retracted laterally, a flat plane of tissue marked by a central vertical line of adhesion obstructs the view (Fig. 9.13). Treatment is not indicated for asympto-

matic girls with labial adhesions because the condition spontaneously remits early in puberty. If the parents request treatment, estrogen cream (Premarin or Dienestrol) can be dabbed on the adhesions at bedtime for 2 to 4 weeks. After the labia have separated, an inert cream (zinc oxide, Vaseline, Desitin) is applied nightly for an additional 2 weeks.

URETHRAL PROLAPSE

Vaginal bleeding or spotting is the chief complaint of 90% of children with significant urethral prolapses. The bleeding is painless, occasionally misinterpreted as hematuria or menstruation, and accompanied by urinary frequency or dysuria in approximately one-fourth of cases. On examination of the child's vulva, a red or purplish, soft, doughnut-shaped mass is seen (Fig. 9.14). Most prolapses are not tender and measure 1 to 2 cm in diameter. A small central dimple in the

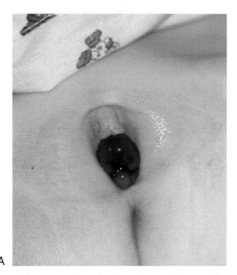

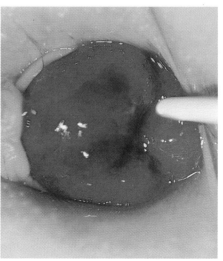

A   B

FIG. 9.15. In this case of urethral prolapse **(A)**, a catheter was placed in the urethra **(B)** to confirm the diagnosis.

mass indicates the urethral lumen. If the diagnosis is in doubt, sterile straight catheterization of the bladder through the mass can be performed to demonstrate the anatomic relationships safely and rapidly (Fig. 9.15). For the symptomatic patient with a small segment of prolapsed mucosa that is not necrotic, warm moist compresses or sitz baths, combined with a 2-week course of topical estrogen cream, may be prescribed.

GYNECOLOGIC DISORDERS OF ADOLESCENCE

Dysmenorrhea

Typical primary dysmenorrhea consists of cramping, dull, midline, or generalized lower abdominal pain at the onset of a menstrual period. The pain may coincide with the start of bleeding or may precede the bleeding by several hours. Many women have associated symptoms including backache, thigh pain, diarrhea, nausea or vomiting, and headache. The discomfort usually abates within 48 hours. Because dysmenorrhea is a hallmark of ovulation, adolescents characteristically do not experience dysmenorrhea until after several months of painless, anovulatory cycles. Patients with straightforward dysmenorrhea have normal physical examinations and no associated abnormalities on routine laboratory evaluation. Nonsteroidal antiinflammatory drugs are the treatment of choice for patients with moderate or severe dysmenorrhea, providing pain relief for 60% to 80% of symptomatic young women. For sexually active adolescents with dysmenorrhea, birth control pills provide both contraception and pain relief.

Dysfunctional Uterine Bleeding

Clinical Manifestations

Dysfunctional uterine bleeding is classically painless, but, occasionally, a patient with active bleeding may experience crampy pain if a large quantity of blood is passed rapidly. Weakness or fainting should alert the examiner to the possibility of significant blood loss. Pertinent questions should include whether the patient is pregnant, whether she uses contraception if she has been sexually active, and whether she has an underlying platelet disorder (e.g., thrombocytopenia, von Willebrand disease). Signs, including pallor, petechiae, or bruises that might indicate a bleeding disorder and hirsutism or obesity consistent with the polycystic ovary syndrome, should be sought. The pelvic examination is likely to be normal.

Management

A determination of the hemoglobin or hematocrit and platelet count is generally appropriate. Sexually active adolescents should have a pregnancy test, a cervical culture for gonorrhea, and an antigen-detection test for chlamydial infection. Patients with menorrhagia beginning at menarche, severe hemorrhage, or a history of bleeding problems should undergo further evaluation for possible disorders of platelet function.

In order of decreasing urgency, management of dysfunctional uterine bleeding includes the identification and treatment of the following problems: shock or acute hemorrhage, moderate bleeding usually accompanied by anemia, and minor bleeding that produces distress but no imminent danger for the patient. Control of the bleeding itself is accomplished with hormonal treatment. (Pregnancy must be excluded in every case before hormonal treatment is begun.) Any of the oral contraceptive pills with 35 or 50 g of either ethinyl estradiol or mestranol and a progestin provides a convenient way to administer the two hormones together. The dose for patients with active bleeding and anemia is one estrogen-progestin tablet orally four times daily for 5 days. In almost every case, bleeding will decrease substantially within 24 hours and stop within 2 to 3 days. A rarely needed alternative treatment for hospitalized patients consists of 20 to 25 mg conjugated estrogens intravenously every 4 hours until the bleeding stops, with a maximum of six doses. This treatment must be accompanied by a progestational agent (10 to 20 mg medroxyprogesterone orally per day for 5 to 12 days). If hormonal treatment fails to arrest the bleeding, dilation and curettage should be performed, but the procedure is almost never necessary. For patients with light but prolonged bleeding and a normal hemoglobin, the oral regimen can be reduced to one estrogen-progestin tablet twice daily for 5 days. A progestin alone in higher doses (10 to 20 mg norethindrone acetate per day for 5 to 12 days) can be used if estrogen is contraindicated or not tolerated, but the resulting hemostasis is less prompt and less predictable.

GENITAL TRACT INFECTIONS

Trichomonal Vaginitis

Clinical Manifestations

The classic vaginal discharge of trichomonal vaginitis after puberty is pruritic, frothy, and yellowish. The so-called strawberry cervix with multiple punctate areas of hemorrhage is pathognomonic for trichomoniasis but is visible without colposcopy in only approximately 2% of infected patients. The diagnosis is made easily and rapidly if characteristically motile, flagellated trichomonads are seen in a saline suspension of discharge examined microscopically within approximately 15 minutes after the specimen has been obtained; however, false-negative rate for wet mount examinations can be as high as 40% (Fig. 9.16). A single oral dose of 2 g metronidazole is prescribed for adolescents. Recent data indicate that metronidazole is not a teratogen, but some clinicians prefer to postpone treatment of pregnant patients until the second trimester. Intravaginal clotrimazole (2 intravaginal tablets at bedtime for 7 days) can provide

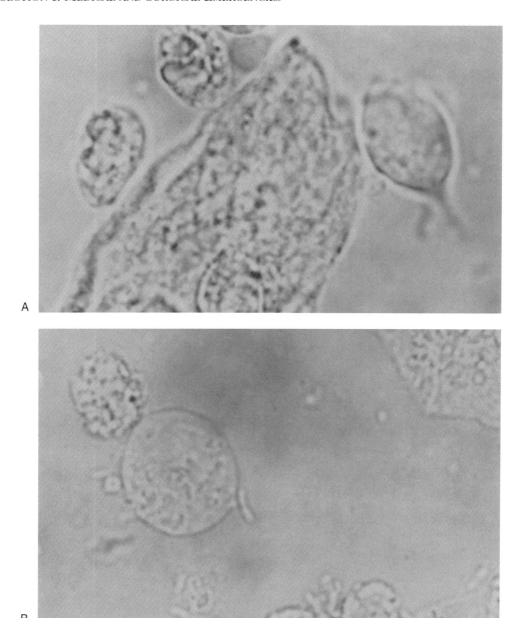

FIG. 9.16. A: Trichomonad in the vaginal discharge of a 17-year-old patient with gonococcal pelvic inflammatory disease. The flagellated protozoan is elliptical and somewhat larger than the adjacent polymorphonuclear leukocytes (225× magnification). **B:** After suspension in saline solution for microscopy, trichomonads gradually become swollen and immobile. This balloon-shaped trichomonad is barely recognizable (225× magnification).

symptomatic relief for pregnant patients but will cure only 10% to 20%.

Candidal Vulvovaginitis

The most common clinical manifestation of vulvovaginal candidiasis is vulvar pruritus. In severe infections, vulvar edema and erythema can occur. External dysuria is produced when urine comes in contact with the inflamed vulva. In severe cases, the vaginal vault is red and dry and has a whitish, watery, or curdlike discharge that may be relatively scanty. Patients with mild disease may have only intermittent itch-

ing and an unimpressive discharge. Microscopic examination of a sample of vaginal discharge suspended in 10% potassium hydroxide solution to clear the field of cellular debris can provide a rapid diagnosis of candidiasis if hyphae are seen (Fig. 9.17). However, in as many as 50% of cases, wet mounts are falsely negative. The diagnosis and subsequent treatment of this infection should be guided by the presence or absence of clinical disease. Topical imidazoles are available without prescription. The creams are packaged with intravaginal applicators, but many premenarchal and virginal girls can be treated adequately and more comfortably by applying cream to the vulva alone. Effective, nonprescription, short-course treatments for patients with mild to moderate candidal vulvovaginitis include butoconazole 2% cream (one full applicator at bedtime for three nights); 500-mg clotrimazole tablets (one tablet intravaginally as a single dose); 200-mg miconazole suppositories (one suppository at bedtime for three nights); and 6.5% tioconazole ointment (one full applicator as a single dose). For patients with severe discomfort, one of the 5- or 7-day formulations of a topical agent is likely to be more effective. Fluconazole, an oral fungicide, treats candidal vulvovaginitis as effectively as the topical preparations, and many patients prefer oral to topical treatment.

Nonspecific Vaginitis in Children

The term nonspecific vaginitis, referring to a disorder of prepubertal girls, encompasses a variety of genitourinary symptoms and signs that are sometimes caused by poor perineal hygiene but that in other cases have no readily identifiable cause. Genital discomfort, discharge, itchiness, and dysuria are relatively common childhood complaints. When a girl with such symptoms has either a normal vulva and vagina or only mild vulvar inflammation on physical examination, a specific vaginal infection is unlikely, and other possible explanations for the complaint (e.g., smegma, pinworms, urinary tract infection, a local chemical irritant, or sexual abuse) should be sought with appropriate questions and laboratory tests. If, conversely, a vaginal discharge is present on physical examination, specific vaginal infections are diagnostic possibilities, and cultures should therefore be obtained. General measures to promote cleanliness and comfort should be initiated for the girl with nonspecific vaginitis.

Bacterial Vaginosis

The symptoms of bacterial vaginosis (malodor and discharge) are not distinctive and can resemble those of trichomonal infection. The vaginal discharge is moderate or copious, grayish white, and homogeneous. On examination, the vulva, vagina, and cervix are not inflamed, but concomitant infection with trichomonas or gonorrhea can complicate this picture. Compared with the composite criteria, use of single tests (pH, clue cells, or whiff test alone) produces lower positive and negative predictive values for the diagnosis of bacterial vaginosis (Fig. 9.18). When a wet mount of vaginal discharge is examined, epithelial cells are seen to be studded with large numbers of small bacteria and have a granular appearance with shaggy borders. Lactobacilli (long rods) are sparse. The standard treatment for bacterial vaginosis is oral metronidazole. Regimens are 500 mg twice daily for 7 days in nonpregnant women and 250 mg three times daily for 7 days in pregnant women. Oral clindamycin (300 mg twice daily for 7 days) is an alternative treatment regimen for pregnant patients with bacterial vaginosis.

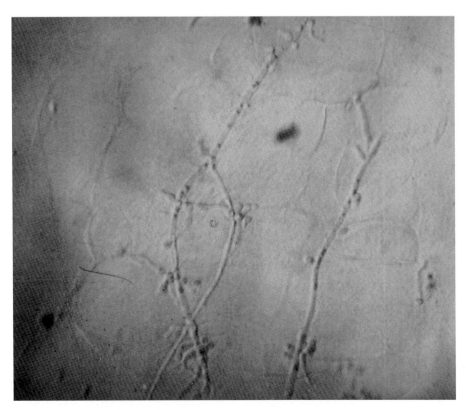

FIG. 9.17. Branching hyphae of *Candida albicans* in vaginal discharge suspected in 10% potassium hydroxide. Ghosts of vaginal epithelial cells are also visible (100× magnification).

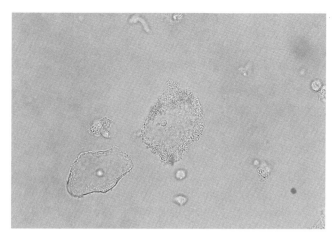

FIG. 9.18. A clue cell. The vaginal epithelial cell on the right has shaggy borders obscured by coccobacilli (100× magnification).

Gonococcal Infections

Clinical Manifestations

Prepubertal girls with vaginal gonorrhea uniformly have an obvious whitish to greenish purulent discharge that can be pruritic. Because the child's vaginal flora is normally fairly sparse, a Gram-stained smear of the vaginal discharge can provide a rapid presumptive positive diagnosis if, on microscopic examination, at least eight pairs of typical gonococci can be seen in each of at least two polymorphonuclear leukocytes. After puberty, infection is localized to the cervix and/or urethra. A vaginal discharge, excessive menstrual bleeding, or symptoms of cystitis may prompt an infected patient's emergency department visit, but most infections will produce no symptoms at all. On examination of the cervix, there may be marked central erythema, a purulent discharge, or no abnormality. A culture of a single specimen taken from the endocervical canal with a cotton-tipped swab, plated on a selective medium, and incubated properly will identify approximately 85% of women with uncomplicated gonorrhea.

Management

Prepubertal girls with culture-proven gonococcal vaginitis should be treated with a single intramuscular dose of ceftriaxone. Treatment for *Chlamydia trachomatis* should not be given presumptively for children but rather should be withheld pending the results of screening chlamydial cultures. Pharyngeal and rectal swabs for culture of *Neisseria gonorrhoeae* should be obtained from every child in whom gonococcal vaginitis is confirmed by culture. The finding of gonorrhea in a child mandates detailed psychosocial evaluation and a report to the state child protective services agency for suspected sexual abuse in every case. Adolescents with uncomplicated genital gonorrhea should receive one of the treatments listed in Table 9.1. The oral treatment regimens have the advantages of easy administration and avoiding painful intramuscular injection and the risk of accidental needle stick. Since 1982, the Centers for Disease Control and Prevention have suggested that every adolescent patient treated for lower genital tract gonorrhea also be treated presumptively for coexisting chlamydial infection because of the substantial likelihood of dual infection.

Chlamydial Infections

Most prepubertal children with urethral, vaginal, and rectal infections are asymptomatic, although a few complain of

TABLE 9.1. *Summary of treatment regimens for lower genital tract gonorrhea and chlamydial infection*

Patient circumstance	Drug	Dose, route	Comments
Treatment for gonorrhea			
In children <45 kg	Ceftriaxone	125 mg IM	
In children >45 kg and adolescents	Ceftriaxone or	125 mg IM	Regimens other than ceftriaxone may not treat incubating syphilis
	Cefixime or	400 mg PO	
	Ciprofloxacin or	500 mg PO	
	Ofloxacin	400 mg PO	
Penicillin allergy			
In children	Spectinomycin	40 mg/kg IM	Maximal dose 2 g
In adolescents	Spectinomycin	2 g IM	May not treat incubating syphilis
Treatment for chlamydial infection			
In children <45 kg	Erythromycin base	50 mg/kg PO in 4 doses for 10–14 d	Effectiveness ~80%
In children ≥45 kg and in adolescents	Azithromycin	1 g PO	Single-dose regimen obviates compliance problems
In children ≥8 yr old and in adolescents	Doxycycline	100 mg PO b.i.d. for 7 d	
During pregnancy	Erythromycin base or erythromycin ethylsuccinate	500 mg PO q.d. for 7 d 800 mg PO q.d. for 7 d	

Adapted from Centers for Disease Control and Prevention. 1998 guidelines for treatment of sexually transmitted diseases. *MMWR Recomm Rep* 1998;47:79–86.
IM, intramuscularly; PO, orally; b.i.d., twice daily; q.d., every day.

dysuria, enuresis, or vaginal discharge. The diagnosis should be suspected in prepubertal girls with vaginal discharge that persists after therapy for a prior gonococcal infection and in girls with urethritis or vaginitis who have had sexual contact. Culture of a urethral or vaginal sample is advisable to confirm the diagnosis in children because the rapid antigen-detection tests can yield false-positive results and because the social and legal implications of a positive test are serious. In adolescents, *C. trachomatis* can cause dysuria–pyuria syndrome and mucopurulent cervicitis but is often asymptomatic. Untreated lower genital tract infection can result in bartholinitis, perihepatitis, pelvic inflammatory disease (PID), and infertility. On speculum examination, the cervix may be erythematous and friable when swabbed. Infected secretions collected from the cervical os may appear yellowish on a cotton swab. The diagnosis in an adolescent should be confirmed by an antigen or DNA detection test of the cervix or urine. Antibiotic treatment regimens for children and adolescents with lower genital tract chlamydial infections are summarized in Table 9.1.

Bartholin Gland Abscess and Cyst

The patient with a Bartholin gland abscess presents with a painful, tender, fluctuant mass bulging on the involved side of the vestibule inferior to the labium minus. Pus can sometimes be milked upward from the gland to the duct orifice. The patient with a cyst complains of vulvar discomfort; the unilateral mass is typically 1 to 3 cm in diameter and mildly tender. Cyst fluid is usually sterile. Abscesses and symptomatic cysts are treated similarly, generally with incision, drainage, and placement of a Word catheter.

Pelvic Inflammatory Disease

Although the constellation of symptoms and signs associated with PID (abdominal pain, irregular uterine bleeding, abnormal vaginal discharge, and lower abdominal and pelvic tenderness) is well known, no single symptom or sign or combination of symptoms and signs is both sensitive and specific. The Centers for Disease Control publishes standard criteria for the diagnosis of PID. Perihepatitis (Fitz-Hugh–Curtis syndrome), consisting of right upper quadrant pain and tenderness produced by inflammation of the liver capsule in association with PID, occurs in 5% to 10% of patients with either chlamydial or gonococcal PID. On transvaginal ultrasonography, approximately one-third of patients with PID will have visible fallopian tubes and approximately one-fifth will have a demonstrable tuboovarian abscess. The Kahn approach to the clinical diagnosis of PID is recommended for the emergency physician (Fig. 9.19). The Centers for Disease Control guidelines for the treatment of PID are summarized in Table 9.2. Hospitalization is recommended for any patient with PID whose diagnosis is uncertain, particularly if ectopic pregnancy or appendicitis seems likely, for patients with severe clinical illness, including those with fever or suspected

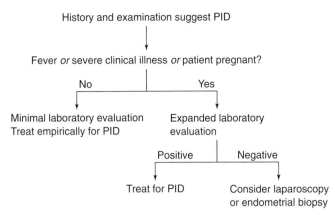

FIG. 9.19. Strategy for diagnosis of pelvic inflammatory disease (PID). Minimal laboratory evaluation should include tests for gonococcal and chlamydial cervicitis. Expanded laboratory investigation may include, in addition to the minimal evaluation, complete blood count, C-reactive protein or erythrocyte sedimentation rate, and pelvic or transvaginal ultrasonography. (Adapted from Kahn JG, Walker CK, Washington E, et al. Diagnosing pelvic inflammatory disease. *JAMA* 1991;266:2594–2604.)

pelvic abscess, and for patients who are either immunodeficient or pregnant.

Genital Warts

Clinical Manifestations

Most patients with genital warts either have no complaint or report noticing bumps in the genital area. Uncommonly, large perianal warts can be painful and interfere with defecation. Prepubertal girls with vulvovaginal warts may have a bloody vaginal discharge. Warts can occur anywhere on the perineum, but their growth seems to be encouraged by moisture. The most common locations in females are the posterior fourchette, adjacent areas of the labia minora and majora, and the lower vagina. Single warts, 1 cm or more in diameter, and clusters of seedlings, each a few millimeters across, are both common. Warts can be velvety and flat or papillomatous (Fig. 9.20). Large warts often contain distinct cauliflower-like lobulations (Fig. 9.21).

Management

Podophyllin resin, in solutions of as much as 25% concentration in tincture of benzoin, and trichloroacetic acid (TCA) 80% solution are applied by the clinician. Podofilox in a 0.5% gel or solution and 5% imiquimod cream, an immune response modifier that induces cytokines, are available for self-application by patients. Safe maximal doses of 10% podophyllin solution are 4 mL for patients weighing more than 40 kg and 0.1 mg/kg for children. TCA can be applied to mucosal surfaces and can be administered to pregnant patients. However, TCA has a viscosity lower than water and

TABLE 9.2. *Treatment regimens for pelvic inflammatory disease*

	Initial therapy	Subsequent therapy	Comments
Regimen A Extended parenteral treatment	2 g cefotetan IV q 12 hr or 2 g cefoxitin IV q 6 hr with 100 mg doxycycline PO or IV q 12 hr	100 mg doxycycline PO b.i.d. to complete 14 d of therapy	Oral doxycycline is preferred to avoid infusion pain Parenteral treatment may be stopped 24 hr after clinical improvement
Regimen B[a] Extended parenteral treatment	900 mg clindamycin IV q 8 hr with 2 mg/kg gentamicin then 1.5 mg/kg IV or IM q 8 hr	100 mg doxycycline PO b.i.d. or 450 mg clindamycin PO b.i.d. to complete 14 d of therapy	Clindamycin is preferred for oral treatment of tubo/ovarian abscess Parenteral treatment may be stopped 24 hr after clinical improvement
Regimen C Combined parenteral/oral treatment	250 mg ceftriaxone IM or 2 mg cefoxitin IM with 1 g probenecid PO	100 mg doxycycline PO b.i.d. for 14 d	Ceftriaxone has better coverage than cefoxitin against *Neisseria gonorrhoeae* Adding metronidazole to this regimen will enhance anaerobic coverage
Regimen D Oral treatment	400 mg ofloxacin PO b.i.d. for 14 d with 500 mg metronidazole PO b.i.d. for 14 d		Ofloxacin is not approved during pregnancy or lactation or for patients <18 yr old

[a] Alternative parenteral treatment combinations include ofloxacin with metronidazole, ampicillin/sulbactam with doxycycline, and ciprofloxacin with doxycycline and metronidazole. Ciprofloxacin has poor coverage against *Chlamydia trachomatis.*

IV, intravenously; q, every; PO, orally; b.i.d., twice daily; IM, intramuscularly.

Adapted from Centers for Disease Control and Prevention. 1998 guidelines for treatment of sexually transmitted diseases, *MMWR Recomm Rep* 1998;47:79–86.

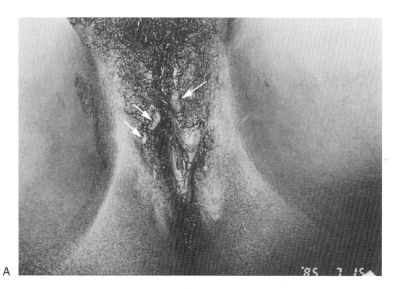

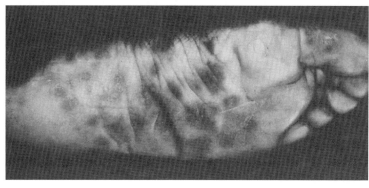

FIG. 9.20. A: Vulvar condylomata lata of secondary syphilis in a 15-year-old patient. **B:** Macular rash on sole of foot of same patient.

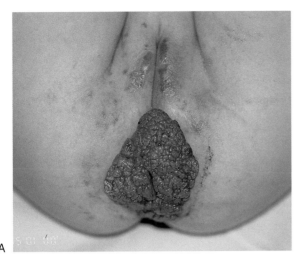
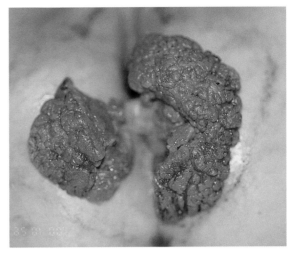

FIG. 9.21. A,B: Large pedunculated condyloma in a 17-month-old girl.

can spread to unaffected skin rapidly, producing patient discomfort during application more often than does podophyllin. Imiquimod commonly produces local itching, erythema, and burning but is generally tolerated well by patients. For extensive or recurrent disease or when repeated applications of podophyllin, TCA, or imiquimod are not successful, alternative treatments include surgical removal, cryotherapy, and intralesional interferon.

SUGGESTED READINGS

Anveden-Hertzberg L, Gauderer MW, Elder JS. Urethral prolapse: an often-misdiagnosed cause of urogenital bleeding in girls. *Pediatr Emerg Care* 1995;11:212–214.

Bayer SR, DeCherney AH. Clinical manifestations and treatment of dysfunctional uterine bleeding. *JAMA* 1993;269:1823–1828.

Brown MR, Cartwright PC, Snow BW. Common office problems in pediatric urology and gynecology. *Pediatr Clin North Am* 1997;44:1091–1115.

Centers for Disease Control and Prevention. 1998 guidelines for the treatment of sexually transmitted diseases. *MMWR Recomm Rep* 1998.

Dowd MD, Fitzmaurice L, Knapp JF, et al. The interpretation of urogenital findings in children with straddle injuries. *J Pediatr Surg* 1994;29:7–10.

Falcone T, Desjardins C, Bourque J, et al. Dysfunctional uterine bleeding in adolescents. *J Reprod Med* 1992;39:761–764.

Glasier A. Emergency postcoital contraception. *N Engl J Med* 1997;337:1058–1064.

Hay PE, Taylor-Robinson D. Defining bacterial vaginosis: to BV or not to BV, that is the question. *Int J STD AIDS* 1996;7:233–235.

Hill DA, Lense JJ. Office management of Bartholin gland cysts and abscesses. *Am Fam Physician* 1998;57:1611–1616.

Kass EJ, Lundak B. The acute scrotum. *Pediatr Clin North Am* 1997; 44:1251–1266.

McAleer IM, Kaplan GW. Pediatric genitourinary trauma. *Urol Clin North Am* 1995;22:177–188.

Mercer LJ, Mueller CM, Hajj SN. Medical treatment of urethral prolapse in the premenarcheal female. *Adolesc Pediatr Gynecol* 1988;1:181–184.

Okur H, Kucukaydin M, Kazez A, et al. Genitourinary tract injuries in girls. *Br J Urol* 1996;78:446–449.

Oosterlinck W. Unbloody management of penile zipper injury. *Eur Urol* 1981;7:365–6.

Paradise JE, Campos JM, Friedman HM, et al. Vulvovaginitis in premenarchal girls: clinical features and diagnostic evaluation. *Pediatrics* 1982; 70:193–198.

Schneider RE. Genitourinary trauma. *Emerg Med Clin North Am* 1993; 11:137–145.

Skoog JS. Benign and malignant pediatric scrotal masses. *Pediatr Clin North Am* 1997;44:1229–1250.

Sobel JD. Vaginitis. *N Engl J Med* 1997;337:1896–1903.

Soifer H. Adhesions of the labia minora in infants and children. *Int Pediatr* 1991;6:347–353.

Spence JE. Vaginal and uterine anomalies in the pediatric and adolescent patient. *J Pediatr Adolesc Gynecol* 1998;11:3–11.

Stone KM, Becker TM, Hadgu A, et al. Treatment of external genital warts: a randomised clinical trial comparing podophyllin, cryotherapy, and electrodesiccation. *Genitourin Med* 1990;66:16–19.

Wolner-Hanssen P, Krieger JN, Stevens CE, et al. Clinical manifestations of vaginal trichomoniasis. *JAMA* 1989;261:571–576.

CHAPTER 10

Hematologic and Oncologic Emergencies

Editor: Stephen Ludwig

DISORDERS OF RED BLOOD CELLS

Severe anemia is a pediatric emergency that requires rapid evaluation and treatment to prevent hypoxia, congestive heart failure, and death. The classification of causes of anemia according to (1) blood loss, (2) increased red cell destruction, and (3) decreased red cell production is familiar to most physicians and provides an excellent starting point for the evaluation of the anemic child.

Increased Red Cell Destruction

Membrane Disorders

The anemia in disorders of the red cell membrane (hereditary spherocytosis, hereditary elliptocytosis, stomatocytosis, liver disease) is rarely severe enough to constitute a hematologic emergency. However, the hemoglobin level may decrease even further when red cell destruction increases (hemolytic crisis) or red cell production slows (aplastic crisis). Hemolytic crises are usually associated with acute infections and are self-limiting. Most aplastic crises accompany parvovirus infection; anemia may be the only manifestation of the infectious process.

Metabolic Abnormalities

Like the red cell membrane disorders, erythrocyte metabolic abnormalities usually do not cause severe anemia. However, episodes of acute and sometimes life-threatening hemolysis can occur in many variants of glucose-6-phosphate dehydrogenase deficiency, including the A variant found in 10% of African-American boys after exposure to drugs or chemicals (Table 10.1) or during an infectious illness. Ingestion of naphthalene-containing mothballs is the most common cause of severe hemolysis in American children with glucose-6-phosphate dehydrogenase deficiency, and parents should be asked about the presence of mothballs as part of the evaluation of any child with acute hemolysis characterized by pallor, malaise, fever, scleral icterus, abdominal and back pain, and dark urine. The anemia is accompanied by an increased reticulocyte count, and diagnostic blister cells are present on the peripheral smear (Fig. 10.1). Treatment should include removal of the offending agent and fluid administration to prevent renal tubular damage.

Autoimmune Hemolytic Anemia

Although this disorder may occasionally be indolent and may go undetected for days or weeks, autoimmune hemolytic anemia (AIHA) is usually associated with the sudden onset of pallor, jaundice, and dark urine. The hemoglobin level may be as low as 1 to 2 g/dL at the time of diagnosis. When the anemia is this severe, the child may appear moribund and desperately ill. Signs of congestive heart failure may be prominent.

The anemia is usually accompanied by reticulocytosis, although the reticulocyte count may be less than 5% during the first few days of the illness. Occasionally, patients remain reticulocytopenic for prolonged periods. Spherocytes are often found on the peripheral smear, and red cell fragments may sometimes be present (Fig. 10.2). Free hemoglobin in the urine produces a positive dipstick reaction for blood in the absence of red cells on microscopic urinalysis. When hemolysis is severe enough to exceed the renal clearance of hemoglobin, the plasma will be pink, and careful inspection of the plasma layer of a spun hematocrit may provide an early diagnostic clue. The direct Coombs test using broad-spectrum Coombs serum (immunoglobulin G and M and complement) is usually positive in childhood AIHA.

Management

The management of the child with AIHA should be aggressive because the hemoglobin level may fall precipitously (Table 10.2). Hospitalization for careful observation and treatment is usually necessary. The immediate institution of corticosteroid therapy (2 to 4 mg/kg prednisone per day or equivalent doses of parenteral preparations) may prevent or

TABLE 10.1. *Drugs and substances associated with acute hemolysis in children with glucose-6-phosphate dehydrogenase deficiency*

Antimalarials (primaquine)
Sulfonamides (including sulfasalazine and trimethoprim–sulfamethoxazole)
Nalidixic acid and nitrofurantoin
Naphthalene (moth balls)
Fava beans
Aspirin (does not cause acute hemolysis with G6PD deficiency in African Americans when used in therapeutic doses)

reduce the need for red cell transfusions. Alternatively, the patient may be treated with 1 g/kg intravenous immunoglobulin by infusion.

Red cell transfusions are hazardous in patients with AIHA and should be reserved for children with severe anemia and signs of hypoxia or cardiac failure.

Nonimmune Acquired Hemolytic Anemia

Acute hemolytic anemia in children may be caused by infections, chemicals, or drugs that damage the red cell directly.

These disorders resemble AIHA in their clinical presentation and should be considered in the child with acquired hemolytic anemia and a negative Coombs test. Treatment is directed at elimination of the offending agent. Red cell transfusions are usually unnecessary unless anemia is severe (hematocrit <15%) or accompanied by signs of cardiovascular compromise.

Decreased Red Cell Production

Aplastic and Hypoplastic Anemias

Hypoplastic anemia may be self-limited, as in transient erythrocytopenia of childhood (Fig. 10.3), or chronic, as in Diamond–Blackfan syndrome. Most of these disorders have a protracted course and, after initial stabilization of the patient, require intensive diagnostic evaluation and careful assessment of chronic therapy rather than emergency management. Transfusion should be used with particular caution in the initial management of patients with hypoplastic and aplastic anemias because exposure to human leukocyte antigen and other antigens may adversely affect engraftment of transplanted bone marrow in patients who might otherwise have benefited from this procedure. If transfusions are required for severe anemia

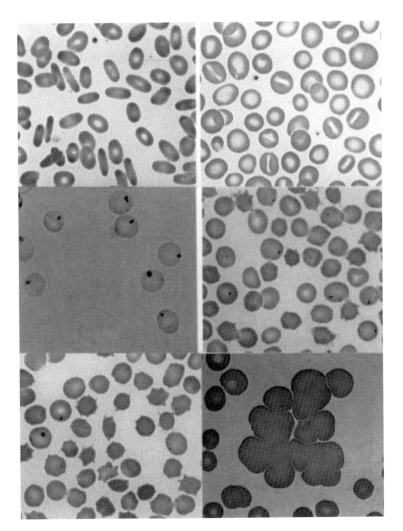

FIG. 10.1. Metabolic abnormalities. Heinz bodies in glucose-6-phosphate dehydrogenase deficiency. Formation of reticulocytes. (From Lee G, Foerster J, Lukens J, et al. *Wintrobe's clinical hematology*, 10th ed. Philadelphia: Lippincott Williams & Wilkins, 1998:1123, with permission.)

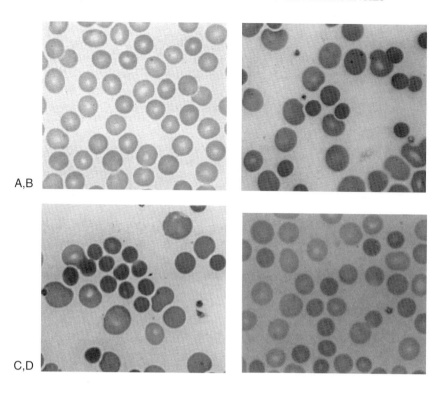

A,B

C,D

FIG. 10.2. Spherocytes in various hemolytic conditions. **A:** Normal cells for comparison. **B, C:** Autoimmune hemolytic anemia. **D:** Hereditary spherocytosis. (From Lee G, Foerster J, Lukens J, et al. *Wintrobe's clinical hematology*, 10th ed. Philadelphia: Lippincott Williams & Wilkins, 1998:1122, with permission.)

(hemoglobin <3 to 4 g/dL) and signs of cardiac failure or poor oxygenation, the goal of treatment should be relief of symptoms, not restoration of a normal hemoglobin level.

Nutritional Anemias

Nutritional anemias in children constitute more of a public health problem than a hematologic emergency. However, on occasion, the hemoglobin level may be very low at the time of diagnosis. Severe iron deficiency occurs mainly in 1- to 2-year-old children who drink 1 qt or more of cow's milk daily and have little room for other foods richer in iron (Fig. 10.4). Adolescent girls make up another group at high risk of iron deficiency because a diet normally marginal in iron content becomes totally inadequate in the face of menstrual blood losses. The presenting complaint in severe iron deficiency anemia is usually pallor, lethargy, irritability, or poor exercise tolerance. In megaloblastic anemias such as vitamin B$_{12}$ deficiency in an infant exclusively breast-fed by a vegetarian mother or in folic acid deficiency caused by impaired

TABLE 10.2. *Treatment of severe autoimmune hemolytic anemia*

Maintain normal or increased urine output with IV fluids.
Immediately begin corticosteroid therapy with 2 mg/kg prednisone per day or a parenteral preparation in an equivalent dose. Alternatively, administer 1 g/kg IV γ-globulin, alone or in combination with corticosteroid.
Administer red cell transfusions when severe anemia is accompanied by signs of hypoxia or cardiac failure.
  Give first 5 mL over 10–15 min and observe for symptoms of acute hemolysis.
  Check plasma layer of a spun hematocrit for pink color indicative of hemolysis of the transfused red cells.
  If symptoms or signs of worsening hemolysis are present, try a different unit of red cells.
If hemoglobin level does not increase after transfusion:
  Increase steroid dose to 4 mg/kg/d or
  Administer IV γ-globulin 1 g/kg or
  Begin plasmapheresis or exchange transfusion or
  Perform splenectomy.

IV, intravenous.

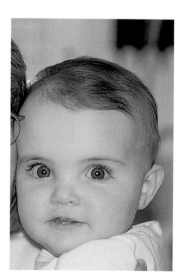

FIG. 10.3. This 8-month-old girl presented with pallor and a hematocrit of 11%. She was diagnosed with transient erythrocytopenia of childhood.

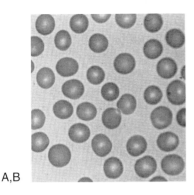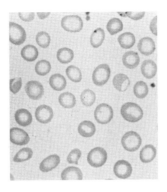

A,B

FIG. 10.4. Nutritional anemia. **A:** Microcytosis and hypochromia in iron deficiency anemia. **B:** Normal blood smear. (From Lee G, Foerster J, Lukens J, et al. *Wintrobe's clinical hematology*, 10th ed. Philadelphia: Lippincott Williams & Wilkins, 1998: 910 and *Atlas of hematology*, 3rd ed. Philadelphia: Lippincott Williams & Wilkins, 44, with permission.)

folate absorption, nonhematologic symptoms such as diarrhea, slowed development, or coma may be more prominent than the symptoms of anemia.

Stabilization and improvement can usually be achieved with replacement of the deficient nutrient. Nucleated red cells or reticulocytes usually appear within 48 hours of replacement therapy in folic acid or vitamin B$_{12}$ deficiency and within 72 hours of therapy in severe iron deficiency anemia.

Iron replacement therapy consists of 3 to 6 mg/kg per day of elemental iron given orally as ferrous sulfate in two or three divided doses.

DISORDERS OF HEMOGLOBIN STRUCTURE AND PRODUCTION

Sickle Hemoglobin Disorders

The diagnosis of sickle cell disease should be considered in African-American children with unexplained pain or swelling (especially of the hands or feet), pneumonia, meningitis, sepsis, neurologic abnormalities, splenomegaly, or anemia (Figs. 10.5 and 10.6). The hemoglobin level and reticulocyte count are inadequate screening tests for the sickle hemoglobinopathies because values in affected

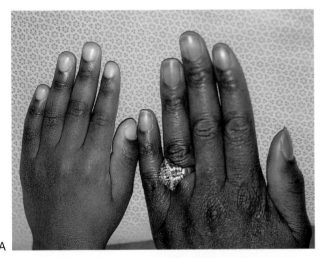

A

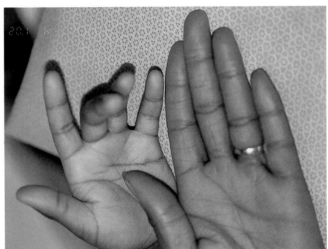

B

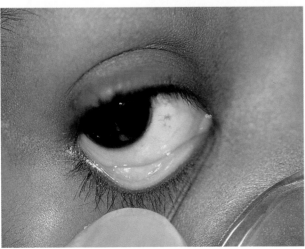

C

FIG. 10.5. **A–C:** Characteristics of Sickle cell.

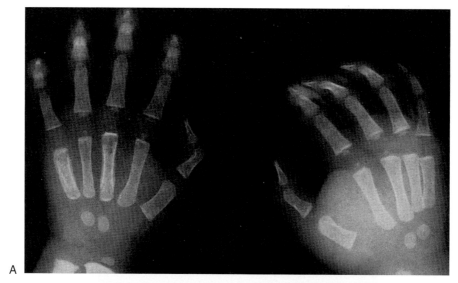

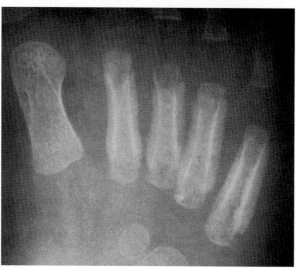

FIG. 10.6. Hand–foot syndrome. **A:** Note extensive swelling of the soft tissues around the thumb and metacarpals of the left hand. **B:** Below, note destructive changes in the third and fifth metatarsals. Also note periosteal new bone deposition. The changes on the right are older than those on the left. (From Swischuk LE. *Imaging of the newborn, infant and young child*, 4th ed. Philadelphia: Lippincott Williams & Wilkins, 1997:781, with permission.)

patients (especially those with hemoglobin sickle cell disease and S-β-thalassemia) may overlap with normal values. Similarly, the peripheral smear may be devoid of sickled cells (Fig. 10.7). Definitive testing for sickling disorders can be accomplished quickly by hemoglobin electrophoresis, isoelectric focusing, or high-pressure liquid chromatography. If these tests are not available, standard solubility tests can be used to identify the presence of sickle hemoglobin. However, solubility tests do not distinguish patients with sickle cell trait, hemoglobin sickle cell disease, or other sickle variants from patients with sickle cell anemia (hemo-

globin SS). Therefore, the results of solubility screening tests must be considered in the context of the clinical presentation and other laboratory studies.

Children with sickle cell disease are affected more often with infections including sepsis compared with their hematologically normal counterparts. Meningitis, pneumonia, septic arthritis, and osteomyelitis may be responsible for substantial morbidity and mortality unless promptly recognized and appropriately treated. The level of suspicion for meningitis should be particularly high in the young, irritable child with sickle cell disease and unexplained fever. Antibiotic therapy

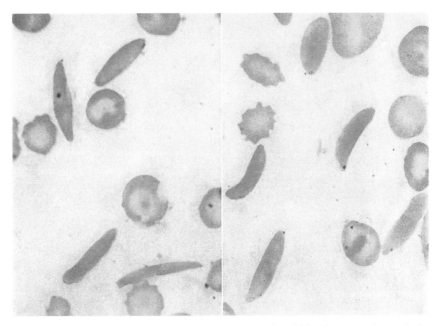

FIG. 10.7. Sickle cell anemia blood film. The bizarre-shaped red blood corpuscles include elongated narrow types with rounded and pointed ends; they are sickle- or oat-shaped and tend to take the stain to a heavier degree than the other erythrocytes. The discrete dark spots present are due to artifact probably caused by precipitation of stain. (From McDonald GA, Dodds TC, Cruickshank B, eds. *Atlas of hematology*, 3rd ed. Edinburgh: E & S Livingstone, 1970:28, with permission.)

of meningitis is similar to that recommended for hematologically normal children with this disorder. Exchange transfusion to lower the percentage of sickle hemoglobin may reduce the risk of intracerebral sickling and infarction in areas of local swelling and possible red cell sludging.

Acute chest syndrome, which includes pneumonia as well as pulmonary infarction, is one of the most common reasons for hospital admission for children with sickle cell anemia. The affected patient is usually tachypneic, even after antipyretic therapy. Rales, rhonchi, and physical findings of lobar consolidation may be present. However, in some children, particularly those who are somewhat dehydrated, physical findings may be far less striking. Rales may be heard only after several hours of rehydration. Because acute chest syndrome may escape detection on physical examination, a chest radiograph should be obtained in children with sickle cell disease and unexplained fever or chest pain. A decrease in oxygen saturation, readily measured in the emergency department and compared with baseline values, may identify patients with early acute chest syndrome.

Septic arthritis and osteomyelitis present particularly difficult diagnostic problems in children with sickle cell disease because the clinical findings so closely resemble those found in infarctions of the bone (Fig. 10.8). Closed or open bone aspiration should precede the institution of antibiotic therapy in the patient with suspected osteomyelitis. Similarly, aspiration of an affected joint should be performed if septic arthritis is strongly suspected. In most instances, swollen, warm, and tender joints are caused by local infarction. The presence of other sites of concurrent infarction and the

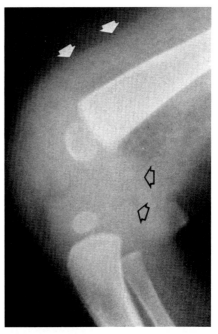

FIG. 10.8. Silent neonatal osteomyelitis and septic arthritis. Note swelling of the soft tissues of the entire leg (mostly around the knee and hip), (arrows) lateral dislocation of the left hip (pus in the joint), and destructive foci in both upper femurs. Clinically, hip abnormality was unsuspected in this infant, although knee swelling was noted. Actually, this patient presented with findings suggesting diabetes insipidus, and the extremity changes for the most part were overlooked. (From Swischuk LE. *Imaging of the newborn, infant and young child*, 4th ed. Philadelphia: Lippincott Williams & Wilkins, 1997:746, with permission.)

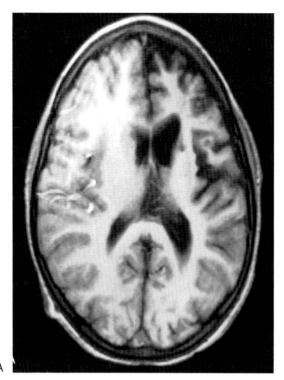
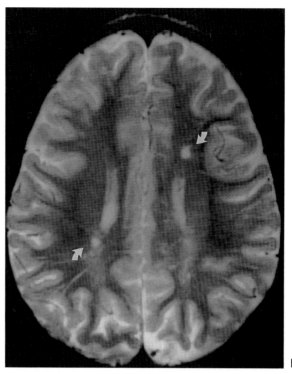

A

B

FIG. 10.9. Vasoocclusive effects in central nervous system. **A:** T1-weighted magnetic resonance imaging in a 6-year-old with HB SS and a history of stroke. There is extensive atrophy involving the distributions of the left anterior and middle cerebral arteries with compensatory enlargement of the left lateral ventricle. **B:** T2-weighted sagittal magnetic resonance imaging in a 4-year-old boy with silent infarcts. Small areas of leukomalacia are seen in deep white matter in frontal and parietal areas. (From Lee G, Foerster J, Lukens J, et al. *Wintrobe's clinical hematology*, 10th ed. Philadelphia: Lippincott Williams & Wilkins, 1998:1360, with permission.)

patient's description of the pain as typical crisis pain may be helpful in identifying the cause as vasoocclusion. The total white blood cell count and differential count of the joint fluid may be similar in both septic arthritis and sterile effusion secondary to infarction. Therefore, the Gram stain and culture are especially important.

Vasoocclusion

Infarction of bone, soft tissue, and viscera may occur as a result of intravascular sickling and vessel occlusion. Children may have only pain or may have symptoms related to the affected organ (e.g., hematuria in papillary necrosis, jaundice in hepatic infarct, seizures or weakness in central nervous system [CNS] ischemia, respiratory distress in pulmonary infarction) (Fig. 10.9). Initial management usually centers on control of pain, general supportive measures, and differentiation of vasoocclusion and disorders unrelated to the hematologic abnormality (Table 10.3).

Several specific areas of vasoocclusion deserve special attention. Between 6 and 24 months of age, dactylitis is a common manifestation of sickle cell disease. Infarction of the metacarpals and metatarsals results in swelling of the hands and feet. These episodes recur frequently. Pain usually resolves after several days, but swelling may persist for 1 or 2 weeks. Treatment is similar to that described for a painful crisis.

Infarction of abdominal and retroperitoneal organs may produce clinical findings that closely resemble the findings in a variety of nonhematologic diseases. The distinction between occlusion of the mesenteric vessels and appendicitis or other causes of an acute abdomen is, at times, particularly difficult. Hepatic infarction may also create a diagnostic dilemma because the acute onset of jaundice and abdominal pain that characterizes this disorder is similar to

TABLE 10.3. *Management of vasoocclusive crisis in sickle cell crisis*

Mild or moderate pain
  Hydration: 1.5 × maintenance with oral fluids or IV D5 in $\frac{1}{4}$ NSS or D5 in $\frac{1}{2}$ NSS
  Analgesia: Acetaminophen with or without codeine
  Disposition: Admit if pain worsens, oral fluid intake is inadequate, or there is a history of repeat visits to the emergency department
Severe pain
  Hydration: 1.5 × maintenance with IV D5 in $\frac{1}{4}$ NSS or D5 in $\frac{1}{2}$ NSS
  Analgesia: 0.10–0.15 mg/kg IV morphine sulfate
  Disposition: Admit unless pain is markedly reduced and patient can take oral fluids

IV, intravenous; D5, 5% dextrose; NSS, normal saline solution.

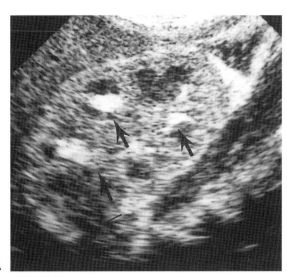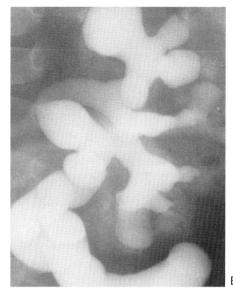

A   B

FIG. 10.10. Papillary necrosis. **A:** Note the echogenic renal papillae (*arrows*). Echogenicity of the kidney in general is increased. **B:** Late stage. With reflux during cystourethrography, marked dilation and blunting of the calyces along with mall diverticula and some pyelotubular backflow are seen. (From Swischuk LE. *Imaging of the newborn, infant and young child*, 4th ed. Philadelphia: Lippincott Williams & Wilkins, 1997:643, with permission.)

the symptoms of hepatitis, cholecystitis, and biliary obstruction. The major emergencies related to vasoocclusion within the genitourinary tract are hematuria, which results from renal papillary necrosis (Fig. 10.10), and priapism. Alkalinization of the urine may reduce bleeding but is difficult to accomplish and usually unnecessary. Administration of antifibrinolytic drugs such as ε-aminocaproic acid (Amicar) (100 mg/kg every 6 hours) or tranexamic acid (25 mg/kg every 6 to 8 hours) may stop bleeding but carries a risk of ureteral clot formation. Priapism is an unusually painful and frightening form of vasoocclusion. The initial treatment consists of fluid therapy and analgesics. Once again, red cell transfusions or exchange transfusion may promote resolution, but these forms of therapy should be reserved for patients without a rapid response to other measures (Tables 10.4 and 10.5).

Splenic Sequestration Crisis

The sudden enlargement of the spleen with resulting sequestration of a substantial portion of the blood volume is a life-threatening complication of sickle cell disease. Because this crisis requires the presence of vascularized splenic tissue, it usually occurs before 5 years of age in patients with homozygous sickle cell disease but may occur much later in children with milder sickling disorders such as sickle cell disease or S-β-thalassemia. The patient undergoing a severe sequestration crisis may first complain of left upper quadrant pain (Table 10.6). Within hours, the patient becomes very pale, lethargic, and disoriented and appears ill. The physical examination shows evidence of cardiovascular collapse; hypotension and tachycardia are often present (Fig. 10.11). The level of consciousness falls. The hallmark of a severe sequestration crisis is a spleen that is significantly enlarged compared with previous examinations and is unusually hard. The hematocrit or

TABLE 10.4. *Management of priapism in sickle cell anemia*

Hospitalize if erection persists or if pain is severe.

Intravenous hydration with D5 in $\frac{1}{4}$ NSS or D5 in $\frac{1}{2}$ NSS at $1\text{-}\frac{1}{2}$–2 × maintenance for 24–48 hr.

Consider aspiration of the corpora.

If swelling does not decrease, transfuse with red cells to raise hemoglobin level to 9–10 g/dL.

If no improvement after simple transfusion, institute exchange transfusion to reduce HbS to <30% of total hemoglobin

Reserve shunting procedures for patients who have failed other forms of therapy in the first 72 hr.

D5, 5% dextrose; NSS, normal saline solution

TABLE 10.5. *Management of stroke in sickle cell anemia*

1. Obtain computed tomography scan or magnetic resonance imaging to identify an area of infarction or to rule out a ruptured cerebral aneurysm or other intracranial bleed.
2. Immediately begin $1\text{-}\frac{1}{2}$–2 volume exchange transfusion to reduce HbS to <30% of total hemoglobin.
   a. Use whole blood <3–5 days old or packed red cells <3–5 days old reconstituted with fresh frozen plasma.
3. Reserve pretransfusion blood sample for characterization of red cell antigens in preparation for long-term transfusion program.

TABLE 10.6. *Splenic sequestration crisis*

Symptoms
    Left upper quadrant pain
    Pallor
    Lethargy
Signs
    Hypotension
    Tachycardia
    Markedly enlarged and firm spleen
Laboratory findings
    Severe anemia
    Increased reticulocytes
    Mild to moderate thrombocytopenia and neutropenia
Management
    Immediate volume replacement
    Transfusion with packed red cells or whole blood

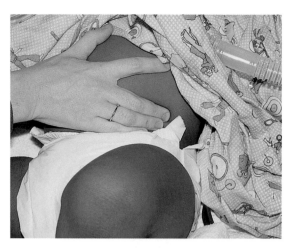

FIG. 10.11. Acute splenic sequestration.

hemoglobin level is much lower than during routine visits, and the reticulocyte count is usually increased. Mild neutropenia or thrombocytopenia may be present.

Recognition of this complication should be immediate so that lifesaving therapy begins without delay. The rapid infusion of large amounts of normal saline or albumin is necessary to restore intravascular volume. Although a sufficient number of red cells to relieve tissue hypoxia may be released by the spleen after initial fluid resuscitation, transfusion with packed red cells (2 to 10 mL/kg) is often required in more severe cases. Whole blood transfusion may help to relieve the dual problems of intravascular volume depletion and impaired tissue oxygenation.

Aplastic Crisis

Increased bone marrow erythroid activity (as reflected by the elevated reticulocyte count and presence of nucleated red cells in the peripheral blood) partially compensates for the shortened red cell survival in sickle cell anemia and other hemolytic disorders. If erythropoiesis slows or ceases, this precarious balance is disturbed, and the hemoglobin level may gradually fall (Table 10.7). The event that most commonly causes erythroid aplasia is a parvovirus infection. Progressive pallor is unaccompanied by jaundice or other signs of hemolysis. If a red cell transfusion is required, a small aliquot is usually sufficient to raise the hemoglobin

concentration to a level that ensures adequate oxygenation until red cell production recovers.

Hemolytic Crisis

Worsening anemia and increasing reticulocytosis may accompany viral and bacterial infections in children with sickle cell disease (Table 10.7). Scleral icterus is more prominent than usual. The findings are consistent with an increasing degree of active hemolysis. The hemoglobin level rarely falls low enough to require specific therapy. Hematologic values return to the usual level as the infection process resolves.

THALASSEMIA MAJOR (COOLEY ANEMIA)

Children with thalassemia major usually develop a sallow complexion and increasing fatigue between the ages of 6 and 24 months. Weight gain and linear growth may be retarded (Fig. 10.12). Physical examination shows pallor and enlargement of the liver and spleen. The hemoglobin level may be as low as 3 or 4 g/dL, and the mean corpuscular volume is usually low. The red cells are hypochromic and microcytic with striking variation in size and shape; nucleated red cells are present in the peripheral smear (Fig. 10.13). Thalassemia major is readily distinguishable from severe nutritional iron deficiency. In the latter disorder, the dietary history is grossly abnormal,

TABLE 10.7. *Comparison of findings in sequestration, aplastic, and hemolytic crises in sickle cell disease*

	Sequestration crisis	Aplastic crisis	Hemolytic crisis
Onset	Sudden	Gradual	Sudden
Pallor	Present	Present	Present
Jaundice	Normal	Normal	Increased
Abdominal pain	Present	Absent	Absent
Hemoglobin level	Very low	Low or very low	Low
Reticulocytes	Unchanged or increased	Decreased	Increased
Marrow erythroid activity	Unchanged or increased	Decreased	Increased

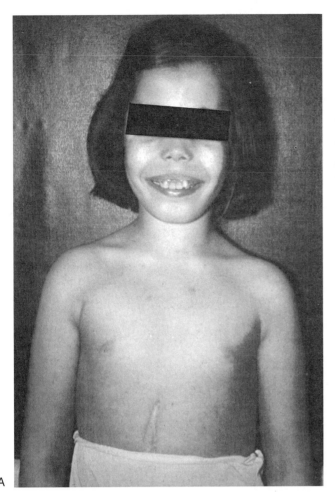

A

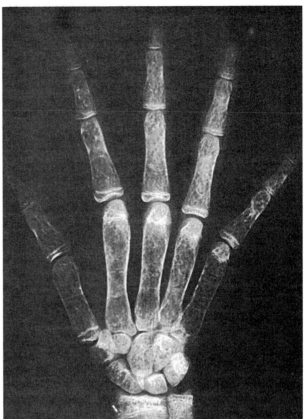

B

FIG. 10.12. Thalassemia major. **A:** Characteristic facies of thalassemia major. Note prominent malar eminences, producing an apparent depression of the nose, and enlargement of the maxilla with upward protrusion of the lip, exposing the upper teeth. **B:** Mosaic pattern produced by trabeculation in the bones of the hand of a patient with thalassemia major. Note the rectangular contour of the metacarpals. (From Lee G, Foerster J, Lukens J, et al. *Wintrobe's clinical hematology*, 10th ed. Philadelphia: Lippincott Williams & Wilkins, 1998:1422, with permission.)

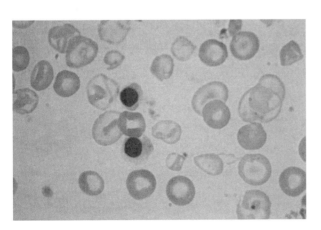

FIG. 10.13. Blood smear from a patient with thalassemia major. Note severe hypochromia, marked anisocytosis, target cells, and nucleated red blood cells. A Howell–Jolly body signifies prior splenectomy. (From Lee G, Foerster J, Lukens J, et al. *Wintrobe's clinical hematology*, 10th ed. Philadelphia: Lippincott Williams & Wilkins, 1998:1424, with permission.)

organomegaly is uncommon, changes in red cell morphology are less impressive, and nucleated red cells are rarely seen in the peripheral smear. The diagnosis of thalassemia major should be considered in a child with severe microcytic anemia and an appropriate ethnic background.

The moderate anemia usually apparent at presentation allows sufficient time for a careful diagnostic evaluation and outpatient transfusion therapy. However, when anemia is severe and congestive heart failure is present or imminent, the need for red cell transfusion may be urgent. In such instances, pretransfusion blood should be saved for appropriate diagnostic studies (hemoglobin electrophoresis) and initial red cell antigen typing. If transfusion is necessary, small aliquots of red cells (2 to 3 mL/kg) should be given. The administration of a rapid-acting diuretic (furosemide 1 mg/kg per dose) may diminish the risk of fluid overload. Partial exchange transfusion has also been recommended for patients with severe anemia to prevent further increases in intravascular volume and myocardial stress.

METHEMOGLOBINEMIA

Symptoms depend on the concentration of methemoglobin (Table 10.8). The diagnosis should be strongly suspected when oxygen administration fails to affect cyanosis. To eliminate an anatomic abnormality as a cause of oxygen-unresponsive cyanosis, an attempt should be made to oxygenate the patient's blood *in vitro*. As a rapid screening test, a drop of blood is placed on filter paper. After the filter paper is waved in the air for 30 to 60 seconds, normal blood appears bright red, whereas blood from a patient with methemoglobinemia remains reddish brown. Arterial blood oxygen saturation is low when measured directly by blood oximetry rather than calculated, even though Po_2 is normal. Although blood oximetry measures oxyhemoglobin as a percentage of total hemoglobin, including methemoglobin that is nonfunctional, pulse oximetry devices measure oxygen saturation of only that hemoglobin that is available for saturation. Thus, a patient with methemoglobinemia and obvious cyanosis may have normal oxygen saturation as measured by pulse oximetry. Spectrophotometric assays can be used for confirmation of methemoglobinemia and for determination of the level of methemoglobin.

The treatment of methemoglobinemia depends on the clinical severity (Table 10.9). In all cases, an attempt should

TABLE 10.8. *Symptoms and signs according to severity of methemoglobinemia*

Methemoglobin level (%)	Symptoms
10–30	Cyanosis
30–50	Dyspnea, tachycardia, dizziness, fatigue, headache
50–70	Lethargy, stupor
70	Death

TABLE 10.9. *Treatment of methemoglobinemia*

Methemoglobin level (%)	Treatment
<30	Not needed
30–70	2 mg/kg of a 1% methylene blue solution, infused intravenously over 5 min[a]
Severely ill and no response to methylene blue	Hyperbaric oxygen or exchange transfusion

[a] If no response to two doses of methylene blue in a noncritically ill patient or a patient with known G6PD deficiency, use 500 mg ascorbic acid orally.

be made to identify an oxidant stress and, once identified, to remove the causative substance. If symptoms are mild after oxidant exposure, therapy is unnecessary. If the symptoms are severe, 1 to 2 mg/kg methylene blue as a 1% solution in saline should be infused over 5 minutes. A second dose can be given if symptoms are present 1 hour later.

DISORDERS OF WHITE BLOOD CELLS

Neutropenia

The most common forms of neutropenia and abnormal neutrophil function are listed in Table 10.10. When the neutrophil count falls below 500/mm^3, the patient exhibits an increased susceptibility to infection.

The management of localized infection or unexplained fever in the child with neutropenia depends in large part on the underlying disorder and on the patient's history of infection. In neutropenic states associated with repeated, severe infections, an aggressive attempt to identify a causative organism should be undertaken. Blood and urine cultures, along with appropriate cultures from identified areas of infection (e.g., skin abscess, cellulitis), should be obtained. The cerebrospinal fluid should be examined and cultured when CNS infection is suspected.

A particularly perplexing problem arises when a child is found to be neutropenic during an evaluation of fever. In most instances, both the fever and neutropenia are the result of a viral illness. Under these circumstances, serious secondary bacterial infections are unlikely to occur, and admission to the hospital and antibiotic therapy are probably unnecessary. However, because the neutropenia usually cannot be attributed with certainty to a viral illness, other causes of neutropenia should be carefully sought.

DISORDERS OF PLATELETS

Idiopathic Thrombocytopenic Purpura

The diagnosis of idiopathic thrombocytopenic purpura (ITP) is made readily in the child with newly acquired pe-

TABLE 10.10 *Causes of neutropenia and disorders of neutrophil function in children*

Congenital neutropenia
    Kostmann syndrome (infantile agranulocytosis)
    Chronic benign neutropenia
    Neutropenia associated with immunoglobulin disorders
    Reticular dysgenesis
    Neutropenias associated with phenotypic abnormalities (metaphyseal chondrodysplasia, cartilage hair hypoplasia)
    Cyclic neutropenia
Acquired neutropenias
    Drugs and chemical toxins
    Infection (bacterial, viral, rickettsial, protozoal)
    Bone marrow infiltration (leukemia, neuroblastoma, lymphoma)
    Nutritional deficiencies (starvation, anorexia nervosa, vitamin B_{12}, folate, copper deficiencies)
    Immune neutropenias (collagen vascular disease, Felty syndrome, neonatal isoimmune neutropenia, autoimmune neutropenia, transfusion reactions)
Disorders of neutrophil function
    Cellular defects of chemotaxis (Job syndrome, "lazy leukocyte" syndrome, congenital ichthyosis, chronic renal failure, diabetes, rheumatoid arthritis, bone marrow transplantation, malnutrition, infection)
    Secondary defects of chemotaxis (Chediak–Higashi syndrome, hypogammaglobulinemia, chronic mucocutaneous candidiasis, Wiskott–Aldrich syndrome, chronic granulomatous disease)
    Complement abnormalities and congenital absence of opsonin system
    Disorders of degranulation (Chediak–Higashi syndrome)
    Defective peroxidative killing of bacteria and fungi (chronic granulomatous disease, myeloperoxidase deficiency)
    Acquired disorders of phagocytic dysfunction (severe iron deficiency, malnutrition, malignancies, severe burns)

common side effects of intravenous γ-globulin is headache, and when this symptom persists despite slowing the rate of infusion, imaging studies of the brain may be necessary to investigate possible intracranial bleeding. An alternative approach to the treatment of the stable patient with ITP is a 4- to 8-week course of prednisone, beginning with 2 mg/kg per day. Some physicians have argued that a bone marrow aspirate to confirm the diagnosis of ITP is unnecessary in the patient with typical findings of the disorder and an absence of neutropenia or anemia.

Currently, the most common option for treatment of acute ITP is the administration of antibody directed against the D antigen of red cells. The effect of this antibody, usually given at a dose of 50 g/kg by intravenous infusion, is slightly de-

techiae (Figs. 10.14 and 10.15) and ecchymoses, thrombocytopenia, normal or increased megakaryocytes in the bone marrow (Fig. 10.16), and the absence of any underlying disease. Epistaxis, gum bleeding, and hematuria occur less commonly than simple bruising and petechiae, but when persistent, these hemorrhagic manifestations can lead to moderate or even severe anemia. In teenage girls with ITP, heavy and prolonged menstrual bleeding can also cause a severe decrease in the hemoglobin level. Fortunately, the development of anemia in children with ITP is gradual; acute, massive blood loss is extremely rare. The major life-threatening complication of ITP is intracranial hemorrhage.

Controversy continues to surround the management of the patient with newly diagnosed ITP who has no serious bleeding. Until recently, the three approaches have included withholding therapy, intravenous γ-globulin, and corticosteroids. In many centers, patients are treated with γ-globulin at a dose of 0.8 to 1.0 g/kg by intravenous infusion, with a second dose 24 hours later if the platelet count remains less than 40,000 to 50,000/mm³. Unfortunately, one of the more

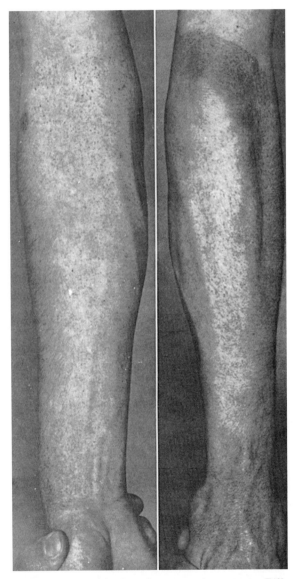

FIG. 10.14. Idiopathic thrombocytopenic purpura. Diffuse petechial rash induced by a tourniquet in a patient with chronic idiopathic thrombocytopenic purpura. (From Lee G, Foerster J, Lukens J, et al. *Wintrobe's clinical hematology*, 10th ed. Philadelphia: Lippincott Williams & Wilkins, 1998:1588 and 1559, with permission.)

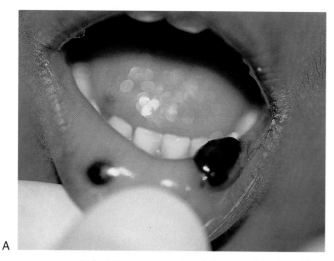

A

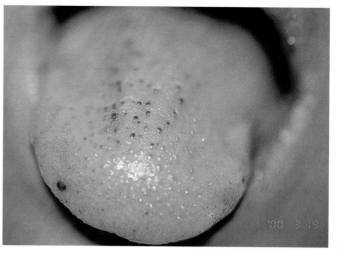

B

FIG. 10.15. Hemorrhagic bullae of the lips **(A)** and petechiae on the tongue **(B)** mark the presentation of this child with idiopathic thrombocytopenic purpura.

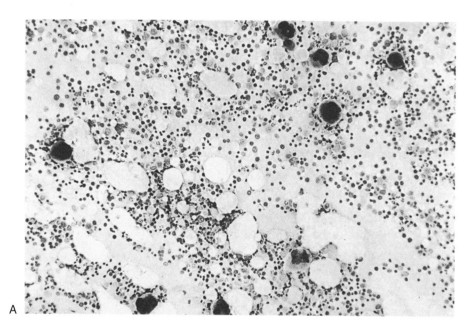

A

FIG. 10.16. Marrow film. **A:** Idiopathic thrombocytopenic purpura. In this condition, there is a marked increase in the number of megakaryocytes which are non–platelet producing. Many young forms of these cells are usually presented. **B:** The illustration is a typical example of the low-power microscopic appearance in this condition. (From McDonald GA, Dodds TC, Cruickshank B, eds. *Atlas of hematology*, 3rd ed. Edinburgh: E & S Livingstone, 1970:141, with permission.)

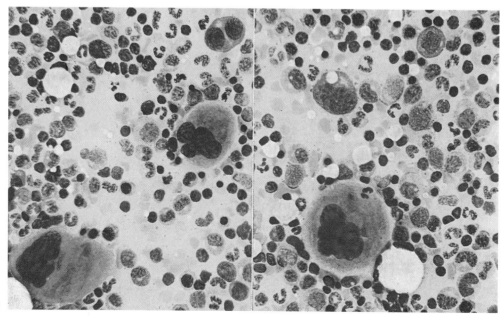

B

TABLE 10.11. *Management of head trauma in idiopathic thrombocytopenic purpura*

Mild head trauma without neurologic findings
  Observe carefully
  Administer 0.8–1.0 g/kg γ-globulin by IV infusion or 50 μg/kg anti-D if:
    Platelet count is 20,000/mm³
    Signs of easy or spontaneous bleeding (e.g., bruises, petechiae)
    Patient is within 1 wk of diagnosis of idiopathic thrombocytopenic purpura
    Follow-up is uncertain
Severe head trauma or neurologic abnormalities
  8–10 mg/kg IV hydrocortisone
  0.8–1.0 g/kg γ-globulin by IV infusion
  Platelet transfusion 0.4 μ/kg
  If neurologic changes are severe or progressive or if no response to earlier measures:
    Perform splenectomy
    Exchange transfusion or plasmapheresis, followed by platelet transfusion

IV, intravenous.

layed compared with γ-globulin, and the peak platelet count may be somewhat lower. However, anti-D antigen antibody has the advantage of being administered over minutes rather than hours, and it rarely causes severe headache. Mild to moderate hemolysis may follow the administration of anti-D antigen antibody with a fall in hemoglobin level of 0.5 to 2.0 g/dL. This therapy is effective only in Rh-positive patients.

If severe head trauma has occurred or if neurologic abnormalities are present, 8 to 10 mg/kg hydrocortisone and 0.8 to 1.0 g/kg γ-globulin should be administered intravenously and random donor platelets (0.4 U/kg; maximum, 20 units) should be infused immediately thereafter. If necessary, the volume of plasma in the platelet preparation can be reduced by centrifuging the platelets, removing a portion of the plasma, and resuspending the platelets. If the platelet count of a patient with ITP and intracranial bleeding does not increase after steroids, γ-globulin, and platelet transfusions or if the initial neurologic changes are severe, the patient should undergo splenectomy and, if appropriate, neurosurgical exploration (Table 10.11).

DISORDERS OF COAGULATION

Inherited Bleeding Disorders

Joint Bleeding

Hemarthroses (Fig. 10.17) and bleeding into the soft tissues (Fig. 10.18) are common complications in hemophilia that often occur in the absence of known trauma in severe disease. Initial replacement therapy should be designed to raise the factor level to 30% to 50% (Table 10.12). Some centers treat all joint bleeds with one or two additional doses of factor replacement, whereas others reserve further treatment for patients with persistent pain or increasing swelling. Initial immobilization of the joint is often helpful and can be easily accomplished with a splint.

Bleeding in the hip is a particularly serious problem. As the joint becomes distended, blood flow to the femoral head may be impeded, resulting in aseptic necrosis. A radiograph of the hip shows widening of the joint space, and ultrasonography may demonstrate fluid (Fig. 10.19). Because of the importance of achieving and maintaining hemostasis in this joint, initial correction to 70% to 100% is usually followed by several days of continuing replacement therapy (30% to 50% correction every 12 hours for factor VIII deficiency or every 24 hours for factor IX deficiency). Hospitalization may be required for immobilization, using either strict bed rest or traction.

Muscle Bleeding

Most muscle bleeding is superficial and easily controlled with a single dose of replacement therapy to achieve 30% to 50% correction. However, emergencies may arise when substantial blood loss occurs or when nerve function is impaired. Extensive hemorrhage is most commonly found in retroperitoneal bleeds (e.g., ilealpsoas) or thigh bleeds (Fig. 10.20). Retroperitoneal bleeds are often accompanied by lower abdominal pain. A mass is sometimes palpable deep in the abdomen, and sensation in the distribution of the femoral nerve may be diminished. Loss of the psoas shadow may be seen on an abdominal radiograph, and a hematoma may be demonstrated by ultrasonography (Fig. 10.21).

Subcutaneous Bleeding

Hemorrhage under the skin may cause extensive discoloration but is rarely dangerous and usually requires no therapy unless compression of critical organs occurs. However, pressure on the airway from a subcutaneous bleed of the neck may be life threatening, requiring steps to ensure airway patency, such as placement of an endotracheal tube, in addition to correction of the factor level to 100%. Careful observation of children with bleeding in the muscles of the neck is mandatory because airway obstruction may be sudden.

Oral Bleeding

Mouth bleeds are particularly common in young children with hemophilia (Fig. 10.22). The site of bleeding should be identified. If a weak clot is present, it should be removed and dry topical thrombin placed on the site. Initial correction should be 70% to 100%. Often, one or more additional treatments are necessary to achieve adequate clot formation and to prevent rebleeding when the clot falls off. The antifibrinolytic agents, ε-aminocaproic acid and tranexamic acid,

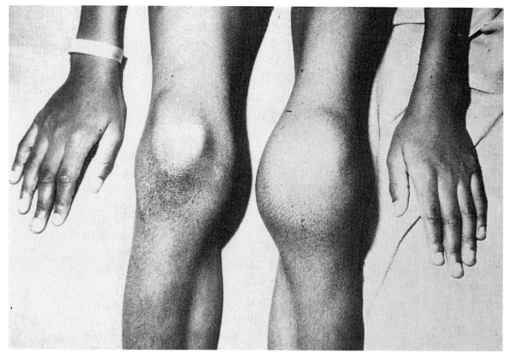

FIG. 10.17. Acute hemarthrosis and its sequelae in a patient with hemophilia B. Note the periarticular swelling in the left leg and the marked atrophy of the thigh muscles as a result of recurrent hemarthrosis. (From Lee G, Foerster J, Lukens J, et al. *Wintrobe's clinical hematology*, 10th ed. Philadelphia: Lippincott Williams & Wilkins, 1998:1560, with permission.)

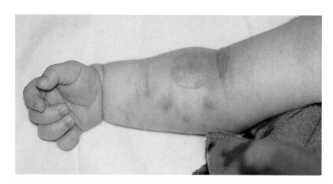

FIG. 10.18. This 4-week-old infant with factor VIII deficiency developed a hematoma of the forearm. Previously, he had experienced prolonged bleeding after circumcision.

TABLE 10.12. *Specific factor deficiencies and replacement therapy*

Factor deficiency	Replacement therapy
Fibrinogen (I) (also dysfibrinogenemias)	Cryoprecipitate Fresh frozen plasma
Prothrombin (II)	Fresh frozen plasma Prothrombin complex concentrates
Factor V	Fresh frozen plasma
Factor VII	Fresh frozen plasma Prothrombin complex concentrates Factor VIIa (recombinant) concentrates
Factor VIII	Factor VIII concentrates DDAVP
Factor IX	Prothrombin complex concentrates Factor IX concentrates
Factor X	Fresh frozen plasma Prothrombin complex concentrates
Factor XI	Fresh frozen plasma
Factor XIII	Cryoprecipitate Fresh frozen plasma
von Willebrand disease	DDAVP Same factor VIII concentrates

DDAVP, 1-deamino-8-D-arginine vasopressin.

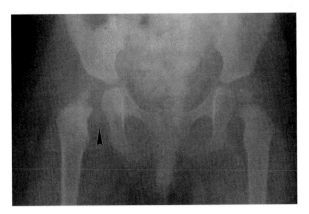

FIG. 10.19. Hip joint widening and joint fluid· Widening of the right hip joint (*arrow*) with congenital dislocation. Note delayed ossification of right femoral head and increased steepness of acetabular roof. Ultrasonographic findings of hip joint fluid. (From Swischuk LE, John SD. *Differential diagnosis in pediatric radiology*, 2nd ed. Philadelphia: Lippincott Williams & Wilkins, 1994:303, with permission.)

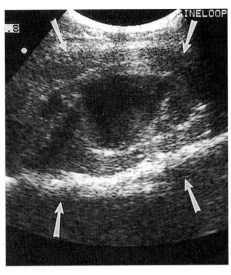

FIG. 10.21. Psoas hematoma. Ultrasonography demonstrates the expanded psoas muscle (*arrows*), which contains a hypoechoic fluid collection (blood). (From Swischuk LE. *Imaging of the newborn, infant and young child*, 4th ed. Philadelphia: Lippincott Williams & Wilkins, 1997:558, with permission.)

are useful adjuncts in the treatment of oral bleeding. ε-Aminocaproic acid should be administered orally for 5 days at a dose of 100 mg/kg every 6 hours, with a maximum of 24 g per day. Tranexamic acid is administered orally at a dose of 25 mg/kg three or four times daily. Because children may swallow a substantial amount of blood, actual acute blood loss may be underestimated by the patient or family, and measurement of the hemoglobin level is helpful.

Gastrointestinal Bleeding

Hemorrhage from the gastrointestinal tract is rarely severe in hemophilia unless an anatomic lesion such as a duodenal ulcer or diverticulum is present. Maintenance of the factor level above 30% to 50% for 2 or 3 days after initial correction to 70% to 100% is usually sufficient. If bleeding persists, appropriate diagnostic studies are necessary. A careful search for infectious causes of gastrointestinal bleeding is important in human immunodeficiency virus (HIV)–positive hemophiliacs.

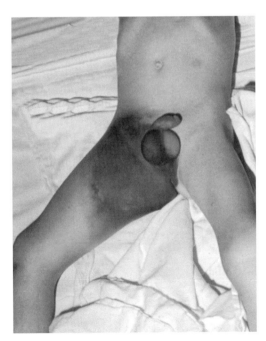

FIG. 10.20. Large dissecting hematoma of thigh in a patient with hemophilia A. The lesion resulted from a slight bump to the inguinal area and spread to involve the entire thigh. (From Lee G, Foerster J, Lukens J, et al. *Wintrobe's clinical hematology*, 10th ed. Philadelphia: Lippincott Williams & Wilkins, 1998:1559, with permission.)

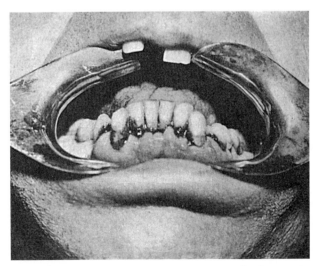

FIG. 10.22. Bleeding gums in a patient with aplastic anemia. (From Lee G, Foerster J, Lukens J, et al. *Wintrobe's clinical hematology*, 10th ed. Philadelphia: Lippincott Williams & Wilkins, 1998:1460, with permission.)

Urinary Tract Bleeding

Atraumatic, painless hematuria is the most common manifestation of renal bleeding in children with hemophilia. In the absence of trauma or a demonstrable lesion, several approaches to ensuring hemostasis seem equally effective. Bed rest without replacement therapy is often successful. In some centers, one or more doses of factor replacement (70% to 100%) are used in combination with bed rest for at least 24 hours after gross hematuria has ceased. A brief course of orally administered prednisone has also been effective. When the child with hemophilia develops hematuria or flank tenderness after trauma, a more aggressive approach to diagnosis and treatment is required.

Intracranial Hemorrhage

In practical terms, however, head trauma in children with hemophilia is common, whereas intracranial hemorrhage is comparatively rare. Thus, the physician must be able to recognize and treat the child at risk without exposing other patients to unnecessary hospitalization, diagnostic studies, or therapy.

Management of the child with hemophilia with head trauma but no neurologic signs requires careful attention to the severity of the bleeding disorder, type of trauma, history of intracranial bleeding, and likelihood of close follow-up. Children with seemingly insignificant trauma may develop the first obvious signs of intracranial bleeding several days later when concern has diminished. To prevent such occurrences, every child with severe hemophilia and reported head trauma is treated with at least one dose of replacement therapy in some centers. However, this approach carries the risk and expense of frequent therapy. Moreover, in an effort to prevent yet another visit to the emergency department, the child or parent may fail to report a serious episode of trauma. Consequently, other centers use an approach that is still conservative, although slightly less rigid. If the trauma is mild (e.g., a light bump on the forehead), the child is observed at home for the usual signs of intracranial hemorrhage or increased intracranial pressure. When the trauma is somewhat more substantial (e.g., falling down two or three carpeted stairs), the child with severe hemophilia is evaluated by the physician, given replacement therapy to achieve a level of 70% to 100%, observed for several hours in the office or emergency department and, if well, is discharged. The child with mild hemophilia usually does not need replacement therapy under these circumstances, whereas the child with moderate hemophilia needs particularly careful attention to the type of trauma and bleeding history for the physician to decide whether to use replacement therapy. A computed tomography scan may be useful in identifying intracranial bleeding that requires more intensive and prolonged treatment (Fig. 10.23). However, the imaging study should not be used to decide on administration of an initial dose of replacement factor that should, in fact, always be given before the study is performed to avoid unnecessary delays.

If more severe trauma (e.g., hitting the head on the dashboard, falling off a changing table onto a hard floor) has occurred in any child with hemophilia, hospital admission and repeated doses of replacement therapy are essential. The initial dose of replacement should be administered as soon as it is available. A computed tomography scan should be performed after initial correction to search for intracranial bleeding and help to determine the duration of treatment.

The management of the patient with hemophilia who has neurologic findings in the presence or absence of head trauma begins with replacement therapy and those measures required for life support and treatment of increased intracranial pressure. Levels of the appropriate factor should be raised to 100%. The indications for surgery are similar to

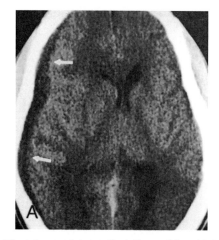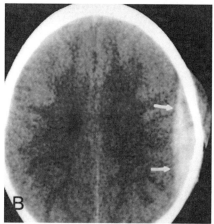

FIG. 10.23. Intracranial manifestations of head injury. **A:** Note the hypodense subdural hematoma (*arrows*). There is ipsilateral compression of the ventricles and contralateral midline shift. **B:** Epidural bleed (*arrows*) with some soft-tissue swelling of the scalp. (From Swischuk LE. *Emergency imaging of the acutely ill or injured child*, 3rd ed. Philadelphia: Lippincott Williams & Wilkins, 1994:595, with permission.)

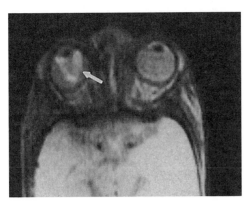

FIG. 10.24. Intraocular hemorrhage. Note the area of increased density within the globe (*arrow*). (From Swischuk LE. *Imaging of the newborn, infant and young child*, 4th ed. Philadelphia: Lippincott Williams & Wilkins, 1997:1015, with permission.)

those for children without coagulation disorders, provided an appropriate correction of clotting abnormalities has been achieved.

Acute neurologic changes, such as decreasing level of consciousness or seizures, may result from direct HIV infection of the brain or from associated infections that affect the immunocompromised host. In the HIV-positive hemo-

philiac patient, these changes may mimic the signs and symptoms of intracranial hemorrhage. Similarly, changes in vision that result from retinitis caused by cytomegalovirus may be similar to visual changes caused by intraocular bleeding (Fig. 10.24). The physician evaluating an HIV-positive hemophiliac patient with new neurologic findings should consider both infectious and hemorrhagic causes, and the absence of demonstrable hemorrhage on imaging studies should prompt careful attention to HIV-related disorders.

Bleeding in von Willebrand Disease

The sites of bleeding in mild von Willebrand disease resemble those found in patients with platelet disorders. Epistaxis, oral bleeding, and menorrhagia are common, whereas joint bleeding is very unusual. Children affected with more severe forms, in which the factor VIII level is very low, may have bleeding problems that resemble those found in both hemophilia and von Willebrand disease.

INHERITED HYPERCOAGULABLE CONDITIONS

Thrombotic events occur rarely in children and only slightly more often in adolescents (Fig. 10.25). The three

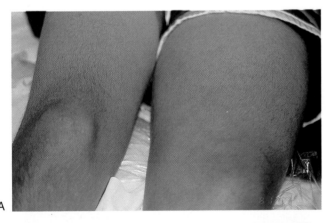

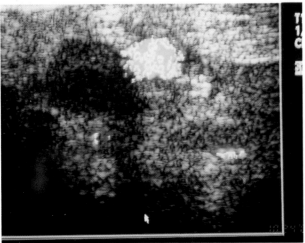

A

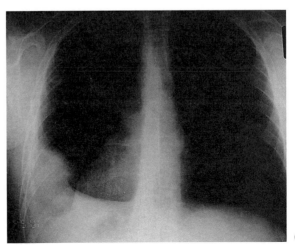

C

FIG. 10.25. A: This 15-year-old boy developed swelling of his left thigh and leg. **B:** Doppler ultrasonography demonstrates a thrombosis in the left iliofemoral vein. **C:** After a 5-day hospitalization and the initiation of an anticoagulation regimen, he developed a pulmonary embolus, manifesting as an infiltrate and a pleural effusion on his chest radiograph.

B

major proteins that serve as brakes on the coagulation pathway are antithrombin III, protein C, and protein S. The most common inherited cause of thrombosis, factor V Leiden, is a single gene mutation that alters the amino acid composition of factor V and makes this coagulation protein resistant to the antithrombotic activity of protein C. Patients who are heterozygous for antithrombin III, protein C, protein S deficiency, or factor V Leiden and who develop a venous thrombosis should be treated with heparin by intravenous infusion. Treatment is usually initiated with a bolus injection of 50 to 100 U/kg body weight followed by a constant infusion of 25 U/kg per hour. The heparin dose should be adjusted to maintain the partial thromboplastin time between 1.5 and 2.0 times normal. Once adequate anticoagulation with heparin has been achieved, warfarin should be given orally.

Newborns with homozygous protein C deficiency and purpura fulminans should receive 8 to 12 mL/kg body weight fresh frozen plasma every 12 hours. Long-term therapy includes regular infusions of fresh frozen plasma or oral anticoagulation. Cryoprecipitate plays an analogous role in the acute and chronic therapy of homozygous protein S deficiency.

ONCOLOGIC EMERGENCIES

Leukemia

Table 10.13 outlines the initial care of patients with acute leukemia. Fortunately, most patients require only general supportive care. However, some patients require immediate intervention for specific life-threatening problems. All patients and their families require emotional support and sensitivity to deal with the fear and disorientation that they feel when confronted with the diagnosis of cancer.

Hematologic Complications

Anemia

At the time of diagnosis, most children with leukemia are anemic. If the hemoglobin is less than 8 g/dL, administration of packed blood cells is advisable because the child is unlikely to have the ability to produce erythrocytes for several weeks; however, if the child is not having symptoms or showing signs of severe anemia, transfusion does not need to take place in the emergency department. If, in the absence of hemorrhage, the child has profound anemia (hemoglobin, 1 to 4 g/dL), transfusions at the usual rate can precipitate heart failure. Blood should be replaced slowly, at 3 to 5 mL/kg over 4 hours, and supplemental oxygen should be given to enhance oxygen delivery to tissues. Furosemide (1 mg/kg) can help avoid fluid overload or heart failure.

Hemorrhage

In most newly diagnosed leukemic children, bleeding problems can be controlled with local measures alone (i.e., pressure and topical thrombin for epistaxis) or in conjunction with platelet transfusions (0.2 U/kg platelets). Epistaxis is sometimes a serious problem that may last for hours and may fail to respond to pressure. If local measures and platelets fail, packing is a necessary but uncomfortable therapy.

In some patients with acute monocytic leukemia, especially those with hypergranular promyelocytic leukemia and some with monoblastic leukemia, a bleeding diathesis may occur at presentation or on initiation of therapy. Bleeding is generally refractory to platelet transfusion.

Patients show prolonged prothrombin and partial thromboplastin times, elevated fibrin split products, and a drastically shortened fibrinogen half-life. The most common form of bleeding in this situation is in the CNS; it may be fatal in the first few days of illness. Fresh frozen plasma (10 mL/kg) and cryoprecipitate can help to maintain levels of fibrinogen and clotting factors. Platelet transfusions (0.2 U/kg) are given to correct thrombocytopenia. Heparinization (loading dose, 50 U/kg; then 5 to 10 U/kg per hour to maintain the partial thromboplastin time at approximately 1.5 times normal) is often given to patients who show no improvement with aggressive blood product support.

Extreme Leukocytosis

In acute leukemia, extreme leukocytosis predisposes patients to early bleeding and thrombosis in the CNS. Hydration and alkalinization often result in a substantially lower white blood cell count (Table 10.13).

Infectious Complications

Although fever is a symptom of leukemia in 25% of patients, more often it indicates infection. Management of fever begins with a thorough physical examination to search for localizing signs of infection. Even an apparently minor swelling or a tear in the skin or a mucosal surface can be a source of disseminated infection. A chest radiograph is needed only if the child has respiratory symptoms or signs (Fig. 10.26). Bacterial meningitis is rare in leukemia, but if symptoms of meningitis are found, spinal fluid should be sent for bacterial, fungal, and viral culture and for cytology to rule out CNS leukemia.

After the appropriate cultures are obtained, intravenous broad-spectrum antibiotics should be started in a patient with leukemia and fever.

TABLE 10.13. *Emergency department care of the patient with probable or certain acute leukemia*

Communication
1. Call referring physician to obtain medical and social histories
2. Call consulting pediatric hematologist/oncologist
3. Review possible diagnoses with family and be available to answer questions
4. Contact support staff (social worker or psychologist) who can assist the family with psychological stress

Initial C diagnostic studies
1. Complete blood count with manual differential
2. Electrolytes, include K, Ca^{2+}, phosphorus
3. Blood urea nitrogen, creatinine, uric acid
4. Coagulation studies (PT and PTT)
5, Blood group, type, antibody screen, complete red blood cell antigen typing
6. Liver function tests to include lactate dehydrogenase
7. Chest radiograph to assess for infection or mediastinal mass
8. Blood cultures if patient is febrile
9. Do not perform bone marrow aspirate

General supportive care
1. In patients with high WBC count, large liver and/or spleen, or mediastinal mass or electrolytes suggesting tumor lysis, obtain intravenous access and start D5W/0.25 NS 40 mEq/L $NaHCO_2$ at 1.5–2 times maintenance (no KCl); stop $NaHCO_2$ after 24 hr.
2. 150 mg/d allopurinol t.i.d. if 6 yr old or 300 mg/d t.i.d if >6 yr old for 3–4 d.
3. Transfuse if symptomatic from hemorrhage, heart failure, shock. Write order for blood products: "All blood products should be irradiated and cytomegalovirus negative (or frozen and reconstituted), and given with an in-line leukocyte-depletion filter until further notice."
4. Begin broad-spectrum antibiotics if patient is febrile and appears toxic or has foci of infection.
5. Do not begin corticosteroid.

Specific problems that require immediate intervention

Problem	Laboratory data	Therapy
Anemia	Hgb 8–10 g/dL 4–6 g/dL <4 g/dL	Transfuse 10 mL/kg PRBCs over 4 hr, if symptomatic and no contraindications (e.g., WBC count >100,000) Transfusions of 5 mL/kg PRBCs until Hgb 8–10 Transfusion of PRBCs = mL/kg Hgb level over 4 hr (e.g., Hgb = 3, then 3 mL/kg initial transfusion) Consider supplemental oxygen
Thrombocytopenia	Platelet count ≥20,000/mm³ <20,000/mm³	No therapy unless signs of hemorrhage Platelet transfusion: 0.1–0.2 U/kg up to 6 units
Hemorrhage	PT, PTT, fibrinogen, and fibrin split products Platelet count <50,000/mm³	Give 5 mg vitamin K intravenously 10 mL/kg fresh frozen plasma Platelet transfusion: 0.1–0.2 U/kg to 6 units
Hyperleukocytosis	WBC count >200,000/mm³ or massive tumor burden (i.e., liver or spleen below umbilicus, multiple nodes >5 cm², anterior mediastinal mass)	Increase intravenous fluids to 2–4 maintenance Allopurinol, as above; follow electrolytes, blood urea nitrogen, creatinine, and uric acid at least every 6 hr until stable Consider radiation therapy for superior vena cava syndrome (see text) Therapy for acute renal failure as needed Consideration of leukocytopheresis
Fever	Blood and urine culture Additional cultures from site of local symptoms; chest radiograph; no lumbar puncture unless meningeal signs present	At diagnosis, consider all patients to be neutropenic despite actual WBC count, empiric broad-spectrum antibiotics; observe closely for signs of poor perfusion and treat for shock as needed
Metabolic	Electrolytes, blood urea nitrogen, uric acid, every 6 hr, until stable	See under hyperleukocytosis; correct specific abnormality
Pain	Search for specific cause (i.e., pathologic fracture) with examination and radiographs	Specific antineoplastic therapy; no aspirin; acetaminophen, codeine, or other narcotics as needed

PT, prothrombin time; PTT, partial thromboplastin time; WBC, white blood cell; D5W, 5% dextrose in water solution; NSS, normal saline solution; t.i.d., three times daily; Hgb, hemoglobin; PRBCs, packed red blood cells.

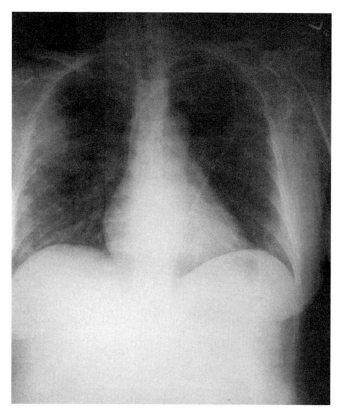

FIG. 10.26. Chest radiograph of a patient with acute leukemia who developed pulmonary *Aspergillus* infection after prolonged chemotherapy-induced neutropenia. (From Lee G, Foerster J, Lukens J, et al. *Wintrobe's clinical hematology*, 10th ed. Philadelphia: Lippincott Williams & Wilkins, 1998:2112, with permission.)

Metabolic Complications

Uric Acid Nephropathy

To prevent urate nephropathy, all children with leukemia should receive the xanthine oxidase inhibitor allopurinol (150 mg per day orally in three doses for those 6 years old or younger; 300 mg per day orally in three doses for those older than 6 years) for at least 24 hours before starting therapy. Hydration at the rate of twice maintenance and alkalinization of urine to pH between 6.5 and 7.5 with sodium bicarbonate (40 mEq/L) facilitates dissolution of uric acid crystals.

Hypercalcemia

Interim supportive management consists of hydration with normal saline (200 mL/m² per hour), followed by diuresis with furosemide (1 to 2 mg/kg intravenously every 4 to 6 hours). Corticosteroids, calcitonin, gallium nitrate, or dialysis may be indicated in symptomatic hypercalcemia (usually greater than 12 to 15 mg/dL).

Tumor Lysis Syndrome

Antineoplastic therapy can cause a potentially fatal tumor lysis syndrome that consists of a rapid increase in serum potassium and phosphorus, a precipitous decrease in serum calcium, and elevations of the serum uric acid, blood urea nitrogen, and creatinine. Hyperkalemia, the most dangerous abnormality, demands prompt treatment with Kayexalate (sodium polystyrene sulfonate), insulin and glucose infusion, or dialysis.

Other Complications

Spinal Cord Compression

Symptoms include radicular pain, back pain, difficulty with urination, paresis, and paralysis. Therapy consists of immediate corticosteroid administration (0.25 to 0.5 mg/kg dexamethasone every 6 hours), prompt irradiation, or both. Leukemia and lymphoma of the spinal cord respond to steroids or radiation therapy and do not require laminectomy.

Thoracic Tumors

Anterior Mediastinum. Hodgkin disease and non-Hodgkin lymphoma are the most common malignant tumors of the anterior mediastinum. Other tumors (Fig. 10.27) include thymoma (Fig. 10.28), thymic cyst, thymic hyperplasia, teratoma, ectopic thyroid, thyroid carcinoma, sarcomas, neuroblastoma (rarely), lymphangiomas, and inflammatory processes such as sarcoid. Half of anterior mediastinal masses are benign. However, almost all large tumors and masses that cause compromise to the great vessels or cause pleural effusions are malignant.

Large tumors in the anterior mediastinum can cause tracheal narrowing, superior vena cava syndrome (Fig. 10.29), or both. Tracheal compression causes tracheal deviation, stridor, cough, dyspnea, and orthopnea. Compression of the vena cava by tumor may cause headache, dyspnea, orthopnea, syncope,

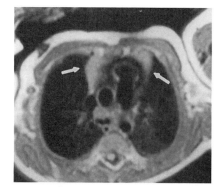

FIG. 10.27. Normal thymus. Axial view demonstrates the anterior position of the thymus. (From Swischuk LE. *Imaging of the newborn, infant and young child*, 4th ed. Philadelphia: Lippincott Williams & Wilkins, 1997:25, with permission.)

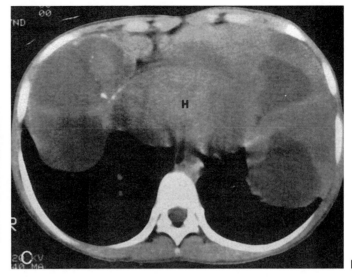

FIG. 10.28. Thymoma. **A:** Plain film demonstrates a large mediastinal mass. **B:** Axial computed tomography demonstrates the anterior position of this large mediastinal mass confirming again the mixed cystic and solid configuration. It encircles the heart (*H*), and small flecks of calcium are seen on the right. (From Swischuk LE. *Imaging of the newborn, infant and young child*, 4th ed. Philadelphia: Lippincott Williams & Wilkins, 1997:24, with permission.)

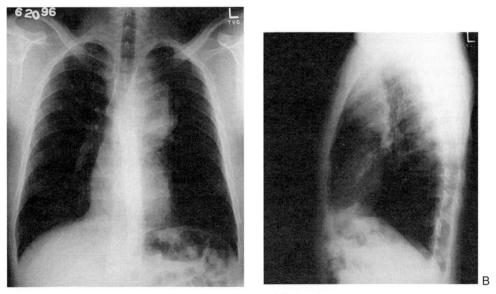

FIG. 10.29. A: A patient with an anterior mediastinal mass due to large B-cell lymphoma developed superior vena cava syndrome. Hematologic neoplasms associated with superior vena cava syndrome include lymphoblastic lymphoma, Hodgkin disease, and large B-cell lymphoma. **B:** Lateral view. (From Lee G, Foerster J, Lukens J, et al. *Wintrobe's clinical hematology*, 10th ed. Philadelphia: Lippincott Williams & Wilkins, 1998:2047, with permission.)

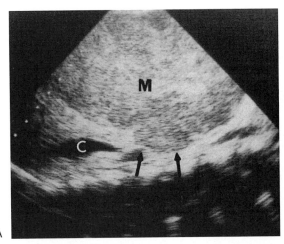
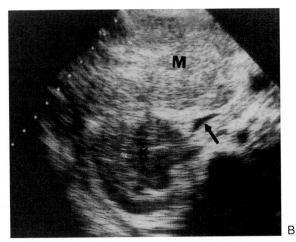

FIG. 10.30. Wilms tumor: caval compression. **A:** Note the large tumor mass (*M*) and a nodule of tumor (*arrows*) compressing the inferior vena cava *C*. **B:** Transverse sonogram demonstrates the large mass (*M*) and the compressed inferior vena cava (*arrow*). (From Swischuk LE. *Imaging of the newborn, infant and young child*, 4th ed. Philadelphia: Lippincott Williams & Wilkins, 1997:607, with permission.)

or cardiovascular collapse (Fig. 10.30). Physical examination may be unremarkable or may show venous distention, plethora, cyanosis, and edema anatomically confined to the head, neck, thorax, and arms. When the arm is involved, the veins will remain full when the arm is raised. Conjunctival and retinal vessels may be engorged. Children with superior vena cava syndrome are often anxious and diaphoretic and will resist efforts to place them in a supine position. When these findings are present, narcotics, sedatives, and any drugs that interfere with venous return are contraindicated. A chest radiograph reveals a mass in the anterior mediastinum (Fig. 10.31). If a tumor is causing superior vena cava syndrome in a child or adolescent, the diagnosis is almost certain to be non-Hodgkin lymphoma or Hodgkin disease.

Neuroblastoma

Treatment of a neuroblastoma is directed toward both the tumor itself and complications of the tumor. Emergency physicians need to recognize special conditions in neuroblastoma.

Massive hepatomegaly in a neonate or infant can cause hepatic failure or respiratory embarrassment (Fig. 10.32). These children need to be admitted for supportive care. Dumbbell tumors can cause cord compression (Fig. 10.33). Treatment may consist of chemotherapy, laminectomy, surgical removal, and irradiation. Children with a neuroblastoma and fever and neutropenia need to be managed similarly to children with leukemia (Fig. 10.34).

Central Nervous System Tumors

The role of the emergency physician in the management of CNS tumors is one of recognizing CNS lesions, performing

the initial diagnostic procedures to establish the presence of the lesion, and stabilizing the patient who has a life-threatening increase in intracranial pressure or spinal cord compression. Lumbar puncture is rarely useful in the initial evaluation of a child with a CNS tumor. If focal neurologic signs or signs of in-

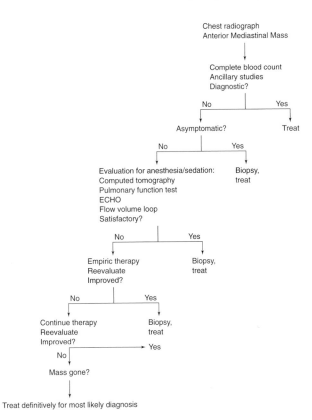

FIG. 10.31. Management guidelines for children with an anterior mediastinal mass who are at risk of superior vena cava syndrome.

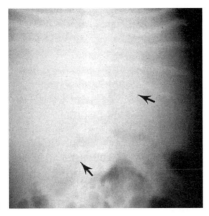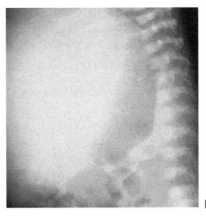

FIG. 10.32. Neuroblastoma in neonate. **A:** Note the large liver (*arrows*). **B:** Lateral view demonstrates similar enlargement. (From Swischuk LE. *Imaging of the newborn, infant and young child*, 4th ed. Philadelphia: Lippincott Williams & Wilkins, 1997:665, with permission.)

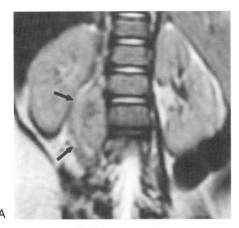

creased intracranial pressure are present, a computed tomography scan should precede any attempt to perform a lumbar puncture. Increased intracranial pressure may be treated with the administration of 0.5 to 1.0 mg/kg dexamethasone per day in four divided doses and diuretics, such as 1 to 2 g/kg mannitol over 30 to 60 minutes. Depending on the severity of the neurologic findings, intubation and hyperventilation may be indicated.

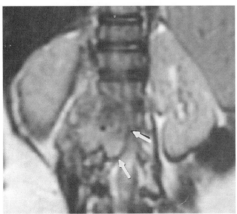

FIG. 10.33. Dumbbell neuroblastoma. **A:** Magnetic resonance T1-weighted coronal image. Note the small adrenal tumor (*arrows*) just medial to the ipsilateral kidney. **B:** A slightly more posterior cut demonstrates the tumor extending into the spinal canal (*arrows*). (From Swischuk LE. *Imaging of the newborn, infant, and young child*, 4th ed. Philadelphia: Lippincott Williams & Wilkins, 1997:674, with permission.)

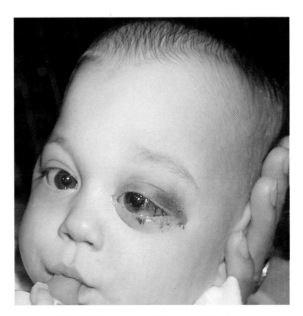

FIG. 10.34. Periorbital neuroblastoma.

SUGGESTED READINGS

Andrew M, Michelson AD, Bovill E, et al. Guidelines for antithrombotic therapy in pediatric patients. *J Pediatr* 1998;132:575–588.

DiMario FJ Jr, Packer RJ. Acute mental status changes in children with systemic cancer. *Pediatrics* 1990;85:353–360.

Ebb DH, Weinstein JH. Diagnosis and treatment of childhood acute myelogenous leukemia. *Pediatr Clin North Am* 1997;44:847–861.

Furie B, Limentani SA, Rosenfield CG. A practical guide to the evaluation and treatment of hemophilia. *Blood* 1994;84:3–9.

Hughes WT, Armstrong D, Bodey GP, et al. 1997 guidelines for the use of antimicrobial agents in neutropenic patients with unexplained fever. *Clin Infect Dis* 1997;25:551–573.

Kelly KM, Lange B. Oncologic emergencies. *Pediatr Clin North Am* 1997;44:809–830.

Lane PA. Sickle cell disease. *Pediatr Clin North Am* 1996;43:639–664.

Lusher J. Approach to the bleeding patient. In: Nathan DG, Orkin SH, eds. *Hematology of infancy and childhood*. Philadelphia: WB Saunders, 1998:1574–1584.

Medeiros D, Buchanan GR. Current controversies in the management of idiopathic thrombocytopenic purpura during childhood. *Pediatr Clin North Am* 1996;43:757–772.

Pizzo PA. Management of fever in patients with cancer and treatment-induced neutropenia. *N Engl J Med* 1993;328:1323–1332.

Pui CH. Acute lymphoblastic leukemia. *Pediatr Clin North Am* 1997;44:831–846.

Sanders JE. Bone marrow transplantation for pediatric malignancies. *Pediatr Clin North Am* 1997;44:1005–1020.

Silverman P, Distelhorst CW. Metabolic emergencies in clinical oncology. *Semin Oncol* 1989;16:504–515.

Vichinsky EP, Styles LA, Colangelo LH, et al. Acute chest syndrome in sickle cell disease: clinical presentation and course. Cooperative Study of Sickle Cell Disease. *Blood* 1997;89:1787–1792.

Young NS, Alter BP. *Aplastic anemia: acquired and inherited*. Philadelphia: WB Saunders, 1994.

CHAPTER 11

Infectious Disease Emergencies

Editor: Gary R. Fleisher

INFECTIOUS SYNDROMES

Bacteremia and Sepsis

Bacteremia

By definition, occult bacteremia causes few symptoms and signs. The complaints are usually malaise or an upper respiratory infection. Fever, without evidence of a source, may be the only physical finding, or the patient may have a minor focus of infection, such as otitis media. The white blood cell (WBC) count is usually elevated in children with bacteremia. The likelihood of bacteremia in a highly febrile (39°C, 102.2°F or higher) infant between 3 and 6 months of age (or in a child 6 to 24 months of age who has not received immunizations against *Haemophilus influenzae* and *Streptococcus pneumoniae*), coupled with the difficulties of clinical assessments in these children, makes obtaining a WBC count and blood culture useful in many cases but rarely mandatory (Fig. 11.1). In these situations, the finding of a WBC count of 15,000 to 20,000/mm^3 or more suggests a role for presumptive antibiotic therapy. For this group, 50 mg/kg intramuscular ceftriaxone has been demonstrated to be effective. In managing highly febrile, young children not thought to be at higher risk, observation at home without antibiotic therapy represents the usual choice of treatment.

Sepsis

Clinical Manifestations

Some children with sepsis are febrile for several days during a preceding bacteremia (Figs. 11.2 and 11.3), but others develop a sudden dramatic illness (Fig. 11.4). The interval between the initial fever and death may be less than 12 hours in fulminant meningococcemia. Although fever is the cardinal sign of infection, children younger than 2 to 3 months of age may remain afebrile. The child with continued sepsis progresses from malaise to profound lethargy and, finally, to obtundation. Tachycardia is an early finding, and hypotension

occurs later in the course. The skin becomes cold and poorly perfused (Fig. 11.5); additionally, petechiae and purpura may appear, particularly with *Neisseria meningitidis*.

Leukocytosis usually accompanies sepsis, but an overwhelming infection occasionally produces neutropenia. As the infection progresses, the platelet count decreases. A Gram stain of a petechial scraping shows the etiologic agent in one-third of cases.

Management

Although the initial therapy for sepsis is directed at the preservation of vital functions, every effort must be made to obtain the appropriate diagnostic studies (Table 11.1). Blood should be drawn for culture, and a complete blood count (CBC), platelet count, prothrombin time, partial thromboplastin time, electrolytes, chemistries, and hematologic analyses should be done in conjunction with the immediate insertion of an intravenous catheter. As initial therapy, normal saline, with or without 5% dextrose, is given at 20 mL/kg per hour or more rapidly depending on the response.

For children younger than 2 months of age, 200 mg/kg ampicillin and 7.5 mg/kg gentamicin per day are administered; 150 mg/kg cefotaxime per day may be used in place of gentamicin for the newborn (Table 11.2). Cefotaxime (200 mg/kg per day) or 100 mg/kg ceftriaxone per day alone provides effective monotherapy for the child older than 2 months of age. Vancomycin (40 mg/kg per day) may be added for patients who are critically ill or at particular risk of infection with penicillin-resistant *S. pneumoniae*, as in the case, for example, in a patient with sickle cell anemia on daily prophylactic penicillin. In the presence of a focus of infection likely to be staphylococcal, 150 mg/kg oxacillin per day can be used together with cefotaxime; alternatively, the combination of clavulanic acid and ampicillin (200 mg/kg per day) may be administered. Meropenem (60 to 120 mg/kg per day) should be kept in mind for children with allergies to penicillins and cephalosporins.

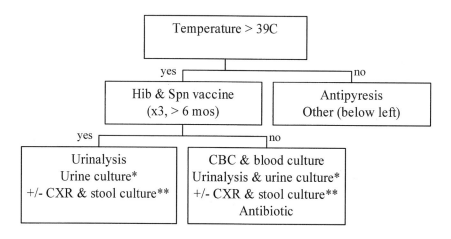

* Urine culture for (a) females < 24 months; (b) for males < 6 (12) months or + urinalysis
** CXR & stool culture for symptoms; CXR if WBC >20,000/mm³

Hib = Haemophilus influenzae type B
Spn = Streptococcus pneumoniae
CBC = complete blood count
CXR = chest x-ray

FIG. 11.1. Algorithm for the approach to the febrile child younger than 2 years of age. The concern for occult bacteremia and urinary tract infection prompts the use of testing for selected patients, particularly those who are youngest, highly febrile, and not immunized against bacterial pathogens. As discussed, antibiotic treatment (ceftriaxone) should be considered when leukocytosis (>15,000/mm³) is found.

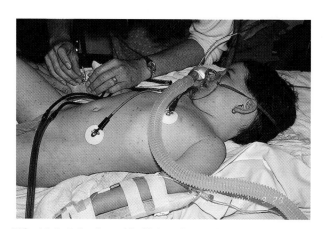

FIG. 11.2. Infection with *Neisseria meningitidis*. This young boy is in the early course of a meningococcal infection. He has scattered petechiae, some of which have reached the size of small purpura. Unlike the child in Figure 11.3, this patient does not have diffuse, confluent lesions. Although he was not critically ill on presentation, his treatment included aggressive supportive care and monitoring. Meningococcemia progresses rapidly in many cases.

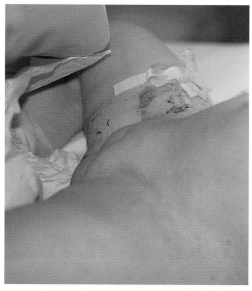

FIG. 11.3. Infection with *Neisseria meningitidis*. This infant has a meningococcal infection that is more severe than that in the child in Figure 11.2. In addition to the purpura, the skin is poorly perfused. A femoral line has been placed for fluid resuscitation.

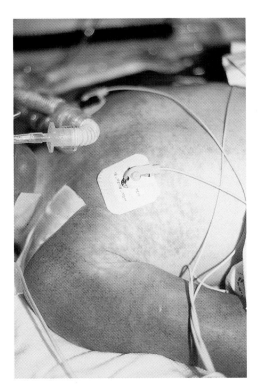

FIG. 11.4. Purpura fulminans in a child with pneumococcal sepsis. The syndrome of purpura fulminans occurs in severe sepsis caused by *Neisseria meningitidis* most commonly but may be seen with other organisms, as illustrated by this patient. The characteristic appearance consists of blotchy, confluent purple discoloration, superimposed on gray, poorly perfused skin. Patients with purpura fulminans have more pronounced findings than the children in the previous figures and are critically ill. Note the endotracheal tube and monitoring devices in this case.

TABLE 11.1. *Immediate management of sepsis*

1. Ensure adequate ventilation and cardiac function.
2. Obtain laboratory studies (simultaneously with step 3):
    Complete blood count, platelet count, PT, PTT, electrolytes, BUN, creatinine, glucose, arterial blood gas, blood culture, fibrin degradation products, AST, ALT.
3. Initiate hemodynamic monitoring and support:
    Peripheral venous access, urinary catheter, central venous and arterial catheters (as indicated), cardiorespiratory monitors.
    Normal saline, starting at 20 mL/kg.
4. Administer drugs and other therapeutic agents:
    Antibiotics: <2 mos: 50 mg/kg ampicillin and 2.5 mg/kg gentamicin
    >2 mos: 50 mg/kg ceftriaxone or 50 mg/kg cefotaxime or 40 mg/kg meropenem
    Sodium bicarbonate (pH <7.0) 1–2 mEq/kg
    Glucose (serum glucose <50 mg/dL) 0.25–1 g/kg
    Packed red blood cells (Hgb <10 g/dL) 10 mL/kg
    Platelet concentrates (platelet count <50,000/mm^3) 0.2 U/kg
    Fresh frozen plasma (elevated PT/PTT) 10 mL/kg.

PT, prothrombin time; PTT, partial thromboplastin time; BUN, blood urea nitrogen; AST, aspartate aminotransferase; ALT, alanine aminotransferase.

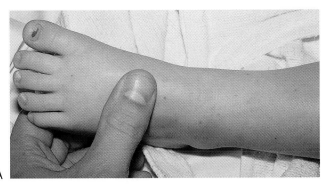

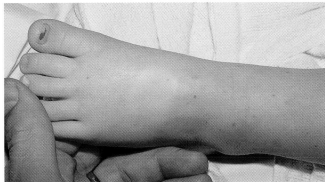

A

B

FIG. 11.5. Delayed capillary refill. **A:** The physician is pressing on the foot of a child with meningococcemia. **B:** A thumbprint remains visible several seconds later, during which time the physician released the foot, picked up a camera, and took the photograph. Note as well the scattered petechiae.

TABLE 11.2. *Intravenous antibiotic dosing for newborn infants*

	Based on age and weight (mg/kg/d)				
	Weight <2,000 g		Weight >2,000 g		
Antibiotic	0–7 d	8–28 d	0–7 d	8–28 d	>28 d
Ampicillin	100 mg q 12 hr	150 mg q 8 hr	150 mg q 8 hr	200 mg q 6 hr	200 mg q 6 hr
Cefotaxime	100 mg q 12 hr	150 mg q 8 hr	100 mg q 12 hr	150 mg q 8 hr	150 mg q 8 hr
Ceftriaxone	50 mg q.d.	50 mg q.d.	50 mg q.d.	75 mg q.d.	100 mg q.d.

	Based on gestational age (mg/kg/dose)			
	Age (wk)			
Antibiotic	≤26	27–34	35–42	>43
Gentamicin	2.5 mg q 24 hr	2.5 mg q 18 hr	2.5 mg q 12 hr	2.5 mg q 8 hr

q, every; q.d., every day.

Central Nervous System Infections

Meningitis, an inflammation of the membranes lining the central nervous system, results from an infection or irritation on a noninfectious basis. Table 11.3 lists those organisms that are the more frequent invaders of the meninges.

Bacterial Meningitis

Background

The most common organism varies with the age of the child. In the first month of life, *Escherichia coli* and group B streptococci are usually isolated; *Listeria monocytogenes*, a Gram-positive rod, accounts for 1% to 3% of the cases. At 30 to 60 days of age, group B streptococci continue to be re-

TABLE 11.3. *Organisms that cause meningitis*

Viruses
  Enteroviruses
  Herpes simplex
  Lymphocytic choriomeningitis
  Mumps
  Other
Mycoplasma
Bacteria
  Streptococcus pneumoniae
  Neisseria meningitidis
  Escherichia coli
  Group B streptococci
  Haemophilus influenzae
  Salmonella spp
  Listeria monocytogenes
  Mycobacterium tuberculosis
  Spirochetes (Lyme, syphilis)
Fungi
  Candida albicans
  Cryptococcus neoformans
Parasites
  Cysticercosis
  Amoebae

covered frequently, followed by *S. pneumoniae* and *N. meningitidis*; *H. influenzae* occurs rarely. After the first 2 months of life, *S. pneumoniae* and *N. meningitidis* cause most meningeal infections; *H. influenzae* remains a consideration primarily among children not immunized with conjugated *H. influenzae* type b vaccine or recent immigrants from a Third World country.

Clinical Manifestations

The signs and symptoms of meningitis vary with the age of the child (Table 11.4). Before 3 months of age, there is a history of irritability, an altered sleep pattern, vomiting, and decreased oral intake. In particular, paradoxical irritability points to the diagnosis of meningitis. A bulging fontanelle, an almost certain sign of meningitis in the febrile, ill-appearing infant, is a late finding. It is only in the child older than 2 to 3 years of age that meningitis manifests reliably with complaints of headache and neck stiffness.

The physical examination in the very young infant rarely provides specific corroboration, even when the history suggests meningitis. Fever is often absent in these children, despite the presence of bacterial infection. After 3 months of age, increasing, but not absolute, reliance can be placed on the physical findings; fever is almost inevitably noted. Specific evidence of meningeal irritation is often present, including nuchal rigidity (Fig. 11.6) and, less frequently, Kernig and Brudzinski signs. In those instances in which a lumbar puncture fails to confirm the diagnosis of meningitis despite the presence of meningeal signs, other conditions must be pursued that can mimic the findings on physical examination. Conditions capable of producing meningismus (irritation of the meninges without pleocytosis in the cerebrospinal fluid) include severe pharyngitis, retropharyngeal abscess, cervical adenitis, arthritis or osteomyelitis of the cervical spine, upper lobe pneumonia, subarachnoid hemorrhage, pyelonephritis, and tetanus. Complications of meningitis are frequent.

TABLE 11.4. *Signs and symptoms of meningitis*

Age (mo)	Symptoms	Signs	
		Early	Late
0–3	Paradoxical irritability, altered sleep pattern, vomiting, lethargy	Lethargy, irritability, fever (±), hypothermia (<1 mo)	Bulging fontanelle, shock
4–24	Irritability, altered sleep pattern, lethargy	Fever, irritability	Nuchal rigidity, coma, shock
>24	Headache, neck pain, lethargy	Fever, nuchal rigidity, irritability	Coma, shock

Management

Several studies have shown the average elapsed time between arrival in the emergency department and the delivery of antibiotics averages 2 to 3 hours, but every effort should be made to reduce this interval to enhance the theoretical advantages of early therapy (Table 11.5). In the first 30 days of life, the most likely organisms include the Gram-negative enteric rods, such as *E. coli*, and group B streptococci. Ampicillin and a third-generation cephalosporin (cefotaxime) or an aminoglycoside (gentamicin) provide appropriate coverage. Between 30 and 60 days of age, group B streptococci remain the predominant pathogen, but the Gram-negative enteric bacilli decrease in frequency. *S. pneumoniae* and *N. meningitidis* occur sporadically, as does *H. influenzae* because these children are too young to be immunized against *H. influenzae* type b. The usual antibiotic combination is vancomycin to cover penicillin-resistant pneumococci and either ceftriaxone or cefotaxime.

After the first 2 months, the predominant pathogens that cause meningitis are *S. pneumoniae* and *N. meningitidis*. As for the child between 30 and 60 days of age, initial antibiotic therapy includes vancomycin and either ceftriaxone or cefotaxime. Chloramphenicol or meropenem are options for patients with a history of serious reactions to penicillin. In addition to the antibiotic administration aimed at the eradication of the offending organism, supportive therapy for complications is an essential component in the care of the child with meningitis.

Aseptic Meningitis

Aseptic meningitis is defined here as an inflammation of the meninges that occurs in the absence of bacterial growth on routine culture media (Table 11.6). The signs and symptoms of aseptic meningitis resemble those of bacterial infections of the central nervous system but are not usually as severe. Nuchal rigidity in a patient who is alert and conversant suggests aseptic rather than bacterial meningitis. An altered level of consciousness or focal neurologic deficit points to meningoencephalitis rather than aseptic meningitis. Treatment of the common viral infections does not extend beyond supportive care at present; however, a new antiviral agent, pleconaril, is currently under investigation for enteroviral meningitis.

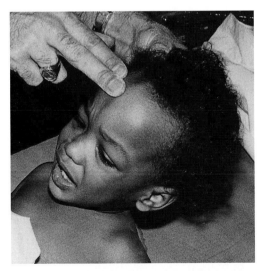

FIG. 11.6. Nuchal rigidity. This young girl has bacterial meningitis. She resists flexion of her neck, instead lifting her shoulders off the table. Additionally, the child grimaces in response to the attempt because stretching the inflamed meninges causes pain.

TABLE 11.5. *Immediate management of bacterial meningitis*

1. Ensure adequate ventilation and cardiac function
2. Obtain laboratory studies (simultaneously with step 3):
   - CSF: Cell count, glucose, protein, Gram stain, culture, latex agglutination (as indicated)
   - Blood: CBC, platelet count, PT, PTT, electrolytes, BUN, creatinine, glucose, arterial blood gas, blood culture
3. Initiate hemodynamic monitoring and support:
   - Achieve venous access, cardiorespiratory monitors
4. Administer drugs:
   - Treat septic shock, if present
   - Consider 0.15 mg/kg dexamethasone before or shortly after antibiotic administration
   - Antibiotics: <1 mo: 50 mg/kg ampicillin and 50 mg/kg cefotaxime
     - >1 mo: 15 mg vancomycin and either 50 mg/kg ceftriaxone or 75 mg/kg cefotaxime[a]
   - Glucose (if serum glucose <50 mg/dL) 0.25–1 g/kg
   - Treat acidosis and coagulopathy, if present

[a] Chloramphenicol (25 mg/kg) may be used in place of cephalosporins for children allergic to those agents.

TABLE 11.6. *Aseptic meningitis syndrome*

Infectious
  Viruses
  Early or partially treated bacterial meningitis
  Parameningeal infection
  Unusual bacteria
    Leptospirosis
    Syphilis
    Tuberculosis
    Ehrlichia canis
    Borrelia burgdorferi (Lyme)
  Mycoplasma
  Rickettsia
  Fungi
    Cryptococcus
    Candida
  Parasites
    Trichinosis
    Toxoplasmosis
    Cysticercosis
    Malaria
    Naegleria
Noninfectious
  Neoplasm
  Hemorrhage
  Hypersensitivity reactions
  Heavy metal poisoning
  Collagen-vascular disease
  Sarcoidosis
  Kawasaki disease (?infectious)

Upper Respiratory Tract Infections

Nasopharyngitis

Nasopharyngitis or the common cold is a viral illness of the upper respiratory tract in children. Fever of less than 39°C (102.2°F) and coryza characterize the illness. Therapy is limited to a recommendation for rest, adequate hydration, saline nose drops, and antipyretic agents.

Stomatitis

Stomatitis, an infection of the mouth, is caused by herpes simplex virus (Fig. 11.7) and the coxsackieviruses, at any age, and by *Candida albicans* (thrush) in the infant or the immunosuppressed child. Viral infections cause vesicular lesions initially and ulcerations and plaques subsequently. Some coxsackieviruses may involve the hands and feet (Fig. 11.8A) and the mouth (Fig. 11.8B) (coxsackie hand-foot-and-mouth disease), and herpetic stomatitis may be complicated by the spread of infection to the digits, which is referred to as herpetic whitlow (Fig. 11.9). For otherwise healthy patients, treatment is limited to systemic antipyretic and analgesic drugs, and the local application of topical analgesics, such as 2% viscous Xylocaine or the combination of Kaopectate and diphenhydramine. Oral acyclovir hastens the resolution of herpetic lesions in immunosuppressed patients. *C. albicans* produces white plaques on the mucosa that bleed

if scraped. Nystatin (200,000 U four times daily) leads to a prompt resolution of this condition.

Pharyngitis

In the immunocompetent child, several viruses, perhaps *Mycoplasma pneumoniae* and *Chlamydia trachomatis*, and only a few bacteria cause pharyngitis. Three bacteria, the latter two quite rare, have well-defined roles: group A streptococci, *Corynebacterium diphtheriae*, and *Neisseria gonorrhoeae*. For practical purposes, isolated pharyngitis can be considered as streptococcal (bacterial) or nonstreptococcal (viral). Streptococcal infections more often have an abrupt onset with fever and sore throat; examination of the pharynx reveals an erythematous mucosa, often with exudate (Fig. 11.10) and petechiae on the posterior palate. Additionally, the tongue may be inflamed ("strawberry tongue") and cervical lymph nodes often become enlarged and tender. Oral phenoxymethyl penicillin (250 mg per dose for children and 500 mg per dose for adolescents, given two to three times per day) or ampicilin provides excellent therapy, if prescribed for 10 days. Erythromycin, (40 mg/kg per day) is used for penicillin-allergic children; azithromycin for 5 days (10 mg/kg on the first day and 5 mg/kg on subsequent days) represents a more expensive alternative.

Otitis Media

Clinical Manifestations

Otitis media (OM) refers to inflammation within the middle ear. The disease is divided into two broad categories (Table 11.7): acute otitis media (AOM) and otitis media with effusion (OME). AOM may produce minimal symptoms, being detected only on examination, or it may cause obvious localizing pain. In the young child, the initial manifestations are often not otologic but rather fever, irritability, or diarrhea. Children older than 3 years of age generally, but not invariably, complain of pain in the ear. Less frequent symptoms include vertigo and hearing impairment. Fever, occurring in 25% to 35% of children with AOM, serves only to arouse suspicion of infection in the middle ear. The diagnosis rests in the usual clinical settings on the accurate interpretation of the otoscopic findings (Fig. 11.11).

The tympanic membrane in AOM typically bulges out at the examiner as a result of the positive pressure generated by the production of purulent material in the middle ear cavity. Although the drum is sometimes red, it more often appears yellow because of the exudate behind it. Difficulty arises in differentiating AOM from OME and in diagnosing "early" AOM, particularly in the child with a preexisting middle ear effusion. The tympanic membrane has decreased mobility in both AOM and OME; however, it is usually retracted in the latter condition. It is safer to assume a bacterial etiology when the findings are equivocal.

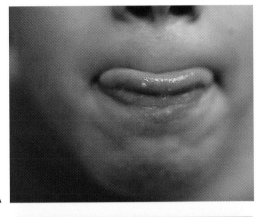

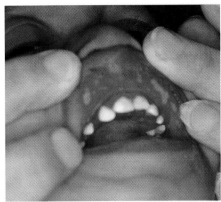

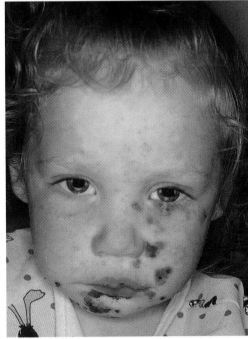

FIG. 11.7. Herpetic stomatitis. These three children demonstrate the spectrum of oral infection with herpes simplex virus, which ranges from asymptomatic to severe. **A:** The first patient has a single vesicle on his tongue, **B:** the second manifests widespread labial lesions, **C:** the third patient shows dissemination to the face. In the young girl with facial involvement, fluorescein dye is dripping from the right eye after its instillation in an attempt to identify the typical dendritic ulcer seen with herpetic keratitis.

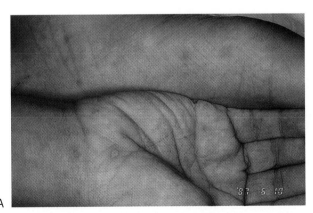

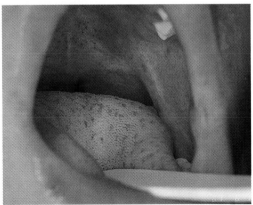

FIG. 11.8. Coxsackie hand-foot-and-mouth disease. **A:** A hand and a foot of this child show isolated vesicles compared with the grouped vesicles seen in the patient in Figure 11.7 with a herpetic infection. The child also had palatal lesions. **B:** Scattered petechiae appear centrally, and there is a vesicle posteriorly at the junction of the hard and soft palates. Coxsackievirus produces lesions toward the posterior of the oropharynx, whereas herpes simplex virus appears anteriorly.

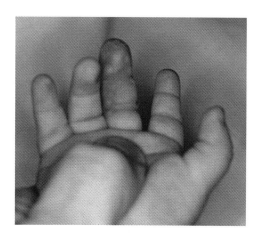

FIG. 11.9. Herpetic whitlow. Herpetic whitlow is an infection of a digit by herpes simplex virus, characterized by grouped vesicles on an erythematous base. Extensive swelling, erythema, and discharge from ruptured lesions may lead to confusion with bacterial cellulitis or suggest secondary bacterial infection, which rarely occurs.

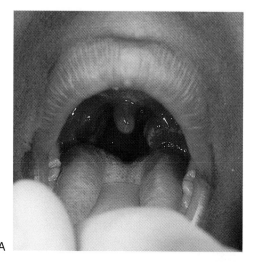

A

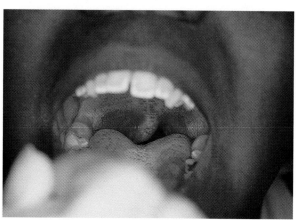

B

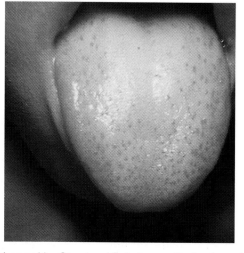

C

FIG. 11.10. Streptococcal pharyngitis. Streptococcal pharyngitis is characterized by an erythematous posterior pharynx **(A)**, palatal petechiae **(B)**, and a white strawberry tongue **(C)**. Each of these findings suggests streptococcal, not viral, infection. Many cases are not as obvious.

TABLE 11.7. *Classification of otitis media*

Type	Duration	Bacteriology	Tympanum	Signs and symptoms
Acute otitis media	Days to weeks	Isolates in 70%	Erythematous or purulent, bulging	Fever (30%), earache (older child), irritability
Otitis media with effusion	Weeks to months	Occasional isolates	Dull, retracted, fluid level	Asymptomatic, decreased hearing, fullness

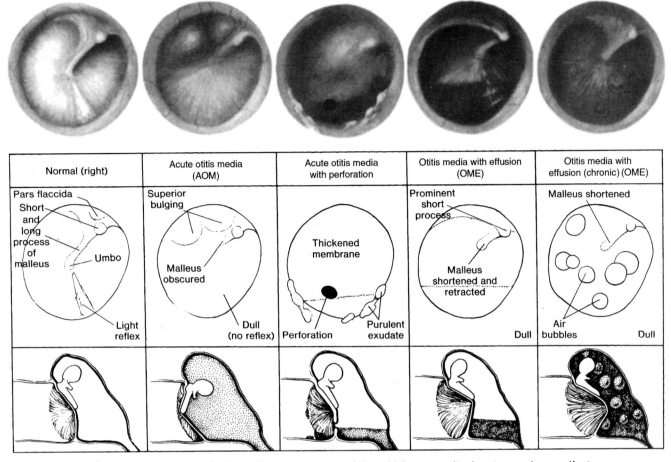

FIG. 11.11. Otitis media. Otitis media, inflammation of the middle ear cavity, has two major manifestations. Acute otitis media (AOM) is a bacterial infection that classically causes an erythematous, bulging tympanic membrane. During an episode of otitis media with effusion (OME), the tympanic membrane may be dull, rather than erythematous, and more often assumes a retracted position. Decreased mobility of the membrane occurs with both AOM and OME. Unfortunately, the findings represent a spectrum and are not always typical.

Management

Uncomplicated OM in the child older than 1 month of age should be treated with oral antibiotic therapy on an outpatient basis. Amoxicillin (80 to 90 mg/kg per day in three divided doses) is the drug of choice in the United States. If unusual local resistance patterns dictate initiating therapy with a drug other than amoxicillin, reasonable second choices include (1) amoxicillin fortified with clavulanic acid in a 14:1 formulation, 90 mg/kg amoxicillin per day in two divided doses, (2) 10 mg/kg azithromycin per day on the first day and 5 mg/kg per day thereafter once daily for 5 days, and (3) 50 mg/kg ceftriaxone intramuscularly as a single dose. Antihistamines and decongestants are not indicated.

If a child younger than 1 month of age presents with fever or irritability and is found to have OM, admission for intravenous antibiotic therapy provides the safest course pending the outcome of cultures of the blood, urine, and spinal fluid (Fig. 11.12). Afebrile infants in the first month of life may be treated as outpatients with the usual oral antibiotics used for older patients and with careful follow-up. Infants between 4 and 12 weeks of age with OM can be managed as outpatients because *S. pneumoniae*, *H. influenzae*, and *Moraxella catarrhalis* are the predominant organisms. However, other sources of infection, including meningitis, must be considered in the febrile child before attributing the source of a temperature elevation to OM alone.

Otitis Externa

Otitis externa (OE), or swimmer's ear, is an infection of the auditory canal and external surface of the tympanic membrane that spares the middle ear. The first symptom is itching of the ear canal. The child complains subsequently of an earache that may be unilateral or bilateral, and purulent material often drains from the ear. Fever is never present unless there is an associated cellulitis or other illness. Unlike AOM, pulling on the ear lobe to straighten the canal in preparation for otoscopic examination elicits marked tenderness. A cheesy white or gray-green exudate fills the canal in more than 50% of patients, often obscuring the tympanum.

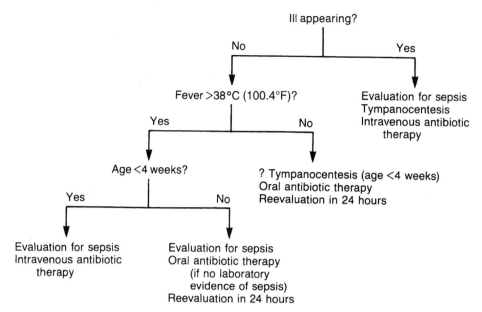

FIG. 11.12. Algorithm for the management of otitis media during the first 2 months of life. Infants younger than the age of 2 months are at risk of unusual pathogens and the development of disseminated disease compared with older children. Those who are ill appearing, febrile, or younger than 4 weeks of age demand careful evaluation, for which this algorithm provides a set of guidelines. The role of tympanocentesis varies between centers.

Treatment consists of removing the inflammatory debris from the ear canal, eliminating pathogenic bacteria, symptomatic measures, and control of predisposing factors. Usually, dry-mopping of the canal with a cotton-tipped wire applicator serves to cleanse the canal adequately; occasionally, gentle suction is also necessary. Specific therapy is with antibiotic/corticosteroid preparations (Cortisporin), four drops instilled four times daily, or ofloxacin otic, five drops instilled twice daily. For the occasional patient with a very edematous canal and thick exudate, a wick should be inserted 10 to 12 mm into the canal after cleansing to facilitate entry of the medications. All patients should be instructed to avoid swimming until cured. The occurrence of a local cellulitis or adenitis requires the addition of an antistaphylococcal antibiotic, such as 50 mg/kg dicloxacillin per day or 100 mg/kg cephalexin per day.

Sinusitis

Sinusitis is an inflammation of the paranasal sinuses: maxillary, ethmoid, frontal, or sphenoid. The predominant pathogens in acute sinusitis are the same organisms causing AOM. Two features that distinguish sinusitis from a viral upper respiratory infection include persistent (>10 days) and/or severe (temperature >39°C, 102.2°F for more than 3 days) symptoms. A cough occurs in 75% of the patients. Unlike adolescents, young children do not often complain of a headache or facial pain. Fever is noted in approximately half of children with sinusitis. Nasal discharge occurs in almost all these infections and is often the symptom that prompts a visit. The area of the face that overlies the sinus

swells in 10% to 20% of the patients with maxillary disease, and periorbital or orbital edema and cellulitis even more commonly accompany ethmoiditis. The child with chronic sinusitis complains only of a chronic cough and rhinorrhea. The sinus radiograph is abnormal in almost every child with sinusitis (Fig. 11.13); there may be an air-fluid level, complete opacification, or mucosal thickening (>4 mm). A

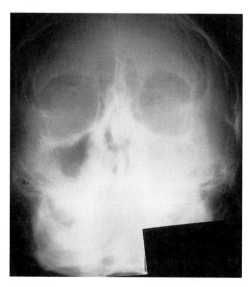

FIG. 11.13. Maxillary sinusitis. This radiograph demonstrates a pronounced case of maxillary sinusitis, with an air-fluid level on the left and complete opacification of the sinus cavity on the right. Milder infections may produce only mucosal thickening.

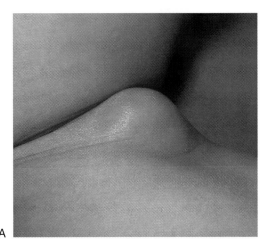
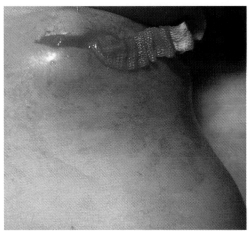

A   B

FIG. 11.14. Supraclavicular lymphadenitis. This child has an infected supraclavicular node **(A)** that has developed fluctuance. The node shows the characteristic taut, shiny, red appearance that occurs when pus accumulates under pressure. *Staphylococcus aureus*, the most frequent pathogen in pediatric lymphadenitis, was the causative agent. A fluctuant node requires treatment either by aspiration or incision and drainage **(B)**.

computed tomography scan is more sensitive for diagnosis than a plain radiograph but is not needed in routine cases.

Management

Children suspected of acute sinusitis with severe symptoms or an uncertain clinical picture should have a radiographic evaluation of their sinuses. Among this group of patients clinically thought to be at risk of an infection, any abnormality (air-fluid level, opacification, or mucosal thickening) suffices to confirm the diagnosis. Afebrile children with chronic sinusitis diagnosed based on persistent nasal discharge need no laboratory or radiographic evaluation. Amoxicillin (80 to 90 mg/kg per day for 10 to 14 days) effectively treats the common pathogens *S. pneumoniae* and *H. influenzae* in most cases. Alternative drugs are the same as those listed for AOM.

Peritonsillar Abscess

A peritonsillar abscess, or quinsy, which results from the accumulation of purulent material within the tonsillar fossa, is more common in adolescents. Group A streptococci, various anaerobic organisms, and, occasionally, *S. aureus* are the usual pathogens. The complaints of trismus and difficulty in speaking separate a peritonsillar abscess from the far more common pharyngitis. The voice sounds muffled, and the child drools profusely. Both tonsils may swell, but the enlargement of one is more pronounced. Usually, the abscessed tonsil becomes sufficiently large as to push the uvula to the opposite side of the pharynx.

All children with a peritonsillar abscess should have the lesion drained in the emergency department or after admission to the hospital and receive treatment with antibiotics. Clindamycin is the drug of choice. In the unusual child with

respiratory compromise, drainage or aspiration of the abscess can be life saving. Aspiration is accomplished by using an 18-gauge needle mounted on a 10-mL syringe.

Cervical Lymphadenitis

Cervical lymphadenitis is a bacterial infection of the lymph nodes in the neck (Figs. 11.14, 11.15, and 11.16). This condition must be distinguished from lymphadenopathy, an enlargement of one or more lymph nodes that occurs with viral infections or as a reaction to bacterial disease in structures that drain to the nodes (Fig. 11.17). *S. aureus* causes lymphadenitis in most of those children with an identifiable pathogen. Other organisms that may play a role rarely

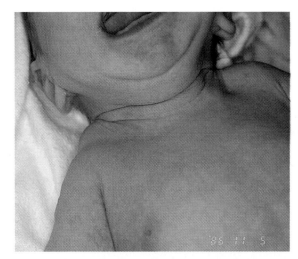

FIG. 11.15. Supraclavicular lymphadenitis in an 8-day-old infant. The lymph node in this child was less inflamed than that of the child in Figure 11.14 but yielded abundant pus on incision and drainage. Group B streptococci were isolated.

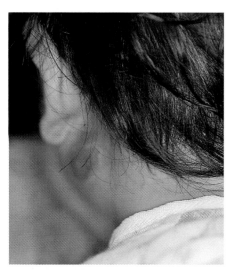

FIG. 11.16. Mycobacterial lymphadenitis. This young girl, who had recently returned from India, presented with an inflamed lymph node and additional signs of systemic disease. An excisional biopsy showed caseating granulomas.

include mycobacteria, *Bartonella henselae* (cat scratch disease), anaerobic bacteria, *Yersinia pestis* (plague), Gram-negative bacilli, *H. influenzae*, *Francisella tularensis*, *Actinomyces*, and *Nocardia*. Fever occurs only occasionally, more often in children younger than 1 year old. The infected node may vary in size from 2 to more than 10 cm. Initially, it has a firm consistency, but fluctuance (Fig. 11.14) develops in approximately 25%. The skin overlying the node becomes erythematous, and edema may surround it.

Management

Figure 11.18 outlines the management of the child with cervical lymphadenitis. Children with cervical adenitis who are otherwise healthy should receive an antibiotic effective

FIG. 11.17. Lymphadenopathy from tularemia. This boy has posterior cervical lymphadenopathy **A:** secondary to the ulceroglandular form of tularemia. **B:** Cutaneous lesions. *Francisella tularensis* was isolated from the lesions.

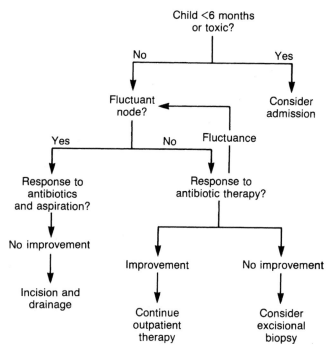

FIG. 11.18. Algorithm for the approach to management of the child with presumed bacterial lymphadenitis.

against *S. aureus* and the group A streptococci. Agents such as dicloxacillin (50 mg/kg per day) and cephalexin (50 mg/kg per day) have activity against both organisms. In more severe infections, 150 mg/kg oxacillin per day in four divided doses can be administered intravenously. If the node is fluctuant, aspiration or incision and drainage (Fig. 11.14B) provide useful etiologic information and speed the rate of resolution. Children younger than 3 months of age and those who appear toxic or have developed a draining sinus are best managed in the hospital.

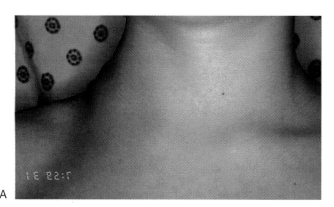

A

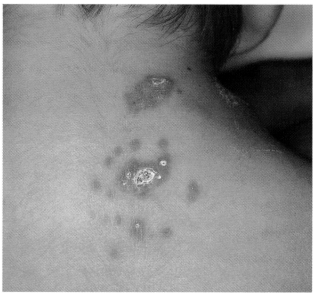

B

Retropharyngeal and Lateral Pharyngeal Abscess

A retropharyngeal abscess fills the potential space between the anterior border of the cervical vertebrae and the posterior wall of the esophagus. The usual pathogens are group A streptococci, anaerobic organisms, and, occasionally, *S. aureus*. These infrequent infections occur most often in children younger than 4 years of age. The child with a retropharyngeal abscess presents with a clinical picture similar to that seen with epiglottitis, but the onset is less abrupt. Fever and a toxic appearance are common. As purulent material collects, the fluctuant mass obstructs the larynx and esophagus, leading to stridor and drooling. The abscess may cause meningismus. Although a retropharyngeal infection can rarely be seen as a midline swelling on examination of the pharynx, it is usually difficult to observe this finding in the uncooperative child. If the diagnosis is suspected and the airway is not threatened, a lateral neck radiograph or computed tomography scan should be obtained.

A lateral pharyngeal abscess causes virtually identical symptoms to an infection in the retropharyngeal area. One important difference is that a lateral pharyngeal abscess, which is not well visualized by radiograph, requires a computed tomography scan for diagnosis.

Unless the airway is in immediate jeopardy, intravenous access should be secured and treatment given with either clindamycin or ampicillin/sulbactam. Some patients require surgical drainage, either transcutaneously with ultrasonography guidance or at surgery, but high-dose antibiotics may suffice, particularly when the computed tomography scan shows cellulitis or only a small collection of pus.

Laryngotracheobronchitis (Croup)

Clinical Manifestations

Croup, or laryngotracheobronchitis, is a viral infection that involves the larynx and may extend into the trachea and bronchi. Children between the ages of 6 months and 3 years are affected most frequently. Croup begins insidiously with the onset of fever and coryza. During the next 1 to 2 days, the infection spreads farther along the airway, producing signs of upper respiratory obstruction. Inspiratory stridor develops at this stage of the illness, and a barking cough is heard. The fever usually ranges from 38° to 39°C, (100.4° to 102.2°F). There are tachycardia and tachypnea, but the respirations rarely exceed 40 breaths per minute. Suprasternal and subcostal retractions frequently accompany croup. On auscultation of the chest, the examiner may hear either stridor alone in mild disease or rhonchi and wheezes with more extensive involvement of the respiratory epithelium.

Ancillary studies are indicated only occasionally. Lateral and anteroposterior neck radiographs show subglottic narrowing ("steeple" sign) from soft-tissue edema in severe disease. However, most radiographic studies of the airway are normal or disclose only ballooning of the hypopharynx. Rather than confirm the diagnosis of croup, radiographic examination more often excludes other illnesses such as epiglottitis and retropharyngeal abscess.

Management

Croup is usually apparent from the history and physical examination. Soft-tissue radiographs of the neck are needed only if the diagnosis is uncertain. Of children with croup who come to the emergency department, most can be managed as outpatients. Clear indications for admission are dehydration and/or significant respiratory compromise. If any of the signs of respiratory failure are noted, hospitalization becomes necessary. Use of a scoring system may be helpful in deciding on disposition (Table 11.8).

A reasonable approach is to tailor therapy to the severity of illness. In rare cases with inadequate gas exchange, management of the airway, at times with endotracheal intubation, takes precedence; tracheal edema may make passage of a tube with the usual diameter impossible, and the physician should

TABLE 11.8. *Scoring system for croup patients*

	Croup score			
	0	1	2	3
Stridor	None	Only with agitation	Mild at rest	Severe at rest
Retraction	None	Mild	Moderate	Severe
Air entry	Normal	Mild decrease	Moderate decrease	Marked decrease
Color	Normal	Not applicable	Not applicable	Cyanotic
Level of consciousness	Normal	Restless when disturbed	Restless when undisturbed	Lethargic

	Croup severity[a]	
Score	Degree	Management
≤4	Mild	Outpatient: mist therapy
5–6	Mild to moderate	Outpatient if child improves in emergency department after mist, is >6 mos, and has a reliable family; consider dexamethasone
7–8	Moderate	Admit: racemic epinephrine and dexamethasone
≥9	Severe	Admit: racemic epinephrine, dexamethasone, oxygen, intensive care unit

Modified from Taussig LM, Castro O, Beaudry PH, et al. Treatment of laryngotracheobronchitis (croup). Use of intermittent positive-pressure breathing and racemic epinephrine. *Am J Dis Child* 1975;129:790–793.

[a] Any one category with score of 3 leads to classification as severe disease.

TABLE 11.9. *Epiglottitis and croup: a comparison*

	Epiglottitis	Croup
Anatomy	Supraglottic	Subglottic
Etiology	Bacterial: *Haemophilus influenzae*	Viral: Parainfluenza
Age range (yr)	3–7, adults	0.5–3
Onset (hr)	6–24	24–72
Toxicity	Marked	Mild to moderate
Drooling	Frequent	Absent
Cough	Unusual	Frequent
Hoarseness	Unusual	Frequent
WBCs	Leukocytosis	Normal

WBCs, white blood cells.

be prepared with one that is a size smaller. Patients with concerning upper airway obstruction in the emergency department and a high likelihood of hospitalization will benefit from prompt administration of both racemic epinephrine by nebulization and steroids [either inhaled budesonide or dexamethasone (0.6 mg/kg orally or intramuscularly)]. For those children with moderately severe croup, when hospitalization is being considered, the response to an initial trial of mist and either intramuscular dexamethasone or nebulized budesonide can be assessed. Most patients who are mildly ill require only instructions for home care.

Epiglottitis

Clinical Manifestations

Epiglottitis is a life-threatening bacterial infection of the epiglottis and the surrounding structures. The duration of ill-ness before presentation is often as short as 6 hours and rarely exceeds 24 hours. As the disease progresses, the supraglottic edema interferes with the ability to swallow secretions; thus, drooling is a complaint in 60% to 70% of cases. Fifty percent of the children with epiglottitis complain of a sore throat. Aphonia, hoarseness, and cough are infrequent. Although both croup and epiglottitis manifest with stridor in a febrile child, the examiner can usually differentiate these two illnesses based on the clinical features (Table 11.9).

The anxious appearance of most children with epiglottitis strikes the examiner immediately (Figs. 11.19 and 11.20). To maximize air entry, these children assume a sitting position with their jaws thrust forward (Fig. 11.19B). Cyanosis may occur in the later stages of the illness. The temperature, almost always elevated, often reaches 40°C, or 104°F. Although the patients are universally tachypneic, the respiratory rate infrequently exceeds 40 breaths per minute. Stridor can be heard without a stethoscope, but auscultation of the lungs reveals no other adventitious sounds. Marked retractions are seen, predominantly involving the suprasternal and subcostal musculature.

Rigorous attempts to visualize the epiglottis are hazardous and should be avoided in the child with suspected epiglottitis. If visualized, the mucosa of the epiglottis is seen to be erythematous (Fig. 11.21), and pooled secretions are present in approximately half the children. Occasionally, a swollen, cherry-red epiglottis protrudes above the base of the tongue and is visible without instrumentation.

Management

When a child is suspected of having epiglottitis, the thrust of the management plan is to make a definitive diagnosis and

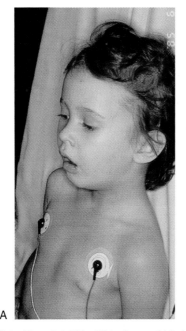
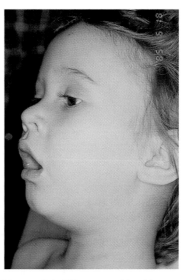

A   B

FIG. 11.19. A child with epiglottitis. This 4-year-old girl has epiglottitis caused by *Haemophilus influenzae* type b. **A:** She prefers to sit and appears anxious. **B:** The child assumes the characteristic sniffing position to maximize the patency of her airway.

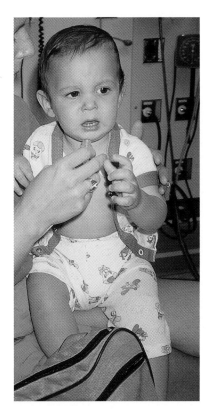

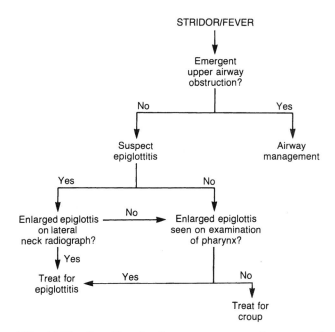

FIG. 11.22. Algorithm for the management of suspected epiglottitis.

FIG. 11.20. Infant with epiglottitis. Although not widely appreciated, epiglottitis caused by *Haemophilus influenzae* type b varies widely along the spectrum of severity. This 1-year-old infant appears mildly anxious but looks much less toxic than the patient in Figure 11.19.

institute therapy before the onset of airway obstruction. The initial steps are based on the degree of respiratory distress and the likelihood of epiglottitis, as judged from the clinical features (Fig. 11.22). Some children with epiglottitis have total or nearly total airway obstruction as the initial presentation of their disease. In this situation, treatment precedes any diagnostic evaluation; steps are taken to maintain an adequate exchange of air. When performed, the lateral neck radiograph either confirms or disproves the clinical diagnosis (Figs. 11.23 and 11.24). Ceftriaxone (100 mg/kg per day in one or two divided doses) or cefotaxime (200 mg/kg per day in four divided doses) serve as single drug alternatives and are useful, particularly for patients allergic to penicillins. Chloramphenicol and meropenem are useful for penicillin-allergic patients.

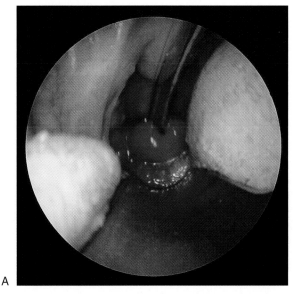

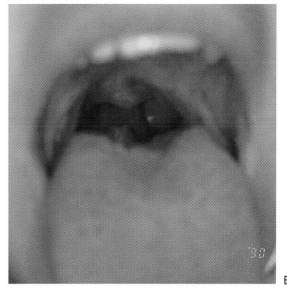

A

B

FIG. 11.21. Epiglottitis. A: A swollen, cherry-red epiglottis with an endotracheal tube passing posteriorly. B: In comparison, this child has a thin, pink, uninfected epiglottis.

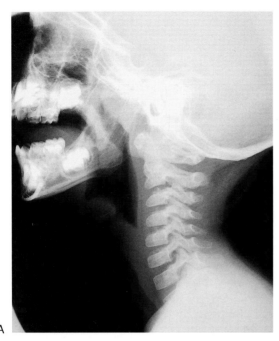
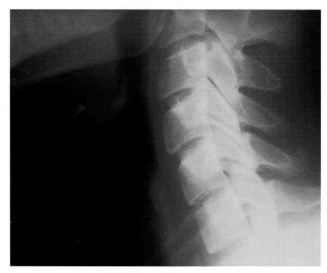

A

B

FIG. 11.23. A: The patient has epiglottitis. The radiograph demonstrates a swollen epiglottis at the level of the hyoid bone, which is convex on both sides and appears in the shape of a thumbprint. Edema anterior to the epiglottis has obliterated the vallecula, which usually appears as an elongated black shadow. Note the marked swelling of the aryepiglottic folds, projecting inferiorly and posteriorly from the epiglottis and the arytenoid cartilages at the base of the folds. Because *Haemophilus influenzae* type b infection involves all the structures in this area, this disease has alternatively been referred to as "supraglottitis." **B:** For comparison, a normal epiglottis is shown, which is thin and fine with a concave surface posteriorly and the appearance of a slightly bent finger.

Bacterial Tracheitis

Bacterial tracheitis is a relatively uncommon infection during childhood. The usual etiologic agent is *S. aureus*. The signs and symptoms of bacterial tracheitis mimic those of acute epiglottitis but with a somewhat slower onset. The fever is usually higher than 39°C, and the patients are stridorous. Toxicity and respiratory distress occur as a rule. On radiography, there is tracheal narrowing, and a pseudomembrane (Fig. 11.25) may be visible within the tracheal lumen; the supraglottic area is normal. The first priority for management is to secure an adequate airway in those few cases with severe respiratory distress. Antibiotic therapy should be initiated with ceftriaxone (100 mg/kg per day in one or two divided doses) or ampicillin/sulbactam (200 mg/kg ampicillin per day in four divided doses).

Lower Respiratory Tract Infections

The most frequent lower respiratory tract infections in childhood include bronchiolitis and pneumonia. Pneumonia is an inflammation of the lung tissue that may follow a noninfectious or an infectious insult. In the emergency department, the febrile child with an acute onset of pneumonia almost always has an infection. The causative organisms in pneumonia vary according to the age of the child. Although viral agents account for 60% to 90% of pneumonia, bacteria, particularly *S. pneumoniae*, play a major role (Table 11.10). *M. pneumoniae* increases in frequency after puberty. Unusual causes of pneumonia in the immunocompetent child include *Legionella pneumophila* (Legionnaires disease), *Mycobacterium tuberculosis*, Hantavirus, rickettsia (Q fever), fungi, and protozoa. Children with neoplasms, human immunodeficiency virus (HIV), and other forms of immunocompromise show susceptibility to a variety of unusual pathogens, including *Pneumocystis carinii*.

Bacterial Pneumonia

Clinical Manifestations

Bacterial pneumonia, which may be caused by a variety of bacterial pathogens (Table 11.10), as a rule generally has an abrupt onset with fever, often accompanied by chills. A cough is a common but nonspecific complaint. Occasionally, pleuritic involvement produces pain with respiratory effort. Tachypnea out of proportion to the fever is frequently the only additional sign, particularly in the first year of life. Grunting respirations in a young child should arouse a strong suspicion of pneumonia. Localized findings, more often seen in the child older than 1 year of age, include inspiratory rales and decreased breath sounds. Gastric dilation may

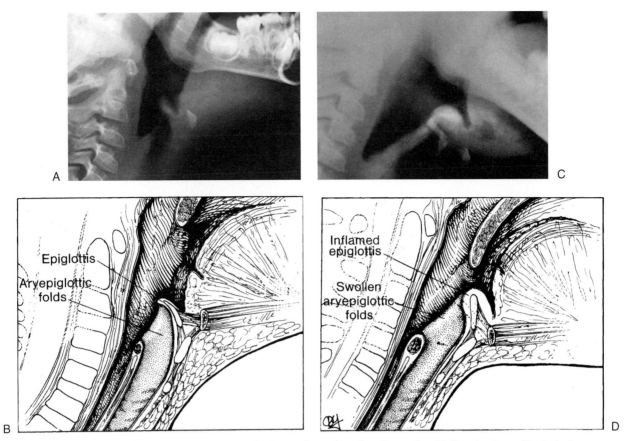

FIG. 11.24. Epiglottitis. **A:** A normal epiglottis on a lateral neck radiograph, with the structures illustrated in **B**. Epiglottitis is similarly depicted radiographically **(C, D)**.

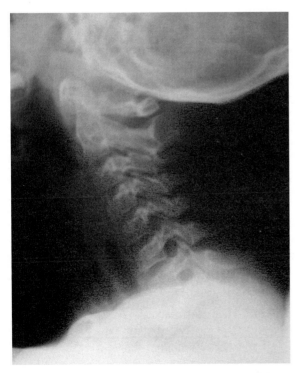

FIG. 11.25. Bacterial tracheitis. The radiograph shows a pseudomembrane in the trachea of a child with bacterial tracheitis. This finding, although not always visualized, is highly suggestive when present.

TABLE 11.10. *Lower respiratory tract infections*

Age	Infecting organism
2 wk	Bacteria
	Group B streptococci
	Gram-negative bacilli
	Viruses
2 wk–2 mo	*Chlamydia*
	Viruses
	Bacteria
	Streptococcus pneumoniae
	Staphylococcus aureus
	Haemophilus influenzae
2 mo–3 yr	Viruses
	Bacteria
	S. pneumoniae
	S. aureus
	H. influenzae
3–12 yr	Viruses
	Bacteria
	S. pneumoniae
	Mycoplasma pneumoniae
13–19 yr	*M. pneumoniae*
	Viruses
	Bacteria
	S. pneumoniae

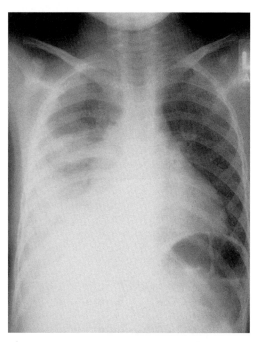

FIG. 11.26. A child with bacterial pneumonia. This radiograph of the chest shows a lobar consolidation and a pleural effusion on the right. Note the meniscus indicating the presence of fluid in the pleural cavity.

accompany pneumonia; occasionally, the abdominal findings in pulmonary infections mimic appendicitis. With upper lobe pneumonia, the pain may radiate to the neck, causing meningismus.

In the emergency department, a chest radiograph often assists in the management of a child suspected of having bacterial pneumonia. A lobar consolidation is assumed to be of bacterial origin, needing treatment with antibiotics (Fig. 11.26). Conversely, a minimal, diffuse interstitial infiltrate in a previously healthy toddler suggests a viral infection that can be managed with symptomatic therapy or in an adoles-

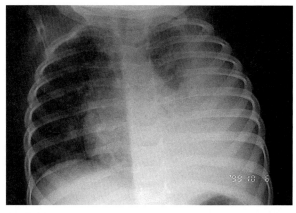

FIG. 11.27. Pneumonia with large pleural effusion. This child presented with bacterial pneumonia and respiratory distress, presumed to be caused in part by the large pleural effusion. In the emergency department, a pleural catheter ("pigtail") was placed for drainage, using the Seldinger technique.

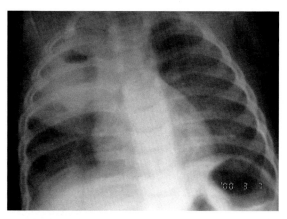

FIG. 11.28. Pulmonary abscess. A small proportion of children with bacterial pneumonia will develop a pulmonary abscess, as shown here. Although pneumococci cause most bacterial infections of the lungs in children, strong consideration must be given to *Staphylococcus aureus* in cases complicated by the formation of an abscess.

cent, *M. pneumoniae*, calling for treatment with erythromycin or azithromycin. Bilateral involvement, pleural effusion, and pneumatoceles point to more severe disease (Figs. 11.27 and 11.28).

Management

Most healthy children with pneumonia respond to outpatient antibiotic therapy. Because most of the infections are caused by *S. pneumoniae*, amoxicillin (80 to 90 mg/kg per day given orally in three divided doses) has been the mainstay of therapy. Ceftriaxone (50 mg/kg) may be administered intramuscularly at the time of diagnosis, especially if there is any concern about oral intake during the first 24 hours. Alternatively, macrolides, including erythromycin (40 mg/kg per day in four divided doses) or azithromycin (10 mg/kg as a single dose on the first day and 5 mg/kg as a single dose on days 2 to 5) may be used in penicillin-allergic children or whenever mycoplasmal infection is suspected based on age or radiographic findings. Indications for admission are listed in (Table 11.11). Effusions if sufficiently large should be cultured by thoracentesis, which requires subsequent observation of the child in the hospital and may require drainage.

TABLE 11.11. *Indications for admission of children with pneumonia*

Age < 1 yr (lobar infiltrate)
Respiratory compromise
Pleural effusion
Pneumatocele
Failure to respond to antibiotic therapy within 24–48 hr
Dehydration

Viral Pneumonia

Viral pneumonia generally has its onset over a 2- to 4-period, being more gradual than with bacterial infection. Cough, coryza, and low-grade fever occur frequently. Particularly with respiratory syncytial virus infections in the first 3 months of life, an apneic spell may be the first sign to draw attention to the illness. Fever in viral pneumonia is usually lower than 39°C, 102.2°F. As with bacterial infections, tachypnea in the undisturbed child may be the only physical finding. Rales are frequently audible diffusely throughout the chest, and wheezing may also be present. With more severe disease, the child shows signs of respiratory failure: grunting, cyanosis, and changes in mental status. Most typically, the radiograph in a child with viral pneumonia shows bilateral air trapping and peribronchial thickening. A diffuse increase in the interstitial markings is also commonly seen. Therapy is symptomatic, although young children or those few with significant respiratory distress may benefit from observation in the hospital.

Mycoplasmal Pneumonia

M. pneumoniae, a common cause of pneumonia in children older than 5 years of age, usually begins insidiously with fever and malaise, followed by hoarseness, sore throat, and, in one-fourth of cases, chest pain. Rales are heard in 75% of these infections, often bilaterally. Pharyngeal inflammation, bullous myringitis, or a rash (maculopapular or vesicular) may occur. Between 10% and 25% of children will have lobar consolidation, but scattered segmental infiltrates, interstitial disease, and combinations of all these patterns may be seen. The diagnosis of mycoplasmal pneumonia is presumptively based on the clinical and radiographic findings and, in some cases, on the cold agglutinin titer. An older child or adolescent with the gradual onset of a mild bilateral pneumonia should be treated for this infection. Conversely, a lobar infiltrate in a 5-year-old child usually is assumed to be of bacterial etiology regardless of the level of the cold agglutinins. Erythromycin (40 mg/kg per day) or azithromycin provides effective therapy for *M. pneumoniae* infections.

Chlamydial Pneumonia

C. trachomatis is the most frequently recovered pathogen from children with afebrile pneumonias between 4 and 12 weeks of age. Infants with chlamydial pneumonia usually have a staccato cough that may resemble the paroxysms seen in pertussis but is usually less prolonged. In 50% of cases, conjunctivitis precedes the onset of respiratory symptoms. Pneumonia with this organism only rarely produces fever. Mild retractions, hyperresonance, and diffuse rales are noted on examination of the chest. Hyperaeration of the lungs depresses the liver, allowing the edge to be palpated 1 to 2 mm below the right costal margin. Although the WBC count is usually in the normal range, the eosinophil count increases slightly (<400/mm^3 or 5% to 10%) in 75% of these patients. Mild hypoxemia is common. The chest radiograph shows hyperaeration of the lungs and a diffuse increase in the interstitial markings. Lobar consolidations and pleural diffusions are not seen. Because of the difficulty in making a definitive etiologic diagnosis and the potential for complications, most young infants with presumed chlamydial pneumonia should be admitted to the hospital. Erythromycin (40 mg/kg per day) may shorten the course and should be given.

Bronchiolitis

Bronchiolitis begins as an upper respiratory illness with cough and coryza. Over a 2- to 5-day period, signs of respiratory distress appear. Fever develops in two-thirds of children with bronchiolitis. Nasal flaring and retractions of the intercostal and supraclavicular muscles increase as the disease progresses. Wheezes and a prolonged expiratory phase are heard in all children with bronchiolitis, at times without a stethoscope; rales are usually minimal. As the ventilatory muscles fatigue, the child will have grunting respirations; only in the most severe cases does cyanosis occur. Usually the chest radiograph shows only hyperaerated lungs, but there may occasionally be areas of atelectasis.

Children with bronchiolitis may benefit from nebulized bronchodilators. For the patient who does not respond to nebulized albuterol or has only mild distress, therapy is limited to antipyretics and the encouragement of adequate oral intake. Dehydration, secondary bacterial infection, and marked respiratory distress necessitate admission to the hospital. An oxygen saturation less than 93% or an arterial PaO$_2$ below 70 torr in room air also suggests the need for hospitalization. Additionally, children with underlying cardiac or pulmonary disease usually require admission. Ribavirin may have some value in ameliorating the course of bronchiolitis, when administered by continuous aerosol for 3 to 5 days to severely ill children who are hospitalized.

Pertussis

The first stage (catarrhal), characterized by a mild cough, conjunctivitis, and coryza, lasts for 1 to 2 weeks. An increasingly severe cough heralds the onset of the second stage (paroxysmal), which continues for 2 to 4 weeks. After a prolonged spasm of coughing, the sudden inflow of air produces the characteristic whoop. Vomiting often occurs after such an episode. When not coughing, the child has a remarkably normal physical examination, except for an occasional subconjunctival hemorrhage. During the third stage (convalescent), the intensity of the cough wanes. The WBC count in children usually reaches 20,000 to 50,000/mm^3 with a marked lymphocytosis, but such changes are not often seen in infants younger than 3 to 6 months old. *Bordetella pertussis* can be identified by fluorescent antibody staining of secretions obtained from the nasopharynx or, less frequently, recovered by culture of this material. Because of the risk of complications, all children younger than 6 months of age with a firm diagnosis of pertussis should be considered for observation in the hospital. Older children who show signs of respiratory compromise, such as cyanosis during paroxysms of coughing, or who develop complications also require admission. Treatment includes 40 mg/kg erythromycin per day for 14 days, maintenance of adequate hydration, and a level of respiratory support appropriate to the severity of the disease.

Tuberculosis

Clinical Manifestations

The onset of primary tuberculosis pneumonia resembles that of bacterial infections of the lungs. It begins with fever and tachypnea; rales and an area of dullness are found on examination of the chest. The WBC count may be elevated with a shift to the left, and the chest radiograph shows a lobar consolidation, accompanied frequently by hilar adenopathy and less often by pleural effusion or cavitation. Although the primary pneumonia often resolves spontaneously, the child occasionally follows a downhill course caused by local progression. Clinical findings, in addition to the epidemiologic risks previously described, that should arouse a suspicion of tuberculous pneumonia in the child otherwise thought to have a bacterial infection of the lung include pleural effusion, cavitation, toxicity, and a failure to respond to antibiotic therapy.

Miliary tuberculosis begins with an abrupt increase in temperature but few other physical findings; it may mimic sepsis. Subsequently, respiratory symptoms and enlargement of the liver, spleen, and superficial lymph nodes occur. The WBC count is usually in the range of 15,000/mm^3. Although the chest radiograph initially shows no lesions, a diffuse mottling of the lung fields appears 1 to 3 weeks after the fever. Miliary tuberculosis is a consideration in a child with persistent fever and hepatosplenomegaly.

Tuberculous meningitis comes on insidiously with low-grade fever, apathy, and, in 50% of patients, vomiting. After 1 to 2 weeks of nonspecific illness, neurologic signs appear, including drowsiness and nuchal rigidity; untreated, the child lapses into coma. The cerebrospinal fluid shows a mononuclear pleocytosis, an elevated protein concentration, and, eventually, a low glucose level.

Management

A child suspected of having pneumonic, meningeal, or miliary tuberculosis should be admitted to the hospital for evaluation and possible chemotherapy. Among inner city populations, where the risk of tuberculosis is greatest, the routine placement of a tine or Mantoux test in children with lobar pneumonia should be considered. The Mantoux test (Fig. 11.29) must be interpreted in accordance with the age of the child and the presence of risk factors (Table 11.12). Current treatment for tuberculosis consists of multiple drugs (isoniazid, rifampin, pyrazinamide, ethambutol, streptomycin, capreomycin, ciprofloxacin, cycloserine, ethion-

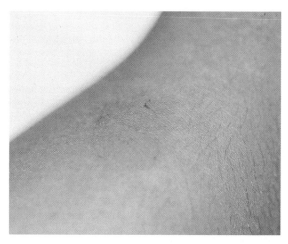

FIG. 11.29. A positive test for tuberculosis. To check a patient for immunity to tuberculous, a Mantoux test is performed. Purified protein derivative, made from the organism, is injected intradermally in a dose of 5 tuberculin units (intermediate strength purified protein derivative). The physician must examine the site 48 to 72 hours after the injection, feeling for induration and ignoring the presence of erythema alone. Traditionally, induration exceeding 10 mm has indicated a positive reaction, although as explained in Table 11.12, the criterion may be as low as 5 mm or as high as 15 mm, depending on the clinical circumstances.

amide, kanamycin, ofloxacin, paraaminosalicylic acid) for a minimum of 6 months.

Hantavirus

The Hantavirus pulmonary syndrome was described in 1994 among 17 adults and has been reported only rarely in children. The syndrome begins with fever, cough, and myalgias

TABLE 11.12. *Definition of positive criteria for the standard Mantoux skin test (5 tuberculin units of purified protein derivative) in children*[a]

Induration >5 mm
    Children in close contact with known or suspected cases of active tuberculosis, if adequate and timely treatment cannot be verified
    Children suspected to have tuberculosis based on consistent chest radiograph or clinical findings
    Children immunosuppressed based on therapy or disease
Induration >10 mm
    Children <4 yr of age
    Children with chronic illness including lymphoma, diabetes mellitus, renal failure, and malnutrition
    Children born in or traveling to regions of the world with a high prevalence of tuberculosis or exposed to adults likely to be infected
Induration >15 mm
    Children ≥4 yr of age without any risk factors

[a]Applies regardless of previous bacillus Calmette–Guérin vaccination.
Modified from 1997 RedBook, American Academy of Pediatrics.

followed shortly thereafter by tachypnea, tachycardia, dyspnea, and, finally, hypotension. Marked leukocytosis is common, along with thrombocytopenia and elevated clotting studies. The initial chest radiograph shows an interstitial infiltrate more often than an alveolar infiltrate, with changes starting or becoming bilateral in most cases. Pleural effusions occur in approximately one-fourth of patients. The diagnosis should be considered when severe pneumonia occurs in combination with systemic deterioration and can be confirmed subsequently by specific viral serology. Treatment is supportive.

Gastrointestinal Infections

Viral Gastroenteritis

Children with viral gastroenteritis are usually brought to the emergency department with a complaint of diarrhea and/or vomiting. Although hematochezia may occasionally occur in viral infections, the presence of blood in the stool should suggest a bacterial gastroenteritis. Vomiting may accompany diarrhea or be the sole manifestation of viral gastroenteritis. Many children with viral gastroenteritis beyond the age of 2 or 3 years complain of crampy abdominal pain. Children with viral gastroenteritis are usually febrile. However, in the child older than 3 years of age, fever higher than 39°C may suggest bacterial enteritis. Tachycardia, hypotension, and lethargy may reflect dehydration in severe episodes. The abdomen is soft and nondistended in most cases. The skin turgor is decreased, and the mucous membranes are dry only in severe gastroenteritis with dehydration. No laboratory studies are indicated in the uncomplicated case of gastroenteritis. The complete blood count and electrolytes and blood urea nitrogen levels usually decrease to within the normal range but may be abnormal when dehydration ensues. Uncomplicated viral gastroenteritis usually remits in 2 to 5 days and does not require treatment in the hospital. The vomiting will generally respond to a brief cessation of oral intake. After 2 to 4 hours of abstinence, the diet should be resumed gradually. The diarrhea may persist for several days, but hydration can usually be maintained orally after the vomiting has subsided. Antiemetic and antidiarrheal agents are generally not recommended; however, recent studies suggested that ondansetron may be useful in children with emesis severe enough to require intravenous hydration.

Bacterial Gastroenteritis

Clinical Manifestations

Five pathogens commonly produce gastroenteritis: *Salmonella*, *Shigella*, *Yersinia*, *Campylobacter*, and pathogenic *E. coli*. Together, these organisms cause 10% to 15% of the diarrheal illnesses seen in children coming to an emergency department. In general, features suggestive of a bacterial rather than a viral gastroenteritis include (1) more than 10 stools per day or diarrhea lasting for more than 4 days, (2) blood in the stool, (3) fever of 39.5°C, 103.1°F or higher, (4) clinical toxicity, and (5) polymorphonuclear leukocytes in the stool. Unless protracted diarrhea has led to clinically apparent dehydration, the physical examination is unremarkable. Methylene blue staining of the stool may show the presence of polymorphonuclear leukocytes.

Management

Salmonella gastroenteritis is usually a self-limiting illness. The treatment should be directed toward the maintenance of adequate hydration. As with viral infections, limitation of the diet to electrolyte solutions (clear liquids) suffices in most children. Antibiotic therapy neither ameliorates the course of the gastroenteritis nor eradicates the organism from the intestinal tract. If bacteremia is suspected, intravenous therapy with 200 mg/kg cefotaxime per day in four divided doses or 100 mg/kg ceftriaxone per day in two divided doses should be initiated. Ciprofloxacin (20–30 mg/kg/day) provides an alternative for cephalosporin-allergic patients. When oral therapy is indicated, trimethoprim-sulfamethoxazole (8 mg/kg per day of trimethoprim and 40 mg/kg/day of sulfamethyrazole in two divided doses) is the drug of choice.

Shigellosis stands alone as the only form of bacterial gastroenteritis for which antibiotics have proved efficacious. Trimethoprim-sulfamethoxazole (8 mg/kg trimethoprim and 40 mg/kg sulfamethoxazole per day) is the initial drug of choice, while the results of sensitivity tests are pending. Fluoroquinolones and ceftriaxone are alternatives.

Most children with yersiniosis can be treated as outpatients. Suspected or proven sepsis merits intravenous administration of antibiotics such as gentamicin (5.0 to 7.5 mg/kg per day in three divided doses beyond the neonatal period).

Campylobacter enteritis is a self-limited but prolonged illness; diarrhea persists for more than 1 week in one-third of children. These organisms exhibit almost universal sensitivity to erythromycin, which can be given orally at a dose of 40 mg/kg per day; 1 gm po twice daily ciprofloxacin is an alternative for adolescents.

Skin, Soft-tissue, and Bone Infections

Impetigo

Impetigo is a frequent infection in children, particularly during the summer months, usually caused by group A streptococci or *S. aureus*. Typically, a parent will bring a child to the emergency department complaining of sores of the body. Physical examination shows a healthy child with a normal temperature. The lesions usually ooze serous fluid but may be bullous or crusted as well (Figs. 11.30, 11.31, and 11.32). Surrounding erythema is minimal, and the regional lymph nodes often do not enlarge noticeably. Erythromycin (40 mg/kg per day in four divided doses) provides effective oral treatment for the usual pathogens. Other acceptable oral drugs include dicloxacillin (50 mg/kg per day) or cephalexin

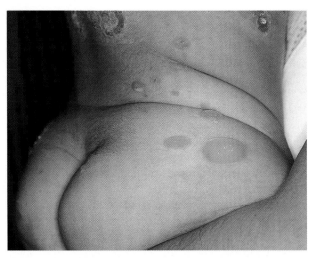

FIG. 11.30. Bullous impetigo. This 6-year-old girl developed widespread impetigo after a visit to Central America. Lesions appear crusted, scabbed, bullous, or covered with calamine lotion. *Staphylococcus aureus* causes almost all cases of bullous impetigo.

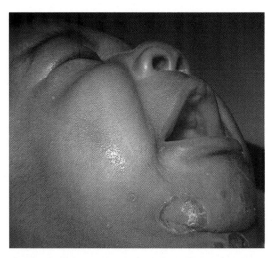

FIG. 11.32. Facial impetigo in an infant. This infant has a single patch of impetigo on her cheek. Because of the circular appearance of the lesion, it was thought to be a cigarette burn from child abuse on initial evaluation. Gram stain yielded abundant segmented neutrophils and Gram-positive cocci, followed by the isolation of *Staphylococcus aureus* in culture.

(50 mg/kg per day). Mupirocin applied locally is able to eradicate most cases of impetigo, particularly if the disease is limited in distribution.

Cellulitis

Background

Facial cellulitis includes buccal, periorbital, and, less frequently, orbital lesions (Figs. 11.33, 11.34, and 11.35). Before the introduction of a vaccine against it, *H. influenzae* type b caused 50% of these infections. At present, the organisms involved are most commonly *S. aureus* and group A streptococci. *S. aureus* causes most cases of nonfacial cellulitis (Figs. 11.36 and 11.37).

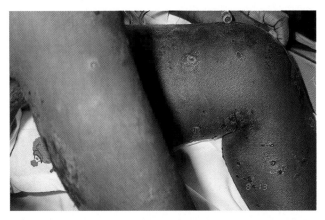

FIG. 11.31. Impetigo. This child has primarily crusted and scabbed as opposed to bullous lesions. Both group A streptococci and staphylococci may produce lesions with this morphology.

Clinical Manifestations

The child with cellulitis develops a local inflammatory response at the site of infection with erythema, edema, warmth, pain, and limitation of motion. There may be a history of a wound, animal bite, or insect sting (Figs. 11.38 and 11.39). Only 10% to 20% of children with cellulitis have fever. The lesion itself is erythematous and tender but not fluctuant; red streaks may radiate proximally along the course of the lymphatic drainage. The regional lymph nodes usually enlarge in response to the infection.

With cellulitis caused by *S. aureus* or group A streptococci, the WBC count is normal in most children. Plain radiographs of an extremity should be obtained when osteomyelitis or a foreign body is a consideration, and a computed tomography scan is indicated when it is not possible to distinguish between orbital and periorbital cellulitis (Fig. 11.34D).

Management

Most children with nonfacial cellulitis can receive antibiotic therapy as outpatients, as long as bacteremic disease is unlikely (Fig. 11.40). Acceptable alternatives include a semisynthetic penicillin, such as dicloxacillin (50 mg/kg per day), cephalexin (50 mg/kg per day), and amoxicillin-clavulanic acid (50 mg/kg amoxicillin per day); *S. aureus* is generally resistant to penicillin and ampicillin. A complete blood count, blood culture, and aspirate culture are not necessary in afebrile patients.

If a child with nonfacial cellulitis has a high fever (39°C, 102.2°F or higher), the likelihood of a bacteremic infection or lymphangitic spread increases. A WBC count and culture of the blood should be obtained, along with consideration of a culture from the lesion. In cases in which the WBC count is

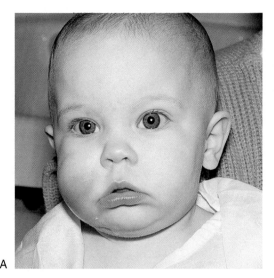
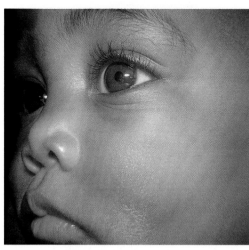

FIG. 11.33. A, B: Buccal cellulitis. Both of these infants have buccal cellulitis caused traditionally by a bacteremic infection with *Haemophilus influenzae* type b. The lesions of this disease are indurated and range from erythematous to reddish purple. In a child immunized against *H. influenzae* type b, *Streptococcus pneumoniae* may still cause buccal cellulitis with bacteremia.

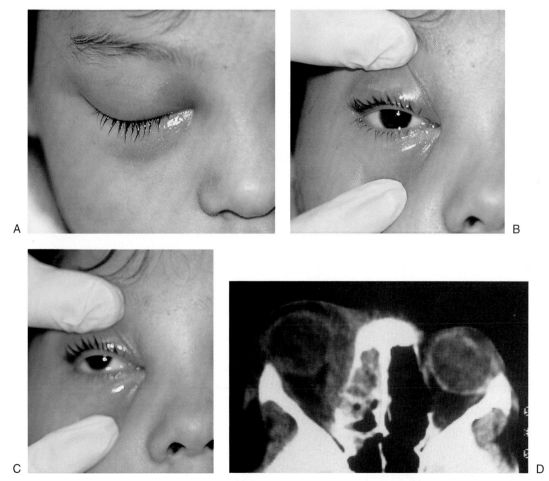

FIG. 11.34. Orbital cellulitis. This young girl has erythema and edema in the periorbital area **(A)**, which could be caused by either orbital or periorbital infection. However, she has limitation of the extraocular muscles, which characterizes orbital cellulitis, as shown when she is staring straight ahead **(B)** and gazing upward **(C)**. **D:** A computed tomography scan of the orbits demonstrates a mass lesion along the medial wall of the orbit in a child with ethmoid sinusitis and orbital infection. No abscess cavity is seen, suggesting that the infection is at the stage of a cellulitis that will respond to intravenous antibiotic therapy without drainage.

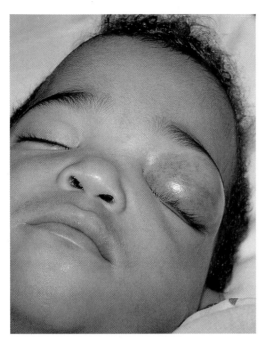

FIG. 11.35. Periorbital cellulitis. This boy has pronounced erythema and edema of the periorbital region. Without checking for proptosis and limitation of extraocular movements, periorbital cellulitis and orbital cellulitis appear indistinguishable. In some cases, a computed tomography scan is required to make the differentiation.

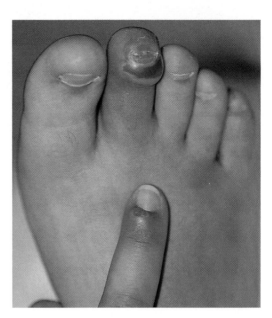

FIG. 11.37. Cellulitis of the toe. This infection began adjacent to the nail as a paronychia but has spread proximally to involve the shaft of the toe as cellulitis. Treatment requires both drainage and antibiotics.

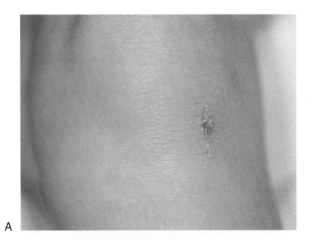

A

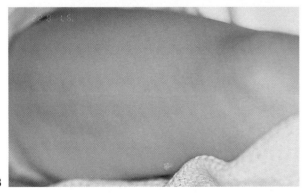

B

FIG. 11.36. Cellulitis of the knee. Cellulitis in this patient developed at the site of a minor wound **(A)**. The child was presented with fever and lymphangitic streaking **(B)**.

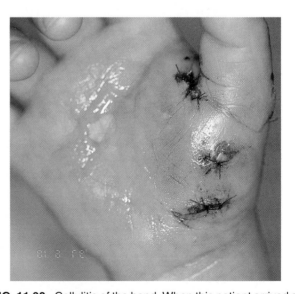

FIG. 11.38. Cellulitis of the hand. When this patient arrived at the emergency department, he had developed cellulitis, or wound infection, of the hand after the repair of a laceration that was secondary to a dog bite. In many cases, bite wounds of the extremities are not managed with primary closure because of the risk of infection, particularly with *Pasteurella multocida*. His sutures were removed to allow drainage he received and treatment with intravenous antibiotics.

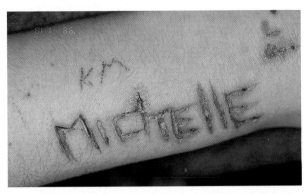

FIG. 11.39. Cellulitis of the arm. This young man developed cellulitis of his arm. Carvings, piercings, and tattoos all predispose to infection.

less than 15,000/mm³, antibiotic therapy is given as described for afebrile children. Leukocytosis in association with fever of 39°C or higher points toward intravenous treatment, usually on an inpatient basis, with 200 mg/kg cefotaxime per day in four divided doses, 100 mg/kg ceftriaxone per day in a sin-

gle dose, or ampicillin-clavulanic acid (200 mg/kg ampicillin per day in four divided doses). Children allergic to penicillins and cephalosporins can be given 40 mg/kg clindamycin per day in four divided doses and 75 to 100 mg/kg chloramphenicol per day in four divided doses or meropenem.

Fasciitis

Fasciitis is a deep soft-tissue infection. Unlike cellulitis, it involves the fascial and muscle layers as well as the skin and subcutaneous tissues but does not extend per se to the bones or joints. In recent years, the most common cause by far has been group A streptococci; other etiologic agents include *S. aureus* and anaerobic organisms.

As occurs with cellulitis, the child with fasciitis develops a local inflammatory response at the site of infection, characterized by erythema, edema, warmth, pain, and limitation of motion (Fig. 11.41). Fever develops in almost every case, often exceeding 39°C, 102.2°F. In contrast to the usual patient with cellulitis, those with fasciitis usually appear toxic with a marked tachycardia and, not infrequently, hypoten-

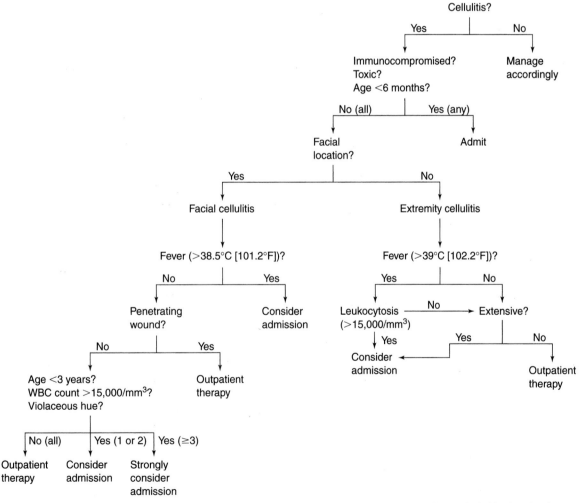

FIG. 11.40. Algorithm for the management of cellulitis. A young child with high fever, facial lesion, and elevated white blood count is at particular risk of a bacteremic infection.

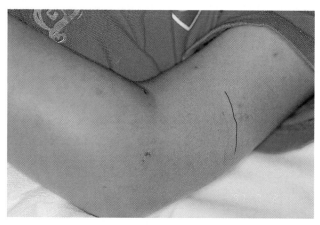

FIG. 11.41. Fasciitis. This child with varicella developed fasciitis of the forearm. He has several crusted lesions of varicella on the forearm and arm. The widespread, profound swelling points to involvement of the fascial planes rather than cellulitis.

sion. The local lesion is often described by the family as progressing rapidly and generally exhibits marked induration and erythema. Particularly in the presence of varicelliform lesions, the physician should maintain a high index of suspicion for fasciitis, as opposed to cellulitis, in children with extensive local disease, high fever, and any degree of prostration. The WBC count generally reflects leukocytosis, and blood cultures yield an organism in most cases. Appropriate antimicrobial therapy includes 500,000 U/kg penicillin per day in four divided doses and 40 mg/kg clindamycin per day in four divided doses intravenously. Surgical debridement is often necessary.

Omphalitis

Omphalitis is an infection of the umbilical cord and surrounding tissues by *Streptococcus pyogenes* (group A streptococci) and *S. aureus*; group B streptococci or Gram-negative enteric rods may also be isolated. Children are at risk during the first 2 weeks of life. Omphalitis is characterized first by drainage and later by erythema and induration (Fig. 11.42) around the umbilical cord stump. Late in the course of infection, infants manifest the signs of sepsis. Appropriate therapy is 150 mg/kg oxacillin per day in four divided doses and 7.5 mg/kg gentamicin per day in three divided doses for term infants.

Neonatal Mastitis

Mastitis is an infection of the breast tissue that affects prepubertal children only during the first 2 to 5 weeks of life. In most cases, *S. aureus* is the offending organism, although 5% to 10% of the infections are caused by Gram-negative enteric bacteria. The primary finding in neonatal mastitis is a warm, erythematous, enlarged breast bud (Fig. 11.43). With disease progression, purulent drainage from the nipple may occur and there is tenderness to palpation. Only 25% of infants are febrile or appear ill. Mastitis in the infant must be distinguished from physiologic hypertrophy, which resolves spontaneously. The normal breast bud that enlarges in response to stimulation by ma-

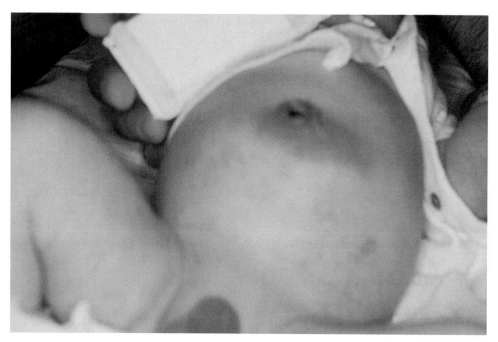

FIG. 11.42. Omphalitis. This 2-week-old (cord not yet detached) infant has omphalitis, characterized by induration and erythema encircling the umbilicus.

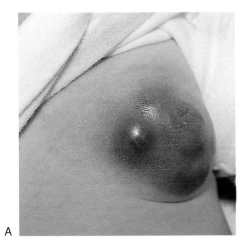
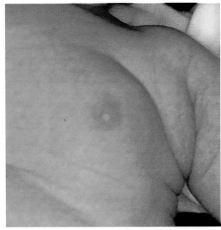

A B

FIG. 11.43. Mastitis. **A:** This infant has mastitis. The breast is swollen and erythematous, with some areas suggesting abscess formation. **B:** In contrast, this newborn has physiologic gynecomastia and lactation ("witch's milk"). Note that the breast shows no erythema.

ternal hormones is neither red nor tender; if any drainage is present, the material is milky white, rather than yellow, and does not contain polymorphonuclear leukocytes or bacteria on Gram stain. Oxacillin (150 mg/kg per day in four divided doses) and gentamicin (7.5 mg/kg per day in three divided doses) provide appropriate coverage for the expected pathogens.

Septic Arthritis

Background

Septic arthritis is an infection within a joint space. During the first 2 months of life, group B streptococci and *S. aureus* predominate. Gram-negative enteric bacilli, *Candida* species, and *N. gonorrhoeae* are seen sporadically. Between 3 months and 3 years of age, *S. aureus* emerges as the single most common pathogen, being isolated from 80% to 90% of children with septic arthritis. In most studies, *N. gonorrhoeae* has been the most common cause of septic arthritis among adolescents, followed closely by *S. aureus*.

Clinical Features

Infection within a joint produces pain and limitation of motion. Ninety percent of children have a monoarticular arthritis that involves the lower extremity (hip, knee, and ankle). Thus, limp is the most common initial manifestation. If a joint in the arm is involved, there will be decreased mobility of the upper extremity. With infections in deeper joints, the pain may radiate to contiguous anatomic structures. Children with a septic hip often complain of an ache at the knee, and sacroiliac arthritis may mimic appendicitis, pelvic neoplasm, or urinary tract infections.

Most children with septic arthritis have fever of 38.5°C, 101.3°F. The absence of fever occurs most commonly in the adolescent with a gonococcal infection or the neonate. Chil-

dren with a septic hip tend to maintain the affected extremities in a position of comfort (Fig. 11.44). An erythematous swelling may surround a superficial joint that is infected (Fig. 11.45).

The erythrocyte sedimentation rate is the most consistently abnormal laboratory study. The peripheral WBC count usually varies from less than 5,000 to more than 20,000/mm³. Although leukocytosis with a shift to the left occurs commonly, as many as 20% of children will have a WBC count less than 10,000/mm³. The first radiographic alteration to be noted is edema of the adjacent soft tissues, which is not

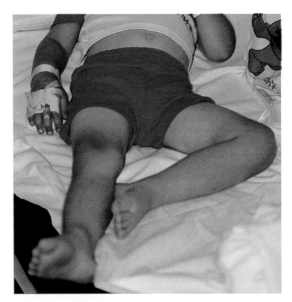

FIG. 11.44. Septic hip. This boy presented with fever and refusal to bear weight. He is holding his left lower extremity flexed and externally rotated at the hip, as is characteristic with bacterial infection of the joint. Ultrasonography-guided aspiration yielded purulent fluid from which *Staphylococcus aureus* was isolated.

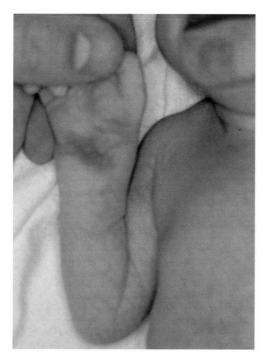

FIG. 11.45. Septic arthritis of the wrist. This 8-day-old infant presented with multiple foci of infection, including his knee and wrist, which is quite swollen. Purulent fluid obtained from the joint grew group B streptococci.

pathognomonic of inflammation in the joint. Later, distention of the capsule becomes visible (Fig. 11.46), and bony destruction may be seen late in the course of the infection. The hip may actually dislocate with intraarticular infection in the young infant, but this is an unusual radiographic finding in older children. Ultrasonographic examination is useful for the detection of a small effusion not apparent on radiography. No constellation of laboratory and radiographic results can

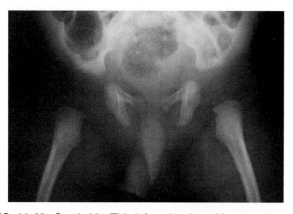

FIG. 11.46. Septic hip. This infant developed fever and paradoxical irritability. On examination, movement of his right hip caused marked discomfort. The radiograph shows dislocation of the head of the femur out of the acetabulum, secondary to the presence of pus under pressure in the joint. This finding occurs only during infancy, when the joint capsule has less strength.

rule out the diagnosis of septic arthritis; an analysis of the joint fluid is mandatory if the index of suspicion is high.

Management

The initial treatment is aimed at relieving the pressure within the joint and controlling the infection. Prompt surgical intervention is needed for hip infections. The initial choice of antimicrobials depends on the age of the child and the Gram stain. If no organisms are apparent on examination of the joint fluid, presumptive antibiotic therapy is begun as follows: (1) 2 months of age or younger: 150 mg/kg oxacillin per day in four divided doses and 7.5 mg/kg gentamicin per day in three divided doses; (2) older than 2 months to 3 years of age: 200 mg/kg cefotaxime per day in four divided doses, ampicillin-clavulanic acid (200 mg/kg ampicillin per day in four divided doses); (3) older than 3 years of age: 150 mg/kg oxacillin per day to a maximum of 6 g per day. Ceftriaxone (100 mg/kg once daily) may be used as a single agent for children older than 2 months; as further experience confirms the virtual disappearance of *H. influenzae*, 150 mg/kg oxacillin per day in four divided doses will probably prove to be sufficient as monotherapy after infancy.

Osteomyelitis

Background

Osteomyelitis is an infection of the bone; a variant, discitis, affects the intervertebral disc space. *S. aureus* causes osteomyelitis in most children regardless of age. During the neonatal period, group B streptococci are the second most frequent isolate; *N. gonorrhoeae* and Gram-negative enteric bacilli are also found. Group A streptococci cause 5% to 10% of cases of osteomyelitis in childhood.

Clinical Features

Osteomyelitis causes bone pain as the infection progresses. The femur and tibia are the most common bones infected, making limp a common presentation. Osteomyelitis affects the bones of the upper extremity in 25% of cases. These children complain of pain on motion of their upper extremities.

Fever exceeds 38.5°C, 101.3°F in 70% to 80% of children with osteomyelitis. The infant with a long bone infection often manifests pseudoparalysis, an unwillingness to move the extremity. Movement may also be decreased in the older child, but to a lesser degree. Point tenderness is seen almost always in osteomyelitis; however, it is found in other conditions such as trauma, may be difficult to discern in the struggling infant, and does not always occur early in the course of the infection. Percussion of a bone at a point remote from the site of an osteomyelitis may elicit pain in the area of infection. Rarely, purulent material ruptures through the cortex and causes diffuse local erythema and edema.

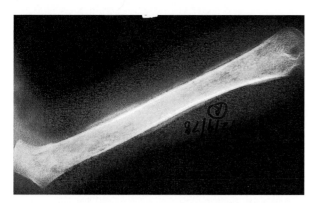

FIG. 11.47. Osteomyelitis. Osteomyelitis caused by *Salmonella* species progressed rapidly in this child with sickle cell anemia, leading to periosteal elevation (one of the earlier bony changes) and bony erosions (a late finding).

The erythrocyte sedimentation rate provides a useful screening test for osteomyelitis because bony infection usually leads to an elevation. Although the WBC count may reach 20,000/mm³, it falls within the normal range in two-thirds of cases. If osteomyelitis is suspected, radiographs of the affected area should always be obtained, even though they are often normal early in the course. The first change, noted after 3 to 4 days, is deep soft-tissue swelling seen as a subtle shift of the lucent deep-muscle plane away from the bone. Late findings include lytic lesions and periosteal elevation (Fig. 11.47). Radionuclide scanning provides a useful diagnostic tool for the clinician. When scintigraphy is not diagnostic and clinical suspicion persists, magnetic resonance imaging should be obtained.

Management

All children strongly suspected or known to have osteomyelitis require admission to the hospital for intravenous antibiotic therapy. Infants should subsequently receive 150 mg/kg oxacillin per day in four divided doses and 7.5 mg/kg gentamicin per day in three divided doses; older children can be treated with oxacillin alone.

Genitourinary Infections

Urethritis/Cervicitis

Urethritis, caused by *N. gonorrhoeae* (p. 209) and/or *C. trachomatis*, produces dysuria and discharge in the male. Mucopurulent cervicitis, caused by *C. trachomatis* in the adolescent female, is characterized by an erythematous friable cervix and the accumulation of purulent yellow endocervical secretions. In prepubertal girls, *C. trachomatis* is a rare cause of vaginitis, usually with scant or no discharge. If an etiologic diagnosis is not possible based on the clinical findings and the results of Gram stain, treatment should be given for both *N. gonorrhoeae* (see later) and *C. trachomatis*. Infections with *C. trachomatis* in adolescents and children older than 8 years of age are treated

with 100 mg doxycycline twice daily or a single dose of 1 g azithromycin. Children younger than 8 years of age may be given 20 mg/kg azithromycin as a single dose or 40 mg/kg erythromycin per day in four divided doses for 10 days.

Urinary Tract Infections

Clinical Manifestations

The manifestations of urinary tract infections vary with age, being particularly nonspecific in infancy. During the neonatal period, a septic appearance or fever is often the only finding. Urinary tract infections in infants may also cause vomiting, diarrhea, irritability, and, reportedly, meningismus. Beyond 2 to 3 years of age, symptoms more often point to the urinary tract. Typically, children with cystitis appear relatively well and complain of dysuria and suprapubic pain. On examination, they have low-grade fever and tenderness in the suprapubic area. In contrast, patients with pyelonephritis may be toxic and usually have additional symptoms, including vomiting and flank pain. The physician is often able to elicit tenderness to percussion in the costovertebral area. The mainstays of diagnosis are the urinalysis and culture of the urine. A schema for the use of urinalysis and urine culture is presented in Figure 11.48.

Management

Most patients respond to oral antibiotic therapy. Indications for intravenous administration of antibiotics include (1) clinical toxicity; (2) age younger than 3 to 6 months; (3) vomiting, refusal to drink, or other factors making the delivery of oral medications unreliable; (4) adverse anatomic factors, such as an obstruction to urinary flow; and (5) a known positive culture for a pathogen resistant to oral agents. For ill-appearing patients, 200 mg/kg intravenous ampicillin per day in four divided doses plus 7.5 mg/kg gentamicin per day in three divided doses, adjusted for gestation age and weight (Table 11.2) are given. Options for oral therapy include 8 mg/kg trimethoprim and 40 mg/kg sulfamethoxazole per day in two divided doses. Or 8 mg/kg cefixime per day as a single daily dose. If the pathogen is susceptible to ampicillin, amoxicillin 40 mg/kg/day in 2–3 divided doses provides effective oral coverage.

SPECIFIC INFECTIONS

Sexually Transmitted Diseases

Gonorrhea

Clinical Manifestations

The most common form of infection with *N. gonorrhoeae* seen among children is infection of the genitals. Prepubertal girls develop vaginitis rather than cervicitis as seen in adult women because of differences in the vaginal mucosa. Vaginal irritation, dysuria, and a discharge are the most frequent complaints. Boys have a urethral discharge and, occasionally, swelling of the penile shaft (Fig. 11.49) or

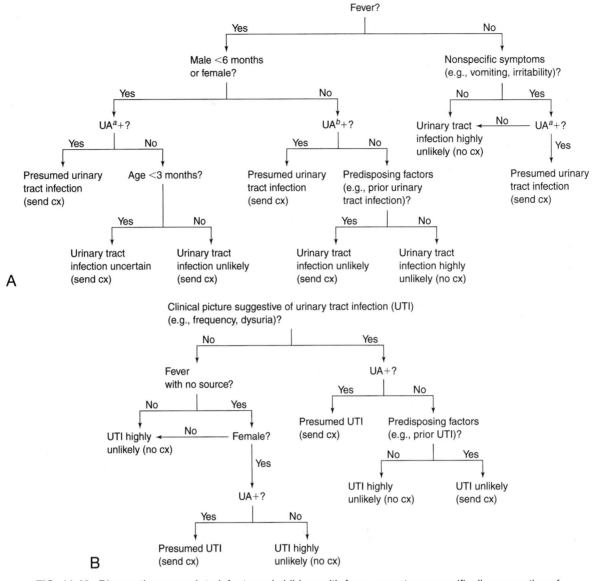

FIG. 11.48. Diagnostic approach to infants and children with fever, symptoms specifically suggestive of urinary tract infection, and/or non-specific symptoms and signs compatible with urinary tract infection. Use of urinalysis and culture in the diagnosis of UTI **(A)** in children 2 years or younger and **(B)** in those older than 2 years

ᵃUA obtained by catheterization or suprapubic aspiration
ᵇUA (only) may obtained using a urine collection bag
UA = urinalyisis
cx = culture

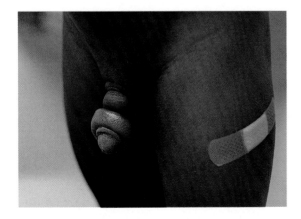

FIG. 11.49. Penile venereal edema. This 2-year-old boy developed a urethral discharge (positive for *Neisseria gonorrhoeae*), followed by painless swelling of the distal penile shift, or penile venereal edema. This condition is more common in adolescent and young adult males.

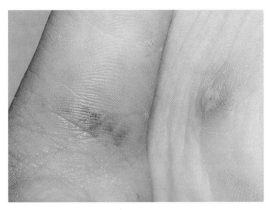

FIG. 11.50. Disseminated gonococcemia. *Neisseria gonorrhoeae* may disseminate from mucosal surfaces via the bloodstream and produce arthritis/arthralgia and a rash. The most characteristic lesion is the hemorrhagic vesicopustule seen in the web space of the teenage girl's hand. There is a pustule on the sole of her foot.

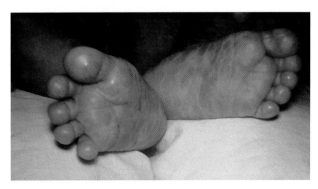

FIG. 11.51. Congenital syphilis. Congenital syphilis has many manifestations, including the pigmented lesions on the soles, as seen in this infant.

urinary retention. Despite the widespread use of prophylactic solutions in the eyes of newborns, gonococcal conjunctivitis continues to appear sporadically. A thick, purulent discharge quickly replaces the initial mild erythema from chemical irritation. Gonorrhea may spread systemically, causing joint pain (or frank septic arthritis) and a hemorrhagic, vesiculobullous rash (Fig. 11.50).

Management

All children with suspected genital gonorrhea should have cultures of the genitals, pharynx, and rectum as well as serologic tests for syphilis and HIV. When possible, treatment should be delayed in prepubertal children until the diagnosis is confirmed by culture because of medicolegal considerations. If the results of sensitivity testing are not available, 125 mg ceftriaxone intramuscularly is used for therapy. Alternatives for adolescents include single-dose oral therapy with 400 mg cefixime, 500 mg ciprofloxacin, or 400 mg ofloxacin. Spectinomycin is an acceptable alternative for penicillin-allergic patients in a dose of 40 mg/kg (maximum, 2.0 g) intramuscularly. Because the usual mode of acquisition often involves sexual contact, a report must be made to the appropriate community department that deals with child abuse. Concomitant therapy should be provided for *C. trachomatis*, with either 20 mg/kg azithromycin (maximum, 1 g) or doxycycline (in children older than 8 years) 100 mg twice daily.

Syphilis

Congenital syphilis usually presents as jaundice and hepatosplenomegaly in an ill-appearing newborn. However, some infants have only minimal findings, and the diagnosis is often overlooked in the nursery. These children may turn up in the first months of life with skin lesions (Fig. 11.51), a persistent nasal discharge, and/or painful extremities

(pseudoparalysis of Parrot). Dark-field examination of cutaneous lesions can identify the spirochetes, and the serologic test for syphilis is positive. Additionally, radiographs may show lesions of the long bones. Diagnostic criteria are provided in Table 11.13.

TABLE 11.13. *Criteria for diagnosis of neonatal and early congenital syphilis*

I. Diagnostic criteria
  A. Absolute
    1. *Treponema pallidum* seen by dark-field microscopy
  B. Major
    1. Condylomata
    2. Osteochondritis, perichondritis
    3. Snuffles
  C. Minor
    1. Fissures of lips
    2. Cutaneous lesions
    3. Mucous patches
    4. Hepatomegaly, splenomegaly
    5. Lymphadenopathy
    6. Central nervous system signs
    7. Hemolytic anemia
    8. Elevated cell count or protein level in spinal fluid
  D. Serologic
    1. Reactive serologic test for syphilis
    2. Reactive immunoglobulin M fluorescent treponemal antibody absorption test
    3. Nonreactive serologic test for syphilis
    4. Reactive serologic test for syphilis (standard test for syphilis) that does not revert to nonreactive within 4 mo
    5. Rising serologic test for syphilis over 3 months
II. Certainty of diagnosis
  A. Definite: absolute diagnostic criterion
  B. Probable: any of the following: (1) serologic criterion 4 or 5, (2) one major or two or more minor clinical criteria and serologic criterion 1 or 2, (3) one major and one minor clinical criterion
  C. Possible: serologic criterion 1 or 2 with only one minor or no clinical criterion
  D. Unlikely: serologic criterion 3, maternal history of adequate treatment for syphilis during pregnancy

Modified from Mascola L, Pelosi R, Blount JH, et al. Congenital syphilis revisited *Am J Dis Child* 1985;139:575–580.

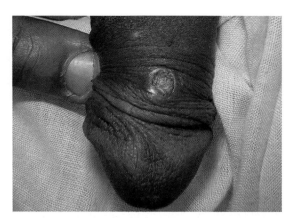

FIG. 11.52. Syphilis. This sexually active teenager developed the characteristic, painless chancre on the shaft of his penis. Serologic testing was indicative of syphilis.

Acquired syphilis appears in the teenager, as in the adult, in the first stage with a chancre (Fig. 11.52) and in the second stage with cutaneous or mucosal manifestations. The rash of secondary syphilis may resemble pityriasis rosea (Fig. 6.23), and all sexually active patients diagnosed with this disease, particularly with involvement of the palms or soles, should have a serologic test for syphilis. Other lesions include white patches on the mucous membranes and flat-topped warts (condyloma lata) around moist areas.

Congenital syphilis is rarely diagnosed in the emergency department, and the delay involved in confirmation moves the treatment out of the realm of the emergency physician. All such children require admission to the hospital. In acquired disease, 2.4 million U benzathine penicillin is given intramuscularly in a single dose for early syphilis and in three doses 1 week apart for syphilis of more than 1 year's duration.

Herpes Genitalis

Herpes simplex is the most common cause of genital ulceration seen in adolescents and adults at venereal disease clinics. Genital pain is a frequent complaint and may precede the appearance of the lesions. Characteristically, the virus produces grouped vesicles on an erythematous base (Fig. 11.53); however, erosion of the overlying skin often leaves only painful ulcers at the time of the first visit. Particularly with a primary infection, the inguinal lymph nodes enlarge. Oral acyclovir therapy is indicated for primary infections; the dose is 80 mg/kg per day in four divided doses.

Systemic Viral Infections

Viral Syndrome

The term nonspecific viral syndrome is used to refer to a generalized illness, presumed clinically to be caused by a virus and characterized by malaise and, usually, fever. Particularly with influenza, children who are able to verbalize their discomfort complain of diffuse aching. There may be a cough or an occasional bout of emesis. Signs of mild inflammation

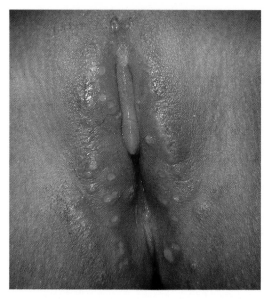

FIG. 11.53. Herpetic vulvovaginitis. These painful vesicles occurred in a 6-year-old girl who had been sexually abused.

may be seen in the upper respiratory tract. Treatment is limited to antipyresis with acetaminophen (15 mg/kg per dose) or ibuprofen (10 mg/kg per dose).

Erythema Infectiosum (Fifth Disease)

Erythema infectiosum, or fifth disease, is an exanthematous illness of childhood caused by parvovirus B19. It occurs most commonly between 2 and 12 years of age. The appearance of a rash marks the onset of the disease; fever or other prodromal symptoms are infrequent. The rash involves the face initially, conferring on the child a "slapped-cheek" appearance. Maculopapular lesions erupt 24 hours later, initially on the upper portion of the extremities, and they then spread both proximally and distally. Fading of the central portion of the lesions gives a lacelike appearance to the rash. Adolescents in particular may develop arthralgia or arthritis, and patients with chronic hemolytic anemias, such as sickle cell disease, are at risk of aplastic crisis. There is no specific therapy.

Human Immunodeficiency Virus

Primary Infection

Clinical Manifestations. Most children are infected prenatally. If not detected at birth by screening programs, they may present with failure to thrive, diarrhea, stomatitis (candidiasis), hepatosplenomegaly, respiratory symptoms due to *P. carinii* pneumonia, or frequent and/or unusual infections (Fig. 11.54). Adolescents who acquire HIV later in life may remain asymptomatic at the time of acquisition or manifest an infectious mononucleosis-like illness with fever, fatigue, and lymphadenopathy; the complete blood count may show thrombocytopenia.

Management. A primary diagnosis of HIV does not constitute an emergency, with the exception of *P. carinii* pneu-

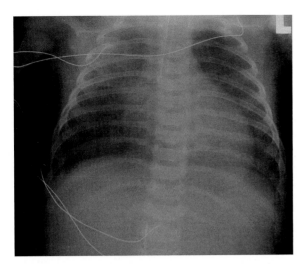

FIG. 11.54. *Pneumocystis carinii* pneumonia. This infant with congenital human immunodeficiency virus presented with pneumonia caused by *P. carinii*.

monia. In all cases, consultation with experts to decide on subsequent antiretroviral therapy is appropriate. Of more immediate concern in the acute care setting is exposure to blood and secretions, either through sexual contact, needle stick, or other types of trauma. Prophylaxis with antiviral therapy is indicated, although the effectiveness remains unproven.

Complications in Patients with Established Infections. The range of complications and the various presentations for patients with known HIV infection are protean. Particularly serious manifestations include, but are not limited to, sepsis, pneumonia, and meningitis caused by various viral, bacterial, fungal, and protozoal agents. In addition, the standard antiviral drugs may cause hepatitis, pancreatitis, nephrolithiasis, bone marrow suppression, and neuropathy. All patients complaining of new symptoms (e.g., fever, headache, respiratory distress, diarrhea, rash) require a careful evaluation with therapy directed to any specific etiology that is identified.

Infectious Mononucleosis

Infectious mononucleosis begins insidiously with fever and malaise. Three-fourths of children with this illness complain of a sore throat (Fig. 11.55). Occasionally, the onset resembles that of infectious hepatitis. Although a child may recover from infectious mononucleosis in 7 to 10 days, the symptoms usually last for 2 to 4 weeks. Enlarged lymph nodes are uniformly palpable. Although the lymphadenopathy may be limited to the cervical region (Fig. 11.56), involvement of the axillary and inguinal areas occurs commonly. In 75% of

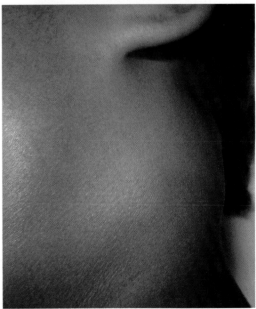

A

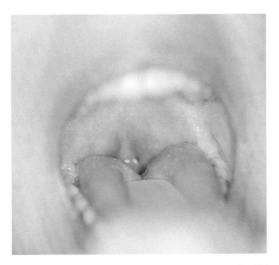

FIG. 11.55. Pharyngitis in infectious mononucleosis. This girl has inflamed, bilaterally swollen tonsils with a diffuse exudate, as is often seen with infectious mononucleosis.

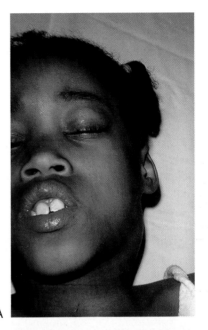

B

FIG. 11.56. A, B: Cervical lymphadenopathy in infectious mononucleosis. Cervical adenopathy occurs in most patients with infectious mononucleosis. As in this case, the nodes of the posterior chain are involved primarily and the appearance is one of enlargement rather than fluctuance.

cases, the pharynx is inflamed, often with an exudate. The spleen enlarges in 60% of children and the liver in 25%. Periorbital edema and a diffuse maculopapular rash are seen occasionally. There is an absolute lymphocytosis with many atypical mononuclear cells. The mainstay for the diagnosis of infectious mononucleosis in the adult is the heterophil antibody test, but these antibodies reach levels detectable by routine assays in only 50% of young children. Confirmation of a heterophil-negative case of infectious mononucleosis requires Epstein–Barr virus–specific serologic assays.

Specific therapy is not available. Adequate rest and nutrition should be maintained, and antipyretic agents will increase the child's comfort. The treatment of a child with uncomplicated infectious mononucleosis does not require the administration of corticosteroids, but the duration of the illness can be shortened and the patient made more comfortable by judicious use of a short course of 2 mg/kg prednisone for 7 to 10 days.

Measles

Fever and malaise herald the onset of measles. Within 24 hours, coryza, conjunctivitis, and cough develop. Koplik spots appear on the buccal mucosa by the third day of fever. These are seen as fine white spots on an erythematous background and have been likened to grains of sand. The rash erupts on the fourth or fifth day. The exanthem is maculopapular in appearance and begins on the face and neck. The lesions are heaviest on the upper portion of the body, often coalescing. As the rash advances down the trunk, the prodromal findings (cough, coryza, and conjunctivitis) and the Koplik spots resolve. The rash involves the extremities on its third day but has already begun to fade on the face. Leukopenia accompanies uncomplicated measles. Specific antibodies, initially absent from the serum, reach detectable levels 2 weeks after the onset of illness. Measles runs a self-limited course. Bed rest and antipyretic therapy help to keep the child comfortable. Measles is a preventable disease. Otherwise healthy, susceptible contacts should receive 0.25 mL/kg immune serum globulin; the dose is increased to 0.5 mL/kg for immunocompromised patients.

Roseola

Roseola infantum, or exanthem subitum, is a common, self-limiting, viral infection of infants caused in most cases by human herpesvirus 6. The child, usually younger than 3 years old, presents with high fever, as high as 40.5°C, (104.9°F) and few physical findings. There may be mild irritability but no coryza, pharyngeal infection, or conjunctivitis. After 2 to 4 days of illness, the fever drops precipitously and a rash appears. The lesions are discrete, pink maculopapules 2 to 3 mm in diameter. They fade with pressure and do not coalesce. The exanthem appears on the trunk initially and spreads outward. Roseola resolves without complications other than an occasional febrile convulsion. The

diagnosis of roseola is made based on the clinical course, often in retrospect. If a WBC count is obtained, leukopenia will be seen. Treatment is limited to antipyretic agents.

Rubella

Rubella is a childhood infection caused by a specific togavirus. Rubella traditionally occurs in children 5 to 9 years of age, but the incidence among teenagers is increasing. Only 10% of children experience prodromal symptoms such as fever, malaise, cough, and mild conjunctivitis. However, such complaints are frequently voiced by the adolescent. The rash begins on the face and spreads downward, reaching the extremities by the end of the second day. The lesions are pink maculopapules that may coalesce. The lymph nodes in the postauricular, suboccipital, and posterior cervical chains enlarge and become somewhat tender. During the first 2 days of illness, fever usually rises but remains less than 39°C or 102.2°F. The WBC count often decreases in rubella, and a few atypical lymphocytes may appear. Rubella is difficult to diagnose clinically because of its infrequent occurrence and the plethora of exanthems that have a similar appearance. Situations that require a definite etiologic diagnosis, such as pregnancy in an adolescent, demand serologic confirmation. Children with rubella can be managed as outpatients with antipyretic therapy.

Varicella/Zoster

Clinical Findings

Varicella. A mild prodrome that lasts 1 to 3 days frequently precedes the exanthem of varicella; however, the first sign of illness may be the rash. A fever, usually lower than 39.5°C or 103.1°F, develops in most children, and they may complain of malaise. Lesions erupt initially on the upper trunk, neck, or face and spread centripetally. Pruritus is universal. The abnormal findings on physical examination are limited to the elevated temperature and the skin and mucous membrane lesions. Initially, the exanthem consists of erythematous papules that evolve into vesicles and then pustules over 6 to 8 hours (Figs. 11.57 and 11.58). The early vesicles have a diameter of 2 to 4 mm and a "dewdrop-like" appearance. Because new lesions erupt in crops for 2 to 4 days, papules, vesicles, and pustules are usually seen together. An exanthem involves the mucosa of the oropharynx and, occasionally, the vagina. The severity of the cutaneous manifestations varies widely, and there may be from one to more than 1,000 lesions. Varicella runs a self-limited course in most cases but is occasionally a more serious illness with complications, including encephalitis, bacterial superinfection, bullous varicella (caused by either viral proliferation or cutaneous superinfection) (Figs. 11.59 and 11.60), pneumonia (Fig. 11.61), hepatitis, Reye syndrome, medication overdoses, exacerbation of an underlying disease, and dehydration. Starting in approximately 1990, several authors reported an increasing incidence of group A streptococcal coinfection with varicella, including primarily sepsis and necrotizing fasciitis (Fig. 11.41).

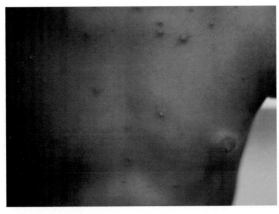
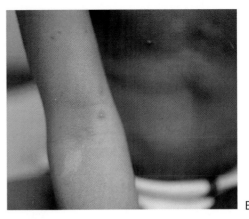

FIG. 11.57. (A, B) Varicella. This patient displays the typical findings in varicella. Lesions occur in different stages. Most characteristic are vesicles and "dewdrops" (2- to 3-mm fine vesicles on a 4- to 5-mm base of erythema).

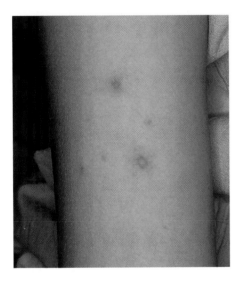

FIG. 11.58. Varicella. This child also displays typical lesions.

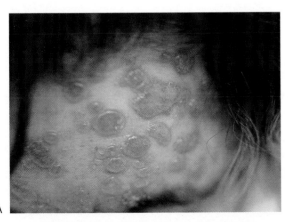
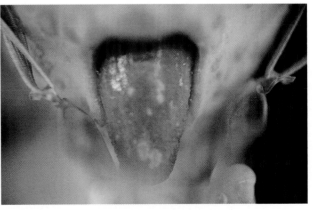

FIG. 11.59. A, B: Bullous varicella. This teenager began with an ordinary case of varicella. By the third day, the lesions had become bullous, on both the skin (exanthem) and mucosa (enanthem). She developed severe pneumonia.

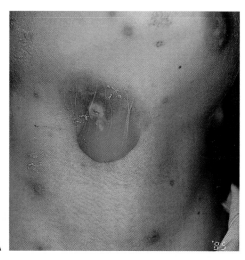

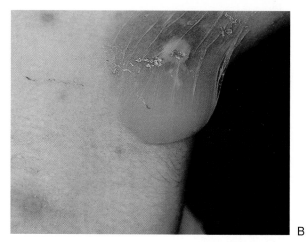

FIG. 11.60. A, B: Bullous varicella. Large bullae appeared in this child with varicella that became secondarily infected with *Staphylococcus aureus*.

Zoster. Zoster appears suddenly in most children without any warning symptoms (pain or pruritus). The lesions are grouped vesicles on an erythematous base in a dermatomal distribution. Zoster varies from mild (Fig. 11.62) to severe (Fig. 11.63) and may involve any portion of the body, including the face (Fig. 11.64). In 15% to 20% of cases, extradermatomal cutaneous dissemination is seen. Severe local disease, extradermatomal spread, and visceral dissemination are particularly likely in the immunocompromised host (Fig. 11.65). However, spread to the viscera does not occur in the immunocompetent child. If the eruption follows the ophthalmic branch of the trigeminal nerve, the cornea may be involved. The appearance of vesicles on the tip of the nose should evoke suspicion of ocular involvement that can be best seen after fluorescein staining of the eye.

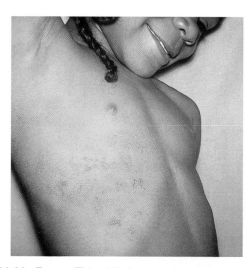

FIG. 11.62. Zoster. This child has a mild outbreak of zoster of the chest. The lesions are virtually identical to the exanthem of primary varicella, other than being confined to a single dermatome.

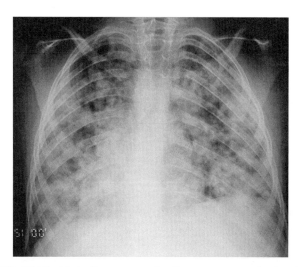

FIG. 11.61. Varicella pneumonia. Severe pneumonia developed in this patient shortly after she developed vesicular skin lesions that were positive for varicella-zoster virus by direct fluorescent antibody. Varicella causes a diffuse, miliary pattern.

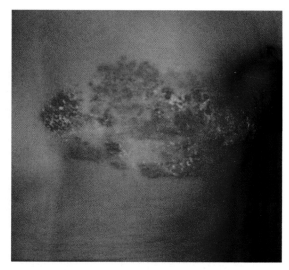

FIG. 11.63. Zoster. This case of truncal zoster is quite severe. Many areas are confluent.

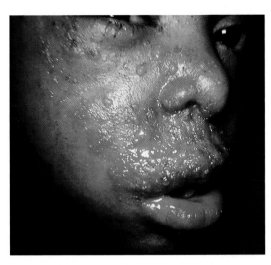

FIG. 11.64. Zoster. Not uncommonly, zoster involves the face. This child has an eruption along the maxillary branch of the mandibular nerve.

Management

Visual inspection suffices for the diagnosis of varicella; no laboratory studies are indicated. Acetaminophen is given to control the fever, and antihistaminic drugs provide some relief from the pruritus. Aspirin is contraindicated because of an association with Reye syndrome. Treatment to decrease pruritus includes 5 mg/kg diphenhydramine per day, 2 mg/kg hydroxyzine per day, or other antihistamines. The child cannot attend school for 1 week after the eruption of the first lesion. For immunocompetent children, 20 mg/kg oral acyclovir per day, given within 24 hours of the onset of the rash, reduces the duration of fever and the number and dura-

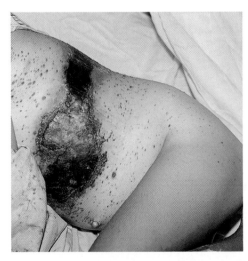

FIG. 11.65. Zoster in a child with relapsed leukemia. This unfortunate girl developed zoster in the era before the development of effective antiviral therapy, when the fatality rate was approximately 10%. The lesions became confluent and hemorrhagic because of the combination of immunodeficiency and thrombocytopenia. Note the scattered extradermatomal spread, which occurs in 25% of immunocompetent patients.

tion of skin lesions. Indications for use have not been formalized, but consideration is warranted for patients who are at some risk of a particularly severe course: infants younger than 6 months old, adolescents (older than 12 years of age), children receiving long-term aspirin therapy or being treated with oral/inhaled steroids, patients with chronic cutaneous (e.g., atopic dermatitis) or pulmonary (e.g., cystic fibrosis) disorders, and those with fever higher than 40°C or 104°F and a large number of lesions noted as early as the first day of the eruption (particularly if the case follows a household contact). Immunosuppressed children with varicella require hospitalization to receive intravenous acyclovir.

Zoster usually requires no specific therapy. Although famciclovir and valacyclovir are recommended for adults, they have not been shown to be efficacious in children. Antipruritic and antipyretic agents provide symptomatic relief. Immunocompromised children should be admitted to the hospital. Intravenous acyclovir therapy benefits immunocompetent children with unusually severe disease and reduces the incidence of dissemination in immunocompromised patients. Ocular involvement merits consultation with an ophthalmologist.

Miscellaneous Infections

Babesiosis

Babesia species, particularly *Babesia microti*, are protozoa transmitted by the bite of an *Ixodes* tick, which also serves as a vector in Lyme disease. The clinical picture of babesiosis resembles that of malaria and is characterized by anorexia, malaise, fatigue, and intermittent chills, sweats, and fever as high as 40°C or 104°F. Other than an elevated temperature, physical findings are absent or limited to mild hepatosplenomegaly. Patients with asplenia or immunocompromise are susceptible to severe or even life-threatening disease. Laboratory findings include hemolytic anemia with reticulocytosis, a normal or slightly decreased leukocyte count, mild thrombocytopenia, and elevated liver enzymes in half the cases. Microscopic examination of a peripheral smears confirms the presence of intra- and extracellular ring forms (Fig. 11.66), similar to those of *Plasmodium falciparum*; specific serologic assays are available as well but the results are often unavailable for several weeks and do distinguish between acute infection and asymptomatic seropositivity. Therapy is reserved for patients with mild to moderate infections or a predisposition to severe disease. The treatment of choice is 40 mg/kg clindamycin per day in four divided doses and 25 mg/kg quinine per day in three divided doses given orally for 7 days.

Botulism

Children with food-borne botulism complain of weakness and a dry mouth; constipation and urinary retention may occur. Paralysis is noted within 3 days, usually affecting the cranial nerves first and then the extremities. Abnormalities

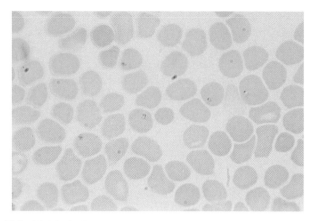

FIG. 11.66. Babesiosis. Babesiosis should be suspected in the setting of fever and anemia occurring in a patient living in an endemic area, such as Cape Cod. This girl, splenectomized during an episode of abdominal trauma years earlier, has a large number of ring forms in her erythrocytes.

of the neurologic examination include ptosis, extraocular palsies, fixed dilated pupils, symmetric weakness, and hyporeflexia. Infantile botulism occurs during the first 6 months of life. Constipation is the first symptom of the disease but may not be sufficiently severe to draw attention to any underlying illness. After several days, mild lethargy, weakness, and a decreased appetite are noted. On examination, the infant is quiet, with little discernible movement, and has a weak cry. The absence of a gag reflex, profound hypotonia, and hyporeflexia are important findings. The profound bulbar weakness in infantile botulism often prevents adequate fluid intake; dehydration occurs frequently. Respiratory failure is a potential life-threatening complication in botulism of any variety, and ventilatory support is often required. All require admission to the hospital; antitoxin is available from the Centers for Disease Control and Prevention.

Catscratch Disease

Catscratch disease is an infection caused by *B. henselae*. The most complete form of the illness begins with the appearance of a pustule at the contact site 7 to 10 days after exposure. Lymphadenopathy follows within 1 to 6 weeks. In one third of cases, the glands become fluctuant. The epitrochlear, axillary, inguinal, and cervical nodes are commonly affected (Fig. 11.67). Manifestations of atypical catscratch disease include encephalitis, aseptic meningitis, neuroretinitis (blindness and stellate macular lesions of the retina), Parinaud syndrome (conjunctivitis and preauricular adenitis), hepatitis, osteolytic lesions, and fever of unknown origin. The only controlled study of patients with typical catscratch disease found that 10 mg/kg azithromycin in a single dose on day 1, followed by 5 mg/kg once daily on days 2 through 5 shortened the duration of adenopathy. Nodes that persist and become fluctuant usually resolve after needle aspiration.

Ehrlichiosis

At least two *Ehrlichia* species cause two similar infectious illnesses, human monocytic ehrlichiosis and human granulocytic ehrlichiosis. *Ehrlichia* species are transmitted by a number of tick vectors throughout the United States. Both forms of the disease resemble Rocky Mountain spotted fever and are characterized by fever, chills, malaise, myalgias and headache. Unlike Rocky Mountain spotted fever, a rash occurs in only 40% of patients with human monocytic ehrlichiosis and rarely with granulocytic ehrlichiosis. The infection may spread to involve the meninges. Laboratory findings include anemia, thrombocytopenia, hyponatremia, and mildly elevated liver enzymes. Examination of the peripheral smear may show inclusions (morulae) in monocytes or granulocytes (depending on the species), but a definitive diagnosis relies on serology, which is available only from reference laboratories. The treatment of choice is 3 mg/kg doxycycline

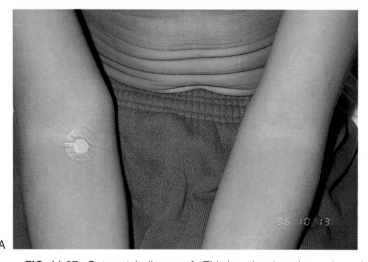
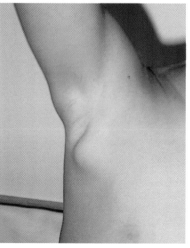

FIG. 11.67. Catscratch disease. **A:** This boy developed an enlarged, epitrochlear lymph node on the medial aspect of his upper extremity and axillary involvement. **B:** Neither node is tender or erythematous.

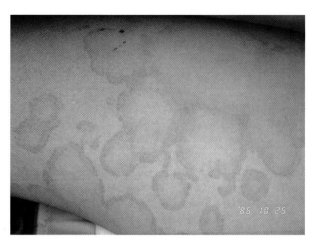

FIG. 11.68. Lyme disease. The characteristic eruption in Lyme disease is erythema migrans, formerly erythema chronicum migrans. Patients may develop a rash limited to the site of the tick bite, consisting of one or several lesions, or may have more diffuse involvement.

per day in two divided doses, even for children younger than 8 years of age; 75 to 100 mg/kg chloramphenicol per day in four divided doses is an alternative.

Kawasaki Disease

Children with Kawasaki disease initially appear to have a nonspecific, febrile viral syndrome. Beginning on approximately the third day of illness, more characteristic symptoms usually begin to evolve, including conjunctivitis, mucositis, anterior cervical lymphadenopathy, peripheral extremity changes (edema/erythema/desquamation), and a rash (Fig. 2.21). The conjunctivitis is bilateral and not purulent. Mucositis manifests as erythematous and/or fissured lips, at times with a "strawberry" tongue. The least constant finding is lymphadenopathy, which requires a node 1.5 cm or larger in diameter to meet criteria. Inflammation of the coronary arteries may be present at the time of diagnosis and detectable by echocardiography, but it does not usually cause clinical symptoms other than tachycardia out of proportion to the fever. Leukocytosis, thrombocytosis, and electrocardiographic signs of myocarditis are variably present at this stage. The diagnosis should be made based on clinical suspicion, without placing undue reliance on ancillary studies for confirmation. Treatment includes intravenous immunoglobulin, aspirin, and specific therapy for complications.

Lyme Disease

Lyme disease, an infection with *Borrelia burgdorferi* transmitted by the bite of a tick, has three stages. Stage 1 (localized disease) present in most but not all patients, consists primarily of erythema migrans. These lesions begin as small, red papules at the site of the bite of an infected tick, and expand centrifugally for weeks, often reaching 10 to 15 cm in diameter with central clearing (Fig. 11.68). In stage 2 (acute disseminated disease), findings may include fatigue, diffuse erythema migrans, headache, meningismus, cranial neuritis (particularly Bell palsy), and arthritis. In patients with neurologic signs, cerebrospinal fluid pleocytosis is common. In approximately 5% of cases, myocarditis occurs, often manifesting as heart block on electrocardiography (Fig. 11.69).

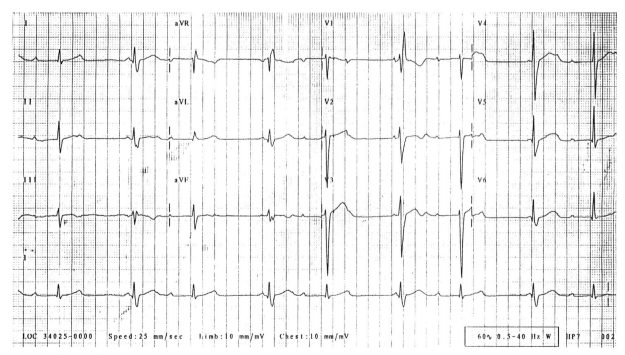

FIG. 11.69. Heart block in Lyme disease. Lyme disease has protean manifestations, including the cardiac and central nervous systems. This electrocardiogram shows heart block in a teenage boy with a tick bite, fever, aseptic meningitis, and positive serology.

Stage 3 (chronic disseminated disease) manifests, as does stage 2, but with more prolonged abnormalities and may include subtle neurologic dysfunction. Laboratory confirmation requires serologic testing with a delayed turnaround time. Patients with stage 1 and 2 disease usually respond to oral antibiotic therapy with either 100 mg doxycycline twice daily for 14 to 21 days or 50 mg/kg amoxicillin per day three times daily for 14 to 21 days. Meningitis, myocarditis, and persistent involvement of other organ systems are treated with ceftriaxone parenterally in a dose of 100 mg/kg per day for 14 to 28 days.

Malaria

Malaria, a protozoal infection, should be considered in recent immigrants from tropical areas and in travelers. The typical attack starts with a chill and tachycardia. Within 1 hour, fever develops and rises to 40°C (104°F) or higher. A profuse diaphoresis follows and lasts for several hours. Hepatosplenomegaly is a common finding. The febrile episodes may be accompanied by hypotension and jaundice. Laboratory findings include anemia, leukocytosis, thrombocytopenia, and hyperbilirubinemia. Complications of malaria caused by *P. falciparum* include massive hemolysis (blackwater fever), renal failure, pulmonary edema, and cerebral dysfunction. Neurologic signs of cerebral malaria include decreased level of consciousness, behavioral changes, hallucinations, seizures, and, rarely, focal signs. The cerebrospinal fluid is usually normal. Thick and thin blood smears should be done and, if positive, will confirm the diagnosis.

Children with suspected or proven malaria from areas without resistant *P. falciparum* should be given chloroquine phosphate (updated information on the geographic prevalence of resistance is available at www.cdc.gov). The initial dose is 10 mg/kg of base (maximum, 600 mg) followed by 5 mg/kg at 6, 24, and 48 hours. Patients unable to take oral medication require intravenous quinidine, beginning with a loading dose of 10 mg/kg infused over 1 hour with cardiac monitoring. Uncomplicated infections with chloroquine-resistant *P. falciparum* can be treated with 30 mg/kg oral quinine sulfate per day in three divided doses plus oral pyrimethamine-sulfadoxine (Fansidar) (younger than 1 year old, one-fourth tablet; 1 to 3 years, one-half tablet; 4 to 8 years, one tablet; 9 to 14 years, two tablets; older than 14 years, three tablets). Fansidar should not be used in patients with known sensitivity to sulfa drugs. An alternative regimen for chloroquine-resistant *P. falciparum* is 15 to 25 mg/kg mefloquine (maximum, 1,250 mg) as a single oral dose, but this drug should not be used in children who weigh less than 15 kg, pregnant women, or patients with epilepsy or psychiatric disorders. In life-threatening infections with known or suspected resistant organisms, quinidine should be administered intravenously, as already described; this drug carries a significant risk of adverse reactions and is thus reserved for emergencies.

Parasitic Infestations of the Gastrointestinal Tract

Various parasites can infest the gastrointestinal tract or invade the body via this route. These infestations may be asymptomatic, being detected on screening examination of the stool. In the emergency department, the diagnosis is usually entertained when a parent reports observing a worm [small pinworm (*Enterobius vermicularis*), large (*Ascaris lumbricoides*)] (Fig. 11.70) or in acute diarrheal diseases, particularly among patients who are immunosuppressed or recently lived in or traveled to underdeveloped countries. Two pathogens deserve particular consideration in the United States among immunocompetent children. *Cryptosporidium parvum*, first described as a cause of human disease in 1976 and well known as a pathogen in children with HIV, has been reported to be the responsible pathogen in 2% to 5% of cases of nonspecific, watery diarrhea and has been implicated in several large, waterborne outbreaks, one affecting an estimated 400,000 persons in Milwaukee, Wisconsin, in 1993. *Giardia lamblia* is also a waterborne parasite that can survive even in running waters and has been described as a cause of diarrhea among campers and hikers who have ingested water from streams. Both cryptosporidiosis and giardiasis merit consideration in daycare settings. Table 11.14 summarizes the clinical symptomatology and treatment of gastrointestinal parasites in children.

Rabies

Rabies is a viral infection of the brain that is almost invariably fatal. Although the actual disease is extremely rare in the United States, potential exposure in the form of animal bites occurs frequently. The decision of whether to give prophylaxis for rabies is influenced by the species of animal, the condition of the animal, the ability to study the animal, the type of exposure, and the prevalence of rabies in the region

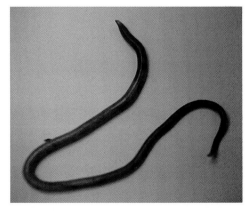

FIG. 11.70. Ascaris. Ascaris, a round worm, is usually 20 to 25 cm in length. As in this case, a typical specimen on visual examination provides sufficient evidence to institute treatment with mebendazole.

TABLE 11.14. *Parasitic diseases*

Parasite	Disease	Clinical manifestations	Treatment (uncomplicated disease)
Ancyclostoma braziliense	Cutaneous larval migrans	Serpiginous rash	Thiabendazole topically or 50 mg/kg/d in 2 divided doses
Ascaris lumbricoides	Ascariasis	Abdominal pain, passage of large (20-cm) worm	100 mg mebendazole b.i.d. for 3 d
Balantidium coli	Balantidiasis	Abdominal pain, vomiting, blooding diarrhea	35–50 mg/kg metronidazole daily in 3 divided doses
Cryptosporidium parvum	Cryptosporidiosis	Diarrhea	No proven therapy
Entamoeba histolytica	Amebiasis	Abdominal pain, bloody diarrhea, extraintestinal abscesses	35–50 mg/kg metronidazole daily in 3 divided doses
Enterobius vermicularis	Enterobiasis (pinworms)	Perianal pruritis, observation of small (1-cm) worm	100 mg mebendazole once; repeat in 2 wk
Giardia lamblia	Giardiasis	Diarrhea, malabsorption, abdominal pain	8 mg/kg furazolidone daily in 4 divided doses or 15 mg/kg metronidazole daily in 3 divided doses
Necator americanus	Hookworm	Initial pedal rash, then diarrhea and eosinophilia, later anemia	100 mg mebendazole b.i.d. for 3 d
Taenia saginatum/solium	Taeniasis (adult)/ cystercicosis (larvae)	Diarrhea, tapeworm segment in stool, seizures (cystercicosis)	Taeniasis: 10 mg/kg prazaquantil once; cystercicosis: 50 mg/kg prazaquantil daily in 3 divided doses
Toxocara canis	Visceral larval migrans	Hepatosplenomegaly	50 mg/kg thiabendazole daily in 2 divided doses
Trichinella spiralis	Trichinosis	Abdominal pain, vomiting, myalgias, periorbital edema, eosinophilia	300 mg mebendazole 3 t.i.d.

b.i.d., twice daily; t.i.d., three times daily.

(Fig. 11.71). If a sleeping or preverbal child has had close exposure to a bat in an area where rabies is endemic in this species, prophylaxis is indicated even in the absence of a visible bite wound because of the occurrence of several pediatric cases occurring in this circumstance. When the physician determines that prophylaxis is necessary, then 20 IU/kg human rabies immunoglobulin and human diploid cell vaccine are used. After cleaning the wound, as much human rabies immunoglobulin as possible is given locally and the remainder at a distant site. Vaccine must be given in the deltoid muscle (not the thigh or buttock) in a different extremity than that used for the human rabies immunoglobulin.

Rocky Mountain Spotted Fever

Clinical Manifestations

The incubation period of Rocky Mountain spotted fever ranges from 2 to 10 days but usually lasts 1 week. The initial symptoms of headache and malaise are followed by fever. The rash erupts on the third or fourth day of illness. In more than half the cases reviewed by Vianna, the exanthem appeared first on the wrists and ankles and then spread inward toward the trunk. The initial lesions are maculopapular but become hemorrhagic in the ensuing 24 to 48 hours if the disease remains unchecked (Fig. 11.72). Early in the course of the illness, the child remains alert. Conjunctivitis and a rash may be the only signs. Edema begins in the periorbital regions and involves the extremities as the vasculitis progresses. Mild splenomegaly is found in one-third of cases. Although the sensorium is clear initially, obtundation, and finally coma develop after several days of illness. The WBC count remains normal or increases slightly with Rocky Mountain spotted fever. Thrombocytopenia occurs in 75% of patients during the first stages of the disease; later, Disseminated Intravaccular Coagulation may develop with a prolonged prothrombin time and partial thromboplastin time as well as elevated fibrin split products. Most patients have hyponatremia but no other electrolyte abnormalities.

Management

The mildly ill child with fever, maculopapular exanthem, and a history of a tick bite can be treated as an outpatient. Chloramphenicol (50 mg/kg per day) is the drug of choice for patients younger than the age of 8 years and 50 mg/kg tetracycline per day in older youths. Admission is indicated in several situations: (1) clinical evidence of toxicity, (2) encephalitis, (3) thrombocytopenia (platelet count <150,000/mm^3) or derangements in the clotting studies, and (4) hyponatremia (sodium <130 mEq/L). In the emergency department, an intravenous infusion should be started and sufficient fluids administered to maintain an adequate blood pressure as discussed in the sepsis section. Chloramphenicol (50 mg/kg per day) can be given alone if the illness is clearly

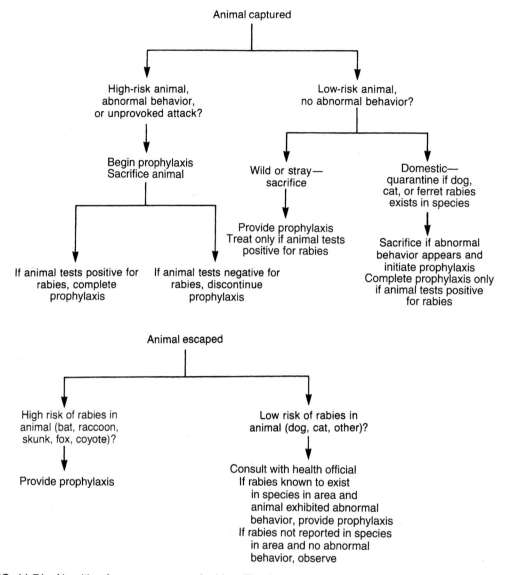

FIG. 11.71. Algorithm for management of rabies. The decision to administer prophylaxis (immunoglobulin and vaccine) against rabies depends on the species of the biting animal, the local epidemiology of rabies, and the ability to observe or study the animal.

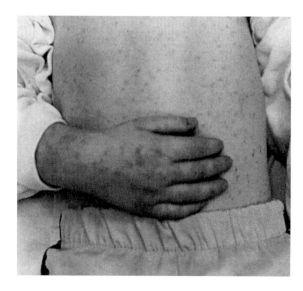

FIG. 11.72. Rocky Mountain spotted fever. This boy, recently returned from a camping trip during which he sustained numerous tick bites, presented with fever, headache, and rash. He has the typical exanthem of Rocky Mountain spotted fever, which begins on the ankles and wrists, spreads to the palms and soles, and evolves from maculopapular to petechial.

thought to be Rocky Mountain spotted fever; in practice, however, broader antibacterial coverage (e.g., chloramphenicol plus ampicillin or oxacillin) is often used because bacterial sepsis cannot be excluded.

Tetanus

Clinical tetanus is caused by the toxin produced by *Clostridium tetani*. The disease is rare in the United States (approximately 50 cases annually) because of widespread use of the vaccine. Neonatal tetanus from infections of the umbilicus by the organism continues to be reported occasionally. However, the more common problem for the emergency physician is the use of prophylaxis after traumatic wounds. Both 0.5 mL tetanus toxoid and 250 U human tetanus immunoglobulin may be indicated, depending on the wound and the immunization history (Table 11.15). Tetanus-prone wounds include punctures, crush injuries, and injuries contaminated by animal excreta or those left untreated for more than 24 hours.

Toxic Shock Syndrome

Toxic shock syndrome is characterized by severe, prolonged shock and is caused by a toxin produced by *S. aureus*. The illness begins suddenly with high fever, vomiting, and watery diarrhea. Pharyngitis, headache, and myalgias may also occur, and oliguria rapidly develops. Within 48 hours, the disease progresses to hypotensive shock. The patient has fever, usually 39° to 41°C (102.2° to 105.8°F, a diffuse, erythematous maculopapular rash, and hyperemia of the mucous membranes. Marked disorientation often evolves. The WBC count is elevated, with a shift to the left. Thrombocytopenia occurs frequently. Most patients develop DIC and have an elevated prothrombin time and partial thromboplastin time. Additional abnormalities in the laboratory studies may include elevated aspartate aminotransferase, alanine aminotransferase, blood urea nitrogen, creatinine, and creatinine phosphokinase levels. The management

of toxic shock syndrome is the same as that for shock caused by other organisms.

SUGGESTED READINGS

Abramson JS, Givner LB. Should tetracycline be contraindicated for therapy of presumed Rocky Mountain spotted fever in children less than 9 years of age? *Pediatrics* 1990;86:123–124.

Bass JW, Chan DS, Creamer KM, et al. Comparison of oral cephalexin, topical mupirocin and topical bacitracin for treatment of impetigo. *Pediatr Infect Dis J* 1997;16:709–710.

Bass JW, Freitas BC, Freitas AD, et al. Prospective randomized double blind placebo-controlled evaluation of azithromycin for treatment of cat-scratch disease. *Pediatr Infect Dis J* 1998;17:447–452.

Berman S. Otitis media in children. *N Engl J Med* 1995;332:1560–1565.

Book I. Microbiology of necrotizing fasciitis associated with omphalitis in the newborn infant. *J Perinatol* 1998;18:28–30.

Dagan R. Management of acute hematogenous osteomyelitis and septic arthritis in the pediatric patient. *Pediatr Infect Dis J* 1993;12:88–93.

Davis JP, Chesney PJ, Wand PJ, et al. Toxic shock syndrome: epidemiologic features, recurrence, risk factors, and prevention. *N Engl J Med* 1980;303:1429–1435.

Doctor A, Harper MB, Fleisher GR. Group A beta-hemolytic streptococcal bacteremia: historical overview, changing incidence, and recent association with varicella. *Pediatrics* 1995;96:428–433.

Finkelstein JA, Schwartz JS, Torrey S, et al. Common clinical features as predictors of bacterial diarrhea in infants. *Am J Emerg Med* 1989;7:469–473.

Fleisher G, Grosflam J, Selbst S, et al. Management of lymphadenitis in childhood. The role of percutaneous needle aspiration. *Ann Emerg Med* 1984;13:908–911.

Fleisher G, Ludwig S, Campos J. Cellulitis: bacterial etiology, clinical features, and laboratory findings. *J Pediatr* 1977;94:355.

Fleisher GR, Rosenberg N, Vinci R, et al. Intramuscular vs. oral antibiotic therapy for the prevention of meningitis and other bacterial sequelae in young, febrile children at risk for occult bacteremia. *J Pediatr* 1994;124:504–512.

Fries SM. Diagnosis of group A streptococcal pharyngitis in a private clinic: comparative evaluation of an optical immunoassay method and culture. *J Pediatr* 1995;126:933–936.

Harper MB, Bachur R, Fleisher GR. Effect of antibiotic therapy on the outcome of outpatients with unsuspected bacteremia. *Pediatr Infect Dis J* 1995;14:760–767.

Hoberman A, Wald ER, Reynolds EA, et al. Pyuria and bacteriuria in urine specimens obtained by catheter from young children with fever. *J Pediatr* 1994;124:513–519.

Huskins WC, Griffiths JK, Faruque AS, et al. Shigellosis in neonates and young infants. *J Pediatr* 1994;125:14–22.

Jones RN, Milazzo J, Seidlin M. Ofloxacin otic solution for treatment of otitis externa in children and adults. *Arch Otolaryngol Head Neck Surg* 1997;123:1193–1200.

Kaplan KM, Fleisher GR, Paradise E, et al. Social relevance of genital herpes simplex in children. *Am J Dis Child* 1984;138:872–874.

Kozyrskyj AL, Hildes-Ripstein E, Longstaff SE, et al. Treatment of acute otitis media with a shortened course of antibiotics. *JAMA* 1998;279:1736–1742.

Krauss PJ, Feder HM. Lyme disease and babesiosis. *Adv Pediatr Infect Dis* 1994;9:183–209.

Kuppermann N, Fleisher GR, Jaffe DM. Predictors of occult pneumococcal bacteremia in young febrile children. *Ann Emerg Med* 1998;31:679–687.

Lee GM, Harper MB. Risk of bacteremia for febrile young children in the post-*Haemophilus influenzae* type b era. *Arch Pediatr Adolesc Med* 1998;152:624–628.

Lieu TA, Fleisher GF, Schwartz JS. Cost-effectiveness of rapid latex agglutination testing and throat culture for streptococcal pharyngitis. *Pediatrics* 1990;85:246–256.

Lieu TA, Fleisher GF, Schwartz JS. Clinical performance and effect on treatmet rates of latex agglutination testing for streptococcal pharyngitis in the emergency department. *Dis J* 1986;5:655–9.

Lieu TA, Schwartz S, Jaffe JM, et al. Strategies for diagnosis and treatment of children at risk for occult bacteremia: clinical effectiveness and cost-effectiveness. *J Pediatr* 1991;118:21–29.

Nagy M, Pizzuto M, Blackstom J, et al. Deep neck infections in children: a new approach to diagnosis and treatment. *Laryngoscope* 1997;107:1627–1634.

TABLE 11.15. *Guidelines for tetanus prophylaxis*

No. of primary immunizations	Years since last booster	Type of wound	Recommendation
2	Irrelevant	Low risk	T
		Tetanus prone	T + TIB
3	10	Low risk	T
		Tetanus prone	T
3	5–10	Low risk	No treatment
		Tetanus prone	T
3	5	Low risk	No treatment
		Tetanus prone	No treatment

T, tetanus toxoid; TIG, human tetanus immunoglobulin.

Paradise JL. Short-course antimicrobial treatment for acute otitis media: not best for infants and young children. *JAMA* 1997;278:1640–1642.

Peña BM, Harper MB, Fleisher GR. Occult bacteremia with group B streptococci in an outpatient setting. *Pediatrics* 1998;102:67–72.

Peter J, Ray CG. Infectious mononucleosis. *Pediatr Rev* 1998;19:276–279.

Pichichero ME, Gooch M, Rodriquez W, et al. Effective short-course treatment of acute group a beta-hemolytic streptococcal tonsillopharyngitis. Ten days of penicillin V vs. 5 days or 10 days of cefpodoxine therapy in children. *Arch Pediatr Adolesc Med* 1994;148:1053–1060.

Ruuskanen O, Nohynek H, Ziegler T, et al. Pneumonia in childhood: etiology and response to antimicrobial therapy. *Eur J Clin Microbiol Infect Dis* 1992;11:217–223.

Schuchat A, Robinson K, Wagner JD, et al. Bacterial meningitis in the United States in 1995. *N Engl J Med* 1997;337:970–976.

Schwartz GR, Wright S. Changing bacteriology of periorbital cellulitis. *Ann Emerg Med* 1996;28:617–620.

Shaw KN, Gorelick M, McGowan KL, et al. Prevalence of urinary tract infection in febrile young children in the emergency department. *Pediatrics* 1998;102:e16.

Siegel RM, Schubert CJ, Myers PA, et al. The prevalence of sexually transmitted diseases in children and adolescents evaluated for sexual abuse in Cincinnati: rationale for limited STD testing in prepubertal girls. *Pediatrics* 1995;96:1090–1094.

Torrey S, Fleisher G, Jaffe D. Incidence of *Salmonella* bacteremia in infants with *Salmonella* gastroenteritis. *J Pediatr* 1986;108:718–721.

Vianna NJ, Hinman AR. Rocky Mountain spotted fever on Long Island. Epidemiologic and clinical aspects. *Am J Med* 1971;51:725–30.

Waisman Y, Klein BL, Boenning DA, et al. Prospective randomized double-blind study comparing L-epinephrine and racemic epinephrine aerosols in the treatment of laryngotracheitis (croup). *Pediatrics* 1992;89:302–306.

Wald ER. Sinusitis in children. *N Engl J Med* 1992;326:319–323.

CHAPTER 12

Musculoskeletal Emergencies

Editor: Marc N. Baskin

Osteomyelitis and septic arthritis are discussed in Chapter 11 (Infectious Disease Emergencies).

TOXIC SYNOVITIS

Toxic or transient synovitis is a benign, self-limiting inflammatory process of the hip and is the most common cause of acute hip pain in children 3 to 10 years of age. The underlying cause is unknown, although a postinfectious inflammatory response has been suggested. Its presentation can mimic that of septic arthritis of the hip, a distinction that is crucial in management.

Clinical Findings

The onset of symptoms is abrupt with unilateral hip pain and limp. Fever is rare, occurring in fewer than 10% of cases and, when present, is usually low grade. Although patients complain of discomfort with movement of the limb, it generally remains possible to put the hip through a full range of motion. This contrasts with the septic hip in which pain and spasm are more extreme, and patients resist a full range of motion.

Laboratory

The white blood cell count and erythrocyte sedimentation rate are generally normal or only slightly elevated. The mean white blood cell count and erythrocyte sedimentation rate are significantly lower than in septic arthritis; however, sufficient overlap exists between values in toxic synovitis and septic arthritis such that they cannot be relied on to distinguish between them in individual patients.

Radiographs may demonstrate an effusion, but their principal role is to exclude pathologic osseous conditions. Ultrasonography is more sensitive than plain films for detecting joint effusions. Reports of an effusion of the hip by ultrasonography in toxic synovitis vary from 50% to 95%. Although patients often report relief of pain after hip aspiration, the procedure is unnecessary except to exclude the presence of a bacterial infection. When obtained, synovial fluid is sterile.

Management and Prognosis

Treatment occurs on an outpatient basis and emphasizes rest and analgesics. Nonsteroidal antiinflammatory medications are the first-line therapy for pain. Pain duration is typically 3 to 4 days but may last as long as 2 weeks.

RADIAL HEAD SUBLUXATION

Nursemaid's elbow is the most common joint injury in pediatric patients, usually occurring in children between 6 months and 4 years of age. Subluxation of the radial head occurs as a result of abrupt traction on a pronated hand. The annular ligament slides over the radial head and becomes interposed between the radius and capitellum.

The child holds the arm slightly flexed and against his or her body. When left alone, the child does not appear to be in significant pain. Parents may report a problem with the wrist or shoulder because, in their attempts to check these joints, inadvertent movement of the elbow causes pain.

Point tenderness of the clavicle, humerus, radius, and ulna can be excluded with a deliberate examination that does not move the elbow at all. True tenderness and swelling at the elbow are usually absent. When disuse of the elbow is present without a history of trauma or swelling or bone tenderness on examination, the clinician should perform the reduction maneuver to confirm the diagnosis of radial head subluxation. Radiographs of the elbow are unnecessary unless the physician suspects another injury. Swelling and localized tenderness are usually apparent with supracondylar fractures, the next most common elbow injury in this age group.

Reduction of a subluxed radial head is a gratifying procedure for physicians and parents alike. Several effective maneuvers are described. The clinician holds the elbow with his or her thumb over the radial head. Supination of the affected arm with either flexion or extension of the elbow snaps the annular ligament back to its original position with a telltale click. If no click is felt, a second attempt can be made. Voluntary use of the arm will return in less than 15 minutes in almost 90% of patients.

Recurrent radial head subluxations are common, occurring in approximately one-third of cases. Caretakers should be counseled to lift the child from the axillae, avoiding traction on the extremities.

SLIPPED CAPITAL FEMORAL EPIPHYSIS

Although most cases of slipped capital femoral epiphysis present with chronic pain, a minority present acutely. Several studies have suggested that structural weakness is present in the capital femoral physis during the onset of puberty. This malady occurs predominantly in children 9 to 15 years of age, with a male/female predominance of approximately 2:1. Obese and African-American children are particularly susceptible.

The diagnosis of slipped capital femoral epiphysis should be considered in any preadolescent or adolescent complaining of hip, thigh, or knee pain. The history is often one of minimal trauma, causing pain in the hip, thigh, or knee region. Vague hip or knee pain and a limp in the preceding weeks are common. The diagnosis is made by the physical and radiographic examination. At rest the patient may lie with the hip slightly flexed with some external rotation. Range of motion abnormalities of the hip, in particular limitation of internal rotation, and abduction, and flexion, are almost universal. Range of motion in all directions may be painful.

The radiographic examination should include anteroposterior and frog-leg views of the pelvis. The affected femoral head is displaced inferior to the femoral neck. An imaginary line running along the superior femoral neck should intersect at least a small part of the femoral head. The slip is often seen more easily on the frog-leg view (Fig. 12.1). Comparison with the normal side may assist in the diagnosis. However, 10% to 25% of slips may be bilateral.

After the diagnosis has been made, treatment should consist of strict non–weight bearing and an urgent orthopedic consultation. Prompt pinning is required to prevent further slippage. This may be performed within 24 hours of assessment or shortly thereafter, depending on the availability of anesthesia.

LEGG–CALVÉ–PERTHES DISEASE

Legg–Calvé–Perthes disease is a hip disorder involving avascular necrosis of the capital femoral epiphysis that generally has onset between the ages of 4 and 9 years. Males outnumber females by a ratio of 4:1 and the incidence is increased in family members of patients. Most children with Legg–Calvé–Perthes disease are short, with delayed bone age.

The onset of symptoms in Legg–Calvé–Perthes disease is usually insidious. Presentation as an acute emergency is rare. Mild hip pain and limp have usually been present for weeks to months before diagnosis. Pain is often referred in the distribution of the obturator nerve to the knee, anteromedial thigh, or groin. Physical findings include decreased hip abduction and internal rotation. Thigh muscle atrophy may be noted.

Early in the disease, radiographs show widening of the articular cartilage with a small, dense proximal femoral epiphysis. Subchondral fracture may be visible. Irregularity and flattening of the epiphysis develop over time. The differential diagnosis includes various bone tumors and skeletal dysplasias (Figs. 12.2 and 12.3).

Management of Legg–Calvé–Perthes disease requires a pediatric orthopedist who will follow and treat the child through the various stages of the disease. Older children, obese patients, girls, and those with more severe disturbance of the epiphysis on radiographs have a poorer prognosis.

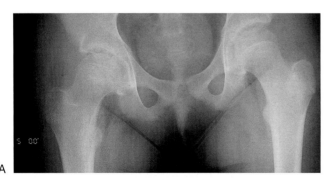
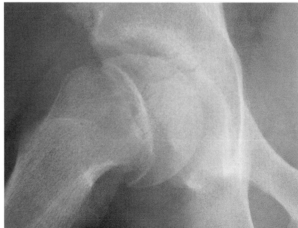

FIG. 12.1. This 12-year-old boy had knee and thigh pain for 2 weeks; however, on examination, he had pain with internal hip rotation. **A:** His anteroposterior films show subtle signs of slipped capital femoral epiphysis on the right. **B:** The frog-leg views show the slip clearly.

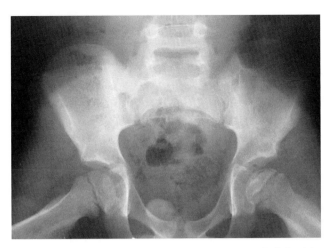

FIG. 12.2. Legg–Calvé–Perthes disease of left hip. Epiphysis is narrowed and radiodense. A subchondral fracture is also visible.

DISCITIS

Discitis is an inflammatory condition involving the intervertebral disc space. The pathophysiology of this condition is poorly understood. Vertebral osteomyelitis with involvement of the disc space is a distinct diagnostic entity with different epidemiology and pathophysiology from discitis.

Discitis is a disease of childhood, with approximately 75% of patients younger than 10 years of age. The involved disc space is usually lumbar or lower thoracic. Most authorities believe that discitis results from infection. A history of trauma is obtained in some patients with discitis, but whether the injury plays a role in cause or is a red herring is unclear.

Diagnosis

Children with discitis are a diagnostic challenge for clinicians. Symptoms are often nonspecific and vague, especially in the younger child. They have usually been present for more than 1 week at the time of diagnosis. Back pain is not always described. Limp, refusal to walk, leg pain, hip pain, and abdominal pain are common presenting complaints. Low-grade fever and irritability may be reported.

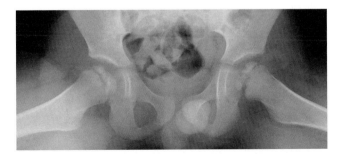

FIG. 12.3. Legg–Calvé–Perthes disease. This 3-year-old boy had an abnormal gait for 1 month. His hip examination was normal. Both of his femoral heads are irregular and sclerotic.

Many children assume a recumbent position of comfort from which they do not want to be moved. Decreased range of motion of the spine and tenderness to palpation of the disc space are usually present. Range of motion of the hips is essentially normal, but inadvertent movement of the lumbar spine during hip examination may cause pain that is misinterpreted to suggest hip pathology. Abnormalities in strength, sensation, and/or deep tendon reflexes suggest a spinal cord lesion, tumor, epidural abscess, or herniation of the disc (rare).

Plain radiographs are initially normal. Intervertebral disc space narrowing develops after 2 to 3 weeks of illness. A bone scan is the most sensitive imaging modality early in the course of this disease. Increased uptake at the level of the involved disc can confirm the diagnosis. Magnetic resonance imaging and computed tomography may help to define bony erosion of the vertebral end plates and paravertebral soft-tissue involvement.

Laboratory testing plays a minor role. Elevation of the white blood cell count and erythrocyte sedimentation rate is sometimes noted at the time of diagnosis. If the presentation is atypical, the signs and symptoms are severe, or the response to therapy is unsatisfactory, obtaining a guided needle aspiration can be helpful.

Management

Discitis is a self-limited disease, and virtually all children in reported series return to normal function in a few months. Resting the spine usually results in improved symptoms in days to weeks. Although there are no data to suggest that they speed recovery or improve outcome, antistaphylococcal antibiotics seem prudent, given the frequency of documented staphylococcal infection. Orthopedics consultation should be obtained.

SPONDYLOLYSIS AND SPONDYLOLISTHESIS

Spondylolysis and spondylolisthesis occur in 2% to 5% of children, but most are asymptomatic. In older children with low back pain, especially adolescents, it is a condition that should be considered. Spondylolysis is a defect in the pars interarticularis of the vertebral body. Spondylolisthesis is displacement of the vertebral bodies, usually involving L5 slipping anteriorly on S1.

The cause of the defect of the pars interarticularis in spondylolysis is not fully understood. Repeated stress, such as occurs in gymnasts with frequent hyperextension of the spine, causes stress fracture. One side of the pars interarticularis fractures overtly, which adds to the stress on the contralateral side. Fracture becomes bilateral. Displacement may or may not occur. Children who play sports that stress the spine, such as gymnastics, football, rowing, diving, weight lifting and high jumping, are at particular risk.

Patients who develop symptoms generally present during the adolescent growth spurt. Back pain worsens with

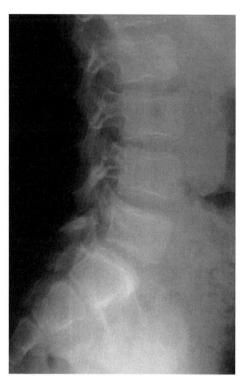

FIG. 12.4. Spondylolisthesis with slippage of L5 anteriorly on S1.

activity, improves with rest, and usually has an insidious onset. Over time, there may be pain in the buttocks and posterior thighs. Symptoms radiating down the legs suggest significant nerve root irritation. Parents may describe an increase in the lumbar lordosis or a change in the child's gait.

Physical examination shows tenderness with hyperextension of the lumbar spine in the prone position and with deep palpation. Children seldom have motor (10%), sensory (15%), or reflex (10%) deficits in the legs.

Plain radiographs should include anteroposterior, lateral, and oblique views. The "scotty dog" of the oblique view will have a collar on the neck if spondylolysis is present. Spondylolisthesis can be diagnosed on the lateral view (Fig. 12.4).

Treatment varies depending on symptoms and degree of displacement, if any. Most cases of asymptomatic spondylolysis and spondylolisthesis with mild displacement will not progress. Children with displacement greater than 25% should avoid rough sports. Symptomatic children with displacement may benefit from immobilization. Decisions about treatment should be made in consultation with an orthopedic surgeon.

OVERUSE SYNDROMES

Overuse syndromes is a general term that encompasses a variety of injuries that result from excessive and repetitive forces on susceptible structures. Children are at unique risk of such injuries, which are particularly common in adolescent athletes. There is an increased susceptibility during the growth spurt when skeletal growth exceeds the growth of the muscle–tendon unit. This results in increased stress at the apophysis, the musculotendinous origin or insertion.

General therapy for these injuries must emphasize several areas. Rest is crucial for the specific area involved until pain has completely resolved. The role of inflammation in overuse injuries is controversial, but the application of ice and use of antiinflammatory agents is generally recommended. Directed stretching exercises are encouraged. Biomechanics should be assessed and corrected when necessary. An appropriate training regimen should emphasize a slow, gradual buildup in intensity and duration.

Little Leaguer's Elbow

Little Leaguer's elbow refers to a group of disorders resulting from repetitive valgus stress applied to the skeletally underdeveloped elbow. Its cause is a combination of excessively repetitive pitching and poor throwing biomechanics. Valgus force places tension on the medial collateral ligaments, which is translated to the medial epicondyle. A medial epicondylitis or apophysitis is the most commonly resulting lesion. An avulsion fracture of the medial epicondyle may result. Little Leaguer's elbow occurs most commonly in boys ages 9 to 12. Patients complain of elbow pain that is exacerbated by throwing. Tenderness is localized over the medial elbow. Flexion of the wrist against resistance also elicits pain, and extension of the elbow may become limited.

Osgood–Schlatter Disease

Osgood–Schlatter disease is an apophysitis of the tibial tubercle. Repetitive stress imposed by the patellar tendon on its site of insertion results in a series of microavulsions of the ossification center and underlying cartilage. The condition is most common in running and jumping athletes between the ages of 11 and 15. Most cases are bilateral, although symptoms are commonly asymmetric.

The physical examination is notable for localized tenderness at the tibial tubercle. Any action that applies tension to the patellar tendon elicits pain. Maneuvers likely to cause pain include forced extension of the knee, jumping, or squatting. In advanced cases, callus formation occurs, resulting in further prominence of the tubercle. The diagnosis is based on the clinical features. Radiographs are not indicated in typical cases (Fig. 12.5).

Management consists first and foremost of avoiding activities that place stress on the tibial tubercle. A brief period of immobilization or non–weight bearing is recommended by some as a means of ensuring compliance. Application of ice and administration of nonsteroidal antiinflammatory medications reduce pain and swelling.

Osteochondritis Dissecans

Osteochondritis dissecans is a lesion involving separation of the osteochondral segment from underlying healthy bone, most commonly seen in adolescents. The primary sites of os-

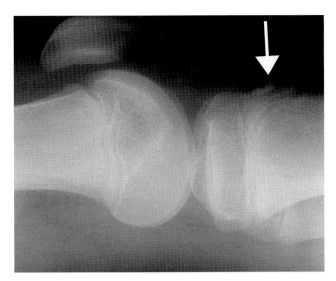

FIG. 12.5. Osgood–Schlatter disease. Radiographs are usually normal, but mild irregularities of the tibial tubercle (arrow) are often present.

teochondritis dissecans are the medial femoral condyle in the knee, the talus in the ankle, and the capitellum in the elbow.

Clinical Findings

The onset of symptoms occurs over several months. Joint pain and swelling typically occur after strenuous exercise and improve over several hours with rest. When a free body is present, patients describe intermittent, abrupt locking of the joint. The physical examination of the joint is often normal.

Occasionally, a small effusion may be detectable. Lesions in the medial femoral condyle may be directly palpated and pain elicited when the knee is held in 90 degrees of flexion.

Diagnosis

A plain film of the joint should be obtained. Radiographs reveal a crescent-shaped defect within the subchondral bone. A free body often includes a portion of dead subchondral bone, which appears as a radiodense object within the joint space. Standard anteroposterior and lateral views, as well as tunnel views, of the knee are recommended for lesions within the femoral condyle (Fig. 12.6). Lateral, anteroposterior, and mortis views of the ankle are adequate when a lesion of the talus is suspected.

Management

Conservative therapy consisting of restricted activity and relief of stress on the joint is the first-line treatment in children who have not reached skeletal maturity and for those diagnosed at an early stage of the disease. Patients should be followed closely by an orthopedic surgeon.

Chondromalacia Patella

Chondromalacia patella is a pathologic diagnosis referring to damage of the articular cartilage of the patella. Specific changes include softening, fissures, and erosions. Patellofemoral pain syndrome, a term often used interchangeably with chondromalacia patellae, more accurately

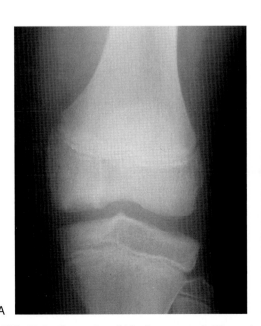

A

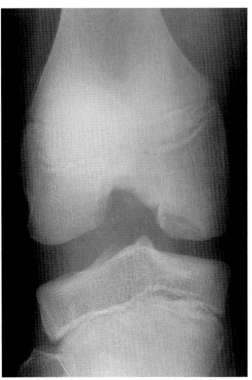

B

FIG. 12.6. Osteochondritis dissecans. **A:** The anteroposterior view in normal. **B:** The tunnel view clearly shows a defect of the subchondral bone.

describes a constellation of symptoms, principally anterior knee pain arising from the patellofemoral joint. Whether the two conditions are actually related is the subject of debate.

Patellofemoral pain syndrome and chondromalacia patellae are first seen in early adolescence. Malalignment of the patella and an abnormal tracking of the patella over the femoral condyles appear to be the major contributors to patellofemoral disorders.

Chondromalacia patellae and patellofemoral pain syndrome are often classified as overuse syndromes because individuals exposed to repetitive trauma are at higher risk of these disorders. Runners are particularly predisposed to develop these conditions.

Symptoms consist mainly of anterior knee pain often described as arising from beneath or on the sides of the patella. Pain is usually of gradual onset and is exacerbated by exercise. Activities that involve loading of the knee when it is in flexion, such as climbing steps, are particularly painful.

The physical examination is notable for tenderness along the patellar margins or posterior surface, which is accessible when the patella is manually displaced. Pain and, occasionally, crepitus are elicited with flexion and extension of the knee or tightening the quadriceps while compressing the patella against the femoral condyles. Range of motion is not limited and swelling is rare. The presence of an effusion is suggestive of significant cartilaginous damage. Provocative tests that reproduce the pain include climbing steps, squatting, or knee extension against resistance.

Radiographs generally lack sensitivity but may show changes in the patella in advanced cases.

Treatment is conservative. More than 90% of cases of patellofemoral pain syndrome resolve after instituting a program of rest, antiinflammatory medications, and ice followed by physical therapy. Exercises that begin once the initial pain has resolved emphasize strengthening of the quadriceps muscles. Recommended exercise regimens include straight leg raises, first without and then with weights.

Osteochondroses

Osteochondroses are idiopathic avascular necrosis or apophysitis syndromes involving various lower extremity bones. Children with limp and foot pain may have avascular necrosis of the tarsal navicular bone (Kohler disease) or second metatarsal (Freiberg disease). Radiographs are diagnostic (Fig. 12.7). Older children with heel pain may have Sever disease, a calcaneal apophysitis occurring at the insertion of the Achilles tendon at the calcaneus. Patients with Sever disease have tenderness at this insertion. Radiographs of the site are usually normal and are unhelpful except to exclude bony injuries such as stress fractures. Management includes rest, ice, and antiinflammatory medications.

Bursitis

Bursa sacs are both the shock absorbers and the ball bearings of the musculoskeletal system. They disperse forces from

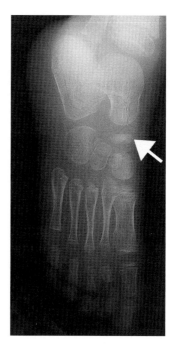

FIG. 12.7. Kohler disease. This 8-year-old child had a limp for 1 week and a nonspecific examination. The radiograph shows collapse and fragmentation of the navicular bone (arrow) caused by Kohler disease.

blows on bony prominences and reduce friction where tendons or ligaments are in frequent motion. Trauma, either in a single blow or by repetitive forces, can inflame the bursa, which responds with increased production of synovial fluid.

Prepatellar bursitis, commonly called "housemaid's knee", results from frequent or prolonged kneeling. Pes anserinus bursitis occurs on the lateral aspect of the knee, where the tendons of the hamstring muscles overlie the tibia. Retrocalcaneal bursitis occurs between the calcaneus and Achilles tendon. Shoulder or subacromial bursitis is often associated with calcifications and produces severe pain with abduction.

An unusual form of bursitis is known as a popliteal or Baker cyst. This occurs in the bursa, which cushions the tendons of the gastrocnemius and semimembranous muscles from the distal femur. In children with a Baker cyst, there is often a congenital opening joining the bursa sac with the knee joint itself. One-way flow of synovial fluid into the bursa produces swelling just below the popliteal fossa on the medial side. The swelling limits full flexion of the knee. Ultrasonography is a useful noninvasive diagnostic modality.

Conservative therapy consisting of restricted activity and regular use of nonsteroidal antiinflammatory medications is successful in most cases.

REFLEX SYMPATHETIC DYSTROPHY

Reflex sympathetic dystrophy (RSD) is a poorly understood disorder characterized by pain, abnormal sensation, and circulatory irregularities. Over time, atrophic changes of the extremity develop.

The average age of children with RSD is approximately 12 years, with girls outnumbering boys by as much as 6:1. Most cases in children involve the lower extremity. RSD usually develops after minor trauma.

The pathophysiology of RSD is not understood. Early theories suggested that abnormal synapses develop between sensory afferent nerves and sympathetic efferents after an injury. Theories of sympathetic receptor hypersensitivity or central, self-exciting pathways in the substantia nigra remain unproved.

Pain is usually the presenting complaint with RSD. The pain is continuous, often burning in quality, with exacerbations but no complete remissions. Abnormal sensitivity is distinctive, with severe pain provoked by normally nontender touching (allodynia). The extremity is usually swollen and cool to the touch. Dusky discoloration of the skin may be present. The arm or leg is not used, and atrophic changes develop in some patients over time.

Psychiatric and personality problems have been suspected in many patients with RSD, but controlled prospective studies are lacking. Factitious illness or conversion reactions may be considered, given that symptoms are out of proportion to the inciting injury.

The characteristic history and physical examination, including pain and evidence of autonomic dysfunction, allow a clinical diagnosis of RSD in most cases. Treatment of RSD focuses on early mobilization of the extremity through physical therapy to avoid atrophic changes. The knee-jerk response to splint for comfort may be counterproductive with RSD. Referral to a pediatric pain program is advisable should symptoms persist.

SUGGESTED READINGS

Causey AL, Smith ER, Donaldson JJ, et al. Missed slipped capital femoral epiphysis: illustrative cases and a review. *J Emerg Med* 1995;13:175–189.

Davidson K. Patellofemoral pain syndrome. *Am Fam Physician* 1993;48: 1254–1262.

Koop S, Quanbeck D. Three common causes of childhood hip pain. *Pediatr Clin North Am* 1996;43:1053–1066.

Lloyd-Thomas AR, Lauder G. Reflex sympathetic dystrophy in children. *BMJ* 1995;310:1648–1649.

Saperstein AL, Nicholas SJ. Pediatric and adolescent sports medicine. *Pediatr Clin North Am* 1996;43:1013–1033.

Skaggs DL, Tolo VT. Legg-Calve-Perthes disease. *J Am Acad Orthop Surg* 1996;4:9–16.

Stinson JT. Spondylolysis and spondylolisthesis in the athlete. *Clin Sports Med* 1993;12:517–528.

CHAPTER 13

Neonatal Emergencies

Editor: Stephen Ludwig

GROWTH

Weight gain serves as an important indicator of general well-being during the newborn period. Failure of a newborn to gain weight appropriately may be a sign of underfeeding or significant underlying illnesses such as heart disease, metabolic problems, or malabsorption. Similarly, gaining weight according to age-specific norms can be one of the best indicators that the infant is well, despite nondescript symptoms such as fussiness.

The average newborn infant weighs 7.7 lb (3.5 kg), is approximately 20 in. (50 cm) long, and has a head circumference of 14 in. (35 cm). The newborn will lose approximately 5% to 10% of his or her birth weight during the first several days of life and then regain this weight by 10 to 14 days of age. Thereafter, the newborn should gain approximately 25 to 35 g per day (approximately 1% of the birth weight per day).

TEMPERATURE

The young infant's immature autonomic thermoregulatory responses, larger body surface area-to-mass ratio, immature sweating response, and limited ability to move away from or modify adverse environments all limit his or her thermoregulatory ability. Temperature instability, either hypothermia or hyperthermia, may be the only sign of significant infectious illness.

HEART RATE

Normal resting heart rate is between 120 to 160 beats per minute. It varies with respiration (increasing with inspiration) and activity (increasing significantly with crying and appreciably slower during sleep). Sinus tachycardia (heart rate greater than 180 beats per minute) is a common response to many types of stress, such as pain, hypovolemia, fever, or cardiac disease. Sinus tachycardia must be differentiated from paroxysmal supraventricular tachycardia. Supraventricular tachycardia is usually associated with a more rapid heart rate (usually greater than 220 beats per minute) than is sinus tachycardia. The development of bradycardia (heart rate less than 80 beats per minute) usually signals the presence of significant cardiorespiratory compromise.

RESPIRATORY RATE

The normal resting respiratory rate is usually between 40 to 60 breaths per minute. During sleep, most newborn infants will exhibit some degree of periodic breathing, in which normal respiration is interrupted with short pauses. This breathing pattern is especially common in premature infants. Periodic breathing must be differentiated from pathologic apnea.

Varying degrees of expiratory grunting, chest retractions, nasal flaring, crackles, or rales are all signs of respiratory distress in the newborn. In addition to a primary pulmonary cause, respiratory distress in the newborn can also be a presenting sign of congestive heart failure. Among term infants, especially those born by cesarean section, a common cause of respiratory distress presenting within the first 24 hours, usually beginning between 2 to 6 hours after birth, is transient tachypnea of the newborn. Symptoms of transient tachypnea of the newborn typically resolve within 72 hours.

BLOOD PRESSURE

Normal systolic blood pressure in the term newborn after the first few days of life ranges between 60 to 90 mm Hg. Blood pressure is lower during the first few days of life and in premature infants is related to weight and gestational age. Congenital renal abnormalities, renal tumors, and complications of umbilical artery catheters are some of the more common causes of hypertension in the neonatal period. Coarctation of the aorta may be diagnosed by the combination of increased upper extremity blood pressure with low blood pressure or diminished pulses in the lower extremities.

COLOR CHANGES

Normal Variants

The skin of a normal Caucasian early neonate is a pink, flushed color. This in itself may be a cause for alarm to some parents but can be dismissed with reassurance if the remainder of the history and physical examination is not remarkable. A hemoglobin or hematocrit determination offers assurance that the baby is not abnormally polycythemic. Racial and ethnic factors may result in variation of the baby's skin color, but this usually can be determined by comparing the baby with the parent's pigmentation.

Alterations of the flushed appearance to blue, deep yellow, orange, or pale may precipitate an emergency department visit. Evaluation and management of these changes are discussed here.

Cyanosis/Acrocyanosis

The presenting complaint may be that "the baby is blue." Relevant questions to be asked include the following: When was the blueness first noted? Is it persistent or does it come and go? Does it involve all the body or only the distal extremities and lips? Does it increase or lessen with crying or feeding? Is there emesis or diarrhea?

Physical examination should be complete. The distribution of the blueness should be carefully noted; particularly, check the color of the tongue. Does the intensity of the blueness decrease or increase with crying or with effort? Are the vital signs normal for a neonate? Is the baby responsive to stimulation? Is mottling present? Is there a cardiac murmur? Are respirations labored? Are the lungs clear? Is the liver enlarged? Are the femoral pulsations palpable?

Acrocyanosis

An otherwise healthy baby has cyanosis confined to the hands, feet, and lips. The tongue is pink; pulse oximetry is normal. It may be associated with cool ambient temperature. Disposition: Parent(s) should be reassured that the acrocyanosis is self-limited.

Cyanotic Congenital Heart Disease

Cyanosis is diffusely distributed and increases with crying. Pulse oximetry shows diminished saturation at rest, worsening with crying; cyanosis responds only minimally to oxygen therapy. A cardiac murmur is usually, but not necessarily, present. Electrocardiography and echocardiography, if accessible, should be performed. Neonates with cyanotic heart disease only rarely go into cardiac failure. Disposition: Very young neonates with a strong suspicion of cyanotic cardiac defect should be admitted if cardiac consultation is not readily available.

Respiratory Disease

Respiratory disease is associated with tachypnea and possibly retractions. Pulse oximetry shows desaturation but usually improves significantly with rest, crying, and oxygenation. The clinician should think of respiratory infection (Fig. 13.1) or congenital intrathoracic defect. A chest radiograph should be done. Disposition: After appropriate emergency treatment, the patient should be admitted.

Hypovolemia, Acidosis, and Shock

Hypovolemia, acidosis, and shock are characterized by cyanosis accompanied by mottling in an extremely lethargic, hypotonic baby with marked tachycardia and possibly

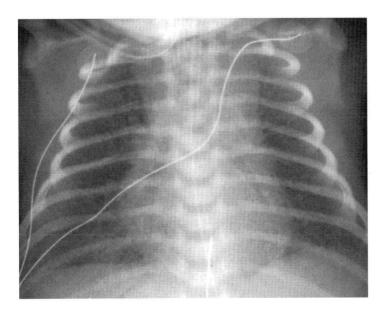

FIG. 13.1. Chest radiograph of infection. A full-term infant of an uncomplicated pregnancy developed respiratory distress, cyanosis, and periods of apnea within 6 hours of life. The blood culture and urine latex particle agglutination assay were positive for group B streptococci. Diffuse reticulogranular pattern, air bronchograms, and right pleural effusion without significant volume loss are consistent with common radiologic features of group B streptococcal pneumonia. (From Avery GB, Fletcher MA, MacDonald MG. *Neonatology: pathophysiology and management of the newborn*, 5th ed. Philadelphia: Lippincott Williams & Wilkins, 1999: 504, with permission.)

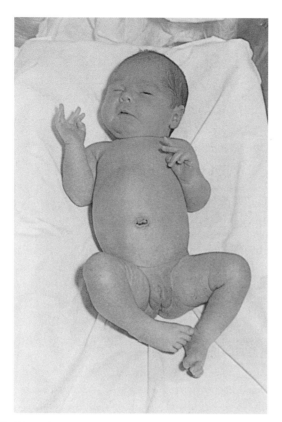

FIG. 13.2. Jaundice. Physiologic jaundice. (From O'Doherty N. *Atlas of the newborn*. Philadelphia: JB Lippincott, 1979:31, with permission.)

hypotension. Pulse oximetry is desaturated. Disposition: After appropriate emergency workup and treatment, the patient should be admitted.

Methemoglobinemia

Methemoglobinemia is characterized by cyanosis diffusely distributed in the absence of cardiac or pulmonary disease. There may be a recent history of gastroenteritis. Pulse

oximetry gives factitiously normal readings. A drop of blood on filter paper remains reddish brown, even after oxygenating it by waving in room air. Disposition: Emergency and laboratory evaluation to determine the intensity of involvement are indicated; treatment with methylene blue and admission should be considered.

Jaundice

The parent may be concerned because the newborn appears yellow or orange. Because this may be a normal variant in Pacific Rim or Native American racial or ethnic groups, the parents' coloring should be compared with the baby's.

The most precise way to determine whether the color change is truly jaundice is by examining the sclerae; yellow color of the sclerae is jaundice. A complete physical examination should be performed, with emphasis on vital signs, intensity and distribution of icterus, presence of cephalohematoma, or hepatosplenomegaly (Fig. 13.2).

The intensity of jaundice is determined by the level of bilirubin in the blood and its distribution. As a rule, jaundice is not discernible in infants at levels less than 5 mg/dL. Jaundice is usually first discerned in the face and becomes more obvious caudally as the total serum bilirubin level increases. Management and disposition can be governed by the recommendations in Table 13.1 and will vary with the baby's age and the bilirubin level.

Pallor

The neonate may be brought to the physician because he or she appears pale to the parents. A careful history and physical examination should be done to consider the possibilities of septic or cardiogenic shock, severe chemical or electrolyte imbalance, or significant anemia. A complete blood count should be done and consideration given to a stat glucose and electrolyte panel and total serum bilirubin level. Normal levels at this age for hemoglobin are in the range of 13 to 20 g/dL with a mean of 16 and for hematocrit, 42% to 65% with a mean of

TABLE 13.1. *Management of hyperbilirubinemia in the healthy term infant according to total serum bilirubin[a] and age*

Age (hr)	Consider phototherapy[b]	Phototherapy	Exchange transfusion if intensive phototherapy fails[c]	Exchange transfusion and intensive phototherapy
≤24	—	—	—	—
25–48	≥12 (170)	≥15 (260)	≥20 (340)	≥25 (430)
49–72	≥15 (260)	≥18 (310)	≥25 (430)	≥30 (510)
>72	≥17 (290)	≥20 (340)	≥25 (430)	≥30 (510)

[a] Total serum bilirubin level, mg/dL (μmol/L).

[b] Phototherapy at these total serum bilirubin levels is a clinical option, meaning that the intervention is available and may be used based on *individual clinical judgment*.

[c] Intensive phototherapy should produce a decrease in total serum bilirubin of 1 to 2 mg/dL within 4 to 6 hours, and the total serum bilirubin level should continue to decrease and remain below the threshold level for exchange transfusion. If this does not occur, it is considered a failure of phototherapy.

Adapted from American Academy of Pediatrics. Management of hyperbilirubinemia in the healthy term infant. *Pediatrics* 1994;94:558–565.

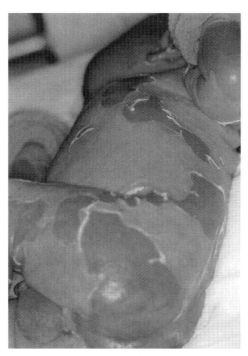

FIG. 13.3. Staphylococcal scalded skin syndrome. A 10-day-old Caucasian boy with staphylococcal scalded skin syndrome. He was treated with fluids, oral dicloxacillin, and wound care. His skin healed completely and without scarring within 2 weeks of this photograph being taken. (From Avery GB, Fletcher MA, MacDonald MG. *Neonatology: pathophysiology and management of the newborn*, 5th ed. Philadelphia: Lippincott Williams & Wilkins, 1999:1199, with permission.)

50%. Diagnostic considerations include the topics discussed in the following sections.

Mottling

Mottling in the neonate is the patchy appearance of the body surface, resulting from prominent dilation of the superficial veins showing through the thin skin and causing a mosaic-like, patchy appearance. Mottling may be a normal variant when it appears in an otherwise normal baby, undressed in a cool ambient temperature. It is more likely to appear in a preterm baby with thin skin.

However, mottling can be an ominous diagnostic sign in a neonate. It may be indicative of hypovolemia and poor perfusion in a baby in shock or a baby with sepsis. A careful history and complete physical examination with cautious evaluation of the vital signs need to be done. If there is doubt about the baby's status, an electrolyte panel and stat glucose should be drawn. Treatment of the underlying cause and restoration of hemodynamic stability should be started in the emergency department.

SKIN FINDINGS

The quality of the newborn's skin varies with gestational age. The premature infant's thin, almost translucent skin is in sharp contrast to the dry, cracked, peeling skin of the postterm infant. Normal peeling of the superficial layers of the skin should be differentiated from the full-thickness skin loss that is associated with staphylococcal scalded skin syndrome (Figs. 13.3, 6.10, and 6.11). Excoriations when noted in an irritable or jittery infant, especially when they are located primarily on the nose or knees, may be a sign of withdrawal in an infant exposed to narcotics prenatally.

Seborrheic dermatitis is a localized scaling or crusting eruption that most commonly involves the scalp (cradle cap), forehead, and area behind the ears. Occasionally, the diaper area may be involved. The eruption may have a greasy appearance, and the lesions are generally nonpruritic.

Hair

Soft, downy, fine body hair (lanugo) located primarily on the back and shoulders, is a normal finding. However, a tuft of coarse, dark hair located in the midline lumbosacral region may be associated with spina bifida occulta (Fig. 13.4).

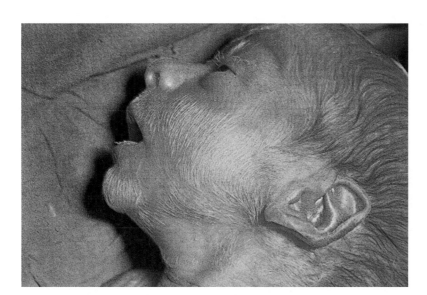

FIG. 13.4. Profuse lanugo hair. (From O'Doherty N. *Atlas of the newborn*. Philadelphia: JB Lippincott, 1979:92–93, with permission.)

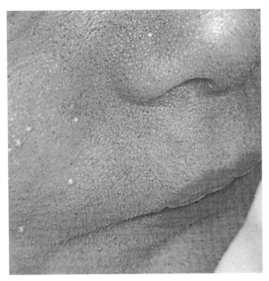

FIG. 13.5. Milia. Some of the larger lesions are cystic. (From O'Doherty N. *Atlas of the newborn.* Philadelphia: JB Lippincott, 1979:33, with permission.)

Papular Rashes

A variety of papular rashes may be observed in the healthy newborn. Characteristic body distribution patterns and age at appearance of these typical rashes may help to differentiate them from more worrisome conditions.

Milia are small 1- to 2-mm ivory or yellow papules located primarily on the forehead, nose, and cheeks of the newborn. Milia are keratin retention cysts that require no treatment because they will spontaneously rupture and disappear during the first 3 to 4 weeks of life (Fig. 13.5).

Erythema toxicum is a more generalized eruption of small papules or pustules on an erythematous base that may occur anywhere on the body (Fig. 13.6). Usually presenting during the first 3 to 4 days of life, these lesions may be noted as late as 2 weeks of age. Herpes simplex infections, although usually vesicular, and impetigo, usually pustular or crusted, may be entertained in the differential diagnosis of this eruption. If the diagnosis is in question, a smear of the papular contents will show a predominance of eosinophils with a relative absence of neutrophils and no organisms.

Erythematous papules or pustules (rarely comedones) confined primarily to the cheeks, chin, and forehead are characteristic of neonatal acne (Fig. 13.7). Lesions are secondary to the influence of circulating maternal hormones and usually appear at 3 to 4 weeks of age and disappear within a few weeks.

Vesicular Rashes

The most important condition to consider when evaluating a vesicular eruption is a herpes simplex virus infection because it has the most significant associated morbidity and

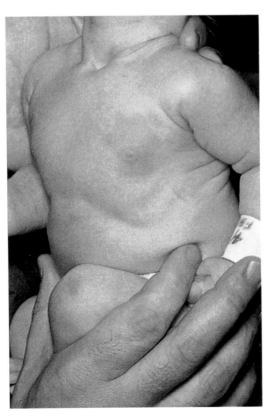

FIG. 13.6. Erythema toxicum. (From O'Doherty N. *Atlas of the newborn.* Philadelphia: JB Lippincott, 1979:32, with permission.)

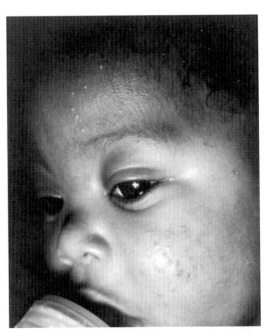

FIG. 13.7. Neonatal acne. Acne neonatorum of the cheeks in a 4-month-old boy; comedones developed at 4 weeks of age. Six miliaria pustulosa lesions are present on the forehead. There was much improvement 1 month after petrolatum was discontinued. (From Avery GB, Fletcher MA, MacDonald MG. *Neonatology: pathophysiology and management of the newborn,* 5th ed. Philadelphia: Lippincott Williams & Wilkins, 1999:1326, with permission.)

mortality. Clinical disease in the newborn may range from localized infection of the central nervous system, skin, eyes, or oropharynx to disseminated viremia with multisystem involvement. The infant generally appears well at birth but then becomes ill at approximately days 4 to 7, at which time a vesicular eruption may be noted (Figs. 11.7C and 13.8).

Neonatal varicella may develop when maternal varicella infection occurs during the last 2 to 3 weeks of pregnancy or the first few days postpartum (Fig. 13.9). The severity of neonatal disease depends on the timing of the maternal infection. If maternal disease onset is 5 or more days before delivery, the infection in the newborn is usually mild because of the transplacental passage of maternal varicella immunoglobulin G antibody. In contrast, if maternal disease onset is within 4 days before delivery or within 48 hours after delivery, the neonate is at risk of developing severe infection with a mortality rate as high as 30% caused by pulmonary or visceral involvement. Diagnosis can usually be made by the history and the characteristic rash of vesicles on an erythematous base (dew drops on a rose petal).

Incontinentia pigmenti is an X-linked dominant disorder with both skin and systemic lesions (affecting the eyes, central nervous system, and bone). It presents at birth or shortly thereafter with an inflammatory vesicular or bullous rash that develops in crops over the trunk and extremities. The cutaneous lesions have four phases (inflammatory vesicles or bullae, verrucous lesions, whorled hyperpigmentation, and hypopigmented patches) that may overlap and occur in an irregular sequence (Fig. 13.10). Suspected cases should be referred to a dermatologist for evaluation because of the potential for systemic involvement.

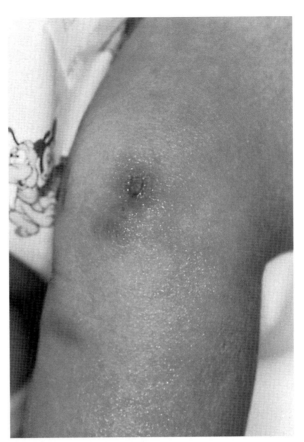

FIG. 13.9. Congenital varicella. Newborn with congenital varicella after maternal infection at approximately week 13 of pregnancy. Notice the ulcerated area with surrounding scars over the knee; a second scar is visible distally over the tibia. Despite an otherwise normal physical examination, computed tomography of the head revealed multiple areas of cerebral infarction and diffuse intracranial calcifications. (From Avery GB, Fletcher MA, MacDonald MG. *Neonatology: pathophysiology and management of the newborn*, 5th ed. Philadelphia: Lippincott Williams & Wilkins, 1999:1162, with permission.)

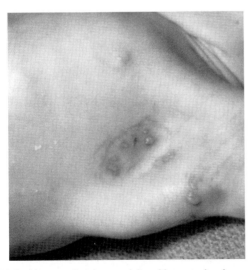

FIG. 13.8. Herpes simplex vesicles. Herpes simplex vesicles in the axilla of a 12-day-old infant with severe type 2 herpes encephalitis of 3 days' duration. The lesions cleared in 12 days. Severe mental retardation developed. (From Avery GB, Fletcher MA, MacDonald MG. *Neonatology: pathophysiology and management of the newborn*, 5th ed. Philadelphia: Lippincott Williams & Wilkins, 1999:1349, with permission.)

Impetigo appears as superficial vesicular, pustular, or bullous lesions on an erythematous base (Figs. 13.11 and 11.32). In the newborn, lesions tend to occur primarily in the diaper area (Fig. 13.12), folds of the neck, and axillae.

VASCULAR LESIONS

The salmon patch (nevus simplex) is the most common vascular lesion of infancy. It is a pale pink macular lesion that is found most commonly on the nape of the neck (often called a stork bite), forehead, nasolabial region, or upper eyelids (Fig. 13.13). With the exception of the lesions on the nape of the neck, most will fade within the first year of life.

Nevus flammeus (port-wine stain) consists of mature dilated dermal capillaries and presents at birth as pink to purple macular lesions that can vary tremendously in size, sometimes involving a significant portion of the body

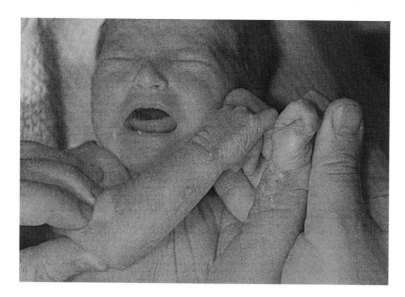

FIG. 13.10. Incontinentia pigmenti. Blistering skin at birth in incontinentia pigmenti. (From O'Doherty N. *Atlas of the newborn.* Philadelphia: JB Lippincott, 1979:393, 396, with permission.)

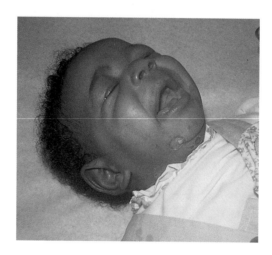

FIG. 13.11. Impetigo.

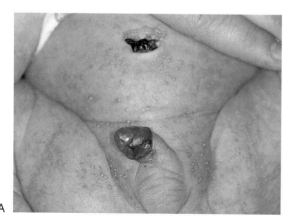
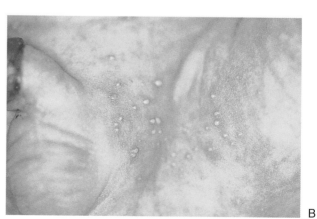

A   B

FIG. 13.12. A–B: This recently circumcised infant has developed staphylococcal pustulosis, a variation of bullous impetigo.

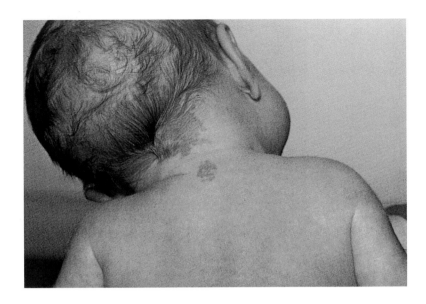

FIG. 13.13. Stork marks. Stork marks at the nape of the neck. (From O'Doherty N. *Atlas of the newborn*. Philadelphia: JB Lippincott, 1979:34, with permission.)

(Klippel–Trenaunay–Weber syndrome should be considered when the port-wine stain involves a lower limb) (Fig. 13.14). Unilateral facial port-wine stains in a trigeminal nerve distribution may be associated with the Sturge–-Weber syndrome (seizures, intracranial calcifications, and hemiparesis). These lesions generally will not fade with time (Fig. 13.15).

Although capillary hemangiomas (strawberry hemangioma) may be present at birth, most develop during the first few weeks of life (Fig. 13.16). Lesions may occur anywhere on the body and typically begin as small, well-demarcated telangiectatic macules that subsequently develop into raised bright red or purple tumors with distinct borders. Most lesions will go through a period of rapid

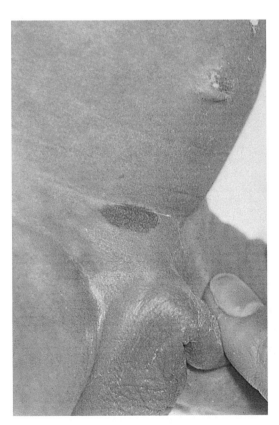

FIG. 13.14. Port-wine stain or nevus flammeus. (From O'Doherty N. *Atlas of the newborn*. Philadelphia: JB Lippincott, 1979:35, with permission.)

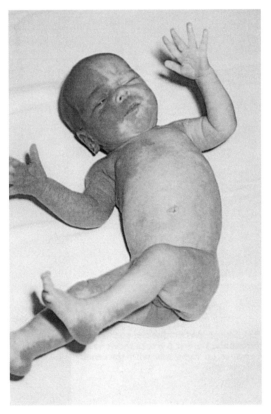

FIG. 13.15. Sturge–Weber disease. Sturge–Weber disease with hypertrophy of the right upper limb. (From O'Doherty N. *Atlas of the newborn*. Philadelphia: JB Lippincott, 1979: 388, with permission.)

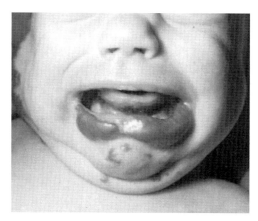

FIG. 13.16. Strawberry hemangiomas. Strawberry hemangiomas of the lip and chin. (From Avery GB, Fletcher MA, MacDonald MG. *Neonatology: pathophysiology and management of the newborn*, 5th ed. Philadelphia: Lippincott Williams & Wilkins, 1999:1342, with permission.)

growth over the first 6 months of life, followed by a static period and then spontaneous involution, usually by 5 years of age (Fig. 13.17).

Cavernous hemangiomas are deep-seated capillary hemangiomas that usually present at birth as a diffuse swelling with little change in the color of the overlying skin or a bluish hue. Most involute spontaneously with time (Fig. 13.18).

Hemangiomas that may require intervention during the neonatal period are those that by location or size may compromise vital structures such as the eyes, nares or auditory

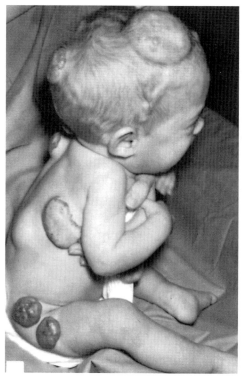

FIG. 13.17. Mixed hemangiomas. A 7-month-old infant with 21 strawberry, cavernous, and mixed hemangiomas. No lesions were seen until 1 month of age. Between 7 and 8 months of age, one new lesion developed. Nine hemangiomas are visible over the scalp, back, and thigh. By 6 years of age, only three involuting lesions remained; these were gone by 12 years of age. (From Avery GB, Fletcher MA, MacDonald MG. *Neonatology: pathophysiology and management of the newborn*, 5th ed. Philadelphia: Lippincott Williams & Wilkins, 1999:1340, with permission.)

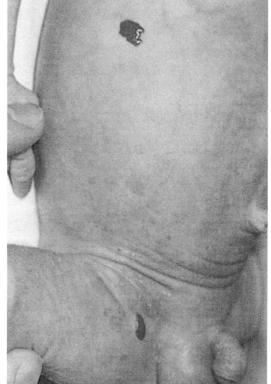

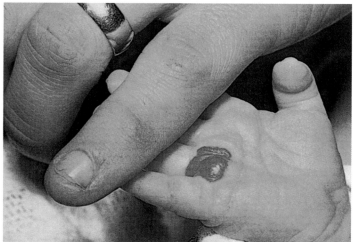

FIG. 13.18. Cavernous hemangiomas. **A:** Multiple cavernous hemangiomas. **B:** Superficial cavernous hemangiomas. (From O'Doherty N. *Atlas of the newborn*. Philadelphia: JB Lippincott, 1979:342–345, with permission.)

A

B

cardiac rhabdomyomas, and renal lesions (hamartomas or cystic kidneys).

HEAD AND NECK PROBLEMS

Head Size and Shape

Microcephaly is usually a sign of a severe underlying abnormality of brain growth or development and is often associated with mental retardation. It may be secondary to a variety of causes, including Down syndrome, congenital TORCH (toxoplasmosis, other infections, rubella, cytomegalovirus infections, and herpes simplex) syndrome, and fetal alcohol syndrome. An excessively large head may be familial or suggestive of hydrocephalus, storage disease, or intracranial hemorrhage.

Molding of the skull bones during the vaginal delivery process is a common cause of temporary asymmetry and scalp edema (caput succedaneum). Caput succedaneum is an ill-defined generalized swelling of the soft tissues of the scalp that extends across suture lines (Fig. 13.20). Generally, both caput succedaneum and skull molding spontaneously resolve by 7 to 10 days of age. Trauma during the birth process may produce a cephalohematoma, a subperiosteal hemorrhage, distinguished from a caput by the fact that the

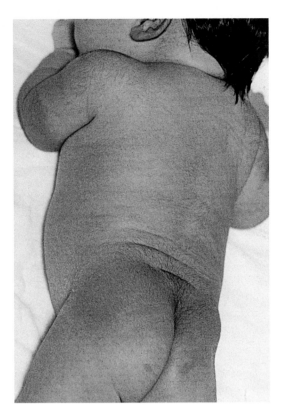

FIG. 13.19. Mongolian spots. Universal Mongolian blue spot. (From O'Doherty N. *Atlas of the newborn.* Philadelphia: JB Lippincott, 1979:37, with permission.)

canals; lesions that by their size or location (e.g., perianal or labial lesions) are susceptible to trauma, ulceration, and secondary infection; and large, rapidly enlarging hemangiomas associated with thrombocytopenia and a consumption coagulopathy (Kasabach–Merritt syndrome).

PIGMENTARY CHANGES

Mongolian spots are poorly circumscribed blue-black, gray, or brown large macular lesions generally located over the lumbosacral region, buttocks, and lower limbs in more than 80% to 90% of African-American, Native American, Hispanic, or East Asian infants (Fig. 13.19). The incidence is less than 10% in Caucasian infants. Lesions will usually fade during the first few years of life.

Café-au-lait macules are round or oval, brown macular lesions varying in size from less than 1 cm to greater than 20 cm. Although normal individuals may have these lesions, they may be a sign of neurocutaneous disease, most commonly neurofibromatosis.

Ash-leaf macules are irregular hypopigmented macules often with an oval or ash leaf appearance found in 70% to 90% of individuals with tuberous sclerosis. This is an autosomal dominant condition characterized by central nervous system lesions, seizures (infantile spasms), retinal lesions,

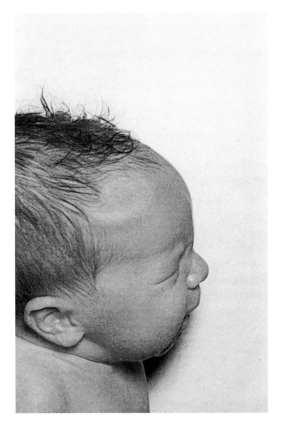

FIG. 13.20. Caput succedaneum. Caput succedaneum shows pitting on pressure. Cephalohematoma is also present in this baby. (From O'Doherty N. *Atlas of the newborn.* Philadelphia: JB Lippincott, 1979:136, with permission.)

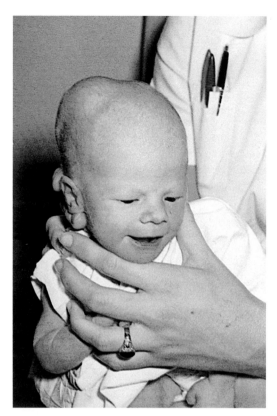

FIG. 13.21. Cephalohematoma. (From O'Doherty N. *Atlas of the newborn.* Philadelphia: JB Lippincott, 1979:117,143, with permission.)

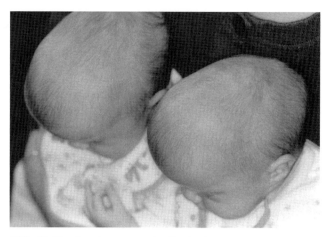

FIG. 13.22. Craniosynostosis. Sagittal synostosis, a far more common type of craniosynostosis, can be detected in the nursery and referred for neurosurgical intervention. Definitive treatment may be delayed for several months. (From Avery GB, Fletcher MA, MacDonald MG. *Neonatology: pathophysiology and management of the newborn,* 5th ed. Philadelphia: Lippincott Williams & Wilkins, 1999:1266, with permission.)

swelling never crosses suture lines (Fig. 13.21). However, the diagnosis can be difficult in the immediate newborn period if overlying scalp edema is present.

Overriding cranial sutures, caused by the pressures exerted on the skull during its descent through the pelvis, may be noted for the first several days of life. Overriding sutures that are palpable beyond this time may be a sign of underlying brain pathology and deserve further evaluation. Ridging or prominence of cranial sutures may be a sign of craniosynostosis (Fig. 13.22), a premature fusion of cranial sutures. Overriding sutures are ballottable, but if the sutures are rigid and have a heaped-up solid closure, radiographs or even a computed tomography scan should be done to rule out craniosynostosis. Soft areas (craniotabes) are occasionally found on palpation of the parietal bones during the first several days of life, especially in premature infants. Soft areas noted in the occipital region may be suggestive of osteogenesis imperfecta or other syndromes and should be investigated.

At birth, the newborn has two fontanelles. The anterior fontanelle, situated at the junction of the coronal and sagittal sutures, usually measures approximately 2 cm (can be as much as 5 to 6 cm in its largest diameter), and normally closes between 9 to 18 months. The posterior fontanelle, situated at the junction of the lambdoidal and sagittal sutures, generally measures between 0.5 to 1 cm (may be closed at birth in some cases) and usually closes to palpation by 3 to 4 months of age. Enlarged fontanelles may be associated with

a variety of conditions, including prematurity, hypothyroidism, or hydrocephalus. Increased intracranial pressure produces a full or bulging fontanelle, whereas dehydration produces a depressed fontanelle. A fontanelle that appears full while the infant is supine or crying should be reassessed while the infant is held upright and sleeping or feeding before it is determined to be full or bulging.

Neck

Congenital muscular torticollis is a positional abnormality of the neck resulting in abnormal tilting and rotation of the head (Fig. 13.23). Although congenital muscular torticollis

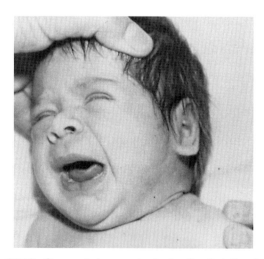

FIG. 13.23. Congenital muscular torticollis. Rotation toward the right is limited by the tightness in the right sternocleidomastoideus muscle. (From Avery GB, Fletcher MA, MacDonald MG. *Neonatology: pathophysiology and management of the newborn,* 5th ed. Philadelphia: Lippincott Williams & Wilkins, 1999:1271, with permission.)

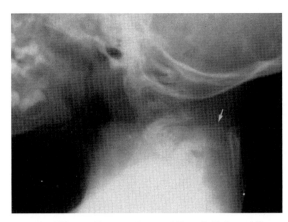

FIG. 13.24. Klippel–Feil syndrome. Klippel–Feil and Sprengel deformity. Lateral view shows multiple fusion-segmentation anomalies of the cervical spine, resulting in marked shortening of the spine. There is also a pronounced kyphosis. The oma vertebral bone (*arrow*) is present as part of the associated Sprengel deformity. (From Swischuk LE. *Imaging of the newborn, infant, and young child*, 4th ed. Philadelphia: Lippincott Williams & Wilkins, 1997:1032, with permission.)

may be noted at birth, it usually manifests at 2 to 4 weeks of age. Unilateral contracture and fibrosis of the sternocleidomastoid muscle result in a characteristic head tilt toward the affected side and the chin pointing toward the opposite side. On examination, a firm, nontender mass may be felt within the body of the sternocleidomastoid muscle. Occipitocervical spine anomalies, such as the Klippel–Feil syndrome (congenital fusion of two or more cervical vertebrae; clinical triad of short neck, limited neck motion and low occipital hairline), are rare causes of torticollis that present in the newborn period (Fig. 13.24).

Congenital neck lesions may present during infancy or sometimes much later in childhood. The most common lesions include, thyroglossal duct cysts (Fig. 13.25A) (midline

in the neck and inferior to the hyoid bone), branchial cleft cysts (along the lateral neck), and cystic hygromas (Fig. 13.25B) (usually located behind the sternocleidomastoid muscle in the supraclavicular fossa; two-thirds of cystic hygromas are present at birth).

Redundant skin on the back of the neck or webbing in a female infant are suggestive of Turner syndrome and may be associated with lymphedema of the dorsum of the hands and feet in the newborn (Fig. 13.26).

EYE PROBLEMS

The newborn is very nearsighted at birth, with a visual acuity of approximately 20/400. The eyelids are closed most of the time, and any attempt to force them open usually meets with marked resistance and causes blepharospasm. Holding the infant upright and gently swaying him or her from side to side or up and down often induces the eyes to open spontaneously.

Leukokoria

The pupillary light reflex is a simple test that takes only minutes and should be performed on all newborns. In the normal newborn, a red reflex is seen when the ophthalmoscope is held 10 to 12 in. in front of the eyes. A white pupillary light reflex, or leukokoria, is never normal in the newborn. Leukokoria may be a sign of several conditions of variable severity and prognosis such as colobomas, cataracts, retinal detachment, retinopathy of prematurity, or retinoblastoma [the most common signs are leukokoria (60%) and strabismus (20%)] (Fig. 13.27). Therefore, all infants with an abnormal pupillary light reflex should be referred to an ophthalmologist for a prompt evaluation.

Excessive Tearing

Dacryostenosis, congenital obstruction of the nasolacrimal duct, is the most common cause of excessive tearing in the

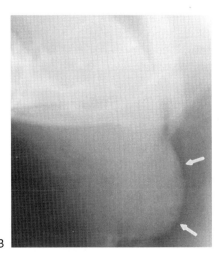
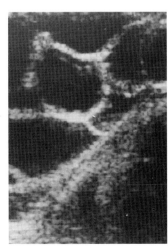

A,B

FIG. 13.25. Common neonate neck lesions. **A:** Thyroglossal duct cyst (*arrows*) encroaching on the airway. Bronchial cleft cyst. **B:** Typical ultrasonographic appearance of multiple anechoic cystic structures separated by echogenic septae. (From Swischuk LE. *Imaging of the newborn, infant, and young child*, 4th ed. Philadelphia: Lippincott Williams & Wilkins, 1997:170,874, with permission.)

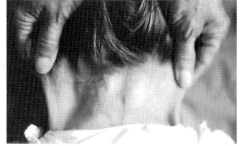

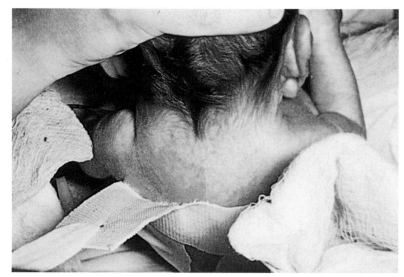

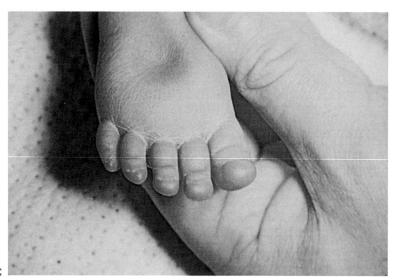

FIG. 13.26. A: Turner syndrome. (From Avery GB, Fletcher MA, MacDonald MG. *Neonatology: pathophysiology and management of the newborn*, 5th ed. Philadelphia: Lippincott Williams & Wilkins, 1999:851, with permission.) **B:** Low trident hairline in Turner syndrome. (From O'Doherty N. *Atlas of the newborn*. Philadelphia: JB Lippincott, 1979:308, with permission.). **C:** Congenital lymphedema and hypoplastic toenails in Turner syndrome. (From O'Doherty N. *Atlas of the newborn*. Philadelphia: JB Lippincott, 1979:309, with permission.)

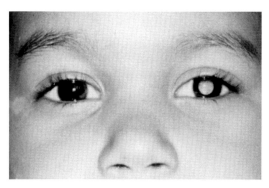

FIG. 13.27. Leukokoria in a child with retinoblastoma of the left eye.

newborn (Fig. 13.28) and should be differentiated from congenital or infantile glaucoma (Fig. 13.29), a serious but fortunately rare cause of excessive tearing. Most cases of infantile glaucoma presenting during the first 3 months of life are bilateral, whereas dacryostenosis is usually unilateral.

Increased wetness of the affected eye relative to the normal eye, excessive tearing, mucoid eye discharge, and crusting along the eyelid margins are the usual presenting symptoms of dacryostenosis. Gentle pressure along the medial canthal region over the lacrimal sac may produce a reflux of tears or purulent material onto the surface of the eye, confirming the diagnosis. In addition to excessive tearing, infants with glaucoma also present with rhinorrhea, photophobia, and corneal haziness. The cornea may be inspected after instillation of fluorescein dye to rule out a corneal abrasion as the cause of the excessive tearing. Uncomplicated cases of nasolacrimal duct obstruction should be managed with gentle cleansing of the eyes with warm water followed by local massage of the nasolacrimal duct several times per day.

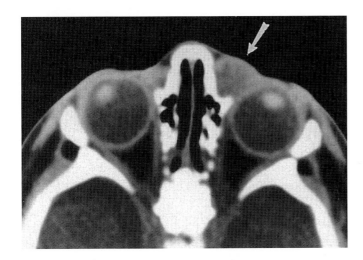

FIG. 13.28. Nasolacrimal duct obstruction. Computed tomography study demonstrates the proximally dilated nasolacrimal duct (*arrow*) in the same area. (From Swischuk LE. *Imaging of the newborn, infant, and young child*, 4th ed. Philadelphia: Lippincott Williams & Wilkins, 1997:1018, with permission.)

Scleral and Subconjunctival Hemorrhage

Scleral and subconjunctival hemorrhage are often noted in the newborn secondary to birth trauma. These lesions are common and spontaneous resolution within 1 to 2 weeks is the rule. If the funduscopic examination is performed, similar hemorrhages may be noted on the retina in approximately 25% of newborns (Fig. 13.30).

MOUTH PROBLEMS

Normal Findings

Common normal findings in the oropharynx include natal teeth and benign gingival cysts. The incidence of natal teeth (teeth present at birth) (Fig. 13.31) is approximately one in every 3,000 livebirths. The mandibular central incisors are the most commonly affected teeth.

Benign gingival cysts are found in 75% of newborns. Epstein pearls are usually single, small, white, keratin-filled cysts found along the midline of the palate (Fig. 13.32). Bohn nodules are mucous gland cysts that appear as multiple, firm, grayish white lesions along the gums and occasionally on the palate. Dental lamina cysts are formed by remnants of dental lamina epithelium and appear as small, cystic lesions along the crests of the mandibular and maxillary mucosa. They are usually larger and more lucent than either Epstein pearls or Bohn nodules. These cysts generally disappear by 4 weeks of age.

Thrush

Thrush is caused by *Candida albicans*. Diagnosis may be based on clinical examination (Fig. 13.33). Creamy white plaques located on the buccal mucosa or tongue that are difficult to remove and may cause bleeding when scraped are characteristic of candidiasis. Treatment consists of local application of nystatin suspension four times daily. Topical application of nystatin ointment to the mother's nipples may be

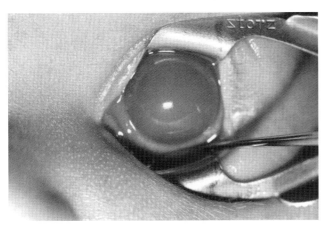

FIG. 13.29. Infantile glaucoma. This cornea is diffusely opacified and enlarged from infantile glaucoma. (From Avery GB, Fletcher MA, MacDonald MG. *Neonatology: pathophysiology and management of the newborn*, 5th ed. Philadelphia: Lippincott Williams & Wilkins, 1999:1287, with permission.)

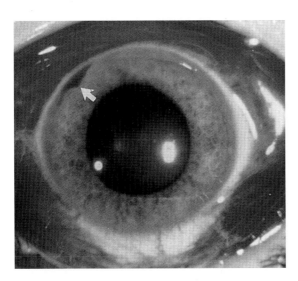

FIG. 13.30. Subconjunctival hemorrhage. Subconjunctival hemorrhage extending for 360 degrees. Note the small hyphema (*arrow*).

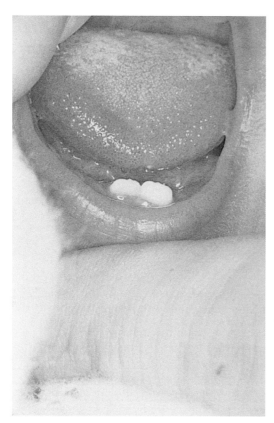

FIG. 13.31. Natal teeth. (From O'Doherty N. *Atlas of the new-born*. Philadelphia: JB Lippincott, 1979:51, with permission.)

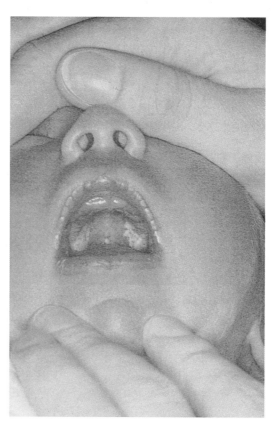

FIG. 13.33. Adherent milk and epithelial pearls, not to be confused with thrush. (From O'Doherty N. *Atlas of the new-born*. Philadelphia: JB Lippincott, 1979:211, with permission.)

indicated in recurrent or refractory cases if the infant is breast-feeding.

CHEST AND BACK FINDINGS

Normally, the term newborn's thorax is symmetric and barrel shaped. It is graced with two nipples anteriorly, each approximately 10 mm in diameter and slightly elevated and stippled. Respiratory excursion should be symmetric and accompanied by simultaneous movement of the abdomen. In the midline of the back, the tips of the vertebrae can be palpated but not visualized. The rib cage is not flared or depressed. There are several variations of this normal anatomy, some normal and some not, which may be striking enough for a parent to bring the child to the emergency department.

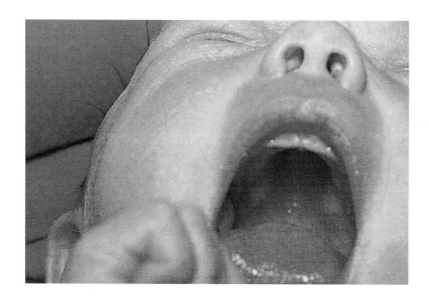

FIG. 13.32. Benign gingival cysts. Epstein pearls. (From O'Doherty N. *Atlas of the new-born*. Philadelphia: JB Lippincott, 1979:49, with permission.)

Fractured or Absent Clavicle(s)

In the course of vaginal delivery, the clavicle may be fractured, resulting in asymmetry at the shoulder girdle area. Palpation of the clavicle may reveal a drop off in the continuity of the bone and possible crepitation when gentle pressure is applied. A confirmatory radiograph should be taken and appropriate reassurance offered for the healing process (Fig. 13.34). Much more rarely, clavicles may be absent bilaterally with resultant low positioning of the shoulders. This positioning may be indicative of the dominant genetic defect known as cleidocranial dysostosis and requires orthopedic and genetic evaluation.

Pectus Excavatum

Relative depression of the lower sternum and rib cage is usually a normal variant unless accompanied by signs of respiratory distress.

Xiphoid Process

Parents may feel a firm, small mass in the midline at the distal end of the sternum. This is the xiphoid process, angled outwardly, and is a normal variant.

Breast

Supernumerary Nipples

A round, possibly slightly elevated or slightly depressed lesion, approximately 10 mm in diameter, lighter in shade than the nipple and located approximately 2 to 3 cm below, is a supernumerary nipple. This is a normal variant and will remain permanently. Uncommonly, these may be associated with renal lesions, but that possibility need not be investigated in a child who is otherwise well.

Breast Buds

Prominent, nontender breast tissue in the neonate of either gender is a normal variant, probably related to maternal estrogen. This subsides with time, and no therapy is indicated. Often, colostrum-like material can be extruded, but efforts to do this should be gentle and conducted under hygienic conditions.

Breast Cellulitis/Abscess

Breast tissue that is hypertrophied, reddened, and tender is probably infected (Fig. 11.43). The child may or may not be febrile. Warm compresses and intravenous antibiotic treatment, including coverage for probable staphylococcal origin, should be started after appropriate cultures are taken. The baby should be admitted for continuing therapy.

SPINAL COLUMN DEFECTS

Spina Bifida

A grossly apparent spina bifida lesion with lower extremity flaccidity and meningeal extrusion in the midline of the back (Fig. 13.35).

Sacral Dimple

A midline dimple of the lower back, with or without a tuft of hair, or a lipomatous intracutaneous or subcutaneous lesion in that area may be clues to the presence of spina bifida occulta, a less obvious form of spina bifida. This may or may not be associated with lower extremity deformity. The dimple may also be the external manifestation of a sinus tract connecting to the intradural space without vertebral anomaly, which would leave the infants susceptible to meningeal infection. Conversely, the dimple may be a normal skin indentation. If in

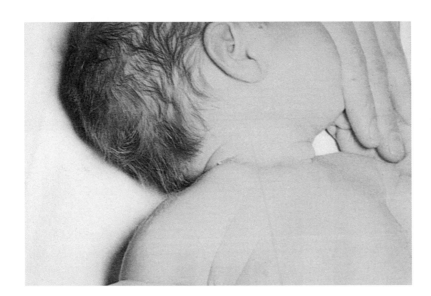

FIG. 13.34. Fractured or absent clavicle. Swelling due to callus formation after fracture of the clavicle. (From O'Doherty N. *Atlas of the newborn*. Philadelphia: JB Lippincott, 1979: 158, with permission.)

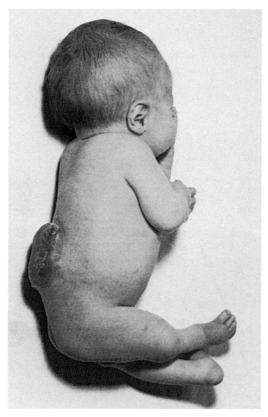

FIG. 13.35. Spina bifida with Chiari–Arnold malformation of the hindbrain causing hydrocephalus. (From O'Doherty N. *Atlas of the newborn*. Philadelphia: JB Lippincott, 1979:254, with permission.)

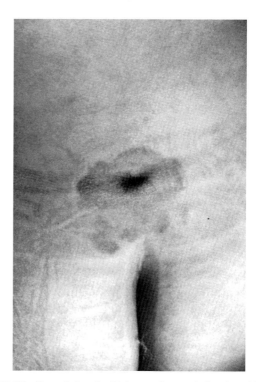

FIG. 13.36. Sacral dimple. This small sacral dimple, with encircling reddened patch, was noted at birth. At surgery, it was found to be a dermal sinus tract into the spinal cord. The gluteal cleft is seen below. (From Avery GB, Fletcher MA, MacDonald MG. *Neonatology: pathophysiology and management of the newborn*, 5th ed. Philadelphia: Lippincott Williams & Wilkins, 1999:1261, with permission.)

doubt, scheduling of magnetic resonance imaging and neurosurgical referral should be considered (Fig. 13.36).

ABDOMINAL AND PERINEAL FINDINGS

The neonatal abdomen is full but is neither distended nor scaphoid. The liver is normally palpable 2 to 3 cm below the right costal margin; the spleen is not usually palpable; the lower edges of the kidneys may be felt with deep palpation. There should be no palpable extraneous masses.

Umbilicus

The umbilical cord is tied or clamped at the time of delivery and usually sloughs off by the 10th day. Careful umbilical care consists of gentle hygienic measures and cleansing with isopropyl alcohol several times daily. Still, the umbilical area may be a source of concern for the parents, who may appear in the emergency department with their neonate.

Discharge from the umbilical area may occur and is benign if it is clear or yellow-tinged and thin. Reassurance and instruction in hygienic measures are all that is necessary. A thick, purulent discharge, accompanied by intense redness and apparent tenderness, however, suggests infection (Figs. 11.42 and 13.37). The discharge should be

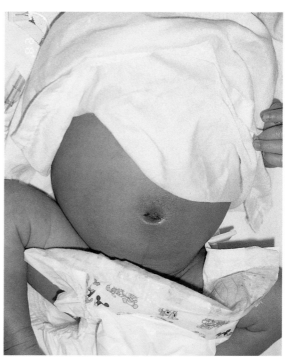

FIG. 13.37. This infant has a milder case of omphalitis than shown in Figure 11.42. Although circumferential erythema is present, the degree of induration is minimal.

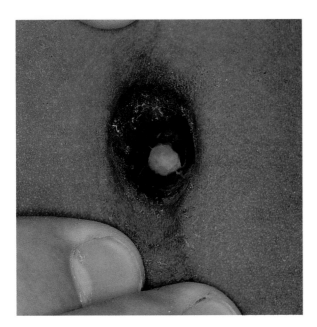

FIG. 13.38. Umbilical granuloma.

cultured and treated vigorously with antibiotics because the umbilical vessels are potential entry points for systemic invasion.

Granulation tissue, lumped into a small ball approximately 1 cm across and attached in the umbilical area, can be cauterized with a silver nitrate stick (Fig. 13.38). The parents should be forewarned that the area will turn transiently black. Often, this treatment has to be repeated in a week or so.

Umbilical Hernia

Umbilical hernia is a result of incomplete merging of the recti muscles at the ring through which the cord had been protruding (Fig. 13.39). It is often accompanied by a larger rectus diastasis extending superiorly, sometimes to as high as the xiphoid process. The size can vary from as small as a few millimeters to as large as 4 or 5 cm. It is covered by skin. With crying or straining, portions of the intestine and omentum can be palpated, but not visualized, within the hernia. No treatment is necessary in the neonatal period because these usually close as the baby becomes ambulant and strengthens the rectus muscles.

Omphalocele

An omphalocele is essentially a large hernia into the base of the cord, but it is covered only by peritoneum, not skin. It contains a significant amount of intestine and, rarely, a lobe of the liver (Fig. 13.40). The child should be admitted for early surgery.

Genital Area

The penis should be at least 1 cm in length with a urethral opening at the tip. The testes are usually palpable within the scrotal sac. The labia majora overlie and cover the labia minora.

Vaginal Discharge and Bleeding

White mucoid discharge, which may be thick, in the vaginal opening is a normal finding. Vaginal bleeding after the first day or two and during the first week is also a normal occurrence. It is the result of postpartum estrogen withdrawal.

Inguinal Mass

A mass palpable in the scrotum may be an inguinal hernia or a hydrocele or a combination of the two (Fig. 13.41). Hernias are usually easily reducible in the neonate. Hydroceles are fluid filled and transilluminate readily. A mass within the

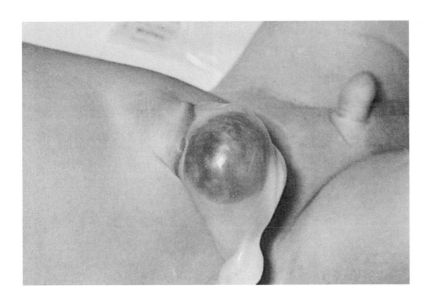

FIG. 13.39. Umbilical hernia. Hernia into the cord. (From O'Doherty N. *Atlas of the newborn.* Philadelphia: JB Lippincott, 1979:259, with permission.)

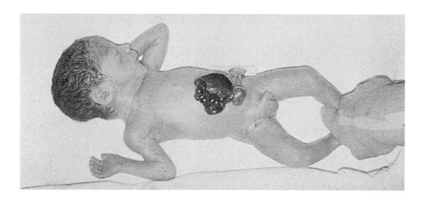

FIG. 13.40. Omphalocele. (From O'Doherty N. *Atlas of the newborn.* Philadelphia: JB Lippincott, 1979:259, with permission.)

labia majora is most likely an ovary or intestine that has passed through an inguinal hernia. These are somewhat more likely to incarcerate than male hernias.

Hypospadias

When the urethral opening is not at the tip of the penis but on the glans, the baby has first-degree hypospadias. When the opening is on the shaft, it is second degree and on the perineum, third degree. Infants with second- and third-degree hypospadias should be referred for urologic evaluation and imaging of the genitourinary tract.

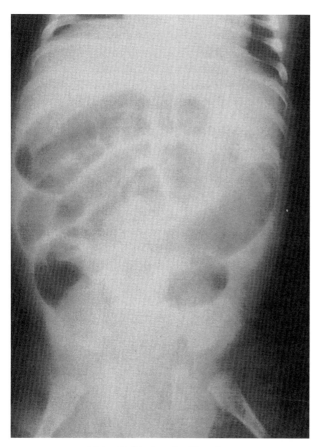

FIG. 13.41. Inguinal hernia.

Ambiguous Genitalia

The possibility of ambiguous genitalia should be considered in a male if the apparent penis is small and there is third-degree hypospadias with a cleft in the scrotum; in the female, genitalia are ambiguous if there appears to be an unusually long clitoris with partial or complete fusion of the labia majora and if there is a firm mass in the labia. In the female, but not in the male, such pseudohermaphroditism may be associated with congenital adrenal hyperplasia, with or without salt-losing symptomatology. To establish gender identity and to evaluate for the possibility of congenital adrenal hyperplasia, electrolyte, imaging, and chromosomal studies need to be done early in the child's neonatal period under the supervision of a urologist and geneticist and possibly an endocrinologist.

Imperforate Anus

An imperforate anus may not be obvious on external examination. The finding of an anus that appears to be located considerably more anteriorly than expected might suggest a fistula from the lower rectum to the skin, detouring around the anus. Meconium may actually pass through this fistula, simulating normal rectal passage. The area should be examined carefully, looking for the normal perianal-anal puckering, which will not be present if the anteriorly placed opening is a fistula (Fig. 13.42). The rectal examination should be carefully performed. The clinician should consider imaging studies and surgical referral.

ORTHOPEDIC CONCERNS

Most neonatal orthopedic problems are deformities secondary to intrauterine positioning. Some problems (e.g., metatarsus adductus) require only parental reassurance and expectant management, whereas others (e.g., congenital clubfoot, hip dysplasia) require early orthopedic attention.

Developmental Hip Dysplasia

Developmental dysplasia of the hip applies to a range of hip pathology, ranging from instability to frank dislocation, that may either be present at birth or develop during infancy (Fig. 13.43). The Ortolani and Barlow maneuvers may be used in the neonatal period to evaluate for hip instability. Both tests are performed with the infant in a supine position and the hips and knees flexed to 90 degrees. Each leg is examined separately, not simultaneously. In the Ortolani maneuver, gentle abduction and lifting of the femoral head anteriorly produces a palpable "thunk" or "clunk" as the examiner relocates a dislocated hip. Nonpathologic processes such as ligamentous snapping can produce hip clicks that differ from the pathologic "clunk" associated with developmental dysplasia of the hip.

Brachial Plexus Injuries

Lateral traction on the head and neck during delivery can result in injury to the brachial plexus (Fig. 13.44). Clinical signs relate to the site of the traumatic injury. Erb palsy, the most common birth injury of the brachial plexus, results from injury to the upper plexus affecting the C5 and C6 roots, the upper trunk, or its divisions (Fig. 13.45). The affected arm is held with the shoulder adducted and internally rotated, the elbow in extension and pronation, and the wrist in flexion ("waiter's tip" posture). On examination, the Moro reflex (allowing the infant's head to drop back suddenly results in abduction and upward movement of the arms followed by adduction and flexion) is asymmetric; there is weakness of shoulder abduction, flexion, and supination; the biceps reflex is decreased; and there is slight weakness of

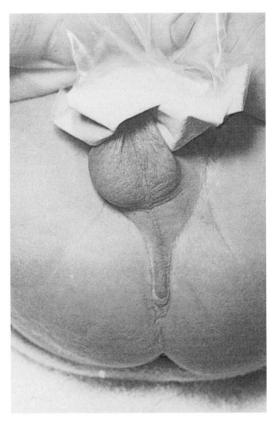

FIG. 13.42. Imperforate anus. (From O'Doherty N. *Atlas of the newborn.* Philadelphia: JB Lippincott, 1979:251, with permission.)

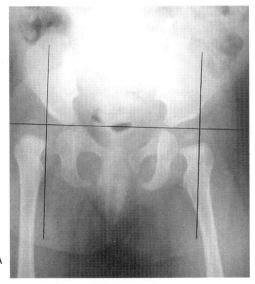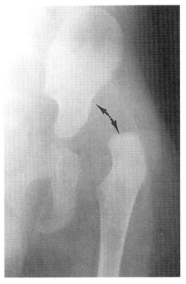

A

B

FIG. 13.43. Congenital dislocating hip (developmental dysplasia of the hip). **A:** Infant beyond neonatal period. Classic findings show lateral displacement of the right femur, delayed ossification of the right femoral head, and increased angulation and underdevelopment of the right acetabular roof. On the left (normal side), the vertical line (Perkins line) runs through the center of the femur. On the right, the femur is displaced lateral to the line. **B:** Chronic dislocating hip with pseudoacetabulum. In this infant, note gross dislocation of the hip with outward and upward displacement. The femoral head is articulating with a pseudoacetabulum (*arrows*) above the normal acetabulum. (From Swischuk LE. *Imaging of the newborn, infant, and young child,* 4th ed. Philadelphia: Lippincott Williams & Wilkins, 1997:699, with permission.)

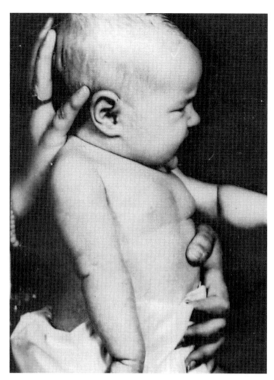

FIG. 13.44. Brachial plexus injury. An Erb–Duchenne type of brachial plexus injury. (From Avery GB, Fletcher MA, MacDonald MG. *Neonatology: pathophysiology and management of the newborn*, 5th ed. Philadelphia: Lippincott Williams & Wilkins, 1999:1282, with permission.)

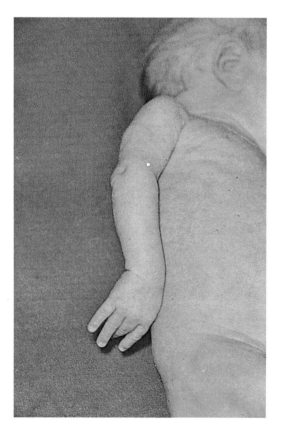

FIG. 13.45. Erb palsy after traction. (From O'Doherty N. *Atlas of the newborn*. Philadelphia: JB Lippincott, 1979:159, with permission.)

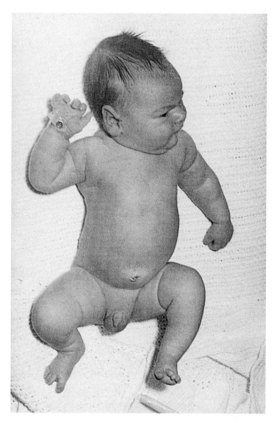

FIG. 13.46. Brachial paralysis. (From O'Doherty N. *Atlas of the newborn*. Philadelphia: JB Lippincott, 1979:159, with permission.)

wrist and finger extensors. In addition, when the C4 root is involved, ipsilateral hemidiaphragmatic paralysis may be appreciated by fluoroscopic examination.

Klumpke paralysis results from injury to the lower plexus affecting the C8 and T1 roots and the lower trunk or its divisions. The injury primarily affects the muscles of the hand. The infant presents with clawing of the affected hand (hyperextension at the metacarpophalangeal joints and flexion of the interphalangeal joints), the elbow is held in flexion and the wrist is usually held in extension, unless there is injury to the middle trunk. On examination, the palmar grasp is decreased, and the triceps reflex is decreased (Fig. 13.46).

Treatment consists of immobilization and appropriate positioning to prevent contractures. Orthopedic referral is indicated.

NEUROLOGIC CONCERNS

Neonatal Seizures

Neonatal seizures may be difficult to recognize clinically because it is rare for newborns to have symmetric, generalized tonic-clonic convulsions. It is much more common to see seizure episodes that present as focal abnormalities or subtle findings. Subtle seizures can be difficult to distinguish from the normal spectrum of newborn behaviors, jitteriness, or

TABLE 13.2. *Clinical differentiation of neonatal seizures from jitteriness*

Clinical characteristic	Seizure	Jitteriness
Stimulus sensitive	No	Yes
Movement ceases with restraint	No	Yes
Accompanied by autonomic changes	Yes	No
Speed of movements	Slower	Faster
Abnormal eye movements	Common	No

TABLE 13.3. *Classification of neonatal seizures*

Seizure type	Electroencephalogram seizure correlation
Subtle	
Sucking or chewing motion	Uncommon[a]
Lip smacking	
Bicycling of legs	
Apnea	
Eyelid fluttering	
Eye deviations	
Laughter	
Tonic posturing	
Tonic	
Focal	Common
Generalized	Uncommon
Clonic	
Focal	Common
Multifocal	Common
Myoclonic	
Focal	Uncommon
Multifocal	Uncommon
Generalized	Common

[a] Except for tonic eye deviation, which often has an electroencephalographic correlation.

benign myoclonic movements. Benign myoclonic movements are isolated jerky movements of an extremity that occur primarily during sleep. Jitteriness may be differentiated from seizures by its disappearance when the affected extremity is touched or held (Table 13.2). Four clinical seizure types are recognized in the newborn (Table 13.3): subtle, tonic, clonic, and myoclonic

Hypotonic Infant

A healthy term newborn normally moves his or her extremities spontaneously and has a dominance of flexor tone. Compared with the term newborn's tone, the premature infant's tone is relatively hypotonic, so corrected gestational age must be taken into consideration during evaluation.

The causes of hypotonia depend on the level of the nervous system that is affected (Table 13.4). Motor dysfunction at any level from the central nervous system to the muscle itself may result in hypotonia. Central hypotonia involves pathology of the cerebral cortex down to the level of the lower motor neuron or can be caused by systemic disease affecting motor function. Neuromuscular disease can be caused by dysfunction at any of four anatomic sites: anterior horn cell (lower motor neuron), peripheral nerve, neuromuscular junction, and muscle.

TABLE 13.4. *Differential diagnosis of neonatal hypotonia*

Central nervous system disease
Perinatal asphyxia (hypoxic-ischemic encephalopathy)
Intracranial hemorrhage
Infection
Hyperbilirubinemia
Neonatal drug withdrawal
Metabolic diseases
   Organic and aminoacidemias
   Hypercalcemia
Chromosomal abnormality
   Down syndrome
   Prader–Willi syndrome
Neuromuscular disease
Anterior horn cell diseases (lower motor neuron)
   Type I spinal muscular atrophy (Werdnig–Hoffmann disease)

Neonatal poliomyelitis
Type II glycogen storage disease (Pompe disease)
Peripheral nerve diseases
   Leukodystrophies
   Guillain–Barré syndrome
Neuromuscular junction diseases
   Infantile botulism
   Neonatal myasthenia gravis (congenital or acquired transient myasthenia)
Muscle diseases
   Congenital myopathies
   Mitochondrial myopathies
Glycogen storage disease
Hypothyroidism

Suggested Readings

American Academy of Pediatrics. Management of hyperbilirubinemia in the healthy term infant. *Pediatrics* 1994;94:558–565.

Cheng JC, Au AW. Infantile torticollis: a review of 624 cases. *J Pediatr Orthop* 1994;14:802–808.

Driscoll DJ. Evaluation of the cyanotic newborn. *Pediatr Clin North Am* 1990;37:1–8.

Elhassani SB, Mease AD. Visible neonatal masses: separating the serious from the benign. *Contemp Pediatr* 1990;11:42–60.

Newman TB, Maisels MJ. Evaluation and treatment of jaundice in the term newborn: a kinder, gentler approach. *Pediatrics* 1992;89:809–818.

Stafstrom CE. Neonatal seizures. *Pediatr Rev* 1995;16:248–255.

Thilo EH, Townsend SF. Early newborn discharge: have we gone too far? *Contemp Pediatr* 1996;13:29–46.

CHAPTER 14

Neurologic and Neurosurgical Emergencies

Editor: Gary R. Fleisher

SEIZURES

Clinical Manifestations

Paroxysmal events other than seizures that involve changes in consciousness or motor activity are common during childhood and may mimic epilepsy (Table 14.1). Breath-holding spells occur in children 6 months to 4 years of age and take one of two forms: cyanotic and pallid. Syncope is a brief, sudden loss of consciousness and muscle tone. The child is typically upright before the event and often senses a feeling of light-headedness or nausea; the child then becomes pale and slumps to the ground. The loss of consciousness is brief, and recovery is rapid. Single episodes of staring, involuntary movements, or eye deviation have been found to occur commonly in the first months of life. Acute dystonia (Fig. 14.1), usually seen as a side effect of some medications, can mimic a tonic seizure. The child having a dystonic reaction, however, does not lose consciousness and has no postictal drowsiness. Several paroxysmal events are associated with sleep. Night terrors usually begin in the preschool years. The sleeping child wakes suddenly, is confused and disoriented, and appears frightened, often screaming and showing signs of increased autonomic activity. Benign myoclonus is characterized by self-limited episodes of sudden jerking of the extremities, usually upon falling asleep.

Pseudoseizures are occasionally seen, often in patients with an underlying seizure disorder or with a relative with epilepsy. Some features suggestive of pseudoseizures are suggestibility, lack of coordination of movements, moaning or talking during the "seizure," lack of continence, autonomic changes, postictal drowsiness, and poor response to treatment with anticonvulsant agents.

Management

Various conditions lead to seizures (Table 14.2). Figure 14.2 provides an algorithmic approach to making an etiologic diagnosis. Management begins urgently on arrival of the actively convulsing patient in most cases and focuses initially on the airway, respiration, and intravenous access. With the exception of simple febrile seizures, control of grand mal convulsions usually requires administration of anticonvulsant medications.

Rarely, a child may enter the emergency department in absence status. In this case, the child may be sitting in a confused or dreamy state. Such attacks may last for hours or even days. The drug of choice in the treatment of absence status is lorazepam or diazepam at the doses already outlined (Fig. 14.3). At times, a child may enter the emergency department with continual focal seizure activity (with or without clouding of consciousness), a condition known as epilepsia partialis continua. In these cases, 18 to 20 mg/kg phenytoin or fosphenytoin can be infused slowly.

ENCEPHALITIS

Clinical Manifestations

Encephalitis is an inflammation of the brain parenchyma. When there is associated leptomeningeal involvement (as often occurs), the term meningoencephalitis may be applied, whereas encephalomyelitis implies involvement of the spinal cord as well. The clinical picture of viral encephalitis ranges from a mild febrile illness associated with headache to a severe, fulminant presentation with coma, seizures, and death. The onset of encephalitis may be abrupt or insidious. Typical features consist of fever, headache, vomiting, and signs of meningeal irritation. Altered consciousness, ataxia, and seizures are also seen. Focal neurologic deficits occur in some types of encephalitis, particularly herpes simplex encephalitis. Flaccid paralysis may be seen in cases of encephalomyelitis, and, rarely, respiratory or cardiac dysfunction results from brainstem involvement. Rash or mucous membrane lesions are often seen with the exanthematous viruses such as measles and varicella; however, cutaneous findings are uncommon with herpes simplex encephalitis. With viral encephalitides, cerebrospinal fluid (CSF) pleocytosis is variable and, if present, is usually fewer than 500 cells/mm^3. These cells may be predominantly polymorphonuclear early in the course of the illness; however, a

TABLE 14.1. *Nonepileptic events that may mimic seizures*

Breath-holding spells	Acute dystonia
Syncope	Gastroesophageal reflux
Migraine	Night terrors
Jitteriness	Sleep paralysis
Benign myoclonus	Narcolepsy
Shuddering attacks	Pseudoseizures
Tics	

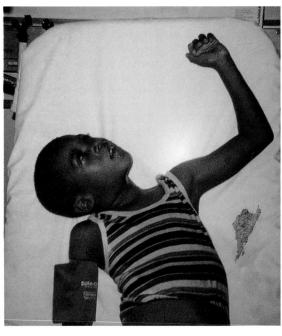 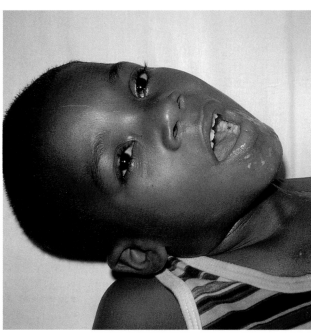

A   B

FIG. 14.1. Acute dystonic reaction manifested by posturing of the upper extremity **(A)** and an oculogyric crisis **(B)**.

TABLE 14.2. *Etiology of seizures*

Infectious	Metabolic
Brain abscess	Hepatic failure
Encephalitis	Hypercarbia
Febrile[a] (nonspecific)	Hyperosmolarity
Meningitis	Hypocalcemia
Parasites (central nervous system)	Hypoglycemia
Syphilis	Hypomagnesemia
Idiopathic[a]	Hyponatremia
Withdrawals	Hypoia
Alcohol	Inborn errors of metabolism
Anticonvulsants[a]	Pyridoxine deficiency
Hypnotics	Uremia
Toxicologic	Vascular
Anticonvulsant	Cerebrovascular accident
Camphor	Hypertensive encephalopathy
Carbon monoxide	Oncologic
Cocaine	Primary brain tumor
Heavy metals (lead)	Metastatic disease
Hypoglycemic agents	Endocrine
Isoniazid	Addison disease
Lithium	Hyperthyroidism
Methylxanthines	Hypothyroidism
Pesticides (organophosphates)	Obstetric
Phencyclidine	Eclampsia
Sympathomimetics	Traumatic
Tricyclic antidepressants	Cerebral contusion
Topical anesthetics	Diffuse axonal injury
Degenerative cerebral disease	Intracranial hemorrhage
Hypoic ischemic injury	Congenital anomalies

[a] Most common causes.

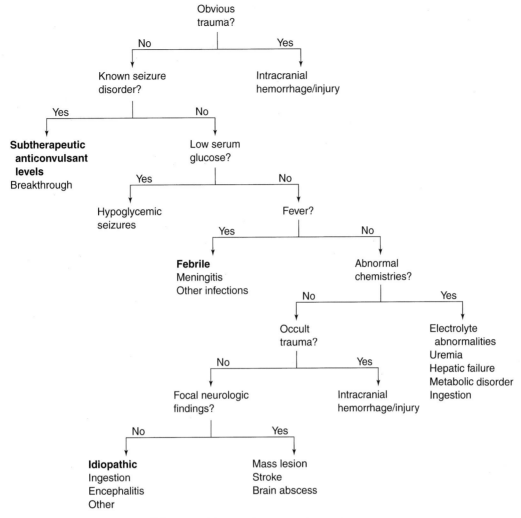

FIG. 14.2. Diagnostic approach to seizures.

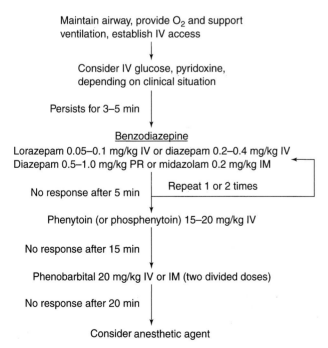

FIG. 14.3. Treatment of status epilepticus. *O$_2$*, oxygen; *IV*, intravenous; *PR*, per rectum; *IM*, intramuscular.

mononuclear predominance is common later. Red blood cells are present in the CSF in approximately 50% of children with herpes simplex encephalitis. Spinal fluid protein and glucose are usually normal in viral encephalitis, but the protein may be greatly elevated in postinfectious encephalomyelitis.

Management

At present, the treatment of nonherpes viral encephalitis is primarily supportive. Herpes simplex encephalitis causes death or neurologic sequelae in more than 70% of patients. Treatment with 30 to 60 mg/kg acyclovir per day in three divided doses for 14 to 21 days has resulted in a decrease in mortality and some improvement in morbidity.

DISORDERS THAT PRESENT WITH HEADACHE

Migraine

Clinical Manifestations

Prolonged (as long as 24 to 48 hours), moderate to severe headache is characteristic of migraine. The headaches may be pulsating and unilateral but assume this pattern less often

TABLE 14.3. *Agents for acute treatment of migraine*

Drug	Usual dose
Analgesics	
Acetaminophen	10–15 mg/kg/dose PO or PR q 4 hr
Ibuprofen	5–10 mg/kg/dose PO q 6 hr
Ketorolac (Toradol)	30 mg initial dose, then 15–30 mg/dose (0.5 mg/kg) IV or IM, or 10 mg/dose PO, q 4–6 hr
Codeine	0.5–1 mg/kg/dose PO q 4–6 hr
Antiemetics	
Metoclopramide (Reglan)	0.5–2 mg/kg/dose PO or IV q 4–6 hr
Prochlorperazine (Compazine)	0.1 mg/kg/dose PO or IM q 6 hr
Promethazine (Phenergan)	0.25–1.0 mg/kg/dose PO, PR, IV, or IM q 4–6 hr
Specific antimigraine agents	
Dihydroergotamine	0.5–1.0 mg/dose IV or IM; may repeat after 1 hr
Sumatriptan (Imitrex)	6 mg SC or 100 mg PO (>12 years of age)

PO, orally; PR, rectally; q, every; IV, intravenously; IM, intramuscularly; SC, subcutaneously.

in children than in adults. Migraine is commonly associated with nausea, vomiting, abdominal pain, and photophobia or phonophobia. Auras occur in less than half of children who experience migraines. Occasionally, the attacks awaken children from sleep. The physical examination usually shows no focal neurologic deficits, although hemiplegia and ophthalmoplegia may occur in complicated migraine. Unless these episodes have occurred previously, their presence warrants further neurologic evaluation, usually in the form of computed tomography (CT) or magnetic resonance imaging (MRI). A family history of migraine is helpful in diagnosis. The diagnosis of migraine is based almost exclusively on the history and is supported by the absence of abnormalities on examination. There are no diagnostic laboratory tests or imaging studies.

Management

Several agents are available for the treatment of acute migraine (Table 14.3). For many children, mild oral analgesics such as acetaminophen or ibuprofen combined with bed rest may provide sufficient relief and should be considered the first-line agents of choice. Ketorolac (Toradol), a nonsteroidal antiinflammatory agent for parenteral use, may be used when nausea or vomiting limits oral intake. A short course of a narcotic analgesic such as codeine may occasionally be needed if nonnarcotic agents have failed, especially if the headache prevents sleep. When nausea and vomiting are severe, antiemetic medications such as metoclopramide (Reglan), prochlorperazine (Compazine), and promethazine (Phenergan) are useful. In addition to their antiemetic effect, these agents often provide some relief of the headache as well and may permit the use of other oral medications.

Ergot preparations act primarily as cerebral vasoconstrictors and are specifically indicated for aborting acute migraine attacks. Ergotamine tartrate is administered orally or sublingually, but it must be used early in the headache to be effective, preferably at the outset of the prodrome. For acute migraine, D.H.E. (dihydroergotamine mesylate) can be given to older children and adolescents in an initial dose

of 0.5 mg intramuscularly or intravenously (no milligram-per-kilogram dose has been established). The initial dose of D.H.E. may be repeated in 1 hour if necessary.

Sumatriptan succinate (Imitrex) is a serotonergic agent available for either oral or subcutaneous administration. The dose for children 12 years and older is 6 mg subcutaneously or 100 mg orally. Sumatriptan is generally well tolerated; side effects include irritation at the injection site, flushing, tachycardia, disorientation, and chest tightness that lasts for several minutes after parenteral administration. Sumatriptan should not be used concomitantly with ergotamines. A reasonable approach is to use sumatriptan after a trial of analgesics in an older child, although an older child or adolescent with recurrent migraine and a history of successful treatment with sumatriptan in the past may benefit from earlier use of this agent.

Idiopathic Intracranial Hypertension (Pseudotumor Cerebri)

Clinical Manifestations

Headache, of variable severity and duration, is the most common presenting symptom. It is typically worse in the morning. Nausea, vomiting, dizziness, and double or blurred vision also occur. If the process is long-standing, decreased visual acuity or visual field deficits can result. Infants often have nonspecific symptoms of lethargy or irritability. Papilledema is seen in virtually all cases. Other neurologic symptoms and signs are often absent; however, cranial nerve palsies, particularly affecting the sixth cranial nerve, may be seen. Diagnosis should be considered when a child with a prolonged history of headache is found to have evidence of papilledema without other neurologic findings. Pseudotumor cerebri is a diagnosis of exclusion, and mass lesions and infectious processes must be ruled out. Because posterior fossa tumors and obstructive or nonobstructive hydrocephalus may mimic pseudotumor early in the course of disease, CT or MRI should be obtained in all children with this constellation of findings. If no mass lesion is present, a lumbar puncture (LP)

TABLE 14.4. *Symptoms and signs of elevated intracranial pressure*

Symptoms	Signs
Headache	Papilledema
Nocturnal, episodic, severe	Cranial nerve palsies
Vomiting	Meningismus
Stiff neck	Head tilt
Double vision	Retinal hemorrhage
Transient visual loss	Macewen (cracked pot) sign
Gait abnormalities	Decorticate/decerebrate posturing
Dulled intellect	Coma
Irritability	Progressive hemiparesis
	Bradycardia

should be performed with a manometer to measure opening pressure. Children with pseudotumor have elevated opening pressure (greater than 200 mm H_2O) but normal CSF cell count, protein, and glucose.

Management

Removal of sufficient CSF to normalize intracranial pressure (ICP) usually leads to relief of symptoms. Treatment may then be started with 60 mg/kg acetazolamide (Diamox) per day in four divided doses to decrease CSF production. In cases resulting from withdrawal of steroid therapy, a course of prednisone or dexamethasone may be beneficial. Patients with mild symptoms and good response to LP may be discharged to home with close follow-up arranged.

Mass Lesions (Increased Intracranial Pressure)

Clinical Manifestations

A careful history must be taken with respect to the timing and severity of headaches, vomiting, changes in behavior, visual changes, and episodic decreases in level of consciousness (Table 14.4). Nighttime and morning headaches that improve on arising are always ominous suggestions of elevated ICP, as is recurrent vomiting without fever, and gait abnormalities.

The clinical examination can help to confirm the presence of intracranial hypertension, but a normal examination cannot reliably exclude it. Funduscopic examination should be performed to look for papilledema or optic atrophy. VisCranial sutures may split in infants and young children with chronic elevation of ICP, resulting in a hyperresonant note when the skull is percussed, a "cracked pot" sound known as the Macewen sign. Cranial nerve palsy may occur, usually affecting the third and/or sixth nerves, resulting in dilated pupil, diplopia, and strabismus. When the fourth nerve is affected, the child may exhibit a "cock robin" head tilt.

Management

The emergency treatment of increased ICP depends on the patient's clinical state and the cause of the intracranial hypertension (Table 14.5). However, the first priority in all patients is to manage airway, breathing, and circulation and to prevent hypoxemia, hypercarbia, and systemic hypotension. Seizures should be prevented if possible and treated aggressively when they occur because the ICP spikes during seizures aggravate intracranial hypertension.

When the clinical picture suggests intracranial hypertension, CT of the head should be performed without contrast material as soon as the patient is stable. LP should be withheld until the scan has been read for fear of precipitating herniation. The temptation to give sedative agents to the agitated patient to accomplish head CT or to facilitate transport should be avoided. Sedative agents given without controlled ventilation may result in hypercarbia, causing an increase in cerebral blood volume and, therefore, in ICP. Sedatives may also block protective airway reflexes, increasing the risk of aspiration. Therefore, inserting an endotracheal tube before CT scan or before transport is often preferable.

In the absence of signs of impending herniation, P_{CO_2} should be controlled by mild hyperventilation in the range of 30 to 35 mm Hg. Acute hyperventilation (hand ventilation) is used as an attempt to reverse the signs of acute herniation. The head of the bed should be elevated to 30 degrees and the head maintained in a neutral position to promote venous

TABLE 14.5. *Treatment of increased intracranial pressure*

Prevent hypoxia and hypercarbia
Tracheal intubation/controlled ventilation
Seizure treatment and prophylaxis
Maintain adequate cerebral perfusion pressure and cerebral perfusion
Treatment of shock
Limitation of excessive hyperventilation
Decrease cerebral blood volume
Acute hyperventilation
Decrease brain tissue volume
Mannitol
Dexamethasone for vasogenic edema
Decrease CSF volume
CSF drainage
Acetazolamide
Removal of mass lesion
Surgical removal/decompression

CSF, cerebrospinal fluid.

drainage. Also, when the child exhibits acute herniation, drainage of CSF, either from a shunt reservoir or by a ventricular tap via an open fontanelle, a split suture, or a bur burn hole, allows controlled reduction of CSF volume. A ventriculostomy catheter may also be used to directly measure ICP, to direct medical therapy, and to allow drainage of CSF. Mannitol (0.25 to 2.0 g/kg) is the most useful drug to acutely decrease ICP in the deteriorating patient. Acetazolamide and furosemide have a limited role in acute management. Dexamethasone (1 mg/kg) is of controversial benefit, has a slow onset, and appears to be most useful in treating vasogenic brain edema associated with tumors and brain abscess and nontraumatic hemorrhage. Surgical removal of collections of blood or pus may be indicated to lower ICP.

Previously Undiagnosed Hydrocephalus

In a child with unexplained headache, chronic vomiting, and irritability, head circumference should be recorded and the fontanelle, if open, evaluated (Fig. 14.4). Dilated scalp veins should be noted. A cracked pot sound may be noted on percussion if the sutures are split. Difficulty with upward gaze ("sunset" sign) may be seen with hydrocephalus. Muscular spasticity, particularly in the lower extremities, may develop as cortical motor fibers are stretched by the ventricular dilation. Noncontrast head CT demonstrates enlarged ventricles. The urgency with which either insertion of a ventricular shunt or ventricular drainage needs to be performed depends on the child's condition. Ventricular puncture through an open fontanelle or coronal suture may be lifesaving in a child with evidence for impending cerebral herniation who is unresponsive to hyperventilation and mannitol.

Previously Shunted Hydrocephalus

Shunt Malfunction

Patients with shunt malfunction commonly present with manifestations of increased ICP. Children may complain of headache (often worse in the morning), screaming episodes, lethargy, and other behavioral changes and/or visual symptoms. Vomiting is common. On physical examination, unilateral or bilateral cranial nerve palsies, especially a nonlocalizing sixth nerve palsy, may be present. Intermittent downward gaze (sunset sign) may be reported or observed. Swelling from CSF tracking along the shunt tract is indicative of obstruction (Figs. 14.5 and 14.6). At times, the tubing from the shunt may erode through the skin (Fig. 14.7). The fontanelle may be full and tense, even when the infant is upright. Rapid enlargement in head circumference or increase in the prominence of scalp veins may occur. Papilledema is uncommon in acute shunt malfunction. Head tilt may be seen as a result of fourth cranial nerve palsy or cerebellar tonsillar herniation. Most shunts have a pumping mechanism, but pumping the shunt correlates poorly with function. The shunt should not be repeatedly pumped because the negative pressure generated in a small ventricle may occasionally result in obstruction. However, if the ventricular catheter is shown on a CT scan to be in the center of a dilated ventricle and the shunt umbilicates on depression with slow refill, shunt obstruction is likely.

If the history or physical examination suggests shunt malfunction, a plain radiographic shunt series should be done (Fig. 14.5B, C, D). A noncontrast head CT scan should also be done and compared, if possible, with previous scans taken when the shunt was functioning. In most cases (more than 80%), these studies identify shunt malfunction. A shunt tap

FIG. 14.4. These two patients **(A, B)** have acute hydrocephalus manifesting as an increased head circumference and dilated scalp veins.

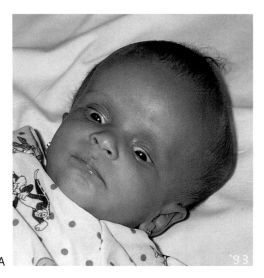

A

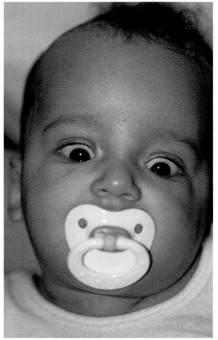

B

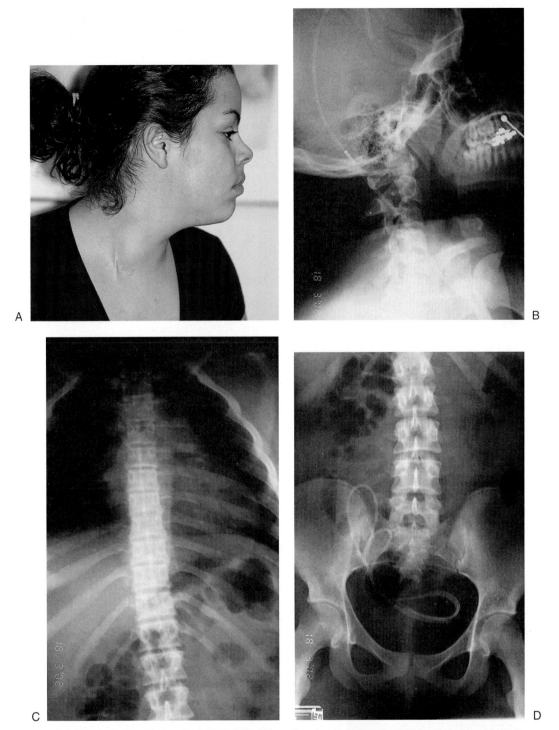

FIG. 14.5. This young girl developed swelling **(A)** at the site of a disconnection of her shunt, which can be seen on the radiographs **(B–D)**. The radiographs show a discontinuity in the shunt, with the distal end coiled in the pelvis.

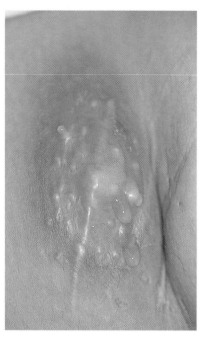

FIG. 14.6. This 16-year-old girl with hydrocephalus developed a cerebrospinal fluid leak at the site of her abdominal scar, where her shunt entered her abdomen. The erythema and blistering aroused suspicion of infection.

may also be useful in patients in whom the function of the shunt is questionable.

The urgency of shunt revision for an obstruction depends on the patient's status. When the distal end of the shunt is blocked, the ICP can be immediately lowered by removing CSF through a shunt tap. There is less need for emergency shunt revision in this setting because the ICP can be easily controlled by tapping the shunt.

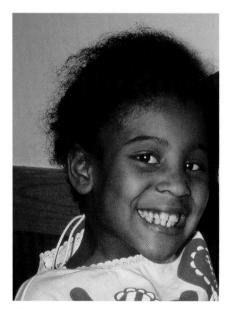

FIG. 14.7. The shunt tube in this child has eroded through the skin on the right side of the neck.

TABLE 14.6. *Causes of hemorrhagic stroke*

Secondary hemorrhage into ischemic brain
Vascular malformations
Arteriovenous malformations
Sickle cell disease
Saccular (berry) aneurysms
Hemorrhage into intracranial tumor
Coagulopathy
Hemorrhagic disease of the newborn (vitamin K deficiency)
Clotting factor deficiency (VIII, IX, XI)
Thrombocytopenia
Arterial hypertension
Renal vascular or parenchymal disease
Coarctation of the aorta
Pheochromocytoma
Drugs with sympathomimetic effect
Amphetamines, cocaine

DISORDERS OF MOTOR FUNCTION

Stroke/Cerebrovascular Accident

Clinical Manifestations

Stroke may result from brain ischemia, hemorrhage, or embolism (Tables 14.6 and 14.7). The presentation of stroke in children is highly variable, influenced by the portion of the cerebral vasculature affected as well as the child's age. Hemiparesis is most often observed, with facial weakness typically ipsilateral to weakness in the rest of the body. Older children often have concomitant headache, whereas children younger than 4 years of age are more likely to have associated seizures. The child with a stroke may also have a diminished level of consciousness. Cranial CT without contrast is the study of choice for identifying acute hemorrhage. However, CT may be normal in the first 12 to 24 hours after an ischemic stroke; MRI, in contrast, may show changes as early as 6 hours after infarction. The usual approach is to obtain a noncontrast CT scan (Fig. 14.8), followed by MRI if no hemorrhage is seen. In a child without a known predisposing condition, ancillary tests may be revealing of the

TABLE 14.7. *Causes of ischemic stroke*

Cardioembolic
  Cyanotic congenital heart disease
  Right-to-left shunts (e.g., patent foramen ovale)
  Congenital or acquired valvular defects
  Contractile dysfunction
  Rhythm disturbance
Vascular disease
  Sickle cell disease
  Arterial dissection
  Homocystinuria
  Vasculitis
  Moyamoya
  Migraine
Thrombotic (arterial and sinovenous)
  Hypercoagulable state, congenital or acquired
  Hyperviscosity (polycythemia, dehydration)
  Genetic/metabolic

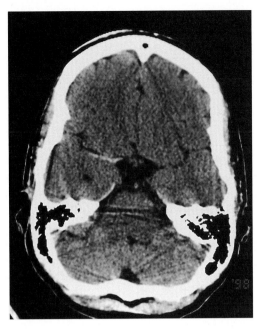

FIG. 14.8. A 21-year-old woman had a syncope episode in the emergency department. Examination revealed a left facial palsy, and her computed tomography scan shows a hyperdense area in the region of the right middle cerebral artery.

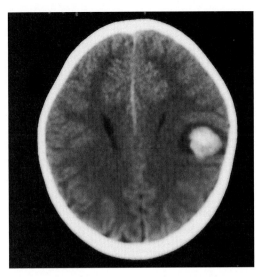

FIG. 14.9. This 4-year-old boy awoke disoriented and was drooling. Shortly thereafter, he had an episode of rhythmic eye blinking and mouth twitching. His computed tomography scan shows a large hemorrhage.

cause of the stroke. Treatments worth considering in such patients, depending on the clinical picture, are listed in Table 14.8.

Management

Initial treatment after an acute stroke is focused on stabilization and supportive care, including control of any seizures. Hypertension, if present, must be treated cautiously, and the blood pressure lowered gradually. Both hypoglycemia and hyperglycemia can exacerbate ischemic stroke, so careful monitoring of serum glucose is important. Fever, which can occur in children with stroke, may also contribute to ischemic damage and should be controlled with antipyretics.

Further therapy is determined by the type of stroke. With hemorrhagic stroke, neurosurgical intervention may be required to evacuate a hematoma or excise a bleeding arteri-

ovenous malformation (Fig. 14.9). Catheter-directed embolization may also be possible in cases of arteriovenous malformation. Children with sickle cell disease and stroke should have an acute transfusion to decrease the level of hemoglobin S to less than 30%. Thrombolytic and anticoagulant therapies have been shown to be effective in adults with ischemic stroke but remain untested in children. Similarly, novel therapies such as calcium channel blockers and free radical scavengers have not been studied in pediatric patients; their use remains experimental.

SPINAL CORD DYSFUNCTION

Background

Dysfunction of the spinal cord may result from any of a variety of disorders, either intrinsic or extrinsic to the spinal cord, with a great deal of overlap in their clinical presentation. Transverse myelitis is an intramedullary disorder, involving both halves of the cord over a variable length, with involvement of motor and sensory tracts. It occurs in chil-

TABLE 14.8. *Studies to consider in the evaluation of the child with acute stroke*

Brain imaging	Erythrocyte sedimentation rate
Computed tomography (noncontrast)	Hemoglobin electrophoresis
Magnetic resonance imaging	Protein C and S quantification
Angiography (standard or magnetic	Antithrombin III level
resonance)	Chemistry
Cardiac	Blood urea nitrogen
Electrocardiogram	Cholesterol and triglycerides
Echocardiogram	Hepatic transaminases
Hematologic	Serum amino acids
Complete blood count	Urine organic acids
Prothrombin and partial thromboplastin times	Toxicology screen
Fibrinogen	Lactate
	Lumbar puncture

dren and adults, although it is rare in the first year of life. Acute spinal cord compression in children usually is caused by trauma, infection, or cancer. Spinal trauma may lead to contusion or concussion of the cord with hemorrhage, edema, and local mass effect or to development of a spinal epidural hematoma. Epidural abscess is the most common infectious cause of spinal cord compression. Neoplastic causes include both primary intraspinal tumors (ependymoma and astrocytoma) and extrinsic lesions such as neuroblastoma or lymphoma.

Clinical Manifestations

Spinal cord dysfunction is characterized by paraplegia below the level of involvement, hyporeflexia, and sensory symptoms such as bandlike pain at the level of compression, and sensory loss or paraesthesias below the area of damage. If the lower spinal cord (the conus) is involved, there usually is early loss of bowel and bladder control. Compression of the cauda equina usually results in asymmetric symptoms, radicular pain, and focal lower extremity motor and sensory abnormalities.

Transverse myelitis may affect any level of the spinal cord, but thoracic involvement is most common. Initial symptoms include lower extremity paresthesia, local back pain, unilateral or bilateral lower extremity weakness, and urinary retention. A preceding respiratory or gastrointestinal illness is usually reported, and at the time of diagnosis, fever and meningismus are sometimes seen in children. Characteristically, the insidious onset of paresthesia or weakness of the lower extremities progresses over days or, rarely, weeks, and then is replaced by the abrupt occurrence of static paraplegia or quadriplegia and, in the cooperative child, a detectable sensory level. In other children, the course of progression may be less than 12 hours. The sensory loss generally involves all modalities, although a spinothalamic deficit (pain) may occur without posterior column dysfunction (vibration). The weakness usually is symmetric but may be asymmetric. After a variable interval, initial flaccidity may be replaced by spasticity. Sphincter disturbance of the bowel and bladder occurs in most patients, bladder distention being the most common initial sign of damage.

Traumatic and infectious spinal lesions are usually accompanied by relatively acute onset of local back pain, which is exacerbated by direct percussion of the area. Pain may precede other symptoms for days. With tumors, however, there may be weakness in the absence of pain. Patients with epidural abscess often have systemic signs of infections such as fever, headache, vomiting, and perhaps neck stiffness. Bony tenderness in such a patient may indicate vertebral osteomyelitis or discitis, which can also present with weakness, although usually less severe than is seen with actual spinal cord involvement.

Diagnosis is confirmed by emergency neuroimaging, with precautions taken to immobilize the patient as much as possible. Plain spine films are useful initially in trauma. MRI of the spine is the procedure of choice to detect compressive mass lesions, but if not immediately available, plain or CT myelography is an alternative. If no mass lesion is noted and transverse myelitis is a diagnostic possibility, LP may be useful, showing a normal or slightly elevated opening pressure and mild pleocytosis in the CSF in nearly 50% of patients at the time of presentation.

Management

Treatment of children with spinal injury from trauma begins with splinting and immobilization of the spine. If trauma is likely, high-dose methylprednisolone, if given within 8 hours of injury at an intravenous dose of 30 mg/kg followed by infusion at 5.4 mg/kg per hour for 23 hours, may improve the quality of neurologic outcome. In cases of possible epidural abscess or tumor-related mass, intravenous dexamethasone at a loading dose of 2 mg/kg (to a maximum of 100 mg) should be given, followed by 1 to 2 mg/kg per day intravenously in four divided doses over the next 24 hours. In patients with a presumed infectious cause and those with cancer of unknown origin, surgical decompression is indicated on an emergent basis to alleviate pressure and pinpoint diagnosis. Treatment of transverse myelitis is supportive, and some degree of recovery occurs in approximately 80% of cases.

ACUTE POLYNEURITIS (GUILLAIN–BARRÉ SYNDROME)

Clinical Manifestations

Weakness, commonly with an insidious onset, is the usual presenting complaint. Paresthesias or other sensory abnormalities such as pain or numbness are prominent in as many as 50% of cases, particularly in older children. The paresthesias and paralysis usually are symmetric and ascending, although variations may occur. Early in the course of illness, distal weakness is more prominent than proximal weakness. Deep tendon reflexes are depressed or absent at the time of diagnosis. Affected children often have an ataxic gait. Cranial nerve abnormalities occur during the illness in 30% to 40% of cases and may be the predominant finding, especially in the Miller–Fisher variant of this syndrome, which is characterized by oculomotor palsies, ataxia, and areflexia without motor weakness of the extremities. As the paralysis ascends, muscles of breathing may become involved, leading to respiratory embarrassment. The primary aid in diagnosis is LP, which demonstrates an elevated protein, normal glucose, and fewer than 10 white blood cells/mm^3, the so-called albuminocytologic disassociation.

Management

Because of the potential for progression to life-threatening respiratory compromise, the child with Guillain–Barré syndrome should be hospitalized and observed closely. Impending respiratory distress must be anticipated, and routine respiratory monitoring should be aided by specific measures of respiratory function, particularly measurement of negative inspiratory force. Because autonomic dysfunction is common, blood pressure must be monitored closely and abnormalities treated vigorously.

Acute polyneuritis is generally self-limiting, with more than 90% of children in most series having complete or nearly complete recovery. In mild cases, in which children retain the ability to ambulate, only supportive care is required. However, immunomodulatory therapy may be of benefit in more severely affected children. Plasmapheresis and intravenous immunoglobulin have both been used.

MYASTHENIA GRAVIS

Clinical Manifestations

The juvenile form of myasthenia clinically mimics the adult disease. The mean age at onset is 8 years, with a female predominance of approximately 4:1. The onset of symptoms may be insidious or acute. Most cases affect the cranial nerves, and any cranial nerve can be involved in combination or isolation. Bilateral ptosis is the most common cranial nerve deficit (Fig. 14.10A), followed in incidence by oculomotor impairment. Generalized truncal and limb weakness is present at onset in as many as one-half of the cases and eventually develops in most children with myasthenia. The diagnosis should be suspected if there is a history of worsening weakness during continual activity or if fatigability of muscle strength is demonstrable.

The Tensilon test is the backbone of diagnosis. In this procedure, the anticholinesterase drug edrophonium (Tensilon), which has a 30-second onset and approximately a 5-minute duration of action, is given slowly intravenously at a dose of 0.2 mg/kg to a maximal dose of 10 mg. Atropine should be immediately available to treat potential severe cholinergic reactions (e.g., bradycardia). Initially, one-tenth of the total dose is given, and if no hypersensitivity or severe reactions are noted, the remainder of the dose is administered. Because the duration of edrophonium is short-lived, interpretation of the response requires close monitoring of a muscle or muscle group in which improvement can be seen clearly, such as the eyelid elevators (Fig. 14.10B).

Management

Although myasthenia gravis is potentially life threatening, specific management usually can be delayed until after the diagnosis is made. If there is evidence of respiratory compromise, ventilatory support is mandatory. Treatment is begun with the use of cholinesterase inhibitors to prolong the availability of acetylcholine at the neuromuscular junction. At present, the anticholinesterase of choice is pyridostigmine (Mestinon) at a starting dose of 1 mg/kg orally every 4 hours, adjusted according to the clinical response. Other agents, such as corticosteroids or antimetabolites, may be beneficial in selected cases. If there is any concern about respiratory compromise or if severe weakness is present, the child should be hospitalized immediately.

INFANTILE BOTULISM

The initial symptom of infantile botulism usually is constipation, followed insidiously by lethargy and feeding difficulties. Physical findings at the time of presentation are hypoactive deep tendon reflexes, decreased suck and gag, poorly reactive pupils, bilateral ptosis, oculomotor palsies, and facial weakness. The diagnosis is confirmed by identification of *Clostridium botulinum* toxin (usually type A or B) in the feces or isolation of the organism in stool culture, which is less sensitive. Management of infant botulism is strictly supportive.

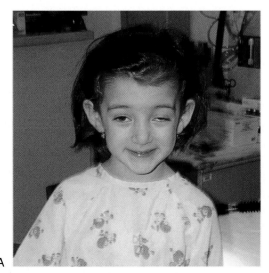 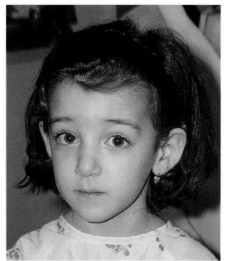

FIG. 14.10. This young girl has myasthenia gravis manifested by bilateral ptosis **(A)**. After a dose of edrophonium (Tensilon) **(B)**, her muscular function has returned.

DISORDERS OF BALANCE

Acute Cerebellar Ataxia

The child develops acute truncal unsteadiness with a variable degree of distal motor difficulty, such as tremor and dysmetria. Dysarthria and nystagmus are variably present. Some children have nausea and vomiting, presumably caused by vertigo. Headache is rare. When acute ataxia follows varicella in a child with no other neurologic findings, the diagnosis may be made on clinical grounds. In atypical cases, CT or MRI may be necessary to rule out a cerebellar mass. LP is not usually necessary in typical cases; if performed, it reveals a mild CSF pleocytosis in approximately one-half of the cases. Treatment is supportive.

Benign Paroxysmal Vertigo

Benign paroxysmal vertigo is an illness that affects children primarily between 1 and 4 years of age, although it can occur any time during the first decade. It manifests with acute episodes of dizziness and imbalance, lasting seconds to minutes. Between episodes, the child is asymptomatic. During the spell, the child characteristically becomes frightened and pale but does not lose consciousness. He or she may have associated nausea, vomiting, or visual disturbance. The physical examination is usually normal except for nystagmus, which may be present. As the name suggests, the course of benign paroxysmal vertigo is self-limiting and benign, and treatment is supportive.

MOVEMENT DISORDERS

Acute Dystonia

Dystonia is marked by involuntary, sustained muscle contractions, typically of the neck and trunk that cause twisting movements and abnormal postures. In generalized dystonia, the head is usually deviated to the side, and there is grimacing of the face. Acute dystonia in children is nearly always the result of exposure to an antidopaminergic agent such as a neuroleptic, or antiemetic. Chronic dystonias are rare but may be seen as isolated disorders or as a manifestation of cerebral palsy. Dystonia must be differentiated from torticollis, an abnormal tilt of the head and neck usually resulting from irritation or spasm of the sternocleidomastoid muscle. Another clinically similar condition is Sandifer syndrome, which involves intermittent arching of the back and neck, observed in infants with gastroesophageal reflux. Acute dystonia resulting from exposure to antidopaminergic drugs is treated with 1 mg/kg diphenhydramine per dose intravenously, orally, or intramuscularly or 1 to 2 mg benztropine (Cogentin) per dose intramuscularly. Because the half-life of many of the precipitating agents is fairly long, treatment should be continued for 24 to 48 hours.

DISORDERS OF CRANIAL NERVE FUNCTION

Optic Neuritis

On examination, decreased visual acuity and decreased color vision are associated with a relative afferent pupillary deficit to light and a central scotoma in the affected eye. The relative afferent pupil defect is demonstrated by the swinging flashlight maneuver, during which the pupil of the affected eye constricts briskly when light is shone into the contralateral eye (the consensual light reflex) and dilates when light is immediately shone into the affected eye. With bilateral disease, the change in pupillary reflexes may not be apparent. Funduscopic examination discloses a hyperemic, swollen optic disk; in the rare cases of retrobulbar optic neuritis, funduscopic examination is normal. If any doubt of increased ICP persists, the patient should undergo evaluation by CT or MRI of the brain and, if normal, CSF analysis. In optic neuritis, the opening pressure is normal, but there may be a mild lymphocytic pleocytosis or elevated CSF protein. Treatment with high-dose systemic corticosteroids, such as 2 mg/kg prednisone per day orally for 7 to 10 days, has not been shown to improve the ultimate prognosis but may result in a slightly faster resolution of symptoms.

Facial Nerve Palsy

Clinical Manifestations

Facial weakness may be partial or complete. On the affected side, there is flattening of the nasolabial fold at rest (Fig. 14.11), and the child has difficulty closing the eye or raising the corner of the mouth to smile. In many cases, pain localized to the ear precedes the paralysis. With upper motor neuron involvement, there will be some residual capacity to furrow the brow because of crossed innervation, whereas the entire face is involved with peripheral disease. There may be bilateral involvement in Lyme disease, in contrast to Bell palsy, which is always unilateral. In children with facial nerve palsy caused by Lyme disease, other manifestations, such as erythema migrans, are rarely seen (27% in one series). Thus, even in the absence of other findings, serologic evidence of systemic Lyme infection should be sought in all children with isolated seventh nerve paresis in endemic areas. An LP should be performed if there is other evidence of meningoencephalitis such as headache; however, the need for LP in a child at risk of Lyme disease with isolated facial nerve palsy is controversial. Other associated neurologic abnormalities, specifically in the other cranial nerves, necessitate further evaluation, including CT or MRI.

Management

Some authors recommend a course of 2 mg/kg prednisone per day in two divided doses for 7 to 10 days if the patient is seen within the first 24 to 48 hours of disease onset. One study suggests that acyclovir may be of benefit. During the

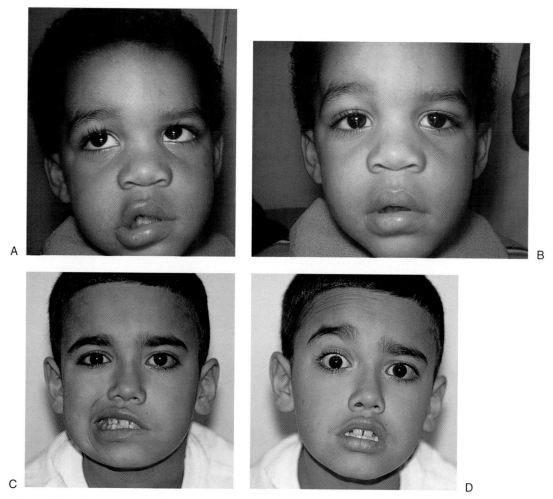

FIG. 14.11. Two patients with facial palsy. The defect appears more obvious when the patient smiles or grimaces **(A, C)** compared with baseline **(B, D)**.

recovery period, special care should be taken to protect the cornea by the instillation of bland ointments (e.g., Lacrilube). Children with clinical or serologic evidence of Lyme disease–associated facial nerve palsy should be treated with oral antibiotics (amoxicillin, tetracycline, or erythromycin) for 21 to 28 days. The effectiveness of steroids in such patients has not been evaluated. Parenteral antibiotic treatment is recommended for children who also have evidence of meningitis.

SHUNT INFECTION

Approximately 70% of all shunt infections occur within 2 months of surgery. In the postoperative period, erythema and warmth along the course of the shunt are highly predictive of early wound infection. Later, signs of indolent infection are often variable and nonspecific. Signs of shunt malfunction occur commonly. The adage "an infected shunt is an obstructed shunt" is well remembered. Although fever raises concern for shunt infection, documented shunt infections

were associated with fever in only 42% of patients in one series. Meningeal signs have been reported in only approximately 33% of patients. Abdominal symptoms from an associated peritonitis may predominate in cases of pseudocyst formation with distal obstruction.

Management

A definite diagnosis of shunt infection is made by tapping the shunt and obtaining a CSF specimen. A definite, although small, rate of infection occurs as a result of a tap, and in a patient with the potential for bacteremia, the blood carried into the shunt reservoir on the tip of the needle may be contaminated and produce a shunt infection. Thus, a shunt tap is not indicated in all children with a shunt who present with fever. Fever without localizing signs in those patients in whom the current shunt was placed or revised many months to years previously and who lack signs and symptoms of shunt malfunction may be appropriately managed with close follow-up and observation without shunt tap.

SUGGESTED READINGS

Adour KK, Ruboyianes JM, Von Doersten PG, et al. Bell's palsy treatment with acyclovir and prednisone compared with prednisone alone: a double-blind, randomized, controlled trial. *Ann Otol Rhinol Laryngol* 1996;105:371–378.

Al Deeb SM, Yaqub BA, Bruyn GW, et al. Acute transverse myelitis: a localized form of postinfectious encephalomyelitis. *Brain* 1997;120:1115–1122.

Albisetti M, Schaer G, Good M, et al. Diagnostic value of cerebrospinal fluid examination in children with peripheral facial palsy and suspected Lyme borreliosis. *Neurology* 1997;49:817–824.

American Heart Association Science Advisory and Coordinating Committee. Guidelines for thrombolytic therapy for acute stroke: a supplement to the guidelines for the management of patients with acute ischemic stroke. *Circulation* 1996;94:1167–1174.

Burton LJ, Quinn B, Pratt-Chaney JL, et al. Headache etiology in a pediatric emergency department. *Pediatr Emerg Care* 1997;13:1–4.

Camfield PR, Camfield CS. Management and treatment of febrile seizures. *Curr Probl Pediatr* 1997;27:6–13.

Chamberlain JM, Altieri MA, Futterman C, et al. A prospective, randomized study comparing intramuscular midazolam with intravenous diazepam for the treatment of seizures in children. *Pediatr Emerg Care* 1997;13:92–94.

Dunn DW. Status epilepticus in infancy and childhood. *Neurol Clin North Am* 1990;8:647–658.

Ferrera PC, Curran CB, Swanson H. Etiology of pediatric ischemic stroke. *Am J Emerg Med* 1997;15:671–679.

Fisher M, Bogousslavsky J. Further evolution toward effective therapy for acute ischemic stroke. *JAMA* 1998;279:1298–1303.

Gurses N, Uysal S, Cetinkaya F, et al. Intravenous immunoglobulin treatment in children with Guillain-Barré syndrome. *Scand J Infect Dis* 1995;27:241–243.

Hamalainen ML, Hoppu K, Santvuori P. Sumatriptan for migraine attacks in children: a randomized placebo-controlled study. *Neurology* 1997;48:1100–1103.

Hamalainen ML, Hoppu K, Valkeila E, et al. Ibuprofen or acetaminophen for the acute treatment of migraine in children: a double-blind, randomized, placebo-controlled crossover study. *Neurology* 1997;48:103–107.

Hesketh E, Eden OB, Gattamaneni HR, et al. Spinal cord compression: do we miss it? *Acta Paediatr* 1998;87:452–454.

Honig P, Charney E. Children with brain tumor headaches: distinguishing features. *Am J Dis Child* 1982;136:121–124.

Hyden D, Roberg M, Forsberg P, et al. Acute "idiopathic" peripheral facial palsy: clinical, serological, and cerebrospinal fluid findings and effects of corticosteroids. *Am J Otolaryngol* 1993;14:179–186.

Iskandar BJ, McLaughlin C, Mapstone TB, et al. Pitfalls in the diagnosis of ventricular shunt dysfunction: radiology reports and ventricular size. *Pediatrics* 1998;101:1031–1036.

Jacobsen FS, Sullivan B. Spinal epidural abscesses in children. *Orthopedics* 1994;17:1131–1138.

Jones HR. Childhood Guillain-Barré syndrome: clinical presentation, diagnosis, and therapy. *J Child Neurol* 1996;11:4–12.

Korinthenberg R, Monting JS. Natural history and treatment effects in Guillain-Barré syndrome: a multicentre study. *Arch Dis Child* 1996;74:281–287.

Madikians A, Conway EE. Cerebrospinal fluid shunt problems in pediatric patients. *Pediatr Ann* 1997;26:613–620.

Nicolaides P, Appleton RE. Stroke in children. *Dev Med Child Neurol* 1996;38:172–180.

Nypaver MM, Reynolds SL, Tanz RR, et al. Emergency department laboratory evaluation of children with seizures: dogma or dilemma. *Pediatr Emerg Care* 1992;8:13–16.

Provisional Committee on Quality Improvement, Subcommittee on Febrile Seizures. Practice parameter: the neurodiagnostic evaluation of the child with a first simple febrile seizure. *Pediatrics* 1996;97:769–775.

Reerink JD, Peters AC, Verloove-Vanhorick SP, et al. Paroxysmal phenomena in the first two years of life. *Dev Med Child Neurol* 1995;37:1094–1100.

Schreiner M, Field E, Ruddy R. Infant botulism: a review of 12 years' experience at the Children's Hospital of Philadelphia. *Pediatrics* 1991;87:159–165.

Selbst SM, Clancy R. Pseudoseizures in the emergency department. *Pediatr Emerg Care* 1996;12:185–188.

Shuper A, Mimouni M. Problems of differentiation between epilepsy and non-epileptic paroxysmal events in the first year of life. *Arch Dis Child* 1995;73:342–344.

Welborn CA. Pediatric migraine. *Emerg Med Clin North Am* 1997;15:625–636.

Whitley RJ. Viral encephalitis. *N Engl J Med* 1990;323:242–247.

Williams JR. Optic neuritis in a child. *Pediatr Emerg Care* 1996;12:210–212.

Working Group on Status Epilepticus. Treatment of convulsive status epilepticus. *JAMA* 1993;270:854–859.

CHAPTER 15

Ophthalmic and Otolaryngologic Emergencies

Editor: Marc N. Baskin

OPHTHALMIC EMERGENCIES

Periorbital and Orbital Cellulitis

The primary concern when making the diagnosis of periorbital cellulitis (preseptal cellulitis) is to rule out the possibility of orbital cellulitis. The cardinal signs of orbital cellulitis include decreased eye movement, pain with eye movements, proptosis, and decreased vision (Figs. 15.1 and 15.2). Both orbital and periorbital infection may be associated with fever, pain, swollen eyelids, and red eye. If orbital cellulitis is suspected, computed tomography (CT) scanning of the orbit is indicated. Ophthalmology consultation is indicated in all cases of orbital cellulitis. Surgical intervention may be required. Otorhinolaryngology consultation should also be considered when orbital cellulitis is secondary to contiguous sinus infection.

One must rule out other conditions that can simulate a periorbital cellulitis. Insect bites and allergic reactions can cause dramatic acute periorbital swelling. However, these conditions are not usually associated with fever. Often, close inspection of the skin can localize the site of an insect bite. Allergic swelling is often bilateral, whereas periorbital cellulitis is rarely bilateral (Fig. 15.3). Underlying sinusitis can also cause periorbital swelling. Severe conjunctivitis, especially adenoviral infection and neonatal gonorrhea conjunctivitis, can also result in significant lid swelling.

A dacryocele (Fig. 15.4) or infected dermoid cyst (Fig. 15.5) may be confused with other periorbital infections.

Management

The appropriate route of antibiotic administration in periorbital cellulitis is controversial. In otherwise well children who are beyond infancy and have mild periorbital cellulitis and no systemic signs or symptoms, particularly when the cause of the cellulitis is believed to be a skin wound, intramuscular and/or oral antibiotics may be tried. The patient should be examined again within 24 to 48 hours, at which time improvement should be documented. If no improve-

ment occurs, the patient should then be admitted for intravenous (IV) antibiotics. Periorbital cellulitis is a potentially fatal disease because complications such as meningitis may develop if inadequately treated. All cases of orbital cellulitis must be treated with IV antibiotics.

The choice of antibiotics should reflect the probable causative organism and is discussed in Chapter 11 (Infectious Disease Emergencies). Before starting IV antibiotics, a blood culture should be taken. Other systemic cultures (e.g., cerebrospinal fluid) may be indicated if signs of systemic toxicity are present. Percutaneous aspiration from the area of cellulitis is not recommended. Conjunctival cultures do not identify the causative agent of the cellulitis.

Acute Hordeolum

Acute red localized eyelid masses may be due to external or internal hordeolum. If the glands of Zeis, adjacent to the eyelid follicles, are involved, the abscess is often small, points at the lid margin (Fig. 15.6), and is called external hordeolum or a stye. If the meibomian glands, within the tarsal plate are involved, the abscess is often larger, may point out through the skin (Fig. 15.7) or inward to the conjunctival surface, and is called internal hordeolum. Internal hordeolum may enter a chronic phase in which there is a nontender, mobile, pea-sized nodule within the body of the eyelid often termed a chalazion.

Management

The treatment for both types of hordeolum is similar. Eyelash scrubs with baby shampoo applied to a washcloth while the eyelids are closed once or twice daily are helpful in mechanically establishing drainage. Warm compresses are also useful. Optimally, warm compresses should be applied four times daily for 10 to 20 minutes at each sitting. Antibiotics probably play a minimal role in the treatment of styes and chalazions. If desired, a topical antibiotic ointment (Table 15.1) can be given twice daily. Chronic chalazions may require excision for cosmetic reasons.

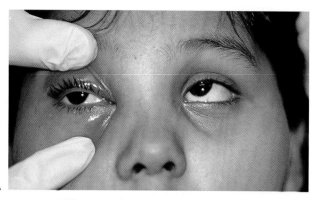 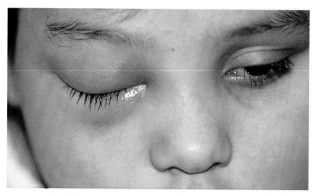

FIG. 15.1. Orbital cellulitis. This 9-year-old girl presented with 2 days of eye pain and swelling. **A:** The patient is attempting to look upward and demonstrates her impaired extraocular movements. **B:** Proptosis and severe upper lid edema are shown.

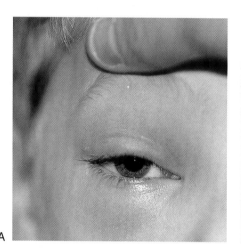 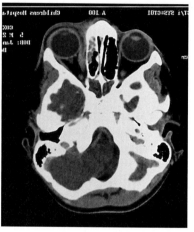

FIG. 15.2. Orbital cellulitis involving the medial rectus muscle. This 5-year-old boy presented with 2 days of fever and eye pain. **A:** When examined, he cried and refused to look to his right. **B:** Computed tomography shows thickening of the left medial rectus muscle and a small subperiosteal fluid collection as well as adjacent sinus disease.

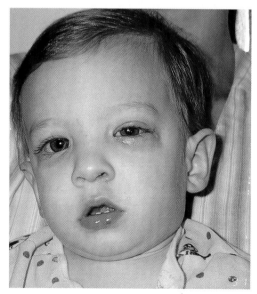

FIG. 15.3. Allergic conjunctivitis. This infant had bilateral lid swelling and rubbing at his eyes without fever or purulent discharge. He improved with oral antihistamines.

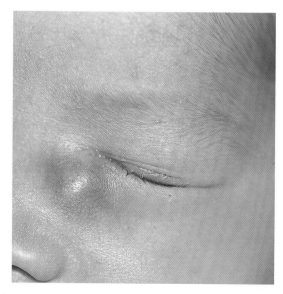

FIG. 15.4. Dacryocele. A 7-day-old neonate with lid swelling for 2 days.

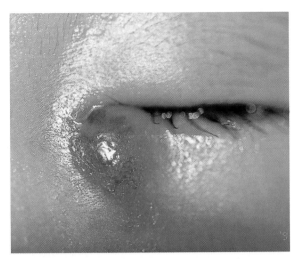

FIG. 15.5. Dermoid cyst abscess. A 10-month-old child presented with 1 week of lid swelling without fever. The swollen area is rather medial for dacryocystitis, although it might be consistent with a lacrimal sac abscess. In this case, pathology was consistent with an infected dermoid cyst.

Chemical Injury

When the child has a clear history of a noxious substance coming in contact with the ocular surface, it is important to determine whether this substance is an acid or an alkali. Alkali injuries tend to be much more severe. It is also important to determine whether particulate matter may have been deposited on the ocular surface. Smoke can also cause chemical conjunctivitis.

Management

Chemical injury to the eyeball is a true ocular emergency. Any patient with sufficient history should be immediately placed in the supine position and ocular lavage started. Although a drop of topical anesthetic can make this procedure more comfortable, the physician should not wait for this

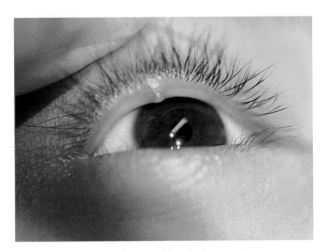

FIG. 15.6. External hordeolum or stye.

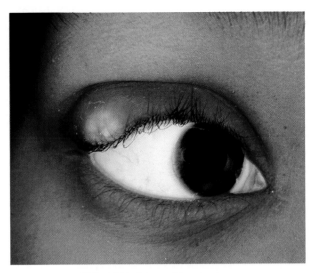

FIG. 15.7. Internal hordeolum.

to become available if it is not immediately handy. If a Desmarres retractor or paper clip is readily available, this may be used to help obtain optimal exposure of the ocular surface. Virtually any IV solution can be used for ocular lavage, although normal saline solution or Ringer lactate is perhaps preferable. A standard IV bag and tubing set is used without a needle on the end. The solution is allowed to flow, with the system at its maximal flow rate, across the surface

TABLE 15.1. *Pediatric emergency department ophthalmic drug guidelines*

Use	Avoid
Dilating drops	Dilating drops
2.5% phenylephrine	Scopolamine
1% tropicamide	Atropine
1% cyclopentolate	Homatropine
	2% cyclopentolate
Antibiotics	Antibiotics
Bacitracin	Neomycin
Erythromycin	Sulfacetamide
Polysporin	Aminoglycosides
Polytrim (trimethoprim/	(except neonate)
polymyxin B)	Quinolones
Lubricants	
Artificial tears/ointment	
Vasoconstrictors/antihistamines	
Naphcon-A, Vasocon-A	
Antiinflammatory agents	
0.5% ketorolac tromethamine	
(Acular)	
Mast-cell stabilizers	
0.1% lodoxamide (Alomide)	
Diagnostic agents	
Topical fluorescein	
Anesthetic agents	
Proparacaine, tetracaine	Cocaine
Avoid all antivirals, miotics, steroids[a], and antiglaucoma agents	

[a] Including steroid-containing preparations, such as combination antibiotic-steroids.

TABLE 15.2. *Differential Diagnosis of Conjunctivitis*

	Bacterial	Viral (nonherpes)	Herpetic	Chlamydial	Allergic
Discharge—purulent	+++	+/−	−	+/−	−
Discharge—clear	−	+++	+++	+/−	+++
Swollen lids	+++	+ to +++	+ to +++	+	+ to +++
Acute onset	++	++	+++	Chronic	Usually
Red eye	+++	+ to +++	Focally or diffuse ++	++	++
Cornea-staining fluorescein	Nonspecific	Nonspecific	Dendrite	−	−
White cornea infiltrates	−	−	Possible	Multiple peripheral	−
Unilateral or bilateral	Uni/bi	Uni/bi	Uni	Usually bi	Usually bi
Contact history	+	+++	−	?STD	−
Preauricular node	++	+++	−	+/−	−
Other associations	Otitis media? *(H influenzae)*	Otitis media? Malaise, fever, pharyngitis	Prior or current skin lesions Recurrent	Genital discharge	Chemosis

STD, sexually transmitted disease symptoms or contact.
Adapted from Levin AV. Ophthalmology. In: Kropt SP, ed. *The HSC handbook of pediatrics,* 9th ed. Toronto: Mosby, 1997.

of the open eye medially to laterally. Lavage should be continued until the involved eye(s) has received either 2 L of fluid or until approximately 20 minutes has elapsed. Lavage should be continued with the lid everted so that the conjunctiva under the upper lid may also be cleansed. Mechanical debridement should be limited to the removal of visible particles from the ocular surface.

The ophthalmologist should be notified while lavage is ongoing. In cases of minor exposure to substances that are clearly not alkaline or strongly acidic and when the eye is not injected, an ophthalmology consultation may be deferred. However, the physician must be cautious about the absence of conjunctival injection because alkali burns can cause blanching of the conjunctiva, which is a poor prognostic sign.

Conjunctivitis

Table 15.2 is designed to help diagnose the causes of conjunctivitis. Neonates presenting in the first 3 days of life can have a chemical conjunctivitis caused by silver nitrate used for ocular prophylaxis perinatally. Most hospitals have now discontinued this practice and are using erythromycin ointment. However, this is not completely effective in eliminating subsequent gonorrheal or chlamydial conjunctivitis in the neonatal period. These two forms of conjunctivitis can be difficult to distinguish clinically. Each can present as either a mild purulent form or chronic purulent conjunctivitis. A dramatically hyperacute conjunctivitis with significant lid swelling and copious purulent ocular discharge is more characteristic of gonorrhea. In view of the risk of spontaneous corneal perforation associated with gonorrheal conjunctivitis, infants should be presumed to have this infection until proven otherwise. Immediate Gram stain should be performed looking for Gram-negative diplococci. If present, treatment for gonorrheal conjunctivitis should be started

while awaiting culture results. *Chlamydia* studies may be useful as well.

In children beyond the neonatal period, a wide range of organisms, both viral and bacterial, as well as *Chlamydia*, can cause conjunctivitis. Clinically, these entities may appear to be similar. In general, purulence is more characteristic of bacterial infections, whereas clear serous discharge is more characteristic of viral infection. Both viral and bacterial conjunctivitis may be unilateral or bilateral. Dramatic lid swelling and intense conjunctival injection, associated with preauricular adenopathy; mucoid or serous discharge; and perhaps an uncomfortable, foreign body sensation that affects one eye followed closely by the other, are strongly suggestive of epidemic keratoconjunctivitis secondary to adenovirus. This fulminant viral infection is easy to recognize (Fig. 15.8). Although most cases of conjunctivitis have a

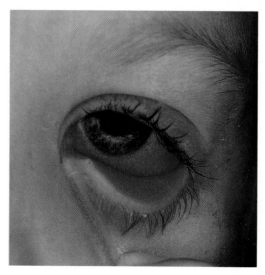

FIG. 15.8. Epidemic keratoconjunctivitis.

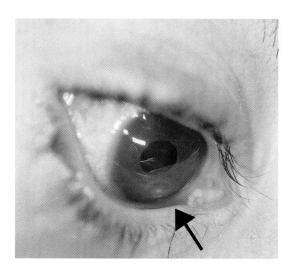

FIG. 15.9. Corneal ulcer and hypophion (*arrow*).

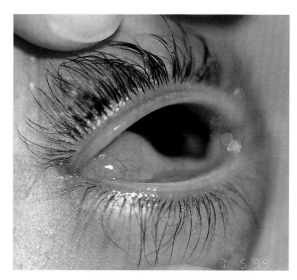

FIG. 15.11. Allergic conjunctivitis with chemosis. Note the swollen conjunctiva extending up to the border of the cornea.

benign course, corneal ulcers (Fig. 15.9) or a hypophion may develop if untreated.

Allergic conjunctivitis is usually an acute bilateral conjunctival infection (Fig. 15.10) associated with swollen lids, itching, tearing and occasionally swelling of the conjunctiva (chemosis) (Fig. 15.11).

Nasolacrimal duct obstruction is often confused with conjunctivitis because discharge may be present and swelling or redness of the adjacent nasal bridge may be absent. However, the conjunctiva is rarely inflamed, indicating the absence of true conjunctivitis.

Management

If the Gram stain demonstrates Gram-negative diplococci, neonatal purulent conjunctivitis should be treated as gonor-

rheal conjunctivitis, pending the results of cultures. The patient should be admitted for antibiotic therapy with 25 to 50 mg/kg ceftriaxone (maximum, 125 mg) intramuscularly or intravenously as a single dose. Ophthalmology consultation is indicated. Saline ocular lavage on an hourly basis may be helpful in decreasing the amount of organisms having access to the cornea. If *Chlamydia* is laboratory proven, then the child must receive a 14-day course of oral erythromycin as well. This is necessary to eradicate carriage of *Chlamydia* in the nasopharynx, which can subsequently lead to pneumonia. The parents should be tested.

Any of the local antibiotics suggested in Table 15.1 would be appropriate for empiric coverage in treating a presumed bacterial conjunctivitis other than gonococcal while awaiting culture results.

If the patient clearly has viral conjunctivitis, antibiotic treatment is probably not needed. Rather, these patients are best soothed with cool compresses and artificial tear preparations.

Allergic conjunctivitis is also helped by topical lubricants and cool compresses. The combination vasoconstrictor/antihistamine preparations, antiinflammatory agents, and mast-cell stabilizers listed in Table 15.1 may also be prescribed.

Any patient with a history of herpetic ocular infection and any patient who wears contact lenses and has conjunctivitis should be referred immediately for ophthalmology consultation. Herpetic corneal infection is usually painful. Patients may or may not have a history of skin lesions. Patients with herpes zoster involving the ophthalmic branch of the trigeminal nerve have pain and skin lesions of the forehead, periorbital area, and nose (Fig. 15.12) and require immediate ophthalmology consultation. Characteristic fluorescein dendritic staining patterns can be seen on the cornea or conjunctiva (Fig. 15.13). Without appropriate antiviral therapy, the infection may extend to the cornea, causing permanent damage. Skin lesions on the lids without

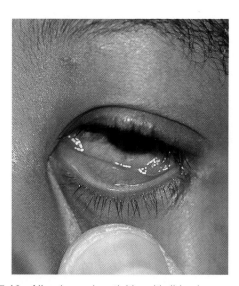

FIG. 15.10. Allergic conjunctivitis with lid edema and conjunctival infection.

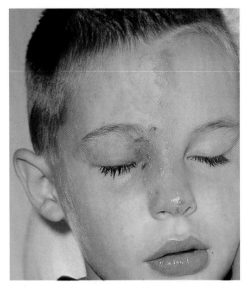

FIG. 15.12. Herpes zoster involving the ophthalmic branch of the trigeminal nerve. The patient presented with 6 days of eye pain and rash that included vesicles on the nose.

conjunctival infection does not require ophthalmology consultation (Fig. 15.14).

Acquired Glaucoma

Although a painful red eye is more commonly caused by a corneal abrasion, severe conjunctivitis (especially herpetic), foreign body, uveitis, or endophthalmitis, the acute onset of a severely painful red eye associated with visual impairment may rarely be due to acquired glaucoma (Fig. 15.15). An ophthalmologic consultation should be obtained.

OTOLARYNGOLOGIC EMERGENCIES

Ear

The tympanic membrane should be evaluated for its appearance, but the examination should not stop there. Part of the

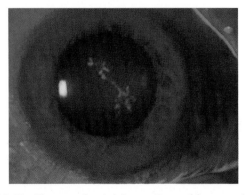

FIG. 15.13. Fluorescein staining pattern of herpes simplex virus corneal infection. The eye is illuminated with blue light to demonstrate the yellow-green branching staining pattern of herpetic dendrite.

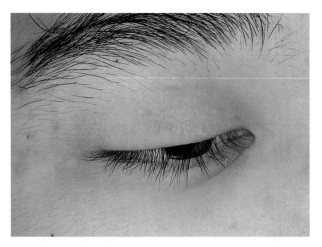

FIG. 15.14. Herpes simplex lesions on upper lid.

middle ear contents can often be seen through a translucent eardrum. Mobility should be assessed with the pneumatic otoscope.

The ear of a neonate requires special attention to perform an adequate otologic examination. The ear canal itself is narrow and collapsible. The neonate's tympanic membrane lies at a more oblique angle to the ear canal (compared with older children) and may make recognition of the tympanic membrane and its landmarks more difficult.

Infections

Acute otitis media and otitis externa are discussed in Chapter 11 (Infectious Disease Emergencies).

Pinna

The pinna may become infected in a fashion similar to skin surfaces anywhere else on the body. If the posterior aspect of

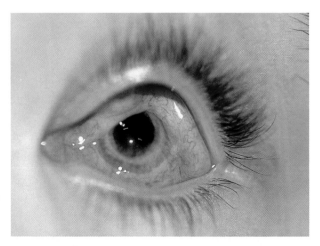

FIG. 15.15. This 17-year-old boy had acute onset of severe eye pain with visual impairment. Note the severe chemosis and conjunctival injection. His globe was very tender to palpation, and his intraocular pressure was elevated to 55 mm Hg.

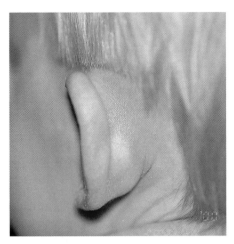

FIG. 15.16. Cellulitis of the pinna. A 19-month-old child with a red, swollen, anteriorly displaced pinna after 10 days of treatment with amoxicillin. The posterior aspect of his pinna was erythematous, but his mastoid process was nontender and his tympanic membrane was normal. Computed tomography demonstrated normal mastoid air cells, and his cellulitis responded to antistaphylococcal antibiotics.

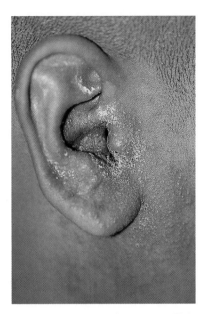

FIG. 15.18. Contact dermatitis of the pinna. This 11-year-old child was referred for worsening ear rash after 2 weeks of "eardrops." The child said the rash was pruritic, and the "eardrops" contained neomycin, an antibiotic commonly implicated in allergic reactions.

the pinna is involved, the pinna may be displaced anteriorly (Fig. 15.16) and mastoiditis may be suspected. In mastoiditis, the tympanic membrane should appear infected, whereas with pinna cellulitis, the tympanic membrane should be normal. CT will demonstrate erosion and infection of the mastoid air cells in mastoiditis.

The pinna is a common site for manifestations of allergic reactions due to bites (Fig. 15.17) or contact with allergens (Fig. 15.18).

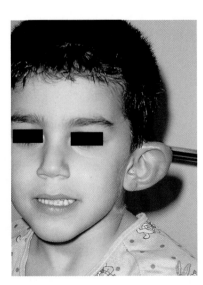

FIG. 15.17. Allergic reaction. This red displaced pinna was warm but nontender, and the tympanic membrane was normal. A small punctum was noted, and the patient responded to antihistamines.

Sudden Hearing Loss

Sudden hearing loss is not a common complaint in the emergency department, but it requires prompt attention, especially if the loss is determined to be sensorineural. Sudden conductive losses almost never occur without a known antecedent event such as head trauma, ear infection, or wax occlusion of the ear canal. History and otoscopy can usually establish the cause of the conductive hearing loss. However, the cause of sudden sensorineural hearing loss is obscure when the history is unrevealing and otoscopy is normal. Tuning fork testing helps to confirm the presence of a sensorineural hearing loss.

Sudden sensorineural hearing loss that occurs after an airplane trip, scuba diving, straining, or head trauma is highly suggestive of a perilymph fistula. A perilymph fistula occurs when inner ear fluid leaks out into the middle ear through a rupture in the round window or stapes footplate (oval window). The leaking fluid causes a fluctuating sensorineural loss and vertigo. Urgent surgical exploration of the middle ear is required for repair.

Sudden sensorineural deafness may occur without a history suggestive of a fistula and without otoscopic abnormalities. This is often secondary to a viral infection of the cochlear labyrinth. Measles, mumps, and cytomegalic viral illnesses are common causes of sudden sensorineural deafness. There may be no systemic symptoms or signs of such a viral infection. These patients may have partial or complete recovery of hearing over several weeks. There is no proven effective treatment for sudden hearing loss. Aspirin has been recommended (in older children) to decrease platelet aggregation and to maintain patency of the cochlear blood vessels, and corticosteroids have been recommended by some authors. Antivertigo medications may be prescribed for patients experiencing dizziness. All patients with a sudden sensorineural hearing loss should be referred to an otolaryngologist.

Vertigo

Sudden vertigo is a disturbing and sometimes confusing symptom. Vertigo may follow dysfunction of any part of the vestibular system from the labyrinth to the vestibular cortex.

Vertigo may be associated with a number of conditions affecting the middle ear:

1. Serous labyrinthitis may develop in a child with otitis media effusion, acute otitis media, or chronic otitis media. Pressure and infection in the middle ear may cause inner ear inflammation and vestibular dysfunction. The conductive hearing loss and dizziness resolve when the middle ear pressure is normalized or the inflammation subsides.
2. Suppurative labyrinthitis may occur when bacteria invade the inner ear. Severe vertigo and a profound sensorineural hearing loss result.
3. When a cholesteatoma arises in association with chronic otitis media, it may invade the bony wall of the labyrinth. Pneumatic otoscopy may produce the sensation of vertigo by transmitting the pressure directly to the inner ear.
4. A common cause of sudden vertigo is vestibular neuronitis. The origin of this entity is uncertain, and the vertigo resolves spontaneously over several weeks. There are no accompanying signs or symptoms.
5. Trauma can be associated with vertigo in several ways. Perilymph fistulae, which occur most often after barotrauma, blunt head trauma, or straining, produce vertigo that fluctuates in severity. However, head trauma may also cause labyrinthine concussion or hemorrhage (hemorrhagic labyrinthitis), resulting in vertigo.
6. Measles and mumps may also infect the inner ear and cause vertigo.
7. Ménière disease is rare in children. Its origin is unknown. The symptoms are intermittent vertigo, tinnitus, and fluctuating hearing.
8. Miscellaneous causes of sudden vertigo in children include benign paroxysmal vertigo of childhood and retrolabyrinthine lesions such as tumors, demyelinating diseases, and temporal lobe seizures.

Neoplasms

Neoplasms of the external ear are as varied as the tissue types of the auricle and are not difficult to diagnose because they are so visible. Neoplasms of the middle and inner ear are rare but are often missed until they are far advanced. External canal and middle ear tumors are most often brought to the physician's attention because of painful secondary infection that does not respond to treatment with antibiotics. The ex-

aminer may overlook a tumor, assuming that it is granulation tissue caused by an infection. If an ear infection does not respond to appropriate treatment or is associated with any abnormal-appearing tissue, a tumor should be suspected; otolaryngologic consultation should be made to obtain a biopsy specimen of the abnormal tissue.

Facial Nerve Paralysis

Facial nerve paralysis is a frightening occurrence in children. Bell palsy (idiopathic facial paralysis) is the most common cause of facial paralysis (see Chapter 14, Neurologic and Neurosurgical Emergencies, for management). Facial paralysis secondary to acute otitis media requires a course of systemic antibiotics (24 to 48 hours of IV followed by oral) and an urgent wide-field myringotomy for drainage. Neoplasms of the middle ear and parotid area can also present with facial nerve paralysis.

NOSE AND PARANASAL SINUSES

Infections

Infections of the nose and paranasal sinuses are discussed in Chapter 11 (Infectious Disease Emergencies).

Complications of acute sinusitis, such as orbital cellulitis, require otolaryngologic consultation and possible operative intervention.

Chronic Nasal Obstruction

Obstruction to the normal passage of air can occur with a variety of conditions and gives the sensation of a blocked or stuffy nose. However, prolonged blockage is not physiologic, and the physician should search for a cause.

A careful examination of the nasal cavities and pharynx is necessary to determine the cause of the obstruction. Septal deviation, turbinate hypertrophy related to allergy and/or infection, or a nasal polyp (Fig. 15.19) are common causes. Nasal polyps are gray, unlike the pink turbinate tissue. Cystic fibrosis may be the most common cause of nasal polyps, and all patients should be tested, even those without respiratory symptoms. Adenoid hypertrophy, nasopharyngeal tumor (lymphoma, rhabdomyosarcoma), and choanal

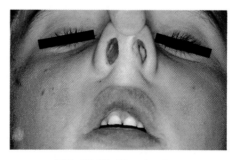

FIG. 15.19. Nasal polyp.

atresia (unilateral or bilateral) can all present with nasal obstruction. Flexible fiberoptic examination and radiographs (usually CT scan) of the nose and nasopharynx may be useful in the evaluation of the blocked nasal airway. If the source of the obstruction is not apparent after these maneuvers, referral should be made to an otolaryngologist to perform a complete examination of the nose and nasopharynx.

Epistaxis

Epistaxis is relatively common in children and may cause significant anxiety in both the child and the parent. The most common cause of epistaxis is the mucosal maceration caused by upper respirator illnesses and nose picking. The usual site of bleeding is the anterior nasal septum (Kiesselbach area).

A complete history is an important step in the proper management of epistaxis. Site of bleeding (one or both sides of the nose), frequency, bleeding from other places, history of trauma, and family history of bleeding are all important factors. Figure 15.20 presents an algorithm for the management of epistaxis. A careful examination of the nose should be performed to identify the site and cause of the bleeding. Good lighting, suction, and material for cauterization and packing should be readily available. Topical vasoconstrictors, such as 0.25% phenylephrine or 0.05% oxymetazoline on a cotton pledget, can be placed in the nose to shrink the nasal mucosa, allowing better visualization of the nasal cavity; vasoconstrictors may slow or even stop the bleeding. Simple pressure by squeezing the nostrils together is usually sufficient to stop most epistaxis. Occasionally, a roll of cotton placed under the upper lip will stop bleeding by compression of the labial artery. If pressure is not successful, cauterization with silver nitrate sticks or packing of the nose is performed. Absorbable packing such as oxycellulose (Surgicel) or gelatin (Gelfoam) is usually adequate for most epistaxis and has the advantage of not requiring removal.

Severe or recurrent episodes of epistaxis require the assistance of an otolaryngologist in their diagnosis and management. Epistaxis that does not stop with simple pressure or oxycellulose or gelatin packing may require a more substantial anterior nasal pack of petroleum jelly–impregnated gauze. A posterior nasal pack (using gauze or a Foley catheter) or commercial balloon epistaxis pack may be necessary in managing severe epistaxis that originates in the posterior nasal cavity or nasopharynx.

If the epistaxis recurs despite the above treatment, an otolaryngologist should be consulted to look for other causes for the epistaxis. Nasal septal perforation, sinusitis, tumor (nasal, nasopharyngeal, or sinus), Rendu–Osler–Weber disease (hereditary hemorrhagic telangiectasia), and nasal foreign body can all present with epistaxis. Blood dyscrasias, such as hemophilia, idiopathic thrombocytopenia purpura, von Willebrand disease, and those hematologic conditions associated with leukemia or the administration of chemotherapeutic agents, may lead to severe epistaxis.

Neoplasms

Neoplasms of the nose and sinuses are uncommon in children. They may present as mass lesions or as chronic/recurrent rhinosinusitis. When a neoplasm is suspected, the child should be referred to an otolaryngologist.

Hemangiomas are the most common benign neoplasms of the head and neck in children and often occur on the skin near or on the nose. Because hemangiomas often go through a period of rapid growth for the first 12 to 18 months of life before they begin to involute, a period of observation is recommended before corticosteroids or surgical excision is considered. Recurrent bleeding, thrombocytopenia, skin breakdown, obstruction to vision, respiratory distress, and cardiac failure are some indications for early intervention. Papillomas are viral-induced verrucous growths that are the most common neoplasms of the aerodigestive tract. When they appear in the nose, they are most often found on the nasal septum.

ORAL CAVITY, PHARYNX, AND ESOPHAGUS

Infections of the oral cavity and pharynx are discussed in Chapter 11 (Infectious Disease Emergencies).

Oral Cavity

A retention cyst or ranula of the sublingual salivary duct can present at any age as a large swelling in the floor of the mouth (Fig. 15.21) The cyst will need excision, and the duct must be exteriorized. Infections of congenital lesions like cystic hygromas of the oral cavity may cause mouth pain and drooling as well (Fig. 15.22). Sialolithiasis is rare in childhood, usually involving the submandibular glands and ducts. The patients present with pain, especially just before meals. The floor of the mouth may be swollen and tender. The stone may be palpable, and 80% are radiopaque (Fig. 15.23).

Adenotonsillar Hypertrophy

Lymphoid hyperplasia (enlarged tonsils and adenoids) can cause airway obstruction that can range from mild snoring to severe sleep apnea with right heart strain. Young children with obstructive sleep apnea often fail to gain weight. Older children with severe obstructive sleep apnea are often obese and present with daytime somnolence (pickwickian syndrome). If right heart strain or daytime somnolence is present, a tonsillectomy and adenoidectomy may be required urgently.

Neoplasms

Benign neoplasms occur in the oral cavity, pharynx, hypopharynx, and esophagus. Minor salivary gland tumors, hemangiomas, lymphangiomas, pyogenic granulomas, and neurofibromas are found in the oral cavity but rarely need emergency treatment.

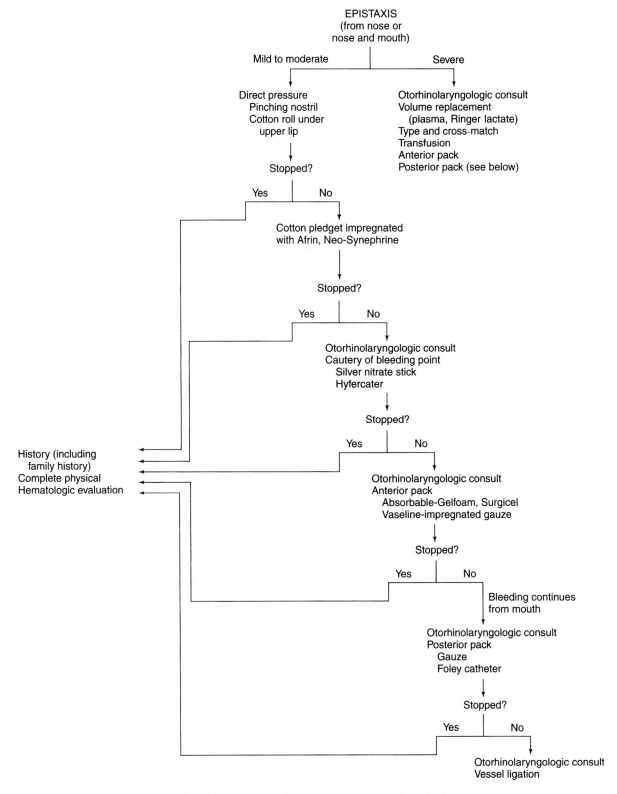

FIG. 15.20. Algorithm for the management of epistaxis.

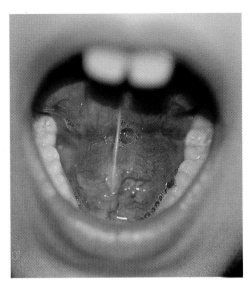

FIG. 15.21. This ranula enlarged over 2 weeks and caused the patient to drool.

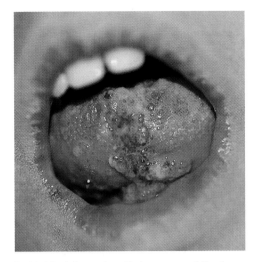

FIG. 15.22. Infected cystic hygroma of the tongue.

Nasopharyngeal angiofibromas occur in prepubescent boys and cause nasal obstruction. They may present to the emergency department with massive epistaxis. Posterior packing is usually required to control the hemorrhage that may be life threatening.

Malignant neoplasms are rare, and rhabdomyosarcoma, lymphoma, and squamous cell carcinoma (lymphoepithelioma) are the most common lesions. They are rarely seen as emergencies unless there is extensive hemorrhage or a compromised airway.

LARYNX AND TRACHEA

Infections are discussed in Chapter 11 (Infectious Disease Emergencies).

Neoplasms

The most common neoplasm of the larynx in children is the laryngeal papilloma. This is believed to be a virus-induced neoplasm that has a predilection for the upper aerodigestive tract and the larynx in particular. The disease is usually diagnosed in the child between 2 and 5 years of age and presents with persistent or worsening hoarseness and, occasionally, airway obstruction. If papillomas are suspected as the source of hoarseness in a child, the otolaryngologist should be consulted to perform the indirect or direct laryngoscopy required to confirm the diagnosis. A lateral neck radiograph may demonstrate a soft-tissue mass in the area of the larynx. The course of the disease is characterized by multiple cycles of growth and regression until a spontaneous remission occurs, usually around puberty.

Hemangiomas may occur in the larynx, primarily in the subglottic area. As with most juvenile hemangiomas, these

FIG. 15.23. A: The floor of this patient's mouth is swollen and tender. **B:** Computed tomography shows an 8-mm stone in the submandibular salivary duct (Wharton duct) and adjacent edema.

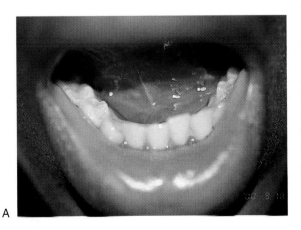

A

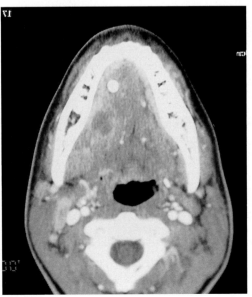

B

lesions present in the second to sixth month of life and can enlarge over several months to cause significant airway obstruction. Episodes of stridor may be precipitated by an upper respiratory infection. Of children with subglottic hemangiomas, 50% have other cutaneous lesions. Therefore, the presence of cutaneous hemangiomas in an infant with stridor should suggest to the emergency physician the possibility of a subglottic hemangioma. If there is severe, persistent, or recurrent respiratory distress, intervention is indicated. Systemic corticosteroids, CO_2 laser or direct surgical excision, and tracheostomy are some of the modes of treatment currently being advocated.

Malignant neoplasms of the larynx are uncommon. They include rhabdomyosarcoma, chondrosarcoma, and lymphoma. These tumors are seen with varying degrees of hoarseness and respiratory obstruction.

NECK AND ASSOCIATED STRUCTURES

Bacterial infections of the neck and associated structures are discussed in Chapter 11 (Infectious Disease Emergencies).

Salivary gland infections should be considered in the differential diagnosis of a cervical mass. Both viral and bacterial agents can be responsible for the infection, with the former being more common. Mumps (endemic parotitis) is the most common salivary infection in children. The infection appears with acute painful swelling of the involved gland or glands, usually involving swelling over the angle of the mandible (Fig. 15.24). There may be erythema around the intraoral orifice of the salivary duct, and the saliva expressed is generally clear. Treatment is supportive with clear fluids, antipyretics, and analgesics as necessary.

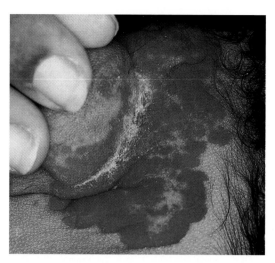

FIG. 15.25. Postauricular hemangioma. This 4-month-old infant presented with a "growing sore".

Bacterial infections of the salivary glands are seen with signs and symptoms similar to those associated with cervical lymphadenitis. The affected gland is swollen, and abscess formation may occur. Purulent material may be expressed from either Stenson duct by massage of the affected salivary gland. The child may be hospitalized for treatment with IV antimicrobials effective against *Staphylococcus aureus* (antistaphylococcal penicillin) and surgical drainage of any collection of purulent material. Recurrent or chronic infections of the salivary glands are usually related to some predisposing factor such as stones, ductal stenosis, and secretory immunodeficiency.

Neoplasms

Neoplasms of the neck, both primary and metastatic, occur in children. If a cervical neoplasm is suspected, an otolaryngologist should be consulted to perform a complete examination of the head and neck, including endoscopy of the nasopharynx, larynx, and hypopharynx.

The hemangioma is the most common neoplasm of the head and neck in children. Although they are more common on the skin of the face and scalp, lesions can occur on the skin of the neck and involve deeper structures, such as the parotid gland. The diagnosis of cutaneous hemangiomas of the cervical skin is usually obvious on physical inspection; the lesions are red to reddish purple, flat or raised, blanch with pressure, and increase in size with crying or straining (Fig. 15.25). Deep-seated lesions without cutaneous manifestations may require special diagnostic aids such as CT or magnetic resonance imaging scans and, rarely, biopsy to confirm the diagnosis.

Lymphangiomas are uncommon benign lesions of the neck. Cystic hygroma is the most common type of lymphangioma found in the neck. These lesions consist of multiple cystic spaces filled with lymph and, occasionally, blood.

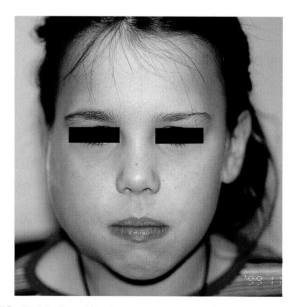

FIG. 15.24. Parotitis. An 8-year-old girl with a 1-day history of right cheek swelling. The swollen area at the angle of the mandible was warm and tender.

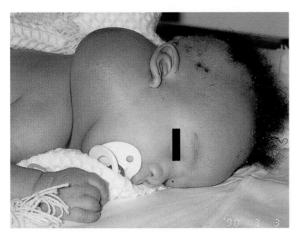

FIG. 15.26. This 3-month-old infant had a small mass that suddenly enlarged when the lymphangioma hemorrhaged.

They appear most commonly as large lateral neck masses in neonates. The diagnosis is often obvious on physical examination of a large cystic lesion that transilluminates. The natural history of these lesions is usually one of progressive growth and enlargement. Lymphangiomas can fluctuate in size secondary to a concurrent infection of the head or neck or hemorrhage into the lesion (Fig. 15.26). Respiratory compromise can be life threatening. Small, stable, asymptomatic lesions can be managed by close observation.

The sternocleidomastoid "tumor" of infancy is an unusual lesion that appears as a discrete mass within the substance of the sternocleidomastoid muscle in a child 4 to 8 weeks old. The cause of this localized area of fibrosis is unknown. The lesion usually resolves with range-of-motion exercises. Surgical intervention is indicated in those cases in which the fibrosis progresses to cause torticollis or if there is suspicion of a malignancy.

The most common malignant neoplasm of the neck in children is lymphoma, being almost equally divided into Hodgkin and nonHodgkin types. The disease may be localized in the neck or be a part of a more generalized disorder. Physical examination often reveals multiple, firm, rubbery, unilateral, or bilateral nodes. If the diagnosis of lymphoma is suspected, otolaryngologic consultation should be obtained for a careful examination of the oral cavity, pharynx, and paranasal sinuses to look for a primary or associated lesion.

This not only aids in the evaluation of the extent of the lymphoma but may also locate a site from which a biopsy specimen can be obtained without the morbidity of a neck exploration.

Cervical lymph nodes may appear as neoplasms metastatic from a nonlymphogenous primary tumor. Thyroid carcinoma, squamous carcinoma (lymphoepithelioma) of the nasopharynx, and malignant melanoma may all be seen first with enlarged cervical lymph nodes. These nodes tend to be hard and singular and may be fixed to underlying structures. Otolaryngologic consultation should be obtained for a complete examination of the head and neck to search for a primary lesion. Biopsy of the node is usually required for diagnosis.

Rhabdomyosarcoma is the most common soft-tissue sarcoma of the head and neck in children. The child usually presents with a history of rapid enlargement of a painless neck mass. The mass itself is hard and poorly mobile. Although the diagnosis of rhabdomyosarcoma may be suspected from the history and physical examination, biopsy is always required for confirmation.

Many other malignant neoplasms can also occur in the neck. These include soft-tissue sarcomas other than rhabdomyosarcoma, malignant fibrous histiocytoma, and neuroblastoma.

SUGGESTED READINGS

Arbour JD, Brunette I, Boisjoly HM. Should we patch corneal erosions? *Arch Ophthalmol* 1997;115:313–317.

Fishman SJ, Mulliken JB. Hemangiomas and vascular malformations of infancy and childhood. *Pediatr Clin North Am* 1993;40:1177–1200.

Gibliotti F, Williams WT, Hayden FG, et al. Etiology of acute conjunctivitis in children. *J Pediatr* 1981;98:531–536.

Handler SD, Raney RB. Management of neoplasms of the head and neck in children: I. Benign tumors. *Head Neck Surg* 1981;3:395–405.

Marcy SM. Infections of the external ear. *Pediatr Infect Dis* 1985;4:192–201.

Leibowitz H. The red eye. *N Engl J Med* 2000;343:345–352.

Lessner A, Stern GA. Preseptal and orbital cellulitis. *Infect Clin North Am* 1992;6:933–952.

Levin AV. Eye emergencies: acute management in the pediatric ambulatory care setting. *Pediatr Emerg Care* 1991;5:367–377.

Levin AV. General pediatric ophthalmic procedures. In: Henretig FM, King CK, eds. *Textbook of pediatric emergency procedures.* Baltimore: Williams & Wilkins, 1997:579–592.

Potsic WP, Handler SD, Wetmore RF, et al. *Primary care pediatric otolaryngology,* 2nd ed. Andover, NJ: J Michael Ryan Publishing, 1995.

Tusa RJ, Saada AA Jr, Niparko JK. Dizziness in childhood. *J Child Neurol* 1994;9:261–274.

Wahrman JE, Honig PJ. Hemangiomas. *Pediatr Rev* 1994;15:266–271.

CHAPTER 16

Pulmonary Emergencies

Editor: Stephen Ludwig

Helpful to the understanding of pulmonary pathology and pathophysiology is a knowledge of pulmonary anatomy and the reflection of that anatomy in the chest radiograph (Fig. 16.1). It is important to be familiar with the normal variations seen in the radiograph of the pediatric patient. There is a normal developmental progression from birth through adolescence.

ACUTE RESPIRATORY FAILURE

Acute respiratory failure represents the severe end of the spectrum of respiratory distress; it signifies an imbalance of O_2 consumption and CO_2 production. Table 16.1 describes the causes of acute respiratory failure by anatomic location, and Table 16.2 outlines the clinical findings and laboratory abnormalities. Few clinical manifestations appear early in the progression of respiratory failure. It is important to remember that prevention of the blood gas–proven respiratory failure should be the goal of the emergency physician. Therefore, in many cases, therapy should be initiated before the laboratory criteria have been fulfilled.

Management

Treatment of respiratory failure is divided into three categories (Table 16.3). First, the physician should always assume that hypoxemia is present and should give sufficient supplemental oxygen (starting at 1.00 FiO_2 in severe situations) to improve arteriolar oxygen levels. The goal of this procedure should be to achieve a minimal acceptable PaO_2 of 60 mm Hg (SaO_2 greater than 90%) in newborns and 70

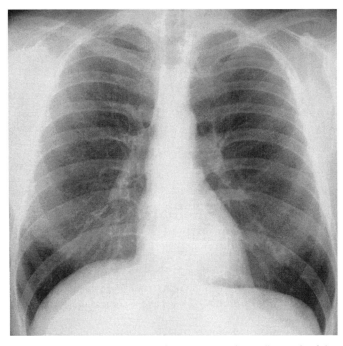

FIG. 16.1. Chest radiograph and anatomy. Normal posteroanterior radiograph of the chest. (From Khan GP, Lynch JP. *Pulmonary disease diagnosis and therapy: a practical approach.* Philadelphia: Lippincott Williams & Wilkins, 1997:2–3, with permission.)

TABLE 16.1. *Causes of acute respiratory failure in children*

Neurologic diseases	
Central nervous system	Status epilepticus
	Severe static encephalopathy
	Acute meningoencephalitis
	Brain abscess, hematoma, tumor
	Brainstem insult
	Arnold–Chiari malformation
	Drug intoxication
	General anesthesia
Spinal/anterior horn cell	Transverse myelitis
	Poliomyelitis
	Polyradiculitis (Guillain–Barré)
	Werdnig–Hoffmann syndrome
Neuromuscular junction	Myasthenia gravis
	Botulism (infant, food, wound)
	Tetanus
	Myopathy
	Neuropathy
	General anesthesia, drugs: succinylcholine, curare, pancuronium Laryngotracheobronchitis (croup), organophosphates
Airway obstruction	
Upper	Acute epiglottitis
	Bacterial tracheitis
	Foreign body aspiration
	Adenotonsillar hypertrophy
	Retropharyngeal abscess
	Subglottic stenosis, web, hemangioma
	Tracheomalacia
	Laryngoedema
	Congenital anomalies
	Static encephalopathy
Lower	Reactive airway disease (asthma)
	Foreign body aspiration
	Cystic fibrosis
	Bronchiectasis
	Tracheobronchomalacia
	Bronchopulmonary dysplasia
	α_1-Antitrypsin deficiency
	Hydrocarbon aspiration, aspiration syndromes
	Congenital lobar emphysema bronchiolitis
Chest wall deformity disorders	Diaphragmatic hernia
	Pneumothorax, hemothorax, chylothorax
	Kyphoscoliosis (severe)
	Restrictive lung disease associated with chest deformity
Pulmonary diseases	Infectious pneumonias
	Tuberculosis (often large airway extrinsic obstruction)
	Pertussis, parapertussis syndrome
	Cystic fibrosis
	Drug-induced pulmonary disease
	Vasculitis, collagen vascular disease
	Pulmonary dysgenesis
	Pulmonary edema
	Near drowning
Other diseases	Cardiac disease
	Anemia (severe)
	Acidemia (severe, i.e., sepsis, renal failure, diabetic ketoacidosis, hepatic disease)
	Oxygen dissociation (methemoglobinemia, carbon monoxide, or cyanide poisoning)
	Hypothermia, hyperthermia
	Sepsis
	Obstructive sleep apnea syndrome (e.g., pickwickian syndrome)

TABLE 16.2. *Diagnosis of acute respiratory failure from pulmonary causes in children*

Clinical findings
  Vital signs: tachycardia, tachypnea
  General appearance: cyanosis, diaphoresis, confusion, restlessness, fatigue, shortness of breath, apnea, grunting, stridor, retractions, decreased air entry, wheezing
Blood gas abnormalities
  $Paco_7$ 50 with acidosis (pH <7.25)
  $Paco_7$ 40 with severe distress
  Pao_2 <60 (or Sao_2 <90%) on 0.4 Fio_2
Pulmonary function abnormalities
  Vital capacity (<15 mL/kg)
  Inspiratory pressure (<25–30 cm H_2O)

mm Hg (Sao_2 greater than 93% to 95%) in older children. If hypoxemia persists after adequate supplemental oxygen is administered, assisted positive-pressure ventilation should be initiated (mask bag reservoir, then proceeding to endotracheal intubation) to improve the efficiency of gas exchange.

Intravenous fluids should be titrated to maintain normal vascular volume as determined by observation of heart rate, blood pressure, peripheral perfusion, and urine output. In severely ill children who require more prolonged therapy in the emergency department, the measurement of central venous pressure may provide a more exact guide.

BRONCHOPULMONARY DYSPLASIA

Bronchopulmonary dysplasia is a chronic lung disorder that may follow moderate to severe hyaline membrane disease (Fig. 16.2) or other acute lung insults around birth. Typically, infants with bronchopulmonary dysplasia are discharged from the nursery initially at 3 to 6 months of age for home therapy, although more severely affected patients may require assisted ventilation for much longer intervals. These children have tachypnea and retractions at rest or during the mildest respiratory infections or fever. Their lungs are hyperinflated (increased anteroposterior chest diameter), and they may have crackles, wheezes, or decreased breath sounds in areas of the thorax. Some patients will manifest dyspnea and moderate to severe failure to thrive. Arterial blood gas (ABG) tensions show Pao_2 less than 60 mm Hg (Sao_2 less than 90% to 92%) and/or $Paco_2$ more than 45 mm Hg in room air, often despite respiratory rates of greater than 60 to 80 breaths per minute. Chest radiographs demonstrate varying amounts of hyperinflation; several patterns occur, including cystic areas with signs of fibrosis, which are often confused with congenital lobar emphysema; and new infiltrates when previous radiographs are not available for comparison (Fig. 16.3).

TABLE 16.3 *Management of acute respiratory failure*

Treatment	
Primary hypoxemia	1. Supplemental oxygen (titrate for cyanosis; use arterial blood gases or pulse oximetry)
	2. Consider endotracheal intubation when Fio_2 0.6 or when decreased lung compliance and Fio_2 >0.4
	3. Use CPAP or PEEP to improve oxygenation
	4. Use assisted ventilation to improve gas exchange (increased inspiratory time, normal respiratory rates, tidal volume: 10–15 mL/kg; pressure cycle ventilation if weight <10 kg, volume cycle ventilation if weight >10 kg)
	5. Treat underlying cause
Primary alveolar hypoventilation	1. Supplemental oxygen (as above)
	2. Support ventilation
	a. Oral/nasal pharyngeal tube or endotracheal intubation
	b. Mask-bag ventilation with high-flow oxygen
	c. Use assisted ventilation (normal to increased respiratory rates; increased expired time, increased flow rates)
	d. Use increased tidal volume (pressure) with obstructive airway disease or atelectasis
	e. Monitor carefully for side effects of ventilation
Adjunctive therapy	1. Intravenous fluid to achieve normal vascular volume (less fluid for child with interstitial lung disease)
	2. Diuretics such as 1 mg/kg furosemide for acute pulmonary edema or fluid overload
	3. Sedatives/analgesics: 0.1–0.2 mg/kg morphine sulfate every 1–2 hr intravenously; 0.1–0.2 mg/kg midazolam every 2–4 hr intravenously
	4. Muscle relaxants: vecuronium bromide (Pavulon), starting at 0.1 mg/kg every 1–2 hr or alternative 0.1–0.2

CPAP, continuous positive airway pressure; PEEP, positive end-expiratory pressure.

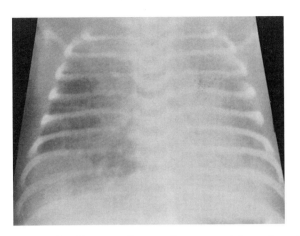

FIG. 16.2. Hyaline membrane disease and bronchopulmonary dysplasia. Hyaline membrane disease. This is one of twins born at 31 weeks' gestation. The chest radiograph shows hypoaeration, diffusely opaque lung fields, air bronchograms, and loss of normal vascular shadows.

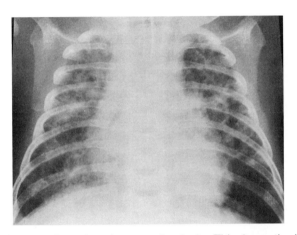

FIG. 16.3. Bronchopulmonary dysplasia. This 2-month-old child was treated with mechanical ventilation during the first days of life for hyaline membrane disease. The chest radiograph shows generalized overaeration and course modularity with multiple cystlike areas throughout both lung fields.

Management

Emergency physicians most often will evaluate children with bronchopulmonary dysplasia accompanied by acute respiratory infections. Management is primarily limited to supportive care: ensuring oral or intravenous intake, providing relief of hypoxemia, and, when necessary, providing assisted ventilation for hypercarbia and acidosis. Pulse oximetry can be beneficial in assessing the degree of oxygen saturation and may obviate immediate arterial puncture in mild illness. An ABG Arreim blood gas (ABG) test should be considered when signs and symptoms may be the result of hypercapnia or when cyanosis, respiratory distress, or deterioration from baseline cannot be easily reversed. A chest radiograph is helpful in most episodes but often merely corroborates clinical changes. Indications for admission include a respiratory rate greater than 70 to 80 breaths per minute (or significant change from baseline), increasing hypoxia or hypercarbia, poor feeding associated with respiratory symptoms, apnea, or significant new pulmonary infiltrates.

ASPIRATION PNEUMONIA

Aspiration pneumonia should be suspected in any at-risk child who has signs of respiratory distress. Most often, after the aspiration of gastric contents, a brief latent period occurs before the onset of respiratory signs and symptoms (Fig. 16.4). More than 90% of patients are symptomatic within 1 hour, and almost all patients have symptoms within 2 hours. Fever, tachypnea, and cough are usually seen. Hypoxia is common. Apnea and hypotensive shock are less common. Sputum production is usually minimal. Diffuse crackles and wheezing are common; cyanosis appears with progression of the disease. Chest radiographs may show either localized or diffuse infiltrates, which are often bilateral. The chest radiograph of a patient who has aspirated stomach contents may evolve suddenly from normal to complete bilateral opacification within 8 to 24 hours (Fig. 16.5).

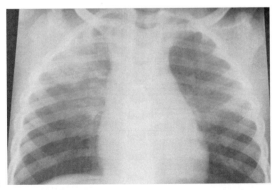

A

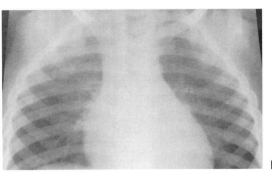

B

FIG. 16.4. Aspiration pneumonia. **A:** Blood aspiration. A 3-year-old boy with tachypnea 1 day after surgery for enlarged adenoids/tonsils. The chest radiograph shows an infiltrate in the right upper and left lower lobe. **B:** Blood aspiration. The chest radiograph 2 days later shows clearing of the infiltrate in the right upper and left lower lobe.

Management

The suspicion of aspiration should be confirmed with a chest radiograph. Children with a significant aspiration pneumonia (lobar infiltrates, moderate to severe respiratory distress) require admission to the hospital. Table 16.4 outlines therapeutic modalities that may be useful.

In the acute care setting, children who aspirate stomach contents require primarily supportive care. Supplemental oxygen should be administered, as determined by pulse oximetry or direct measurement of oxygenation with an ABG test. Another consideration in the therapy of aspiration pneumonias is the role of prophylactic antibiotic administration, which is often given to children with fever and leukocytosis. Community-acquired pneumonias generally involve anaerobes and are adequately treated with penicillin, whereas nosocomial infections require antibiotics effective against both aerobes (including *Staphylococcus aureus* and Gram-negative bacilli) and anaerobes, such as a combination such as clindamycin and gentamicin.

PULMONARY EMBOLISM

The classic presentation of massive pulmonary embolism (Fig. 16.7) with severe circulatory compromise is easily rec-

TABLE 16.4. *Initial treatment of aspiration pneumonia*

A–Proven measures
    Suction
    Airway protection
    Oxygen
B–Optional modalities
    Corticosteroids
    Antibiotics

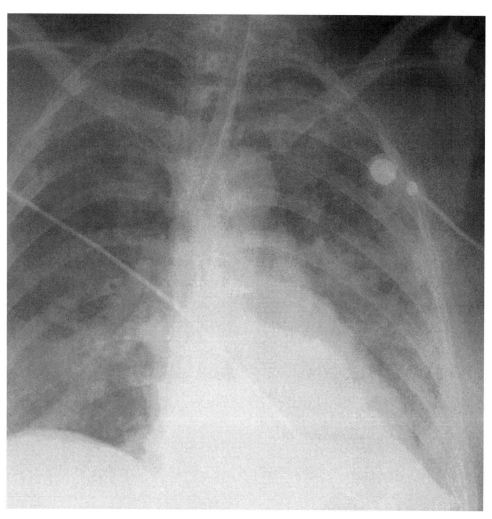

FIG. 16.5. Diffuse opacification of the lungs in a patient who was observed to aspirate gastric fluid before intubation. (From Khan GP, Lynch JP. *Pulmonary disease diagnosis and therapy: a practical approach*. Philadelphia: Lippincott Williams & Wilkins, 1997:83, with permission.)

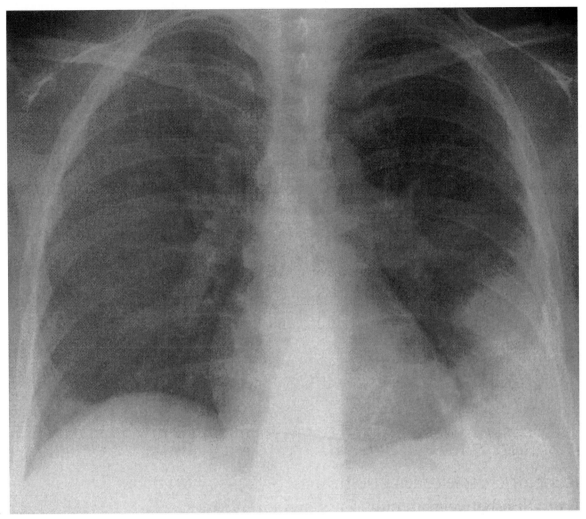

A

FIG. 16.6. Pulmonary embolism. **A:** Parenchymal opacity in the left lower lung zone and prominent left pulmonary artery in a patient with left-sided chest pain, hypoxia, and lower limb deep vein thrombosis. The ventilation–perfusion lung scan showed high probability for pulmonary embolism.

ognized. However, most patients have nonspecific signs and symptoms and no pathognomonic laboratory abnormalities (Table 16.5). The most common presenting abnormalities in children and adolescents are pleuritic pain (which may radiate to the shoulders), dyspnea, cough, and hemoptysis. Additional findings may include apprehension, nonproductive cough, fever, sweats, and palpitations.

Aside from tachycardia, abnormalities on physical examination are often lacking. If a sufficiently large associated infarction is identified, there may be decreased resonance over the lung fields and a pleural friction rub. Breath sounds may be distant or absent, and rales may be heard. The presence of hypoxemia not completely explained by the underlying disease process or clinical state should suggest the possibility of pulmonary embolism.

The diagnosis of pulmonary embolism can be established with high probability based on ventilation–perfusion lung scan findings. The characteristic pattern is normal ventilation of poorly perfused areas of lung. Many physicians consider pulmonary angiography to be the preferred diagnostic method in previously healthy individuals. However, the reliability of this method diminishes with time after the acute embolism. The electrocardiogram is neither a specific nor a sensitive indicator of pulmonary embolism. The S_1-Q_3-T_3 pattern that has been described with pulmonary embolus may be seen in other conditions, including a pneumothorax. Although the presence of a pulmonary infiltrate with an ipsilateral elevated hemidiaphragm is suggestive of a pulmonary embolism, there are no pathognomonic radiographic signs in the acute care setting. ABGs generally indicate a decreased partial pressure of oxygen. However, approximately 15% of patients have a PaO_2 greater than 80 mm Hg and 5% greater than 90 mm Hg. A normal D-dimer levels makes pulmonary embolism unlikely.

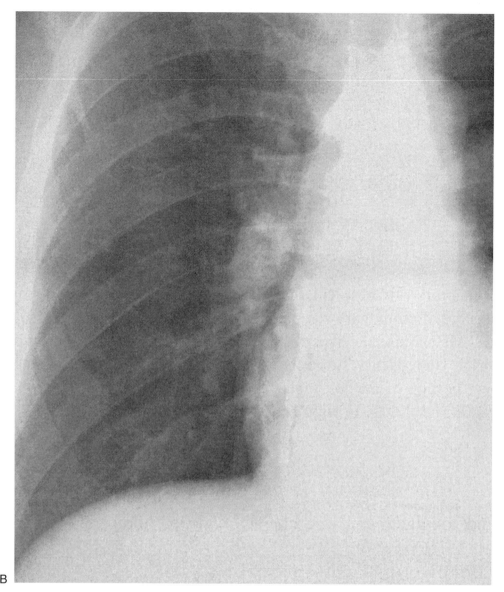

B

FIG. 16.6. *Continued.* **B:** Enlargement of the right hilum from distention of the descending right pulmonary artery from a massive pulmonary embolus. The transverse diameter of the pulmonary artery is 22 mm. The distention is not the result of raised pulmonary artery pressure proximal to the clot but of distention by the thrombus. Note the abrupt change of caliber in the descending pulmonary artery, which is accompanied by diminished vascularity in the lower lobe. (From Khan GP, Lynch JP. *Pulmonary disease diagnosis and therapy: a practical approach.* Philadelphia: Lippincott Williams & Wilkins, 1997:91,15, with permission.)

TABLE 16.5. *Clinical manifestation of pulmonary embolism*

	Nonspecific	Suggestive	Diagnostic
Symptoms	Syncope, sweating, pleuritic pain, dyspnea, cough, apprehension	Dyspnea out of proportion to degree of abnormal findings, hemoptysis	
Signs	Tachypnea, tachycardia, distant or absent breath sounds, rales, fever	Pleural friction rub, unexplained cyanosis, accentuated S_2	
Laboratory/radiography	Decreased Pa_{O_2} ECG abnormalities: R/L axis deviations, ST-T wave changes, ectopic (A & V) beats, right bundle-branch block	Wedged infiltrate with ipsilateral elevated hemidiaphragm, abnormal ventilation–perfusion scan, ECG abnormality: S_1-Q_3-T_3 pattern	Abnormal pulmonary angiography

ECG, electrocardiogram; R/L, right/left; A & V, atrial and ventricular.

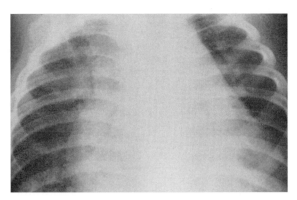

FIG. 16.7. A 2-year-old boy with tachypnea and dyspnea. Secondary to enlarged tonsils and adenoids. The x-ray shows cardiomegaly and mild intestinal edema.

Management

In all patients strongly suspected of having a pulmonary embolism, a chest radiograph, electrocardiogram, and ABG level should be obtained. If the clinical suspicion is high, regardless of the results, the patient should be admitted for initiation of definitive treatment. When the patient is vaguely suspected of having pulmonary embolism, all the aforementioned tests are normal, the patient's clinical condition permits, and the likelihood of pulmonary embolism appears low, the patient may be discharged with close follow-up. When abnormalities are uncovered, further diagnostic workup (i.e., ventilation–perfusion scan) and admission to the hospital should be considered.

Initial therapy includes supplemental oxygen, ventilatory support as indicated, and achievement of venous access. Intravenous heparin remains the mainstay of definitive therapy for pulmonary embolism because its onset of action is immediate and it is rapidly metabolized. However, it should be kept in mind that heparin is a common cause of in-hospital drug-related deaths in reasonably healthy adults, and it has been cited as a source of in-hospital complications in adolescents.

PULMONARY EDEMA

Pulmonary edema refers to the abnormal accumulation of fluid within the alveolar spaces and bronchioles. The onset of pulmonary edema is variable but may be rapid. Tachypnea, cough (often producing frothy, pink-tinged sputum), dyspnea, shortness of breath, and chest pain are commonly seen. Grunting often occurs in an effort to prevent lung collapse. On physical examination, the child may appear pale or cyanotic and have a rapid pulse. Decreased breath sounds and moist (bubbly) rales are the most common auscultatory findings. However, these are generally absent with small increases in lung fluid. Indeed, auscultatory and radiographic findings may not manifest until the interstitial and extravascular fluid has doubled or tripled in volume.

Unless it is massive, acute fluid accumulation may not be detectable by chest radiograph. Lymphatic and interstitial fluid accumulations (Fig. 16.8) may be visible as Kerley A and B lines (septal lines) (Fig. 16.9). Flattening of the diaphragm on radiograph may also be a finding with pulmonary edema. This is presumably caused by air trapping

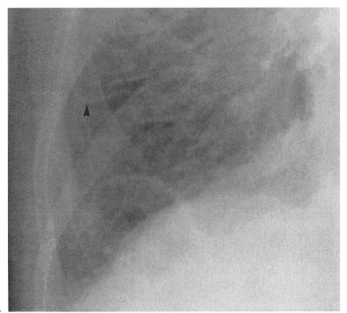

A

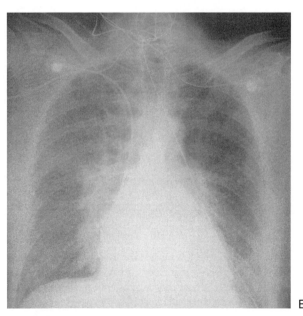

B

FIG. 16.8. Pulmonary edema: radiographic findings. **A:** Kerley B lines in interstitial pulmonary edema. These are short opaque lines (*arrowhead*) seen best along the lateral aspects of the lungs. Thickened interlobular septa from lymphangitic spread of tumor can produce an identical appearance. **B:** Diffuse alveolar pulmonary edema shows ill-defined opacification in both lungs that is most prominent in the perihilar regions.

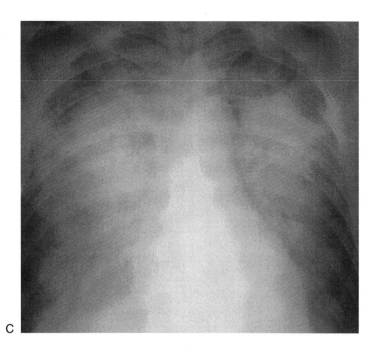

C

FIG. 16.8. *Continued.* **C:** Classical butterfly pattern of pulmonary edema in a uremic patient. (From Khan GP, Lynch JP. *Pulmonary disease diagnosis and therapy: a practical approach.* Philadelphia: Lippincott Williams & Wilkins, 1997:66–67, with permission.)

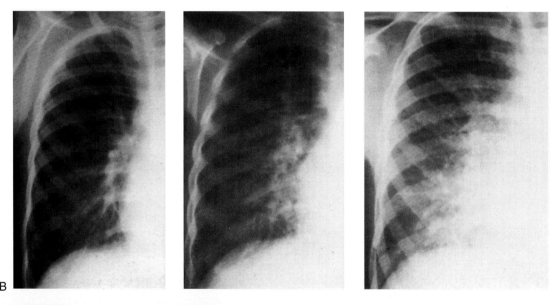

A,B   C

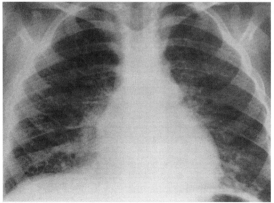

D

FIG. 16.9. Pulmonary edema: interstitial stage. **A:** Note early development of streaky white lines (interstitial septal edema) radiating from the hilar region. In this case, the lines primarily are Kerley A lines. This patient had acute glomerulonephritis. **B:** More extensive reticular pattern of pulmonary interstitial edema in a patient with cardiac failure secondary to aortic stenosis. **C:** Very extensive interstitial edema producing pronounced reticulation through the lung and some underlying parenchymal haziness. Kerley A and B lines are present. This patient had acute glomerulonephritis. **D:** Interstitial fluid from volume overload. This 2-year-old child had a paraspinal sarcoma removed 6 months earlier. Before chest radiation, he received a large fluid load. The chest radiograph shows interstitial edema with Kerley lines and bilateral small pleural effusions. (From Swischuk LE. *Emergency radiology of the acutely ill or injured child,* 2nd ed. Philadelphia: Lippincott Williams & Wilkins, 1986:85, with permission.)

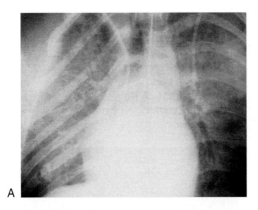

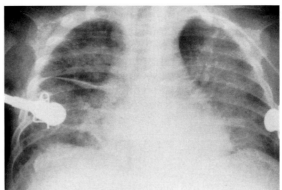

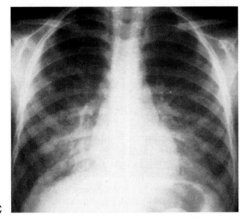

FIG. 16.10. Pulmonary edema: hazy interstitial pattern. **A:** Note diffuse haziness throughout both lungs in this patient with diffuse interstitial pulmonary edema. The cause was iatrogenic fluid overload. **B:** Fluid overload leading to extensively hazy, almost opaque lungs and pleural fluid in the minor fissure on the right. **C:** Hazy almost opaque infiltrates confined more to the lung bases. This patient had acute glomerulonephritis. (From Swischuk LE. *Emergency radiology of the acutely ill or injured child*, 2nd ed. Philadelphia: Lippincott Williams & Wilkins, 1986:85, with permission.)

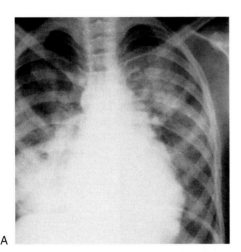

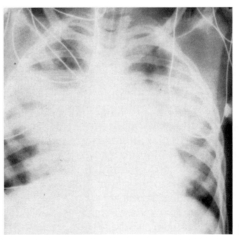

FIG. 16.11. Pulmonary edema: alveolar stage. **A:** Note patchy areas of confluent pulmonary alveolar edema throughout both lungs. The apices and costophrenic angles remain relatively clear. The asymmetric distribution would be difficult to differentiate from widespread pneumonia. **B:** Another patient demonstrates pronounced parahilar and mid-lung field pulmonary alveolar edema. There is more sparing of the apices and costophrenic angles leading to the typical butterfly configuration. This patient was overloaded with fluid during treatment for status asthmaticus. (From Swischuk LE. *Emergency radiology of the acutely ill or injured child*, 2nd ed. Philadelphia: Lippincott Williams & Wilkins, 1986:86, with permission.)

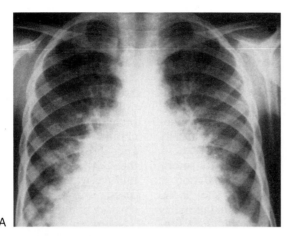

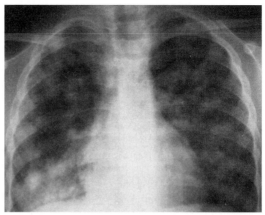

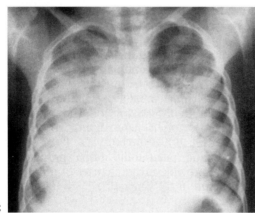

FIG. 16.12. Pulmonary edema: varying causes and configurations. **A:** Acute glomerulonephritis. Note extensive interstitial pulmonary edema, moderate cardiomegaly, and moderate bilateral pleural effusions. The findings would be difficult to differentiate from acute myocarditis with failure. **B:** Near drowning. Note extensive fluffy, nodular infiltrates distributed throughout both lungs. In other patients, the infiltrates may be more diffuse or hazy and less nodular. **C:** Rheumatic pneumonia. This patient was discharged from the hospital after convalescing from acute rheumatic fever. His heart was nearly normal in size at that time. Less than 48 hours later, he returned with severe dyspnea and this radiographic appearance typical of extensive pulmonary interstitial and alveolar edema. Necropsy findings substantiated the diagnosis of rheumatic "pneumonia." (From Swischuk LE. *Emergency radiology of the acutely ill or injured child*, 2nd ed. Philadelphia: Lippincott Williams & Wilkins, 1986:87, with permission.)

that results from airway narrowing as a result of bronchiolar fluid collections (Fig. 16.10). It should be kept in mind that if pulmonary edema is superimposed on another pulmonary process, the clinical and radiographic findings may be obscured by those of the primary illness. Similarly, once pulmonary edema is severe enough, it may be difficult to separate edema, atelectasis, and inflammation on the radiograph (Figs. 16.11, 16.12, and 16.13).

Management

The management of patients with pulmonary edema should ultimately be directed toward treatment of the primary disorder. Initial efforts (Table 16.6) should be directed toward re-

TABLE 16.6. *Treatment of pulmonary edema*

Oxygen	Venodilation
Diuresis	0.1 mg/kg IV morphine
1 mg/kg IV furosemide	Digitalis

IV, intravenous.

versal of hypoxemia by the administration of oxygen and by mechanical ventilation if necessary. Continuous positive airway pressure therapy delivered via face mask has also been shown to be effective in some patients. In addition to satisfying the patient's oxygen demands, reversal of hypoxemia is often useful in relieving chest pain and is important to the metabolism of vasoactive mediators that affect microvascular permeability.

Other therapeutic measures should be tailored somewhat to fit the patient's individual needs. When heart failure is the cause of pulmonary edema, in addition to oxygen and ventilation, diuretics (to decrease plasma volume), digitalis (to improve contractility), and bronchodilators (to improve contractility and afterload and to produce bronchodilation) are useful. Morphine dilates the venous system and may be helpful in relieving anxiety and dyspnea. In patients with acute respiratory distress syndrome, ARDS clinical studies have shown that the use of methylprednisolone does not improve outcome and may in fact increase the mortality and incidence of secondary infections.

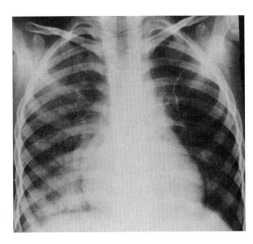

FIG. 16.13. Pulmonary hemorrhage. Idiopathic pulmonary hemosiderosis. A 5-year-old child with repeated bouts of pulmonary hemorrhage. The chest radiograph shows diffuse radiopacities throughout both lungs (more on the right side), with a well-defined alveolar opacity in the right lower lobe. Note the surgical sutures in left upper lobe.

PULMONARY HEMORRHAGE

The hallmark of pulmonary hemorrhage is recurrent intrapulmonary bleeding with lung injury and secondary depletion of body iron stores. Therefore, the symptoms and signs include hemoptysis, recurrent pneumonias (manifested by fever, tachypnea, tachycardia, and coarse or fine crackles), and pallor. Emesis of blood arising in the pulmonary tree may mislead the clinician to investigate the gastrointestinal tract. Associated symptoms of fatigue and poor weight gain are common.

Laboratory findings after recurrent hemorrhage most characteristically include a microcytic, hypochromic anemia with low serum iron. Leukocytosis and eosinophilia may be present, and the stool usually tests positive for blood. Radiographs may show alveolar infiltrates that may be transient, localized processes or diffuse and chronic (Fig. 16.14).

Management

Most children with pulmonary hemorrhage have a chronic disease requiring supportive therapy for hypoxia and anemia in the form of blood transfusions and supplemental oxygen. Occasionally, pulmonary hemorrhage is so severe that it causes respiratory insufficiency or hypotension. Positive-pressure ventilation with positive-end expiratory pressure is the preferred treatment in this situation; bleeding is usually not rapid or well enough localized to be identified and controlled by bronchoscopy. In allergic, vasculitic, and idiopathic hemorrhage, the use of corticosteroids is indicated as either 2 mg/kg methylprednisolone

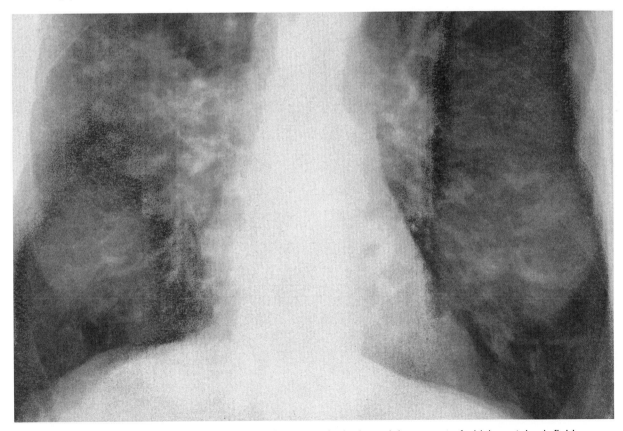

FIG. 16.14. Bronchiectasis. Note the saccular spaces in the lower lobes, many of which contain air-fluid levels. This patient with dyskinetic cilia does not have dextrocardia. (From Khan GP, Lynch JP. *Pulmonary disease diagnosis and therapy: a practical approach.* Philadelphia: Lippincott Williams & Wilkins, 1997:70, with permission.)

per day or 8 mg/kg hydrocortisone per day intravenously in three to four divided doses. When hemorrhage is caused by infection, especially tuberculosis, antimicrobial therapy should be instituted and steroids avoided. Admission is necessary to support the child until the cause of the process has been determined or acutely until the hemorrhage has been controlled. Bronchoscopy can be useful diagnostically to determine infectious causes and may localize bleeding sites. Occasionally, when the bleeding is brisk as in bronchiectasis (Fig. 16.15) with erosion to a bronchial vessel as in cystic fibrosis, embolization of vessels may be needed to stop the bleeding.

PLEURITIS

The causes of pleural inflammation are varied. The determination of the nature of pleural fluid may be helpful from a diagnostic standpoint (Table 16.7). The hallmarks of pleural disease are pain, shortness of breath, fever, and an abnormal chest radiograph. Inspiratory chest pain from pleural inflammation is the most characteristic symptom.

A pleural friction rub is most apt to be heard in pleural inflammation that is associated with little or no effusion. Although symptoms of pleural effusion are varied and relate to the primary cause of the effusion, most patients complain of some degree of dyspnea. Pleuritic chest pain is also a common complaint and can occur before the accumulation of fluid. Characteristic physical findings include restriction of

movement of the chest wall on the affected side, flatness to percussion, diminished to absent tactile and vocal fremitus, and decreased to absent breath sounds.

Pleural effusion is the most common radiographic manifestation of pleural disease (Fig. 16.16). The first radiographic sign of a pleural effusion is usually blunting of the costophrenic angles, producing wedgelike menisci that extend upward along the lateral chest wall. Similar collections are seen in the posterior costophrenic angles on lateral views. Larger effusions may be seen to extend up the entire lateral chest wall or retrosternally.

Management

The management of pleural disease is aimed at determining the cause, treating the primary disorder, and relieving associated functional disturbances. When no effusion is present, relief of chest pain is one of the most pressing issues. Analgesics, bed rest, and/or mild sedatives may be indicated. It should be kept in mind that irritability and restlessness may be a result of pain, which, in dry pleurisy, can occur with every phase of respiration.

The accumulation of pleural fluid usually provides relief from pain. Thoracentesis is indicated when fluid accumulation is extensive enough to cause dyspnea and/or for diagnostic purposes (Fig. 16.17).

TABLE 16.7. *Differential diagnosis of pleural effusion*

A–Transudative pleural effusions
  Congestive heart failure
  Cirrhosis
  Nephrotic syndrome
  Acute glomerulonephritis
  Myxedema
  Peritoneal dialysis
  Hypoproteinemia
  Meigs syndrome
  Sarcoidosis
  Vascular obstruction
  Ex vacuo effusion
B–Exudative pleural effusions
  1. Infectious diseases
    Tuberculosis
    Bacterial infections
    Viral infections
    Fungal infections
    Parasitic infections
  2. Neoplastic diseases
    Mesotheliomas
    Metastatic disease
  3. Collagen vascular diseases
    Systemic lupus erythematosus
    Rheumatoid pleuritis
    Pulmonary infarction/embolization

  4. Gastrointestinal diseases
    Pancreatitis
    Esophageal rupture
    Subphrenic abscess
    Hepatic abscess
    Whipple disease
    Diaphragmatic hernia
    Peritonitis
C–Trauma
  Hemothorax
  Chylothorax
D–Drug hypersensitivity
  Nitrofurantoin
  Methysergide
E–Miscellaneous diseases
  Asbestos exposure
  Pulmonary and lymph node myomatosis
  Uremia
  Postmyocardial infarction syndrome
  Trapped lung
  Congenital abnormalities of the lymphatics
  Postradiation therapy
  Drug reactions

From Light RW. Pleural effusions. *Med Clin North Am* 1977;61:1339, with permission.

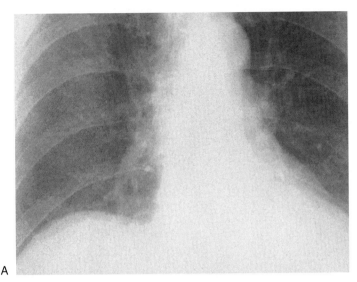

A

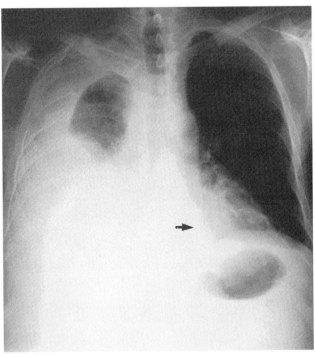

B

FIG. 16.15. Pleural effusion. **A:** Bilateral pleural effusions in a patient with metastatic nodules scattered throughout both lungs, primary unknown. A small left pleural effusion obliterates the left costophrenic angle, with an ill-defined margin. There is a larger right pleural effusion, also with an ill-defined margin, extending along the axillary margin of the lung. There is a little atelectasis in the anterior segment of the right upper lobe, abutting on the outer aspect of the lesser fissure. **B:** Massive right pleural effusion, extending over the apex of the lung onto the mediastinal aspect of the upper lobe. There is no mediastinal shift because of the complete collapse of the middle and lower lobes. The left paravertebral opacity (*arrow*) is the result of right pleural effusion bulging the azygoesophageal recess to the left of the midline. *(continued)*

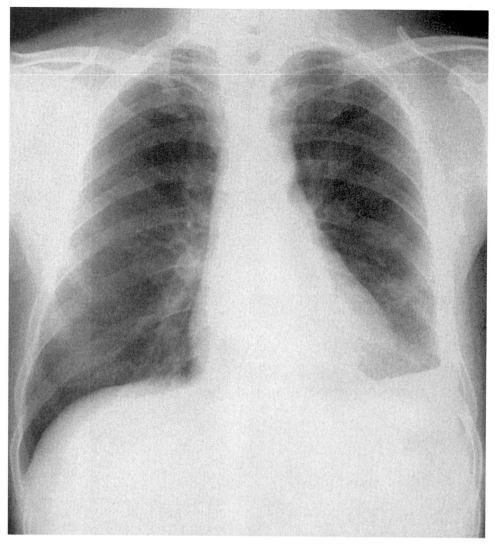

FIG. 16.15. *(Continued)* **C:** Old pleural thickening obliterates the left costophrenic angle. Note the considerable lateral elevation and straightening of the left diaphragm, and the sharpness of the costophrenic angle, indicating an old pleural reaction with adhesions from fibrosis. (From Khan GP, Lynch JP. *Pulmonary disease diagnosis and therapy: a practical approach.* Philadelphia: Lippincott Williams & Wilkins, 1997:36, with permission.)

OBSTRUCTIVE SLEEP APNEA

Most young children have abnormal daytime sleepiness. Other commonly associated behavioral abnormalities include hyperactivity, continuous fighting with peers, crying easily (especially in younger children), short attention span, and quick shifts from hyperactivity to excessive somnolence and withdrawal behavior.

Older children complain of sleepiness, tiredness, and fatigue. Decreased school performance, especially with regard to language acquisition, is seen in some children. One-fourth of patients report morning headaches, and more than half demonstrate signs of failure to thrive. Severe symptoms included massive obesity in 11%, hypertension in 8%, and acute cardiac or cardiorespiratory failure in 17%.

Disordered sleep is the most common symptom of obstructive sleep apnea. All children have continuous snoring, which is interspersed with pauses and snorts. More than 80% have disrupted nocturnal sleep (e.g., nightmares, night terrors, sleepwalking), and 90% sweat profusely during the night. Intermittent or nightly enuresis is also commonly noted (26%). Chronic nighttime cough may also be observed as a result of intermittent aspiration of small amounts of pharyngeal secretions and may aggravate other chronic conditions such as asthma.

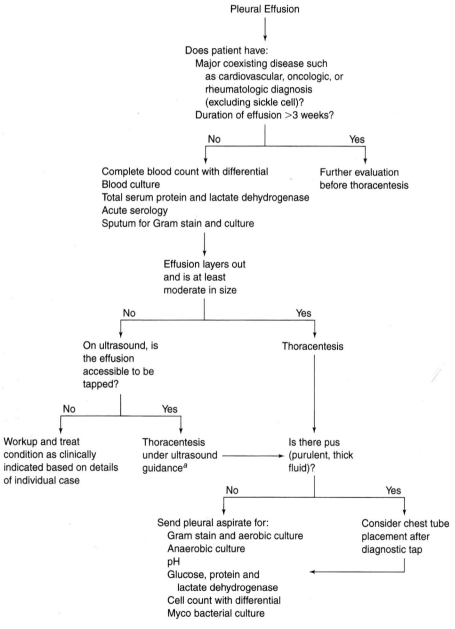

FIG. 16.16. Approach to pleural effusion. Consider simultaneous placement of small-gauge (8 to 10 French) chest tube using the Seldinger technique for large, free-flowing effusions.

Teenagers generally complain of daytime tiredness, fatigue, and sleepiness. Other common symptoms include deterioration of memory and judgment, nausea, headaches, mood swings, and neurotic behavior. Polycythemia, hypertension, cardiac arrhythmias, anoxic seizures, gastroesophageal reflux, and esophagitis are less common associated serious consequences. Two-thirds of one group of adult patients were reported to be overweight (more than 20% more than estimates of ideal weight).

Management

Any child with a definite history of apnea must be managed with caution and concern. Hospitalization in a monitored setting is the rule. At the time of presentation, the child might not appear in extremis, by definition, during wakeful periods. However, this child runs the risk of repeated apnea and the related complication of subsequent hypoxemia. Many children with obstructive sleep apnea have preexisting anatomic airway abnormalities (e.g., facial dysmorphia syndromes, enlarged lymphoid tissue) that require the expertise of an otolaryngologist.

Polysomnography is an accepted method for evaluating apnea; however, it is inconvenient and expensive. This method of evaluation is generally reserved for the most severely obstructed patients. Radiographs of the neck taken with the child lying on his or her back can be helpful but are not a definitive method of diagnosis. Both radiographs and physical examination of the pharynx have similar limitations in that the dynamics of the tissues at night cannot be observed.

SUGGESTED READINGS

Blackmore CC, Black WC, Dallas RV, et al. Pleural fluid volume estimation: a chest radiograph prediction rule. *Acad Radiol* 1996;3:103–109.

Bokulic RE, Hilman BC. Interstitial lung diseases in children. *Pediatr Clin North Am* 1994;41:543–567.

Brook I. Treatment of aspiration of tracheostomy-associated pneumonia in neurologically impaired children: effect of antimicrobials effective against anaerobic bacteria. *Int J Pediatr Otorhinolaryngol* 1996;35:171–177.

Dearborn DG. Pulmonary hemorrhage in infants and children. *Curr Opin Pediatr* 1997;9:219–224.

Fan LL, Lung MC, Wagener JS. The diagnostic value of bronchoalveolar lavage in immunocompetent children with chronic diffuse pulmonary infiltrates. *Pediatr Pulmonol* 1997;23:8–13.

Goddard R, Scofield RH. Right pneumothorax with $S_1Q_3T_3$ electrocardiogram pattern usually associated with pulmonary embolus. *Am J Emerg Med* 1997;15:310–312.

Goldson E. Bronchopulmonary dysplasia. *Pediatr Ann* 1990;19:13–18.

Gouldin CW, DiGiulio GA, Gonzalez del Rey JA. Pulmonary embolism in children and adolescents. *Ambul Child Health* 1997;3:240.

Klein JS, Schultz S, Heffner JE. Interventional radiology of the chest: image-guided percutaneous drainage of pleural effusions, lung abscess, and pneumothorax. *AJR Am J Roentgenol* 1995;164:581–588.

McBride WJ, Gadowski GR, Keller MS, et al. Pulmonary embolism in pediatric trauma patients. *J Trauma* 1994;37:913–915.

Nuss R, Hays T, Chudgar U, et al. Antiphospholipid antibodies and coagulation regulatory pattern in children with pulmonary embolism. *J Pediatr Hematol Oncol* 1997;19:202–207.

CHAPTER 17

Renal and Electrolyte Emergencies

Editor: Marc N. Baskin

DEHYDRATION

Isotonic Dehydration

Appropriate treatment of dehydration requires an understanding of maintenance and deficit fluid and electrolyte calculations.

Weight (kg)	Maintenance fluid/24 hours
<10 kg	100 mL/kg
11–20 kg	1,000 mL + 50 mL for each kg over 10 kg
>20 kg	1,500 mL + 20 mL for each kg over 20 kg

The maintenance requirement for sodium is 2 to 3 mEq/100 mL and 2 mEq/100 mL for potassium. As an example, a 30-kg child would have a daily maintenance fluid requirement of 1,700 mL (1,500 mL + 20 mL/kg × 10 kg). The daily requirement for sodium would be 34 to 51 mEq and 34 mEq for potassium.

Clinical Manifestations

A careful history helps to establish the cause of the fluid loss and to estimate the degree of depletion. The physical examination should begin with weighing the child, the most accurate indicator of dehydration. With a 5% or greater loss of body weight, urine output will be decreased, the patient slightly tachycardic, and the mucous membranes slightly dry, but there are no signs of vascular instability. As fluid losses exceed 10%, changes in mentation, tachypnea secondary to acidosis, cool extremities, abnormal skin turgor (Fig. 17.1), and finally hypotension and shock appear.

Management

In all children with significant dehydration (5% to 10%), an intravenous (IV) infusion should be started and electrolytes, blood urea nitrogen (BUN), creatinine, and glucose measured. A fluid bolus of 20 mL/kg physiologic saline should be given over 30 to 60 minutes. Fluids are administered in the first 24 hours to fulfill the maintenance requirement and correct the total deficit; half the deficit is replaced in the first 8 hours.

ELECTROLYTE DISORDERS

Disorders of Sodium Homeostasis: Hyponatremia

Clinical Manifestations

The multiple causes of hyponatremia are grouped into four categories (Table 17.1). Signs and symptoms are usually seen at serum sodium lower than 120 mEq/L, but specific signs and symptoms do not correlate with specific levels of serum sodium (Table 17.2). It is especially critical to note the presence of edema and hypovolemia. Complications of hyponatremia that require urgent diagnosis and treatment include Cheyne–Stokes respirations and seizures.

Management

Using the clinical history and examination and the few laboratory tests, the emergency physician should be able to diagnose the specific cause of hyponatremia in most cases. A urine sodium concentration is especially helpful. If the urine sodium concentration is more than 20 mEq/L, then renal-mediated etiologies such as sodium-wasting nephropathy, syndrome of inappropriate antidiuretic hormone secretion, adrenal insufficiency, or diuretic use should be suspected. A working schema is outlined in Figure 17.2.

In the patient with hyponatremia in the face of obvious contraction of extracellular fluid (ECF) volume (diarrhea or vomiting), reexpansion with isotonic saline is appropriate. The volume and rate of infusion are dictated by estimates of fluid loss (i.e., weight loss) made from the history and physical examination. Underlying diseases, such as renal tubular acidosis (RTA) and adrenal insufficiency, can be treated most effectively by specific replacement therapy. Diuretics should be discontinued.

In water intoxication, restriction of daily free-water administration by 25% to 50%, depending on the chronicity

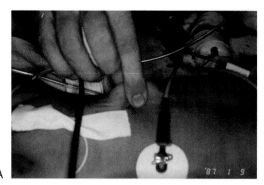
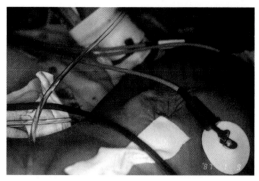

A   B

FIG. 17.1. (A,B) This infant's poor skin turgor is manifested as tenting of his skin.

and severity of the hyponatremia, is the treatment of choice. In the acutely ill patient with neurologic symptoms and signs, immediate relief may be accomplished temporarily by rapidly elevating the serum sodium with the IV administration of 5 to 10 mL/kg of 3% sodium chloride over 1 hour. In adults, the rapid overcorrection of hyponatremia (e.g., an increase in serum sodium of more than 2 mEq/L per hour) may be dangerous, producing the crippling or even fatal osmotic demyelination syndrome. The risk of this is greatest when a rapid overcorrection is made in a case of chronic hyponatremia.

In simple water intoxication, the normal kidney responds with maximal urinary dilution, which, when coupled with restriction of water intake, rapidly restores sodium concentration to normal. In syndrome of inappropriate antidiuretic hormone secretion and the edema-forming states, water

restriction is the initial treatment. Admission is recommended for any patient with symptomatic hyponatremia or hyponatremia per se (less than 130 mEq/L) when the cause is not obvious.

Disorders of Sodium Homeostasis: Hypernatremia

Clinical Manifestations

The causes of hypernatremia can be grouped into four major categories (Table 17.3) based on net changes in total body water and sodium. Symptoms and signs range from lethargy and irritability to muscle weakness, convulsions, and coma. Because ECF volume is defended early in the course of a dehydrating illness associated with hypernatremia, the classic physical sign of decreased skin turgor is absent until total fluid losses are severe (10% to 15% of body weight). The major complications of hypernatremia that require urgent diagnosis are seizures and coma.

Management

The algorithm in Figure 17.3 provides a working schema for evaluation and diagnosis.

In patients who are severely dehydrated, reexpansion with isotonic saline is the appropriate initial therapy. Osmotic diuretics, if previously given, must be stopped. Replacement of water and sodium losses with hypotonic electrolyte solutions is appropriate. Serum sodium should be lowered no more than 10 to 15 mEq/L per 24 hours to guard against brain edema. In hypertonic dehydration, a free-water deficit of 4 mL/kg for every 1 mEq/L of serum sodium greater than

TABLE 17.1. *Cause of hyponatremia*

Normal total body water and sodium (hyperosmolar hyponatremia)
  Hyperglycemia[a]
  Mannitol, glycerol therapy
Increased total body water and sodium (edema-forming states)
  Congestive heart failure
  Nephrosis
  Cirrhosis
  Acute renal failure
Decreased total body water and sodium (hypovolemic states)
  Gastrointestinal losses (vomiting, diarrhea, fistulae)
  Renal losses (diuretics, renal tubular acidosis, primary interstitial disease)
  Adrenal (mineralocorticoid deficiencies)
  Third-space losses (ascites, burns, pancreatitis, peritonitis)
Increased total body water but normal total body sodium
  Syndrome of inappropriate antidiuretic hormone secretion
  Water intoxication
  Miscellaneous (rest osmostat, hypothyroidism, glucocorticoid deficiency)
  Pseudohyponatremia
  Extreme hyperlipidemia or hyperproteinemia

[a] For every 100-mg/dL increase in plasma glucose concentration above normal, there is a corresponding decrease in plasma sodium concentration of approximately 1.6 mEq/L.

TABLE 17.2. *Symptoms and signs of hyponatremia*

Symptoms	Signs
Anorexia and nausea	Clouded sensorium
Muscle cramps	Decreased tendon reflexes
Lethargy	Pathologic reflexes
Disorientation	Cheyne–Stokes respiration
Agitation	Hypothermia
Acute respiratory failure	Seizures—pseudobulbar palsy

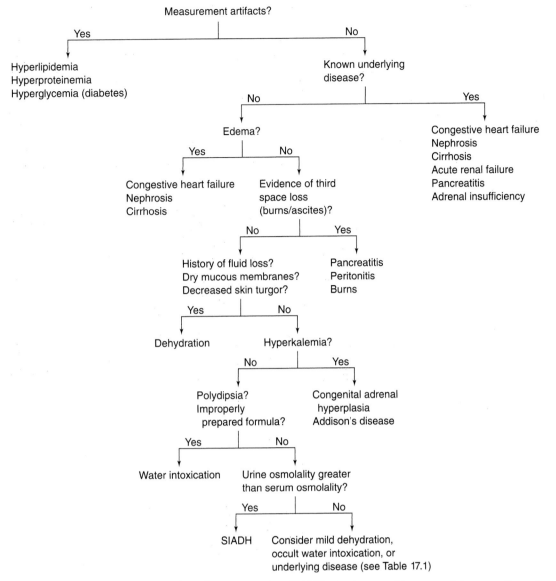

FIG. 17.2. Diagnostic approach to hyponatremia. *SIADH,* syndrome of inappropriate secretion of antidiuretic hormone.

TABLE 17.3. *Causes of hypernatremia*

Increased total body sodium or increased total body sodium greater than increased total body water
  Sodium poisoning (accidental; sodium bicarbonate therapy)
  Hyperaldosteronism (rare in children)
Normal total body sodium; "pure" water loss
  Insensible losses: respiratory and skin
  Renal (central and nephrogenic diabetes insipidus)
  Inadequate access to water
Decreased total body sodium less than decreased total body water
  Extrarenal (gastrointestinal)[a]
  Renal (osmotic diuretics; glucose, mannitol, urea)
  Obstructive uropathy
Normal total body sodium and water with abnormal central osmotic regulation of water balance
  Essential hypernatremia

[a] In diarrheal states, hypernatremia usually results from a combination of relatively greater water than sodium losses coupled with relatively greater sodium than water replacement.

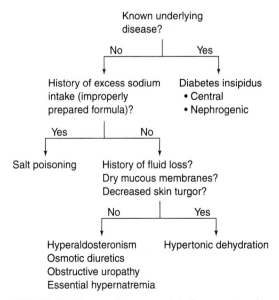

FIG. 17.3. Diagnostic approach to hypernatremia.

145 mEq/L should be replaced over 48 to 72 hours, along with the isotonic deficit, maintenance fluids and electrolytes, and ongoing losses.

The emergency treatment of the diabetes insipidus syndromes is free-water replacement, monitoring vital signs, clinical signs of dehydration, and serum sodium concentration as guides to the rate and volume of replacement.

Children who are victims of acute salt poisoning and are severely symptomatic can safely have serum sodium concentrations lowered rapidly, either by a combination of loop diuretics (0.5 to 2 mg/kg furosemide every 12 hours) and glucose water administration or, rarely, peritoneal dialysis against a sodium-free dialysate. The latter procedure should be carried out only in consultation with a nephrologist. Admission is recommended for any patient with symptomatic hypernatremia or severe hypernatremia per se (greater than 160 mEq/L) when the cause is not obvious.

Disorders of Potassium Homeostasis: Hypokalemia

Clinical Manifestations

The cause of hypokalemia (Table 17.4) can usually be suspected as belonging to one particular diagnostic category after obtaining a careful history. Symptoms are usually not seen at serum potassium concentrations greater than 3 mEq/L.

Nerve impulse propagation and the resultant muscle contraction are impaired in both striated and smooth muscle, leading to ileus, tetany, skeletal muscle weakness, and, if severe enough, paralysis and areflexia. Hypokalemia may cause rhabdomyolysis with myoglobinuria. Alteration of the cardiac action potential leads to conduction abnormalities

TABLE 17.4. *Causes of hypokalemia*

Apparent potassium deficit (transcellular shifts)
  Akalosis
  Familial hypokalemic periodic paralysis
  Insulin
  β_2 catecholamines (e.g. Albuterol)
Decreased intake
  Anorexia nervosa
  Unusual diets (rare in pediatrics)
Extrarenal losses
  Protracted vomitting (e.g., pyloric stenosis, gastric suction)
  Protracted diarrhea
  Ureterosigmoidostomy
  Laxative abuse (rare in pediatrics)
  Increased sweating (cystic fibrosis)
Renal losses
  Diuretic abuse (naturetic, osmotic agents)
  Renal tubular acidosis
  Diabetic ketoacidosis
  Excessive mineralocorticoid effect
Primary or secondary hyperaldosteronism
  Bartter syndrome
  Licorice abuse (rare in pediatrics)
  Cushing syndrome (rare in pediatrics)
Excessive administration of "impermeant anions" (carbenicillin)

and arrhythmias (see Chapter 4, Cardiothoracic Emergencies). Hypokalemia also causes renal-concentrating defects. Complications that require urgent diagnosis include acute respiratory failure from muscle paralysis, cardiac arrhythmias, and myoglobinuria, which can lead to acute renal failure (ARF).

To effectively manage hypokalemia in the emergency department (ED), one must delineate the source of the condition, as shown in Figure 17.4. If the electrolytes reveal a hyperchloremic hypokalemic metabolic acidosis with a normal anion gap and an alkaline urine pH, renal tubal acidosis (RTA) should be suspected. When there is a hypochloremic metabolic alkalosis, the urine electrolytes are helpful. A urine chloride less than 10 mEq/L suggests vomiting, cystic fibrosis, or diuretic abuse as the cause of hypokalemia. A urine chloride greater than 20 mEq/L points to one of the disorders that lead to mineralocorticoid excess. When the urinary potassium is less than 10 mEq/L, several conclusions can be drawn. First, the potassium deficiency has probably been present for at least 2 weeks. Second, the kidney can be excluded as the route of potassium depletion. An elevated urinary potassium concentration, however, suggests either potassium wasting of short duration or a primary renal loss.

Management

When hypokalemia results from simple transcellular shifts in response to alkalosis without an accompanying potassium deficit, correction of the pH is all that is required. In periodic paralysis, potassium supplementation with 2 to 6 mEq/kg per day is recommended with careful monitoring of serum potassium to avoid hyperkalemia as paralysis subsides. Potassium repletion should be slow (over days) and given by the oral route once urine flow is confirmed. IV loading should be avoided except under special conditions. Despite the fact that ECF potassium concentration does not reflect accurately total body potassium deficits, serum potassium concentration is the only practical way to assess adequacy of replacement and avoid unwanted complications. In adults, a serum potassium 1 mEq/L less than normal suggests a deficit of 200 to 300 mEq potassium. In terms of the quantitative rate of repair, this should be no more than 0.2 to 0.3 mEq/kg potassium per hour. However, if potentially life-threatening cardiac arrhythmia or respiratory paralysis is evident, as much as 1 mEq/kg per hour can be given by infusion pump with continuous electrocardiographic monitoring. The child with symptomatic hypokalemia requires admission for therapy and diagnostic workup, as do most children with a serum potassium less than 3.0 mEq/L.

Disorders of Potassium Homeostasis: Hyperkalemia

Clinical Manifestations

The categories of hyperkalemia are shown in Table 17.5. The predominant symptoms and signs are neuromuscular. Paresthesia is followed by weakness and even flaccid paralysis. Major toxicity is reflected in the electrocardiogram.

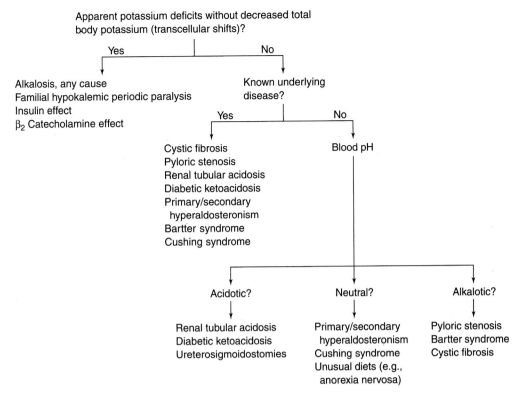

FIG. 17.4. Diagnostic approach to hypokalemia.

Peaked T waves may be seen at serum concentrations exceeding 6 mEq/L (Fig. 17.5). The PR interval increases and the QRS widens at more than 7 mEq/L. At more than 8 to 9 mEq/L, P waves disappear, the ventricular rate becomes irregular, and severe bradycardia or idioventricular rhythms occur (Fig. 17.6). Ventricular fibrillation or asystole occurs at serum concentrations greater than 12 to 14 mEq/L.

Hyperkalemia is often an early and life-threatening consequence of rhabdomyolysis. Elevated BUN and creatinine point to ARF. In acute adrenal insufficiency, urine sodium concentration is inappropriately high due to sodium wasting and urine potassium concentration is inappropriately low for their respective serum concentrations.

TABLE 17.5. *Causes of hyperkalemia*

Pseudohyperkalemia (hemolysis, extreme leukocytosis, or thrombocytosis)
    Apparent potassium excess (transcellular shifts)
    Acidosis
Increased intake
    Endogenous (rhabdomyolysis, massive hemolysis)
    Exogenous (suicide attempt with potassium salts)
Decreased excretion
    Acute or chronic renal failure (oliguria)
    Adrenal corticoid deficiency (acute adrenal insufficiency, hyporeninemic hypoaldosteronism)
    Use of potassium-sparing diuretics in renal failure or in conjunction with dietary potassium supplements
    Beta-blockers angiotensin converting enzyme inhibitors

Management

Determining the origin of hyperkalemia is crucial before managing this life-threatening condition. Figure 17.7 provides an algorithm for ascertaining the cause. Three general techniques are used (Table 17.6) to lower serum potassium levels to normal: (1) reverse the membrane effects, (2) transfer potassium into cells, and (3) enhance renal excretion of potassium. If patients are asymptomatic, serum potassium is less than 6.5 mEq/L and the electrocardiogram is normal or reveals only peaked T waves, all that may be required is discontinuation of potassium intake, removal of potassium-

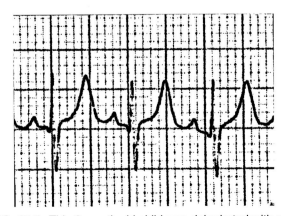

FIG. 17.5. This 6-month-old child was dehydrated with pre-renal azotemia and a serum potassium of 7.5 mEq/L. The V6 lead shows tall T waves.

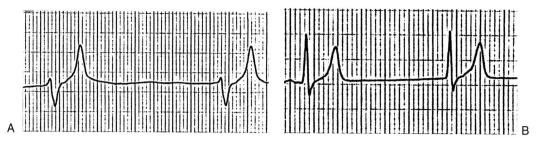

FIG. 17.6. A: This adolescent with end-stage renal disease was "not feeling well" for the past 24 hours. The initial electrocardiogram shows bradycardia, the absence of P waves, tall peaked T waves, and a wide QRS. His serum potassium was 9.0 mEq/L. **B:** Immediately after administration of calcium and sodium bicarbonate, his heart rate, P and T waves, and QRS duration improved.

sparing diuretics if they are being used, and treatment of acidosis. Exceptions to this occur in acute oliguric renal failure and rhabdomyolysis, in which the serum potassium level may rise precipitously to much higher levels, and a more aggressive therapeutic approach is indicated.

When electrocardiographic changes are more widespread and/or serum potassium is greater than 7.0 mEq/L, several available therapies are designed to move potassium into cells acutely, including glucose and insulin combination and sodium bicarbonate.

With the onset of cardiac arrhythmias or a serum potassium level greater than 8.0 mEq/L, urgent therapy is needed. Under continuous electrocardiographic monitoring, IV calcium is given first to reverse potentially life-threatening ar-

rhythmias without altering serum potassium. Calcium accomplishes this by restoring a more normal differential between the threshold and resting transmembrane potentials. This may be followed by glucose and insulin combination and sodium bicarbonate.

For more long-term control of hyperkalemia, the cation exchange resin sodium polystyrene sulfonate (Kayexalate) can be administered. Finally, in patients with oliguric renal failure, peritoneal dialysis removes potassium. The doses of drugs used to treat hyperkalemia, the recommended rates of administration, and onset of action are detailed in Table 17.6.

Any child with symptomatic hyperkalemia or a serum potassium level greater than 6.5 mEq/L on a nonhemolyzed sample deserves admission for therapy and additional workup.

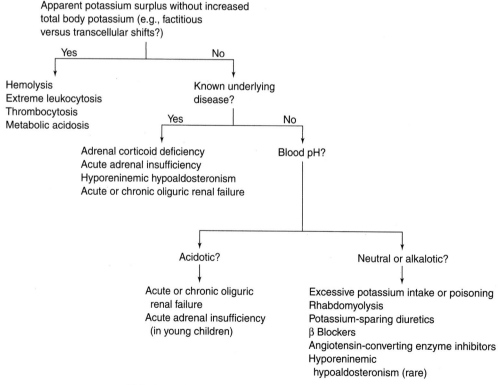

FIG. 17.7. Diagnostic approach to hyperkalemia.

TABLE 17.6. *Emergency treatment of hyperkalemia*

Technique	Agent	Dose	Rate of administration	Onset/duration of action	Comment
Reversal of membrane effects	10% calcium gluconate	0.5 mL/kg	2–5 min IV	Minutes/30–60 min	ECG monitor; discontinue if pulse rate <100
Movement of K into cells	7.5% Na bicarbonate (1 mEq 1 mL)	1–2 mEq/kg	30–60 min	30 min/1–4 hr	May use in the absence of acidosis
	25% glucose plus insulin (regular)	1 unit insulin for every 5 g glucose	Same	Same	Monitor blood glucose
Enhanced excretion of K	Kayexalate	1 g/kg	Can be given in 10% glucose (1 g in 4 mL) every 4–6 hr	Hours/variable	Can be given orally or rectally

IV, intravenous; ECG, electrocardiogram; K, potassium; Na, sodium.

Disorders of Acid-base Homeostasis: Metabolic Acidosis

Clinical Manifestations

Figure 17.8 offers an approach to the diagnosis. The clinical manifestations of metabolic acidosis usually reflect the predisposing illness. Tachypnea and hyperpnea are characteristic of severe lactic acidosis, and coma may ensue if the pH is significantly depressed.

Management

Initial therapy should be directed at the underlying disorder, e.g., saline or other appropriate fluids for dehydration and insulin for diabetic ketoacidosis. For alkali therapy, the preferred agent is usually $NaHCO_3$. Sodium lactate, given as lactated Ringer solution, is an acceptable alternative, provided that liver function is normal and lactic acidosis is ruled out. Patients require treatment if the serum HCO_3 is less than

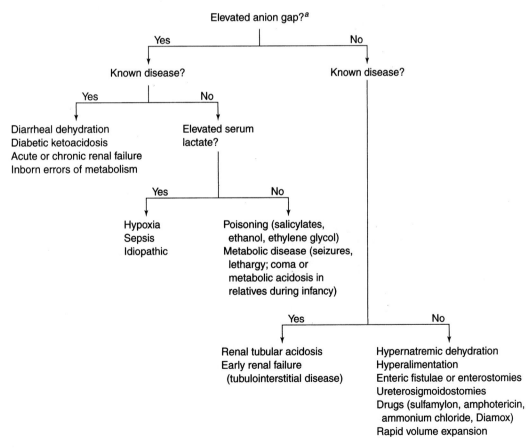

FIG. 17.8. Diagnostic approach to metabolic acidosis (reduced serum bicarbonate for age). *a*, anion gap = serum [Na]mEq/L − [Cl⁻ + HCO₃]mEq/L. Normal range in children is 16 ± 4 mEq/L.

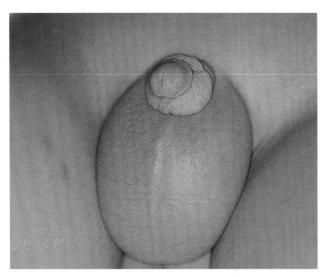

FIG. 17.9. This 7-year-old boy presented with scrotal swelling but had proteinuria and an albumin of 0.9 g/dL.

15 mEq/L and/or the pH is less than 7.20, unless the underlying disorder is simple diarrheal dehydration.

Of equal importance to the choice of alkali therapy is the amount of bicarbonate to use and the rate of repair. Calculations of the HCO$_3$ deficit may be as follows.

Mild/moderate acidosis (pH 7.20 to 7.37):

HCO$_3$ deficit in mEq = [normal serum (HCO$_3$)

− observed serum (HCO$_3$)]

× 20% of total body weight in liters

Severe acidosis (pH less than 7.20):

HCO$_3$ deficit in mEq = [normal serum (HCO$_3$)

× observed serum (HCO$_3$)]

× 50% of total body weight in liters

If the volume of infused solution must be limited, 7.5% NaHCO$_3$ (1 mEq/mL) is used; otherwise, lower concentrations should be used. Full correction of serum HCO$_3$ should never be attempted; a reasonable goal is to increase serum HCO$_3$ in increments of 5 to 10 mEq/L until a level of 15 to 18 mEq/L is achieved or a pH of 7.25 or greater. At this point, maintenance HCO$_3$ therapy can be continued at approximately 2 mEq/kg per day unless the underlying cause of the acidosis has been successfully treated. Overzealous alkali therapy is risky and can lead to a variety of complications including hypokalemia, alkalosis, cerebrospinal fluid acidosis, sodium overload, or hypokalemic tetany. Any child who requires IV alkali therapy should be admitted to the hospital.

SPECIFIC RENAL SYNDROMES

Nephrotic Syndrome

Clinical Manifestations

Nephrotic syndrome is the clinical expression for a variety of primary and secondary glomerular disorders, the hallmarks of which are hypoproteinemia (serum albumin less than 3.0 g/dL), proteinuria, and edema. Primary nephrotic syndrome is the term applied to diseases limited to the kidney. They are further classified according to the response to corticosteroid therapy and histology on renal biopsy. Secondary nephrotic syndrome is the term applied to multisystem disease in which the kidney is involved. Occasionally, nephrotic syndrome develops as a consequence of exposure to environmental agents, including heavy metals and bee venom.

Presentations

The major presenting complaint is edema, which may be localized (Fig. 17.9) or diffuse (Fig. 17.10). Rarely, salt and water retention is abrupt and massive, leading to respiratory

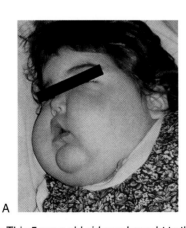

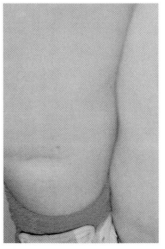

A   B

FIG. 17.10. A,B: This 5-year-old girl was brought to the emergency department with a 3-week history of "allergic" eyes and weight gain. She has diffuse edema, most pronounced either in the areas that are very distensible, such as her eyes and face, or dependent regions, such as her legs, which demonstrate pitting edema.

distress because of a combination of hydrothorax and ascites with elevation of the diaphragm.

Complications

The acute complications of nephrotic syndrome occur in two groups of patients: those who present *de novo* or in relapse but not taking steroids and those who present in relapse or remission while still receiving pharmacologic doses of steroids. Unusual bacterial infections such as peritonitis may occur. The typical signs and symptoms of infection may be masked in the steroid-treated nephrotic child, especially when the dose of steroid is high (e.g., 2 mg/kg prednisone per day). These patients are also at risk of thromboembolic complications due to a hypercoagulability state.

Symptomatic hypovolemia, which can progress to shock despite the presence of edema, results from injudicious fluid restriction, excess diuretic administration, or a combination of both. The problem is not total body water or salt depletion but intravascular depletion that results from the abnormal distribution of what amounts to excess total body salt and water in the interstitial spaces.

In steroid-treated children, acute increases in blood pressure (BP) with symptoms of headache, blurred vision, or frank encephalopathy may occur at any point in the clinical course. Acute mood changes, ranging from euphoria to depression, are associated with the sudden increase or decrease of steroid therapy. Abrupt reductions in steroids may lead to benign intracranial hypertension characterized by headaches, vomiting, and occasional papilledema, which are not associated with hypertension.

Management

Acute management of nephrotic syndrome can be divided into two categories: specific and supportive. In the ED, the primary goal is usually to restore and preserve intravascular volume or to treat symptomatic edema.

Despite the presence of peripheral edema, shock is treated in the usual way, with 20 mL/kg per hour of normal saline until circulation is restored. If the child is clinically dehydrated but not in shock, a trial of sodium-deficient fluids orally at twice maintenance is preferable to an immediate start of hypotonic IV solutions (i.e., 5% dextrose in 0.25 N salt solution). Fluids should be given in small amounts at frequent intervals) to avoid vomiting caused by an edematous gut. Although sodium restriction is indicated for an edematous nephrotic child, water restriction is rarely indicated and only further decreases a usually low urine output.

If the patient is well hydrated but symptomatic from massive edema, a trial of diuretics is warranted. Symptoms include difficulty in ambulating, abdominal discomfort, skin breakdown, and respiratory distress. Furosemide (1 to 2 mg/kg per day in two divided oral doses) can be used. If there is no response, additional diuretics that act at other sites in the tubule (thus enhancing the diuretic effect) may be added. Commonly used agents are spironolactone and hydrochlorothiazide, both starting at 1 mg/kg per day in two doses. Diuretics do not usually work, however, if the serum albumin concentration is less than 1.5 g/dL. When it appears urgent to remove some edema fluid, a combination of albumin infusions followed 30 minutes later by IV furosemide is often effective. The dose of albumin is 0.5 to 1.0 g/kg given as 25% salt-deficient albumin followed by 0.5 to 1.0 mg/kg furosemide. Paracentesis is rarely indicated but may bring prompt relief of severe respiratory distress from massive ascites.

After consultation with a nephrologist, prednisone is generally begun at a dose of 2 mg/kg per day in two divided doses after the workup is initiated and a tuberculin test is placed. If the patient has previously been responsive to prednisone, a return to full therapy is indicated, provided frank relapse is obvious. If not, a quantitative 24-hour urine test should be ordered. Concurrent administration of a low-sodium antacid may reduce the risk of gastric irritation.

Antibiotics are not administered prophylactically but are used when a bacterial infection is suspected. Any child with active nephrotic syndrome and an unexplained fever must be considered to have a bacterial infection until proved otherwise. A blood culture is indicated, and diagnostic paracentesis for Gram stain and culture is appropriate in the presence of obvious ascites. Initial coverage with cefotaxime for possible *Streptococcus pneumoniae* or Gram-negative bacterial infection may be indicated.

Hypertension

Clinical Manifestations

Hypertension reflects an elevation of BP above the upper limits of normal (Table 17.7) and arises from numerous causes (Table 17.8). Hypertension usually presents in one of four ways.

First, there is the asymptomatic or mildly symptomatic child with mild to moderate elevations in BP. Second, malignant hypertension is characterized by marked elevations in systolic and/or diastolic BP (e.g., 160 mm Hg or higher systolic for those younger than 10 years of age; 170 mm Hg or higher systolic for those older than 10 years; 105 mm Hg or higher diastolic for those younger than 10 years; 110 mm Hg or higher diastolic for those older than 10 years) and is often associated with papilledema and hemorrhages and exudates on funduscopic examination. Third, accelerated hypertension is defined as an acute increase in BP superimposed on previously existing hypertension. In both malignant hypertension and acceler-

TABLE 17.7. *Hypertension*

Age (yr)	Upper limit of normal (mm Hg)	
	Systolic	Diastolic
0–2	110	65
3–6	120	70
7–10	130	75
11–15	140	80

TABLE 17.8. *Causes of hypertension*

Primary
  Essential hypertension
Secondary
  Renal
    Acute or chronic glomerulonephritis
      Postinfectious
      Henoch–Schönlein purpura
      Systemic lupus erythematosus
      Membranoproliferative nephritis
    Hemolytic uremic syndrome
    Pyelonephritis (reflux nephropathy)
    Obstructive uropathy (with or without urinary infection)
    Segmental hypoplasia (Ask–Upmark kidney)
    Renal vascular disease (renal artery stenosis, embolus)
    Hemodialysis or renal transplant patients
  Endocrine
    Pheochromocytoma
    Cushing syndrome
    Treatment with adrenocortical steroids
    Hyperthyroidism
  Cardiac
    Coarctation of the aorta
    Congestive heart failure (multiple causes)
  Neurologic
    Central nervous system infection, drugs, tumor
Miscellaneous drugs or poisons

TABLE 17.10. *Differential diagnosis of hypertensive encephalopathy*

Head trauma
Cerebral hemorrhage or infarction
Meningitis, encephalitis
Brain tumor
Uremic encephalopathy

ated hypertension, the patient may present with dramatic symptoms and signs such as heart murmur, congestive heart failure, lower motor neuron facial palsy, and hematuria. Fourth, hypertensive encephalopathy is often seen in malignant hypertension and consists of a combination of symptoms and signs that often vary from patient to patient (Table 17.9). The diagnosis is confirmed by demonstrating a rapid improvement in the symptoms and signs after the BP is lowered.

Ascertaining the cause of increased BP in the acutely hypertensive child with an abnormal neurologic examination presents a difficult challenge (Table 17.10). When there is primary neurologic disease with secondary hypertension, the hypertension is usually mild and predominantly systolic. If signs and symptoms clear rapidly, he or she is probably dealing with true hypertensive encephalopathy. Primary neurologic disease can be screened for by a spinal tap (if a mass lesion is not suspected) or computed tomography scan.

When confronted with newly diagnosed hypertension in the child, the physician should ask three important questions: (1) Is the hypertension primary or secondary? (2) Is there evidence of target organ injury? (3) Are there associated risk factors that would worsen the prognosis if the hypertension were not treated?

TABLE 17.9. *Malignant hypertensive encephalopathy*

Nausea, vomiting
Headaches
Altered mental status or psychiatric symptoms
Visual disturbances (blurry vision, decreased visual acuity, diplopia)
Seizures, stroke

Management

Acute Management of Hypertension

A brief but careful history and physical examination aim to classify the severity of the hypertension. When the hypertension is severe, this evaluation should progress only after airway, breathing, and circulation have been stabilized. Emphasis should be placed on the neurologic examination, searching for any evidence of dysfunction.

The presence or absence of acute end-organ dysfunction, not the height of the BP, distinguishes hypertensive urgency from a hypertensive emergency.

Hypertensive Emergency

In a hypertensive emergency, an IV line should be placed immediately to allow administration of medications and fluid resuscitation if indicated. Many patients in hypertensive crisis have volume depletion caused by vomiting, diarrhea, or a diuresis of unclear origin. A cardiac monitor should be used and the BP monitored continuously, preferably by arterial catheter. Any serious complications must be managed before or while the hypertension is treated (e.g., anticonvulsants should be administered to a seizing patient along with hypertensive medications).

In a hypertensive emergency, the goal is to lower the BP promptly but gradually. The mean arterial pressure should be lowered by 25% over several minutes (e.g., for a patient who is seizing or herniating) to several hours (e.g., for a patient with headache or vomiting). The patient's BP and neurologic status must be assessed frequently. Precipitous decreases in BP can lead to avoidable neurologic deficits. The preferred drugs are those that allow close monitoring of BP reduction. Recommended emergency setting medications are described in Table 17.11.

Hypertensive Urgency

Hypertensive urgency is defined as severe hypertension without evidence of end-organ involvement. Patients with known hypertension who present in an urgent hypertensive crisis may not require hospitalization if the therapy in the ED is successful and adequate follow-up can be ensured. Often, oral antihypertensive agents will be sufficient (Table 17.12), although occasionally parenteral therapy is indicated. A 4- to 6-hour period of observation should follow the administration of the antihypertensive

TABLE 17.11. *Drugs used in hypertensive emergencies*

Drug	Initial dose	Administration	Onset of action	Interval to repeat or dose (min)	Duration of action	Acute side effects
Nitroprusside	0.5 μg/kg/min	IV infusion	Instantaneous	30–60	Only during infusion	Headache; abdominal pain; chest pain, NaCl, H_2O retention
Diazoxide	3–5 mg/kg (max., 150 mg/dose)	Rapid IV push into vein	Minutes	15–30	4–12 hr	Hyperglycemia; hyperuricemia; NaCl, H_2O retention
Hydralazine	0.1–0.5 mg/kg (max., 20 mg)	IV infusion over 15–30 min	20 min	10	4–12 hr	Tachycardia; flushing; headache; vomiting, NaCl, H_2O retention
Labetalol	0.25–0.5 mg/kg (max. initial dose 20 mg)	IV infusion while supine	5 min	10	To 24 hr	GI upset; scalp tingling; headache; sedation
Nifedipine	0.25–0.5 mg/kg (max., 20 mg)	Bite and swallow or sublingual	15–30 min	30–60	6 hr	Dizziness; facial flushing (contraindicated in the presence of intracerebral bleeding)
Phentolamine	0.1 mg/kg	IV	Instantaneous	30	30–60 min	Tachycardia; abdominal pain

max., maximum; IV, intravenous; NaCl, sodium chloride; GI, gastrointestinal.

agent in the ED. This should be done to identify any untoward effects of the medication such as orthostasis. Patients should be discharged on the same medication used in the ED.

When hypertension is discovered by accident and is not the reason for the patient's visit, medical follow-up for repeated BP measurements is indicated before therapy is begun, especially if the elevation is mild (no more than 5 to 10 mm Hg above the upper limits of normal for systolic and diastolic pressures given in Table 17.7). If the BP is moderately elevated but the patient is asymptomatic, two options exist. Arrangements can be made for an outpatient workup in the future and a thiazide diuretic or beta-blocker may be initiated at a low dose. Alternatively, the patient may be admitted to begin an evaluation and therapy under hospital observation.

Acute Renal Failure

Clinical Manifestations

Presentation

The presentation of ARF varies and usually relates to the underlying disorder (Table 17.13). Typical symptoms and signs are given in Table 17.14 together with the likely diagnosis. If solute retention is severe and has persisted for days to weeks before seeking medical attention, the clinical manifestations of uremia may ensue and obscure, for the moment, the underlying diagnosis (Table 17.15). One consideration that must always be raised in a patient with suspected ARF is whether it has occurred *de novo* or is superimposed on preexisting chronic renal failure. Clinical clues that may lead to the latter diagnosis are failure to thrive, a history of polyuria/polydipsia, continued good urine output despite historical and physical evidence of dehydration, and physical evidence of renal rickets.

Complications

The major complications in terms of frequency and threat to life are disturbances in serum tonicity and water balance; severe hyperkalemia with impending or actual cardiac arrhythmia; congestive heart failure with pulmonary edema, usually secondary to hypertension; malignant hypertensive encephalopathy with seizures; urinary tract infection with associated urinary obstruction; and metabolic seizures.

TABLE 17.12. *Drugs used in hypertensive urgencies*

Drug	Dose	Administration	Onset	Duration
Nifedipine	0.25–0.5 mg/kg	Bite and swallow or sublingual	15–30 min	6 hr
Captopril	Age <6 mo, 0.05–0.5 mg/kg; age >6 mo, 0.3–2.0 mg/kg	Oral	15–30 min	8–12 hr
Minoxidil	2.5–5.0 mg	Oral	2 hr	12 hr

TABLE 17.13. *Causes of acute renal failure*[a]

Prerenal
  Decreased cardiac output (cardiogenic shock)
  Decreased intravascular volume (hemorrhage, dehydration, "third-spacing")
Renal
  Primary renal parenchymal disease
    Vascular (acute glomerulonephritis, hemolytic uremic syndrome (HUS))
    Interstitial (pyelonephritis, drug induced)
    Acute tubular necrosis
    Ischemic injury
    Nephrotoxic injury (antibiotics, uric acid)
    Pigmenturia (myoglobinuria, hemoglobinuria)
Postrenal
  Obstructive uropathy
    Posterior urethral valves
    Intraabdominal tumor
    Nephrolithiasis (rare)
      Renal vein thrombosis (rare outside the neonatal period)

[a] Major pediatric causes of acute renal failure are in parentheses.

Laboratory and Radiographic Studies

The urinalysis is most helpful in separating glomerulonephritis from the other causes of ARF. In the typical case of acute glomerulonephritis, the dipstick shows large amounts of blood and protein, and red blood cells (RBC), granular, and cellular (i.e., RBC) casts are in the spun sediment. Patients with prerenal ARF and those with acute tubular necrosis typically have little blood or protein by dipstick and an unremarkable sediment save for hyaline casts.

Typically, the patient with prerenal ARF has a concentrated urine (specific gravity, >1.025), whereas the patient with acute tubular necrosis tends to have an isosthenuric urine (specific gravity, 1.005 to 1.015). Hematuria by dipstick examination without corresponding RBCs in the sediment suggests hemoglobinuria or myoglobinuria as the

TABLE 17.15. *Acute renal failure: clinical uremia*

Gastrointestinal
  Nausea, vomiting, diarrhea
  Hiccoughs, fetid odor
  Hematemesis, melena
Cardiovascular
  Pericarditis
Dermatologic
  Pruritus
  Uremic "frost"
Neurologic
  Apathy, fatigue
  Psychiatric disturbance
  Seizures
  Asterixis
  Coma
  Peripheral neuropathy

cause of ARF, especially if pigmented granular casts are also seen. Renal tubular and bladder epithelial cells and epithelial cell casts are commonly seen in nephrotoxic ARF or drug-induced (hypersensitivity) acute interstitial nephritis. Pyuria supports the diagnosis of acute pyelonephritis.

Fractional excretion of filtered sodium (FENa) assists in differentiating prerenal ARF from acute tubular necrosis. In older children and adults, a FENa percentage $\{[(\text{urine sodium/plasma sodium})/(\text{urine creatinine/plasma creatinine})] \times 100\} < 1.0$ suggests prerenal causes, and a level greater than 1.0 suggests intrinsic pathology such as acute tubular necrosis of various causes. In neonates and very young infants, a cutoff of 2.5% may be more accurate. Other diagnostic studies are outlined in Table 17.16.

Management

When confronted with a child who has ARF, the ED physician should always ask the following questions about therapy: (1) Is this prerenal renal failure and can parenchymal

TABLE 17.14. *Acute renal failure presenting symptoms and signs*

Symptoms	Signs	Likely diagnosis
Nausea, vomiting		Gastroenteritis (ATN)
Diarrhea	Dehydration, shock	Gastroenteritis (ATN)
Hemorrhage	Shock	ATN
Fever	Petechiae, bleeding	Sepsis, DIC (ACN)
Melena		HUS
Sudden pallor		HUS
Grand mal seizures		HUS
Fever, chills	Flank tenderness	Pyelonephritis
Fever, skin rash	Erythema multiforme, purpura	AIN
		HSP nephritis
Sore throat	Hypertension	PSGN
Pyoderma	Edema	PSGN
Grand mal seizures	Congestive heart failure	PSGN
Trauma	Muscle tenderness	Myoglobinuria
Myalgia	Myoedema	Myoglobinuria
Antibiotics, diuretics		Nephrotoxic acute renal failure
Variable urine output	Suprapubic mass	OU

ATN, acute tubular necrosis; DIC, disseminated intravascular coagulation; ACN, acute cortical necrosis; HUS, hemolytic uremic syndrome; AIN, acute interstitial nephritis (hypersensitivity nephritis); HSP, Henoch–Schönlein purpura nephritis; PSGN, poststreptococcal glomerulonephritis; OU, obstructive uropathy.

TABLE 17.16. *Acute renal failure laboratory tests for diagnosis*

Test	Diagnosis
Blood	
Platelet count	HUS, DIC
Blood smear	HUS, DIC
Coagulation profile	HUS, DIC
Streptococcal serologies	PSGN
C3 complement	PSGN
Antinuclear antibody	Systemic lupus erythematosus nephritis
IgE, eosinophil count	AIN
Creatine phosphokinase	Myoglobinuria
Haptoglobin, "pink" plasma	Hemoglobinuria
Urine	
Culture	Acute pyelonephritis
Protein (24 hr)	Acute nephritis
Uric acid (24 hr or Uuric:Ucreatinine ratio)	Uric acid nephropathy
Radiology	
Renal ultrasonogram	Obstructive uropathy
Intravenous pyelogram	Obstructive uropathy, pyelonephritis
Voiding cystourethrogram	Underlying chronic renal disease, obstructive uropathy
Renal flow scan	Acute tubular necrosis (cortical necrosis), renal vascular insult

HUS, hemolytic uremic syndrome; DIC, disseminated intravascular coagulation (bacterial sepsis); PSGN, poststreptococcal glomerulonephritis; IgE, immunoglobulin E; AIN, acute interstitial nephritis (hypersensitivity nephritis).

ARF be prevented by the appropriate fluid therapy? (2) Are there any life-threatening complications evident at this time that must be treated immediately? (3) Is there urinary tract infection with associated obstruction that must be relieved immediately? (4) Are there indications for immediate peritoneal dialysis or hemodialysis?

1. If prerenal ARF is suspected from the clinical history, physical examination, and laboratory tests, fluid resuscitation should be used. Confirmation of this diagnosis requires a resumption of normal urine flow and a decrease in solute retention after restoration of euvolemia. Crystalloid solution (20 mL/kg per hour), such as normal saline, should be administered until urine flow is reestablished. If no urine is produced in 2 or 3 hours, the patient should be catheterized. If no urine is in the bladder, administer 2 mg/kg furosemide intravenously, and if still no urine is produced, treat as though the cause is parenchymal ARF. One exception to this approach might be the patient who is euvolemic or even hypervolemic but in cardiogenic shock.

One clinical condition that demands the use of mannitol and furosemide is myoglobinuria or hemoglobinuria. Here the purpose of therapy is to prevent tubular obstruction by pigmented proteins after ECF volume is restored. IV furosemide (1 to 2 mg/kg) is given initially followed 5 to 10 minutes later by 0.5 g/kg mannitol. After urine flow is established, an infusion of 5% mannitol in one-fourth strength saline can be administered as milliliter-for-milliliter replacement of urine until the pigmenturia has resolved. Finally, failure to respond to a fluid challenge or a fluid plus diuretic challenge has one of three explanations: (1) volume losses have been underestimated, (2) there is coexistent urinary obstruction, or (3) the patient has already developed parenchymal ARF. The major risk of mannitol occurs in a parenchymal ARF because, if not excreted, it will recirculate and may cause ECF volume expansion.

2. Regarding life-threatening complications of ARF, the therapy of hypertensive emergencies has been discussed previously. In euvolemic or clinically edematous patients, the treatment is fluid restoration and no extra sodium. Hypocalcemia is also common but rarely symptomatic in ARF and should not be treated with supplemental calcium until and unless the serum phosphorus concentration is known. Failure to take this precaution may result in increasing the calcium P_i product and risk ectopic calcification or further renal damage. Metabolic acidosis does not need correction unless the serum bicarbonate is less than 15 mEq/L, and only then with slow replacement with 1 mEq/kg bicarbonate per day and frequent monitoring. A sudden shift of the pH toward normal or an alkaline range can convert asymptomatic hypocalcemia into frank tetany. Treatment of hyperkalemia is often the most urgent goal in ARF. Specifics of therapy for varying levels of serum potassium are outlined in Table 17.17.

3. If the clinical picture, urinalysis, and Gram stain suggest urinary tract infection, then coexistent obstructive uropathy must be ruled out rapidly by performing renal ultrasonography. The indications for dialysis are outlined in Table 17.18.

TABLE 17.17. *Acute renal failure: emergency treatment of hyperkalemia*

1. Serum K 5.5–7.0 mEq/L (normal ECG): 1 g/kg Kayexelate orally or rectally[a]
2. Serum K >7.5 mEq/L or >7.0 mEq/L with abnormal ECG[b]:
   Step 1. 0.5 mL/kg calcium gluconate as 10% solution over 2–4 min with ECG monitoring; stop when pulse rate decreases to 20 beats/min or to <100 beats/min
   Step 2. 3.3 mL/kg sodium bicarbonate as 7.5% solution
   Step 3. 1 mL/kg glucose as 50% solution; if hyperkalemia persists, infuse 20–30% glucose solution with 0.5 U/kg regular insulin; keep blood sugar <300 mg/dL
3. Serum K persistently >6.5 mEq/L: dialysis

K, potassium; ECG, electrocardiogram.
[a] Kayexelate exchanges 1 mEq potassium for 1 mEq sodium and lowers serum potassium by approximately 1 mEq/L within 4 hours. It can be administered orally with food or beverage, by nasogastric tube, or rectally in 10% glucose/water (1 g in 4 mL) or in 20% sorbitol (50–100 mL). It must be retained for at least 30 minutes.
[b] Serum potassium >7.0 with a normal electrocardiogram can be treated as outlined in step 1.

TABLE 17.18. *Acute renal failure: indications for peritoneal dialysis*

Uremic syndrome
Blood urea nitrogen >100 mg/dL
Persistent hyperkalemia (serum potassium >6.5 mEq/L)
Persistent metabolic acidosis (serum bicarbonate <10 mEq/L)
Persistent congestive heart failure
Oliguric acute renal failure secondary to hemolytic uremic syndrome or rhabdomyolysis with myoglobinuria

Hemolytic Uremic Syndrome

Clinical Manifestations

Historical features of diarrhea-associated hemolytic uremic syndrome include abdominal pain and often bloody diarrhea. Vomiting may be present, but *Escherichia coli* O157:H7 infection rarely results in fever. Within the first week of symptoms, the patient will experience an abrupt onset of pallor, listlessness, irritability, and oliguria. Physical examination reveals a sallow complexioned, listless, dehydrated child who may have edema, hypertension, petechiae, and/or hepatosplenomegaly. Some degree of encephalopathy is present in most patients, and some progress to obtundation, hemiparesis, seizures, and brainstem dysfunction. The initial impression may be that of a surgical abdomen, primary colitis, or intussusception when hematochezia is the predominant complaint.

Diagnosis of hemolytic uremic syndrome is based on the clinical profile of hemolytic anemia, thrombocytopenia, and ARF. The anemia is severe in many cases with a hemoglobin of 5 to 9 g/dL, and the platelet count can drop as low as 20,000/mm^3. The peripheral smear shows helmet cells, burr cells, and schistocytes, confirming the microangiopathic process. The urinalysis reveals hematuria, sometimes gross, with variable degrees of proteinuria and leukocyturia. Granular and hyaline casts are often seen in the urine sediment. Chemical studies reveal azotemia, metabolic acidosis, hyperbilirubinemia, and an increased lactate dehydrogenase. Specific stool testing for *E. coli* O157:H7 should be sent.

Management

The cornerstone of treatment remains early recognition and supportive care. Oliguric ARF is best managed by dialysis when any one of the following complications occurs: (1) BUN more than 100 mg/dL, (2) congestive heart failure, (3) encephalopathy, and (4) hyperkalemia, particularly if associated with an arrhythmia. The microangiopathic process is managed with transfusions of blood and platelets as clinically indicated. There has been no efficacy demonstrated in the use of fresh frozen plasma or plasmapheresis in the diarrhea-associated form of hemolytic uremic syndrome. However, success has been reported after infusion of fresh frozen plasma in patients with the nondiarrheal form of hemolytic uremic syndrome.

Acute Glomerulonephritis

Clinical Manifestations

Various causes may lead to acute glomerulonephritis. These causes can be divided into conditions that affect the kidney and conditions that are more systemic in nature that may present with renal manifestations. The typical story is that of a 5- or 6-year-old boy who, 1 to 2 weeks after a sore throat, develops the sudden onset of brown, tea-colored, or grossly bloody urine in association with peripheral edema, particularly around the eyes, and a decreased urinary output. On examination, hypertension is found. Some children are completely asymptomatic and present merely with abnormally colored urine. Rarely, patients develop acute congestive heart failure or acute malignant hypertensive encephalopathy. These patients are particularly challenging for the emergency physician because the complications often mask the underlying disease. Seventy-five percent of children have edema and abnormally colored urine.

The emergency physician must always consider an underlying chronic nephritis with an acute exacerbation when making the diagnosis of acute glomerulonephritis *de novo*.

The findings on urinalysis are important in categorizing glomerulonephritis. Proteinuria is almost always greater than 2+ on the dipstick, indicating that the protein present is not merely a result of the hematuria itself. RBC casts are the hallmark of acute glomerulonephritis of any cause. Urinary tract infection can present with proteinuria and hematuria; therefore, in female patients, a urine culture should be obtained.

Management

The goals of the emergency physician are to recognize the diagnosis and to treat life-threatening emergencies secondary to hypertension, as discussed in the Hypertension section. Encephalopathy requires antihypertensive therapy only if the link between severe hypertension and the neurologic abnormalities is noted immediately.

Any child with acute glomerulonephritis who is oliguric or hypertensive should be admitted for close observation. In the mildly affected patient, discharge from the ED is reasonable if the patient is instructed to follow a low-sodium diet. A follow-up appointment within 48 to 72 hours with the primary physician is advised, and instructions are given to the family on following urine output and weight and observing for the signs and symptoms of hypertension.

Henoch–Schönlein Purpura

Antecedent upper respiratory tract infections are frequently noted in patients with Henoch–Schönlein purpura, which is characterized by rash, joint swelling, abdominal pain, and renal involvement. The rash is symmetric and purpuric and most noticeable over the extensor surfaces of the arms, legs, and buttocks (Fig. 17.11). The joint swelling is migratory,

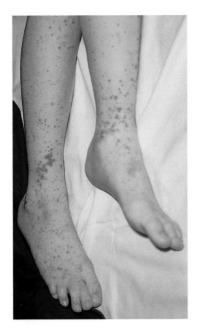

FIG. 17.11. This patient demonstrates the classic appearance of the rash over the lower distal extremity.

affecting the larger joints (Fig. 17.12). The abdominal pain is described as colicky and often severe (Fig. 17.13). Intestinal involvement can result in rectal bleeding or intussusception, as illustrated in Figure 1.14 in Chapter 1 (Abdominal Emergencies). Scrotal pain can be a presenting complaint leading to an evaluation for testicular torsion (Fig. 17.14).

Renal involvement is variable but typically occurs in the first month of illness. Asymptomatic microhematuria occurs most commonly. Azotemia is usually transient. The older the child and the later the onset of renal involvement are, especially if there is nephrosis-range proteinuria and/or renal insufficiency, the worse the prognosis is. Laboratory studies should always include a urinalysis. It the urinalysis is abnormal, a complete blood count, electrolytes, BUN, creatinine, serum proteins, and C3 complement should be obtained. The diagnosis is primarily based on clinical findings. There is no specific therapy for Henoch–Schönlein purpura other than

the possible use of corticosteroids to treat the severe abdominal pain that occurs in some patients.

Renal Tubular Acidosis

RTA is a syndrome characterized by a persistent hyperchloremic nonanion gap metabolic acidosis due to abnormal renal regulation of the bicarbonate reabsorption and/or regeneration. A child with RTA may come to the ED with an acute urinary tract infection, muscle weakness and/or an adynamic ileus of the bowel secondary to profound hypokalemia, or acute renal colic secondary to the passage of renal calculi.

Management

The immediate treatment of RTA in the ED depends on the severity of signs and symptoms of hypokalemia (see section on hypokalemia). Administration of alkali is the treatment of choice for most types of RTA. However, overzealous IV alkali therapy should not be attempted because an increase in blood pH often lowers serum potassium and may exacerbate symptoms of weakness and/or cardiac arrhythmia. Therapy of this disorder is best carried out in conjunction with a nephrologist.

Urolithiasis

Clinical Manifestations

Children with urolithiasis often present with abdominal pain. In infants, such pain may be confused with colic, and a pink-stained diaper may provide a clue. Hematuria, either microscopic or macroscopic, occurs in 90% of children with urolithiasis. A family history of urolithiasis can be elicited in 50% of patients. Abdominal, costovertebral angle, and/or flank tenderness may be present.

Management

If the history and physical examination are suggestive of urolithiasis, one should proceed to the detection of the calcu-

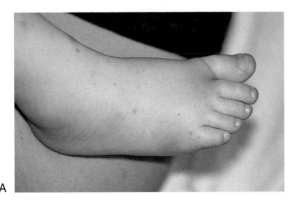

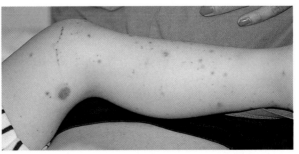

FIG. 17.12. A: The child's ankle and foot appear swollen with minimal discoloration. **B:** The patient's upper leg has a more classic Henoch–Schönlein purpura rash.

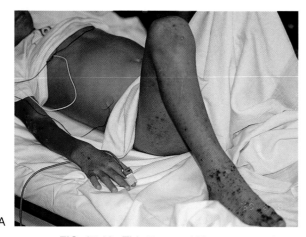
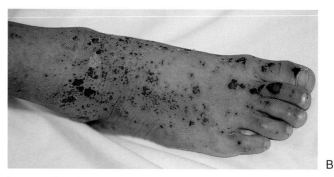

FIG. 17.13. This 7-year-old boy presented appearing very ill with severe pain and abdominal distention **(A)** and skin lesions suggestive of sepsis **(B)**. He developed small bowel obstruction due to jejunal inflammation.

lus and acute management (Fig. 17.15). If a urinary calculus is not found but the history is suspicious of calculus disease, it is likely that the patient has already passed the stone and is currently experiencing the aftermath of stone passage (i.e., spasm and dilation of the ureter). In this scenario, one must carefully examine the urine for crystalluria and hematuria and search for an increased Ca:Cr ratio.

Prompt pain relief with narcotic analgesics such as morphine sulfate or meperidine may be necessary. Nonsteroidal antiinflammatory medication may be used if the patient can tolerate oral medications. IV hydration may be required to ensure an adequate urine flow rate. If there is no evidence of urinary obstruction or renal insufficiency, fluids should be run at twice the maintenance requirement. When an associated urinary tract infection is suspected, appropriate antimicrobials should be initiated after culture. If urinary obstruction is suspected, sonography should be performed and an urologic consultation obtained. All urine should be strained to collect stone particles for analysis. If a patient is known to have renal insufficiency, the management of superimposed urolithiasis should be done in conjunction with a pediatric nephrolo-

gist. Patients with urolithiasis should be admitted if they have urinary obstruction, renal insufficiency, a solitary kidney, or intractable pain or are unable to tolerate oral fluid.

Chronic Renal Failure

Clinical Findings

Many patients are not known to have chronic renal failure when they present acutely to the ED. Clues in the history are excessive fatigue, anorexia, vomiting, skeletal pain, polyuria, and polydipsia. On physical examination, signs of anemia, a fetid breath, chronic changes of hypertension, asterixis, and peripheral neuropathy are clues. Signs and symptoms of chronic renal failure usually begin at a glomerular filtration rate of 20% of normal or less.

Management

Disturbances in fluid, electrolyte, and acid-base balance; calcium and vitamin D metabolism; and cardiovascular and

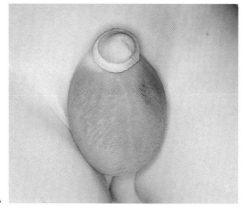
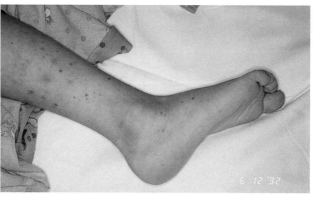

FIG. 17.14. This 6-year-old boy was referred for severe testicular pain and to "rule out" testicular torsion. **A:** The patient's scrotum was swollen with a small area of possible purpura. **B:** The more typical Henoch–Schönlein purpura rash is only seen when the patient's lower extremity is examined.

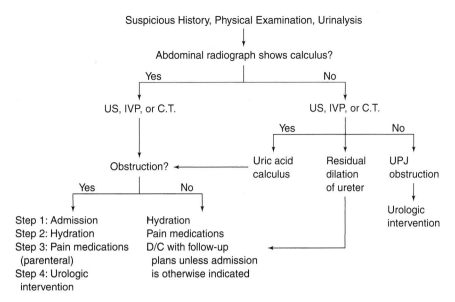

Suspicious History, Physical Examination, Urinalysis

↓

Abdominal radiograph shows calculus?

Yes / No

US, IVP, or C.T. / US, IVP, or C.T.

Yes / No

Obstruction? ← Uric acid calculus / Residual dilation of ureter / UPJ obstruction

Yes / No

Step 1: Admission
Step 2: Hydration
Step 3: Pain medications (parenteral)
Step 4: Urologic intervention

Hydration
Pain medications
D/C with follow-up plans unless admission is otherwise indicated

Urologic intervention

FIG. 17.15. Diagnostic approach for evaluation for urinary calculi. *US*, ultrasonography; *IVP*, intravenous pyelography; *D/C*, discharge; *UPJ*, ureteropelvic junction.

neurologic function predominate in end-stage renal failure and are outlined in Table 17.19. Anemia in end-stage renal failure has been managed successfully with a combination of effective dialysis and recombinant erythropoietin injections. The monitoring of water intake is required to avoid hyponatremia and hypernatremia because the kidneys' ability to modulate urinary water excretion is greatly reduced. Potassium retention is a significant risk in end-stage renal failure, particularly in patients who have not yet started dialysis. Accumulation of organic acids and the inability of the damaged kidney to regenerate new bicarbonate buffer explain the metabolic acidosis of end-stage renal failure.

Of particular note is the dialysis dysequilibrium syndrome, characterized by headache, nausea and vomiting, visual disturbances, disorientation, wide swings in BP, and seizures. This rare condition occurs when initial dialysis (usually hemodialysis) lowers a significantly elevated BUN (150 mg/dL or greater) too rapidly, allowing water to move into brain cells and cause cerebral edema. Rapid infusion of mannitol is often effective in reversing these signs and symptoms.

Rhabdomyolysis

Clinical Manifestations

Rhabdomyolysis may be caused by a number of disorders, including trauma, intoxications, seizures, infections, endocrinopathies, and metabolic defects and may lead to significant injury of skeletal muscle (Table 17.20). The classic triad of complaints in rhabdomyolysis consists of myalgias, weakness, and dark urine. Myalgias may be the predominant manifestation, with or without mild weakness. The emergency physician should inquire about preceding viral infections, exercise, environmental conditions, injuries, bite wounds, ingestions, and medication use.

On examination, findings specific to rhabdomyolysis include tenderness of the muscles to palpation, decreased strength, and, less commonly, edema. If the cause is hyperthermia, the vital signs may be revealing. In some cases, trauma may be apparent, as in the form of a crush injury; however, patients with muscle injury secondary to vigorous exercise may manifest no local signs or only minimal tenderness.

The most reliable test for rhabdomyolysis is elevation of the creatine phosphokinase. The release of creatine phosphokinase occurs rapidly after injury to the muscle, peaks at 24 to 36 hours, and persists for several days. The urine from pa-

TABLE 17.19. *Metabolic and clinical abnormalities in end-stage renal failure*

Anemia
  Decreased erythropoietin production
  Hemolysis
  Blood loss (bleeding tendency)[a]
Cardiovascular
  Congestive heart failure[a]
  Uremic pericarditis[a]
Fluid, electrolyte, acid-base balance
  Reduced free-water clearance, obligatory isothermia[a]
  Potassium balance lost when glomerular filtration rate 10 mL/min, hyperkalemia common[a]
  Metabolic acidosis (increased anion gap)[a]
Vitamin D/Calcium metabolism
  Hypocalcemia, hyperphosphatemia[a]
  Secondary hyperparathyroidism
  Osteomalacia (aluminum bone disease)
Immune function
  Increased risk of infection[a]
  Impaired host defense (white blood cell function)
Neurologic function[a]
  Inability to concentrate, loss of memory
  Headache, drowsiness, coma
  Weakness, tremors, seizures
  Peripheral neuropathy
  Autoimmune dysfunction (sweating, swings in blood pressure)

[a] Improved with dialysis.

TABLE 17.20. *Causes of rhabdomyolysis*

Trauma
Extensive muscle injury
Crush injury
Compartment syndrome
Strenuous exertion
Infections
Influenza
Sepsis
Toxic shock syndrome
Rocky Mountain spotted fever
Tetanus
Hyperthermia
Prolonged seizure
Toxins/medications
Ethanol
Cocaine
Amphetamines
Aspirin
Neuroleptic agents
Monoamine oxidase inhibitors
Succinylcholine
Envenomations
Endocrinopathies
Hyperthyroidism
Hypothyroidism
Diabetic ketoacidosis
Inherited disorders of muscle enzymes
Miscellaneous
Polymyositis

tients with rhabdomyolysis may appear dark and test positive for blood with a reagent strip, but RBCs are not increased on microscopy. Other laboratory abnormalities include hyperphosphatemia, hypocalcemia, acidosis, hyperuricemia, and elevations of BUN and creatinine.

The major potential complication of rhabdomyolysis is ARF, resulting at least in part from myoglobin casts obstructing renal tubules.

Management

Steps should be taken to eliminate the inciting event. For example, anticonvulsants are administered to interrupt status epilepticus and cooling is indicated for the patient with hyperthermia. Initial measurement of muscle enzymes and electrolytes is appropriate. Therapy is directed at facilitating blood flow to the kidneys to preserve renal function. Management begins with the delivery of a 20-mL/kg bolus of normal saline. In more severe cases, diuresis is achieved with either 1 g/kg mannitol or 1 mg/kg furosemide. Depending on their severity, acidosis and electrolyte disorders may need specific treatment. Patients with markedly elevated levels of creatine phosphokinase and/or myoglobinuria require admission to the hospital.

SUGGESTED READINGS

Berry PL, Belsha CW. Hyponatremia. *Pediatr Clin North Am* 1990;37:351–363.
Boineau FG, Lewy JE. Estimation of parenteral fluid requirements. *Pediatr Clin North Am* 1990;37:257–264.
Brem AS. Disorders of potassium homeostasis. *Pediatr Clin North Am* 1990;37:419–427.
Brewer ED. Disorders of acid-base balance. *Pediatr Clin North Am* 1990;37:429–447.
Cetta F, Hurley M, Hatch D, et al. Malignant hypertension. *J Pediatr* 1991;118:981–986.
Chamberlain MC. Rhabdomyolysis in children: a 3-year retrospective study. *Pediatr Neurol* 1991;7:226–228.
Conley SB. Hypernatremia. *Pediatr Clin North Am* 1990;37:365–372.
Gaudio KM, Siegel NJ. Pathogenesis and treatment of acute renal failure. *Pediatr Clin North Am* 1987;34:771–784.
Groshong T. Hypertensive crisis in children. *Pediatr Ann* 1996;25:368–376.
Kaku Y, Nohara K, Honda S. Renal involvement in HSP: a multivariate analysis of prognostic factors. *Kidney Int* 1998;53:1755–1759.
Murphy C. Hypertensive emergencies. *Emerg Med Clin North Am* 1995;13:973–1007.
Remuzzi G, Ruggenenti P. The hemolytic uremic syndrome. *Kidney Int* 1998;66:554–557.
Sinaiko AR. Hypertension in children. *N Engl J Med* 1996;335:1968–1973.
Stapleton FB. Nephrolithiasis in children. *Pediatr Rev* 1989;11:21–30.
Trachtman H. Sodium and water homeostasis. *Pediatr Clin North Am* 1995;42:1343–1463.

CHAPTER 18

Toxicologic Emergencies

Editor: Gary R. Fleisher

GENERAL APPROACH TO THE POISONED CHILD

Initial Life Support Phase

The management approach to the poisoned child attempts to prioritize critical assessment and, at times, simultaneous management interventions (Table 18.1). The initial phase (or primary survey) addresses the traditional basics of securing the airway and cardiorespiratory support, with a slight additional emphasis on emergent toxicologic considerations.

Evaluation

History and Physical Examination

For a known or highly suspected toxin, an attempt is made to estimate the total amount ingested. The best estimate of time elapsed since ingestion is also sought. General historical features that suggest a poisoning include (1) acute onset, (2) age of 1 to 5 years, (3) history of pica, (4) substantial environmental stress, (5) multiple organ system involvement, (6) alteration in level of consciousness, and (7) a puzzling clinical picture. The physical examination should begin with an assessment of vital functions and complete recording of vital signs, including core temperature (Table 18.2). After stabilization, the examination should then focus on the central and autonomic nervous systems, eye findings, changes in the skin and/or mucous membranes, and odors, looking for a constellation of findings that resembles known toxidromes (Table 18.3).

Laboratory Studies

Blood levels should be obtained, when available, for known ingestions (Table 18.4). The comprehensive drug screen of blood and urine samples fails to detect some poisons (Table 18.5) but may be useful for patients who are seriously ill with an occult ingestion or for the occasional adolescent with an intentional overdose whose clinical picture does not fit with the stated history. Metabolic acidosis with a high anion gap is found in many clinical syndromes and toxidromes [MUD-PILES: *m*ethanol and *m*etformin, *u*remia, *d*iabetic, and other ketoacidoses; *p*araldehyde; *i*soniazid, *i*ron, and *i*nborn errors of metabolism; *l*actic acidosis (seen with hypoxia, shock, carbon monoxide, cyanide, and other drugs); *e*thanol and *e*thylene glycol; and *s*alicylates]. Differences between calculated and measured serum osmolarity (calculated = 2[serum sodium] + blood urea nitrogen/2.8 + glucose/18 with normal osmolarity = 290 mOsm/kg) may suggest intoxication with ethanol, isopropanol, or, more rarely in pediatric patients, methanol or ethylene glycol. An immediate determination of quantitative levels is helpful in making management decisions for some drugs. An electrocardiogram may reveal conduction delays that sometimes precede life-threatening cardiac rhythm disturbances.

Detoxification

Gastrointestinal Decontamination

Gastrointestinal decontamination strategies are summarized in Figure 18.1. Emesis is limited for the most part to first aid in the home. Gastric lavage provides a superior alternative. Charcoal administration (Fig. 18.2) is most effective when used in the first few hours after ingestion. Several notable compounds, such as iron and lithium, are not absorbed well by activated charcoal (Table 18.6). The usual dose of activated charcoal is 1 g/kg (maximum, 50 to 100 g). Whole bowel irrigation, with large volumes of a polyethylene glycol–balanced electrolyte solution (GoLYTELY), has proven particularly useful for overdoses of iron and other metals (e.g., lead), sustained-release medications (e.g., lithium, theophylline), and cocaine packets. The usual recommended dosing is 500 mL/hour in toddlers and 2 L/hour in adolescents and adults.

Antidotal Therapy

Those antidotes that should be available for immediate administration are listed in Table 18.7.

TABLE 18.1. *General approach to known or suspected intoxication*

Initial life support phase		
Airway: Maintain patency, assess protective reflexes	Social:	Grandparents visiting
Breathing: Adequate tidal volume?		Holiday parties and so on
ABG:	Physical examination	
Circulation: Secure IV access, assess perfusion	Vital signs	
Disability: Level of consciousness (AVPU or GCS)	Level of consciousness, neuromuscular status	
Pupillary size, reactivity	Eyes–pupils, extraocular movements, fundi	
Drugs: Dextrose (± rapid bedside test)	Mouth–corrosive lesions, odors	
Oxygen	Cardiovascular–rate, rhythm, perfusion	
Naloxone	Respiratory–rate, chest excursion, air entry	
(Other ALS medications)	GI–motility, corrosive effects	
Decontamination: Ocular—copious saline lavage	Skin–color, bullae or burns, diaphoresis, piloerection	
Skin—copious water, then soap and water	Odors	
GI—consider options	Laboratory (individualize)	
Evaluation and detoxification phase	CBC, cooximetry	
History: Brief, focused	ABG, serum osmolarity	
Known toxin: Estimate amount	ECG/cardiac monitor	
Elapsed time	Chest radiograph, abdominal radiograph	
Early symptoms	Electrolytes, BUN/creatinine, glucose, calcium, liver	
Home treatment	function panel	
Significant underlying conditions	Urinalysis	
Suspected but unknown toxin–consider poisoning if:	Rapid overdose toxicologic screen	
Patient: Acute onset of illness, pica-prone	Quantitative toxicology tests (especially acetaminophen)	
age, history of pica, ingestions	Assessment of severity/diagnosis	
Current household stress	Clinical findings	
Multiorgan system dysfunction	Laboratory abnormalities (with consideration of anion,	
Significantly altered mental status	osmolar gaps)	
Puzzling clinical picture	Toxidromes (see Table 18.3)	
Family: Medications at home	Specific detoxification	
Recent illness (under treatment)	Reassess ABCDs	
	Institute appropriate GI decontamination (if not already	
	under way)	
	Urgent antidotal therapy	
	Consider excretion enhancement	
	Continue supportive care	

ABG, arterial blood gas; IV, intravenous; AVPU, alert, verbal, pain, unresponsive; GCS, Glasgow Coma Scale; ALS, advanced life support; GI, gastrointestinal; CBC, complete blood coount; ECG, electrocardiogram; BUN, blood urea nitrogen; ABCDs.

Enhancing Excretion

Urinary alkalinization promotes excretion of salicylate (a weak acid) and may also enhance clearance of phenobarbital, chlorpropamide, and chlorophenoxy herbicides; this can be initiated with sodium bicarbonate at a dose of 1 to 2 mEq/kg intravenously over a 1- to 2-hour period. Dialysis is indicated for selected cases of severe poisoning or when renal failure is present (Table 18.8). Common pediatric poisonings for which repetitive charcoal dosing may be indicated include phenobarbital, carbamazepine, phenytoin, digoxin, salicylates, and theophylline. The dose is of 0.5 to 1.0 g/kg of activated charcoal every 4 to 6 hours. Cathartics, such as sorbitol, should be administered no more frequently than every third dose. Table 18.9 provides a list of nontoxic ingestions.

SPECIFIC POISONS

Acetaminophen

Initially, the signs and symptoms of acetaminophen ingestion are vague and nonspecific but include nausea and vomiting, anorexia, pallor, and diaphoresis. These manifestations usually resolve within 12 to 24 hours, and the patient appears well for 1 to 4 days. Acetaminophen in single doses of less than 150 mg/kg in children is likely to be harmless. However, the only reliable indication of the potential severity of the hepatic damage is the plasma acetaminophen level, taken at least 4 hours after (Fig. 18.3). For most cases of acetaminophen overdose, and particularly for those patients typically seen 2 to 4 hours after ingestion, charcoal alone is effective. In patients who present after 4 hours have elapsed, gastric decontamination is usually not warranted. *N*-acetylcysteine, given orally or intravenously, essentially prevents the occurrence of hepatotoxicity when instituted within 8 hours of ingestion.

Alcohols

Ethanol

After ingesting ethanol, children may develop nausea, vomiting, stupor, and ataxia. Values of 100 to 150 mg/dL are consistent with intoxication and cause mild neurologic findings. Lethal blood alcohol concentrations are generally greater than 500 mg/dL. Infants and toddlers who ingest ethanol have a clinical course that is significantly different from that in adolescents and adults; a triad of coma, hypothermia, and hypoglycemia appears when ethanol levels exceed 100 mg/dL. A rough rule is that ingestion of 1 g/kg of ethanol is sufficient to raise the blood alcohol concentration to 100 mg/dL.

TABLE 18.2. *Clinical manifestations of poisoning*

Vital signs
Pulse
Bradycardia
Digoxin, narcotics, organophosphates, cyanide, plants (lily of the valley, foxglove, oleander), clonidine, beta-blockers, calcium channel blockers
Tachycardia
Alcohol, amphetamines and sympathomimetics, atropinics, tricyclic antidepressants, theophylline, salicylates, phencyclidine, cocaine
Respirations, slow, depressed
Alcohol, barbiturates (late), narcotics, clonidine, sedative-hypnotics
Tachypnea
Amphetamines, barbiturates (early), methanol, salicylates, carbon monoxide
Blood pressure
Hypotension
Cellular asphyxiants (methemoglobinemia, cyanide, carbon monoxide), phenothiazines, tricyclic antidepressants, barbiturates, iron, theophylline, clonidine, narcotics, beta-blockers, calcium channel blockers
Hypertension
Amphetamines/sympathomimetics (especially phenylpropanolamine in OTC cold remedies, diet pills), tricyclic antidepressants, phencyclidine, MAOIs, antihistamines, atropinics, clonidine, cocaine
Temperature
Hypothermia
Ethanol, barbiturates, sedative-hypnotics, narcotics, phenothiazines, antidepressants, clonidine, carbamazepine
Hyperpyrexia
Atropinics, quinine, salicylates, amphetamines, phenothiazines, tricyclics, MAOIs, theophylline, cocaine
Neuromuscular
Coma
Narcotic depressants, sedative-hypnotics, anticholinergics (antihistamines, antidepressants, phenothiazines, atropinics, OTC sleep preparations), alcohols, anticonvulsants, carbon monoxide, salicylates, organophosphate insecticides, clonidine, γ-hydroxybutyrate
Delirium/psychosis
Alcohol, phenothiazines, drugs of abuse (phencyclidine, LSD, peyote, mescaline, marijuana, cocaine, heroin, methaqualone), sympathomimetics and anticholinergics (including prescription and OTC cold remedies), steroids, heavy metals

Convulsions
Alcohol, amphetamines, cocaine, phenothiazines, antidepressants, antihistamines, camphor, boric acid, lead, organophosphates, isoniazid, salicylates, plants (water hemlock), lindane, lidocaine, phencyclidine, carbamazepine
Ataxia
Alcohol, barbiturates, carbon monoxide, anticonvulsants, heavy metals, organic solvents, sedative-hypnotics, hydrocarbons
Paralysis
Botulism, heavy metals, plants (poison hemlock), ticks, paralytic shellfish poisoning
Eyes
Pupils
Miosis
Narcotics, organophosphates, plants (mushrooms of the muscarinic type), ethanol, barbiturates, phenothiazines, phencyclidine, clonidine
Mydriasis
Amphetamines, atropinics, barbiturates (if comatose), botulism, cocaine, methanol, glutethamide, LSD, marijuana, phencyclidine, antihistamines, antidepressants
Nystagmus
Diphenylhydantoin, sedative-hypnotics, carbamazepine, glutethimide, phencyclidine (both vertical and horizontal), barbiturates, ethanol, MAOIs
Skin
Jaundice
Carbon tetrachloride, acetaminophen, naphthalene, phenothiazines, plants (mushrooms, fava beans), heavy metals (iron, phosphorus, arsenic)
Cyanosis (unresponsive to oxygen, as a result of methemoglobinemia)
Aniline dyes, nitrites, benzocaine, phenacetin, nitrobenzene, phenazopyridine
Pinkness to redness
Atropinics and antihistamines, alcohol, carbon monoxide, cyanide, boric acid
Odors
Acetone: acetone, isopropyl alcohol, phenol, and salicylates
Alcohol: ethanol (alcoholic beverages)
Bitter almond: cyanide
Garlic: heavy metal (arsenic, phosphorus, and thallium), organophosphates
Oil of wintergreen: methylsalicylates
Hydrocarbons (e.g., gasoline, turpentine)

Modified from Mofenson HC, Greensher J. The unknown poison. *Pediatrics* 1974;54:336.
OTC, over-the-counter; MAOIs, monoamine oxidase inhibitors.

TABLE 18.3. *Toxidromes*

	Sympathomimetics (Amphetamines, cocaine)	Anticholinergics (Antihistamines, many others)	Organophosphates (Insecticides, nerve gases)	Opiates/ Clonidine	Barbiturates/ Sedative-Hypnotics	Salicylates	Theophylline
Mental status/ Central nervous system (CNS)	Agitation, delirium, psychosis, convulsions	Delirium, psychosis, coma, convulsions	Confusion, fasciculations, coma	Euphoria, somnolence, coma	Somnolence, coma	Lethargy, convulsions	Agitation, tremor, convulsions
Heart rate	Increased	Increased	Decreased (or increased)	Decreased	—	—	Increased
Blood pressure	Increased	Increased	—	Decreased	Decreased	—	Decreased
Temperature	Increased	Increased	—	Decreased	Decreased	Increased	
Respirations	—	—	Increased	Decreased	Decreased	Increased	Increased
Pupils	Large, reactive	Large, sluggish	Small	Pinpoint	—	—	—
Bowel sounds	Present	Diminished	Hyperactive	—	—	—	—
Skin	Diaphoresis	Flushed, dry	Diaphoresis	—	—	—	—
Miscellaneous	—	—	SLUDGE[a]	—	—	Vomiting	Vomiting

[a] SLUDGE is a mnemonic representing *s*alivation, *l*acrimation, *u*rination, *d*efecation, *g*astric cramping, and *e*mesis.

TABLE 18.4. *Frequently useful quantitative toxicology tests in pediatric patients*

Drug/Toxin	Optimal time after ingestion (hr)
Acetaminophen	4
Carbamazepine	2–4
Carboxyhemoglobin	Immediate
Digoxin	4–6
Ethanol	1/2–1
Ethylene glycol	1/2–1
Iron	4
Lithium	2–4[a]
Methanol	1/2–1
Methemoglobin	Immediate
Phenobarbital	1–2
Phenytoin	1–2
Salicylates	2–4[a]
Theophylline	1–2[a]

Modified with permission from Weisman RS, Howland MA, Flomenbaum ME. The toxicology laboratory. In: Goldfrank LR, Flomenbaum NE, Lewin NA, eds., *Toxicologic emergencies.* Norwalk, CT: Appleton & Lange, 1990.

[a] Repeat levels over 6 to 12 hours may be necessary with sustained-release preparations.

TABLE 18.5. *Important drugs and toxins not detected by most drug screens*

Coma-causing	Hypotension-causing
Bromide	Beta-blockers[a]
Carbon monoxide	Calcium channel blockers[a]
Chloral hydrate	Clonidine[a]
Clonidine	Colchicine
Cyanide	Cyanide
Organophosphates	Digitalis[a]
Tetrahydrozoline (in over-the-counter eyedrops)	Iron

Modified from Wiley JF II. Difficult diagnoses in toxicology: poisons not detected by the comprehensive drug screen. *Pediatr Clin North Am* 1991;38:725–737.

[a] Hypotension is often seen with bradycardia.

TABLE 18.6. *Activated charcoal*

Substances poorly (or not) adsorbed
Common electrolytes
Iron
Mineral acids or bases
Alcohols
Cyanide
Most solvents
Most water-insoluble compounds (e.g., hydrocarbons)

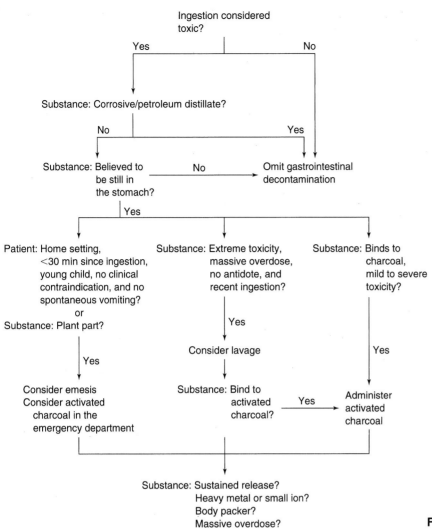

Ingestion considered toxic?

Yes → Substance: Corrosive/petroleum distillate?

No →

Substance: Corrosive/petroleum distillate?
- No → Substance: Believed to be still in the stomach?
- Yes → Omit gastrointestinal decontamination

Substance: Believed to be still in the stomach?
- No → Omit gastrointestinal decontamination
- Yes →

Patient: Home setting, <30 min since ingestion, young child, no clinical contraindication, and no spontaneous vomiting?
or
Substance: Plant part?
- Yes → Consider emesis. Consider activated charcoal in the emergency department

Substance: Extreme toxicity, massive overdose, no antidote, and recent ingestion?
- Yes → Consider lavage → Substance: Bind to activated charcoal? — Yes → Administer activated charcoal

Substance: Binds to charcoal, mild to severe toxicity?
- Yes → Administer activated charcoal

Substance: Sustained release? Heavy metal or small ion? Body packer? Massive overdose?
- Yes → Consider whole bowel irrigation

FIG. 18.1. Approach to gastrointestinal decontamination. For patients in whom the toxin is no longer believed to be in the stomach, activated charcoal administration and/or whole bowel irrigation might still be valid considerations.

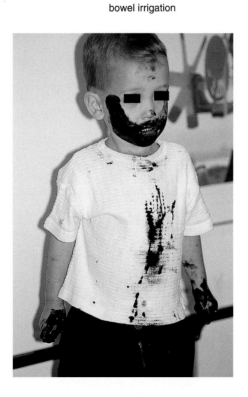

FIG. 18.2. Although this 2-year-old child who ingested a veterinary medication did not readily drink his charcoal, 80% to 90% of children usually cooperate with this therapy.

TABLE 18.7. *Summary of antidotes*

Poison	Antidote
Acetaminophen	*N*-acetylcysteine (Mucomyst): initial dose of 140 mg/kg PO in water, fruit juice, or soda, then 70 mg/kg q 4 hr for 17 doses (see text regarding IV *N*-acetylcysteine)
Anticholinergics	Physostigmine: adult, 2 mg; child, 0.5 mg IV; may repeat in 15 min until desired effect is achieved; subsequent doses q 2–3 hr p.r.n. (caution: may cause seizures, asystole, cholinergic crisis; see text)
Anticholinesterases	Atropine: adult, 2–5 mg; child, 0.05–0.1 mg/kg IM or IV, repeated q 10–15 min until atropinization is evident
Organophosphates	Pralidoxime chloride: adult, 1–2 g; child, 25–50 mg/kg IV; repeat dose in 1 hr p.r.n., then q 6–8 hr for 24–48 hr (consider also constant infusion; see text)
Carbamates	Atropine: as above; pralidoxime for severe cases (see text)
Benzodiazepines	Flumazenil: 0.01 mg/kg IV (estimated pediatric dose; see text)
β-Adrenergic blockers	Glucagon: 50 μg/kg IV
Calcium channel blockers	10% calcium chloride: adult, 10 mL; child, 0.2 mL/kg IV or 10% calcium gluconate: adult, 30 mL; child, 0.6 mL/kg IV; glucagon: 50 μg/kg IV
Carbon monoxide	100% oxygen inhalation, consider hyperbaric for severe cases
Cyanide	Adult: Amyl nitrite inhalation (inhale for 15–30 sec q 60 sec) pending administration of 300 mg sodium nitrite (10 mL of a 3% solution) IV slowly (over 2–4 min); follow immediately with 12.5 g sodium thiosulfate (2.5–5 mL/min of 25% solution) IV. Children: Sodium nitrite should not exceed recommended dose because fatal methemoglobinemia may result:

Hemoglobin (g)	Initial dose 3% sodium nitrite IV	Initial dose 25% sodium thiosulfate IV (mL/kg)
8	0.22 mL (6.6 mg)/kg	1.10
10	0.27 mL (8.7 mg)/kg	1.35
12 (normal)	0.33 mL (10 mg)/kg	1.65
14	0.39 mL (11.6 mg)/kg	1.95

Poison	Antidote
Digitalis	Fab antibodies (Digibind): dose based on amount ingested and/or digoxin level (see text, package insert)
Ethylene glycol	4-Methylpyrazole: load, 15 mg/kg; maintenance, 10 mg/kg q 12 hr for 4 doses, then 15 mg/kg q 12 hr thereafter (little experience in children) (see methanol)
Fluoride	0.6 mL/kg 10% calcium gluconate: IV slowly until symptoms abate, serum calcium normalizes; repeat p.r.n.
Heavy metals/usual chelators	BAL: 3–5 mg/kg/dose deep IM q 4 hr for 2 days, q 4–6 hr for an additional 2 days, then q 4–12 hr for up to 7 additional days
Arsenic/BAL, lead/BAL, EDTA, penicillamine, DMSA, mercury/BAL, DMSA	EDTA: 50–75 mg/kg/24 hr deep IM or slow IV infusion given in 3–6 divided doses for up to 5 days; may be repeated for a second course after a minimum of 2 days; each course should not exceed a total of 500 mg/kg body weight (see text)
	Penicillamine: 100 mg/kg/day (max., 1 g) PO in divided doses for up to 5 days; for long-term therapy, do not exceed 40 mg/kg/d
	DMSA (succimer): 350 mg/m^2 (10 mg/kg) PO q 8 hr for 5 days, followed by 350 mg/m^2 (10 mg/kg) PO q 12 hr for 14 days
Iron	Deferoxamine: 5–15 mg/kg/hr IV; use higher dose for severe symptoms (see text) and decrease as patient recovers
Isoniazid	5–10% pyridoxine: 1 g per gram of INH ingested (70 mg/kg up to 5 g if dose unknown) IV slowly over 30–60 min
Methanol (and ethylene glycol)	Ethanol loading dose: 0.75 g/kg infused over 1 hr; maintenance: 0.1–0.2 g/kg/hr infusion; adjust as needed with target level 100 mg/dL; 1 mg/kg folate IV q 6 hr (methanol); 0.5 mg/kg thiamine and 2 mg/kg pyridoxine (ethylene glycol)
Methemoglobinemic agents	1–2 mg/kg 1% methylene blue (0.1–0.2 mL/kg) IV slowly over 5–10 min if cyanosis is severe or methemoglobin level >40%
Opioids	1–2 mg naloxone IV, IM, sublingual, or by ETT; may repeat up to total 8–10 mg in adolescent/adult (see text)
Phenothiazines (dystonic reaction)	1–2 mg/kg diphenhydramine IM or IV or 1–2 mg benztropine IM or IV (adolescents)
Tricyclic antidepressants	1–2 mEq/kg sodium bicarbonate IV
Warfarin (and "superwarfarin" rat poisons)	Vitamin K: adult, 10 mg; child, 1–5 mg IV, IM, SC, PO
Animals	For envenomation (see Chapter 3) Antivenin[a]
Snake, Crotalidae (all North American rattlers and moccasins)	Antivenin (Crotalidae) polyvalent (Wyeth)
Snake, coral	Antivenin (*Micrurus fulvius*), monovalent (Wyeth)
Spider, black widow	Antivenin *Latrodectus mactans* (Merck, Sharp & Dohme)

[a] See package insert for dose and administration.

PO, orally; q, every; IV, intravenous/intravenously; p.r.n., as needed; IM, intramuscularly; BAL, dimercaprol; EDTA, ethylenediametetraacetic acid; DMSA, ^{99m}Tc-dimercaptosuccinic acid; max., maximum; ETT, endotracheal tube; SC, subcutaneously.

TABLE 18.8. *Drugs and their plasma concentrations for which hemodialysis or hemoperfusion should be considered*

Hemodialysis	Hemoperfusion
4.0 mEq/L lithium	100 mg/L phenobarbital
50 mg/dL ethylene glycol	6–10 mg/dL (60–100 mg/L)
50 mg/dL methanol	theophylline
100 mg/dL salicylates	0.1 mg/dL paraquat
	4 mg/dL glutethimide
	4 mg/dL methaqualone
	15 mg/dL ethchlorvynol
	10 mg/dL meprobamate

Modified from Winchester JF. Active methods for detoxification. In: Haddad LM, Winchester JF, eds. *Clinical management of poisoning and drug overdose.* Philadelphia: WB Saunders, 1983:162–166.

The management of ethanol ingestion in children begins with prompt recognition and evaluation of blood glucose. Because ethanol is rapidly absorbed from the gut and is not adsorbed by activated charcoal, gastrointestinal (GI) decontamination plays no role for patients presenting more than 1 to 2 hours after ingestion, except if congestions are suspected. The institution of hemodialysis may be useful in those patients with impaired liver function or a blood alcohol concentration greater than 450 to 500 mg/dL.

Methanol

Ingestions approaching 100 mg/kg should be considered dangerous. The clinical effects of a methanol ingestion usually occur after a latent period of 8 to 24 hours. In large ingestions, acute methanol poisoning may cause severe central nervous system (CNS) depression, metabolic acidosis, and optic changes. There are three specific treatments for methanol intoxication: sodium bicarbonate, folic acid, and ethanol (or 4-methylpyrazole, see the following). Sodium bicarbonate should be administered aggressively to correct metabolic acidosis. Folate is given at 1 mg/kg intravenously every 6 hours. Serum methanol levels of 20 mg/dL require interventions, such as ethanol or 4-methylpyrazole, to block production of toxic metabolites. Ethanol may be given by continuous intravenous infusion (600-mg/kg bolus followed by 110 mg/kg per hour) or by oral administration. Patients who have a blood methanol concentration of 50 mg/dL or greater require hemodialysis in addition to ethanol administration. During hemodialysis, the infusion rate of the ethanol must be doubled.

Ethylene Glycol

Clinical Manifestations

The clinical syndrome of ethylene glycol intoxication appears in three different stages. The first stage consists predominantly of central nervous system (CNS) manifestations and is accompanied by a profound metabolic acidosis. In this early stage, mild hypertension, tachycardia, and a leukocytosis are often present. Nausea and vomiting commonly occur, and with larger doses, coma and convulsions may appear within a few hours. Hypocalcemia may be severe enough to cause tetany and cardiac conduction disturbances. Urinalysis usually reveals a low specific gravity, proteinuria, microscopic hematuria, and crystalluria. Coma and cardiopulmonary failure usher in the second stage. The third stage usually occurs after 24 to 72 hours, with renal failure as the dominant problem. Findings suggestive of ethylene glycol poisoning include (1) alcohol-like intoxication without the odor of alcohol, (2) large anion-gap metabolic acidosis, (3) an elevated osmolar gap in the absence of ethanol or methanol ingestion, and (4) oxalate crystals in the urine. If the ingested substance is radiator antifreeze, the fluorescein dye in it will fluoresce in urine placed under a Woods lamp.

TABLE 18.9. *Products that are nontoxic when ingested in small amounts*

Abrasives	Corticosteroids	Hydrogen peroxide	Rubber cement
Adhesives	Cosmetics	(medicinal 3%)	Shampoos (liquid)
Antacids	Crayons (marked AP, CP)	Incense	Shaving creams and lotions
Antibiotics	Dehumidifying packets	Indelible markers	Soap and soap products
Baby-product cosmetics	(silica or charcoal)	Ink (black, blue)	Suntan preparations
Ballpoint pen inks	Detergents (phosphate)	Laxatives	Sweetening agents
Bath oil	Deodorants	Lipstick	(saccharin, cyclamates)
Bathtub floating toys	Deodorizers (spray and	Lubricating oils	Teething rings (water
Bleach (less than 5% sodium	refrigerator)	Magic markers	sterility)
hypochlorite)	Elmer's glue	Matches	Thermometers (mercury)
Body conditioners	Etch-a-Sketch	Mineral oil	Thyroid tablets
Bubble-bath soaps	Eye makeup	Newspaper (black and white	Toothpaste
Calamine lotion	Fabric softener	pages)	Vitamins (without iron)
Candles (beeswax or	Fertilizer (if no insecticides	Paint (indoor, latex)	Warfarin (rat poison;
paraffin)	or herbicides added)	Pencil (graphite)	excludes
Caps	Glues and pastes	Perfumes	"superwarfarins")
Chalk	Grease	Petroleum jelly	Watercolors
Cigarettes (<3)	Hair products (dyes, sprays,	Phenolphthalein laxatives	Zinc oxide (Desitin)
Clay (modeling)	tonics; excludes	(Ex-Lax)	Zirconium oxide
Colognes	"relaxers")	Porous-tip marking pens	
Contraceptive pills	Hand lotions and creams	Putty (<2 oz)	

Adapted from Mofenson HC, Greensher J. *Pediatrics* 1974;54:336–342.

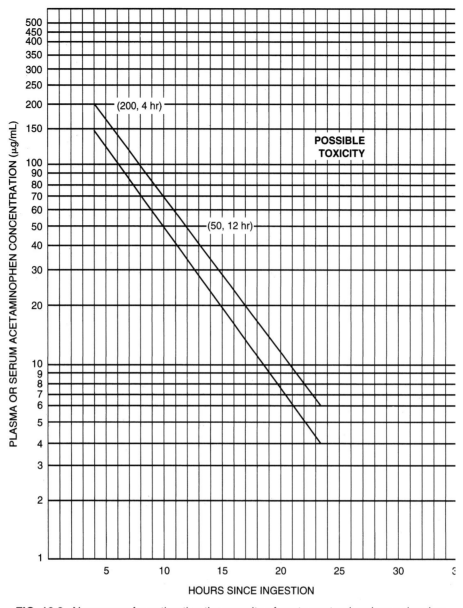

FIG. 18.3. Nomogram for estimating the severity of acute acetaminophen poisoning.

Management

Gastric emptying is the only decontamination measure that is effective after ethylene glycol ingestion and should be performed within 1 hour of ingestion. Pharmacologic therapy employs five drugs: administration of sodium bicarbonate, calcium, pyridoxine, thiamine, and ethanol or 4-methylpyrazole. Correction of acidosis should begin immediately with the administration of sodium bicarbonate. Adverse effects of hypocalcemia may be alleviated by the prompt institution of calcium (e.g., 0.3 to 0.6 mL/kg 10% calcium gluconate). Thiamine (0.25 to 0.5 mg/kg) and pyridoxine (1 to 2 mg/kg) are recommended for the first 24 hours of treatment. Ethanol administration is one option to inhibit ethylene glycol metabolism by alcohol dehydrogenase. As with methanol, ethanol is indicated for ethylene glycol concentrations of 20

mg/dL. For serum ethylene glycol concentrations of 50 mg/dL, both ethanol and hemodialysis are recommended. Hemodialysis is also indicated if there is renal failure or severe electrolyte disturbances. Although the use of ethanol is recommended currently in children, 4-methylpyrazole may be considered. The loading dose is 15 mg/kg intravenously, and the maintenance dose is 10 mg/kg every 12 hours for four doses, then 15 mg/kg every 12 hours thereafter.

Antihistamines

Antihistamines may depress or stimulate the CNS. In children, CNS stimulation causes tremors, hyperactivity, hallucinations, and, with higher doses, tonic-clonic convulsions. Children are also more likely to have signs and symptoms of anticholinergic poisoning: flushed skin, fever, tachycardia, and fixed dilated pupils. Some nonsedating antihistamines, such as astemizole, have caused cardiac arrhythmia after overdose. The treatment of antihistamine overdoses begins with GI decontamination. Patients with seizures require anticonvulsant therapy promptly. Severely agitated patients with a clear anticholinergic syndrome may have improved sensorium after administration of physostigimine (0.5 mg IV slowly over 3 minutes), which should be accompanied by monitoring of the EKG. Meticulous supportive care is essential.

β-Adrenergic Blockers and Calcium Channel Blockers

Typical presentations of both agents include marked bradycardia and hypotension; particularly with the calcium channel blockers, common additional findings are those of abnormal atrioventricular node conduction, with atrioventricular block or accelerated junctional rhythm. The CNS may also be affected, with coma and/or convulsions that occur in either category of overdoses. Metabolic disturbances include hypoglycemia with β-adrenergic blockers and hyperglycemia and metabolic acidosis with calcium channel blockers. Management begins with aggressive gastric decontamination for both types of agents. Bradycardia and hypotension may improve with standard treatment such as atropine, fluid boluses, and pressors. Additional therapy includes calcium infusion for the calcium channel blockers; the recommended initial pediatric dose is approximately 0.2 mL/kg calcium chloride or 0.6 mL/kg calcium gluconate. Glucagon (100-μg/kg boluses) has been used with success to improve heart rate and blood pressure in overdoses of both types of agents.

Digoxin

When the serum digoxin concentration exceeds 4 ng/mL (therapeutic, <2 ng/mL), some evidence of intoxication usually appears. With significant poisoning, symptoms include nausea, vomiting, and visual disturbances. More severe intoxication causes lethargy, disorientation, electrolyte disturbances (especially hyperkalemia), and cardiac arrhythmias. The typical rhythm disturbance starts as heart block, but ventricular or supraventricular escape patterns may ensue. If significant cardiac arrhythmias occur, they are treated initially according to advanced cardiac life support protocols. GI decontamination should include administration of activated charcoal with a cathartic. Electrolyte disturbances require aggressive treatment. Digoxin-specific antibody fragments are indicated in the following circum-

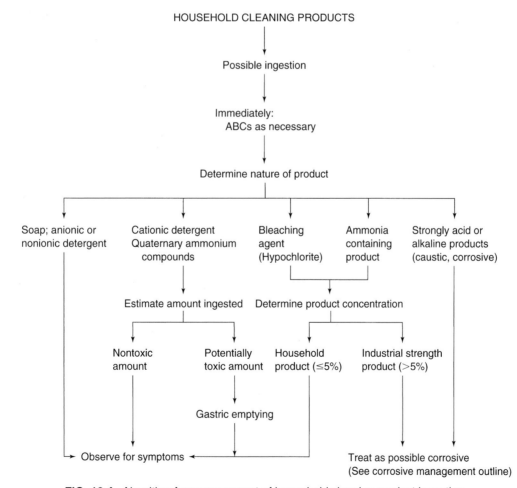

FIG. 18.4. Algorithm for management of household cleaning product ingestion.

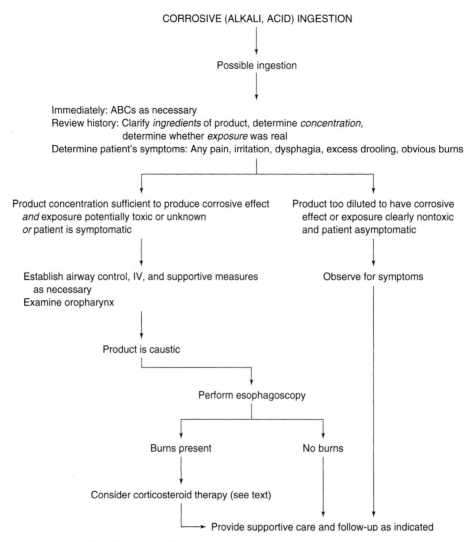

FIG. 18.5. Algorithm for management of corrosive ingestion.

stances after digoxin poisoning: (1) progressive signs and symptoms of intoxication, (2) life-threatening cardiac arrhythmias, or (3) severe hyperkalemia (≥ 5.5 mEq/L). The total dose of Fab antibodies needed (in 40-mg vials) may be estimated by dividing a known ingested dose by 0.6 or calculated for the steady-state context as body load of digoxin: number of vials = [serum digoxin concentration (ng/mL) $\times$ wt (in kg)]/100.

Household Cleaning Products and Caustics

Ingestions of acid and alkali corrosives cause immediate severe burning of exposed surfaces, usually with intense dysphagia. Associated glottic edema may cause airway obstruction and asphyxia. Severe acid ingestions most often cause gastric necrosis and may be complicated by gastric perforation and peritonitis. With alkalis, severe damage is more commonly found in the esophagus; deep-tissue injury may quickly lead to esophageal perforation, mediastinitis, and death. The approach to management of cleaning products and caustic ingestions, as outlined in Figures 18.4 and 18.5,

begins with rapid assessment of cardiorespiratory function, neurologic status, and evidence of GI hemorrhage. Life support measures may be needed emergently to secure the airway and to treat shock or acidosis. Even patients with minimal symptoms and the absence of oral lesions may have significant esophageal injury; thus, all patients with a convincing history of exposure need esophagoscopy.

Hydrocarbons

The low viscosity of hydrocarbons leads to a necrotizing, often fatal chemical pneumonitis when these compounds are aspirated. The high volatility of these substances is responsible for alterations in mental status, including narcosis, inebriation, and frank coma. All these compounds cause significant GI irritation that may be associated with nausea and bloody emesis. Finally, with some hydrocarbons, additional adverse effects may occur, such as cardiotoxicity or as a result of the pharmacologic properties of the other agents contained within these compounds (Table 18.10). Because most hydrocarbons cause clinical toxicity only when aspirated, the

TABLE 18.10. *Classification of hydrocarbons*

Nontoxic (unless complicated by gross aspiration)
  Asphalt, tars
  Mineral oil
  Liquid petrolatum
  Motor oil, axle grease
  Baby oils, suntan oils
Systemic toxicity
  Halogenated (carbon tetrachloride, trichloroethane)
  Aromatic (benzene, toluene, xylene)
  Additives (camphor, organophosphates, heavy metals)
Aspiration hazard (without significant systemic toxicity unless
    ingested in massive quantity)
  Turpentine
  Gasoline
  Kerosene
  Mineral seal oil (furniture polish)
  Charcoal lighter fluid
  Cigarette lighter fluid
  Mineral spirits

mainstay of treatment is to leave ingested compounds in the gut (when possible) and to prevent emesis or reflux. Gastric emptying is generally reserved only for those compounds with the potential for systemic toxic effects. Management of these patients is outlined in Figure 18.6.

Iron

Clinical Manifestations

The clinical effects of iron poisoning are classically divided into four phases. Phase I represents the effects of direct mucosal injury and usually lasts 6 hours. Vomiting, diarrhea, and GI blood loss are the prominent early signs; when severe, the patient may lapse into early coma and shock caused by volume loss and metabolic acidosis. Phase II, which lasts from 6 to 24 hours after ingestion, is marked by diminution of the GI symptoms. However, this remission may be transient, only to be followed by phase III, characterized by profound metabolic acidosis, intractable shock, seizures, and coma. Jaundice, elevated transaminases, a prolonged clotting time, leukocytosis, and hyperglycemia are noted in this phase. Survivors may develop pyloric stenosis in phase IV. Abdominal radiographs may show radiopaque material in the stomach, (Fig. 18.7) but the absence of this finding does not indicate a trivial ingestion.

Management

Usually, iron levels less than 350 μg/dL, when drawn 3 to 5 hours after ingestion, predict an asymptomatic course. Patients with levels in the 350- to 500-μg/dL range often show mild phase I symptoms but rarely develop serious complications. Levels higher than 500 μg/dL suggest significant risk of phase III manifestations. Children who are completely asymptomatic 6 hours after ingestion are unlikely to develop systemic illness. Among laboratory studies, a white blood cell count of 15,000/mm^3 and a glucose level of 150 mg/dL are somewhat predictive of elevated serum iron levels. Radiopaque material on the abdominal radiograph also suggests significant ingestion of iron. Figure 18.8 offers a protocol for the initial management of the patient with a possible iron ingestion. Chelation therapy with parenteral deferoxamine (15 mg/kg per hour; maximal daily dose, 360 mg/kg to as much as 6 g total) provides the mainstay of therapy.

Isoniazid

In overdose, the hallmark of isoniazid poisoning is the triad of seizures, metabolic acidosis, and coma. Isoniazid is not usually detected on routine toxin screens. Pharmacologic treatment for isoniazid intoxication includes sodium bicarbonate, anticonvulsants, and intravenous pyridoxine, given in a dose that equals the estimated dose of isoniazid in milligrams. In cases in which the ingested amount is unknown, the dose is 70 mg/kg in children to as much as 5 g.

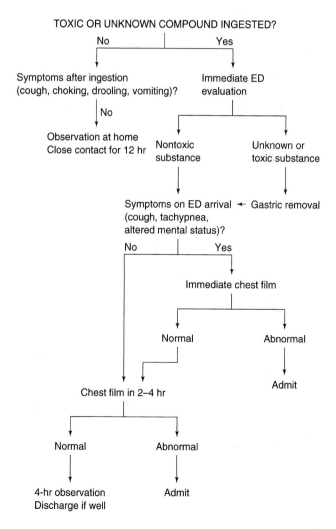

FIG. 18.6. Management of petroleum distillate ingestion.

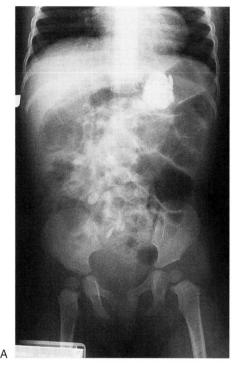
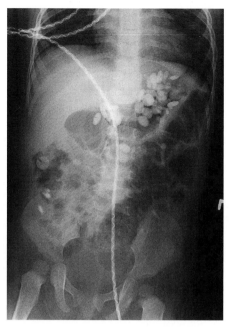

A

B

FIG. 18.7. This child ingested vitamins with iron, which causes the pills to be radiopaque. Radiographs initially show the initial cluster of pills in the stomach **(A)** and, subsequently, the progression through the intestine **(B)**.

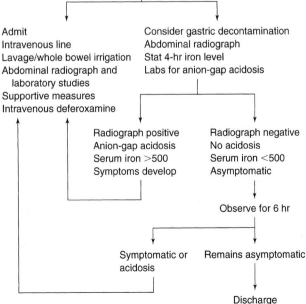

FIG. 18.8. The initial approach to the patient ingesting a possibly toxic dose of iron (500 micrograms/dL).

Lead

Clinical Findings

Early signs and symptoms of plumbism are notably vague and nonspecific. All children between 1 and 5 years of age are suspect if they have (1) persistent vomiting, listlessness or irritability, clumsiness, or loss of recently acquired developmental skills; (2) afebrile convulsions; (3) a strong tendency to pica, including a history of acute accidental ingestions or aural or nasal foreign body; (4) a deteriorating pre–World War II house or a parent with industrial exposures; (5) a family history of lead poisoning; (6) iron deficiency anemia; or (7) evidence of child abuse or neglect. Peripheral neuropathy is rare in children. The kidneys may develop disturbances that range from slight aminoaciduria to full Fanconi syndrome with glycosuria and phosphaturia (in addition to aminoaciduria). The asymptomatic child discovered to have a lead level in the 20- to 44-μg/dL range requires immediate referral. Symptomatic children and those with lead levels higher than 44 μg/dL need urgent treatment.

The child aged 1 to 5 years who comes to the emergency department with an acute encephalopathy presents the physician with a dilemma: lead intoxication requires urgent diagnosis, but confirmation with a blood level is usually not available on an immediate basis. A constellation of features increases the likelihood of lead poisoning, including a prodromal illness of several days' to weeks' duration (suggestive of mild symptomatic plumbism); a history of pica; and a source of exposure

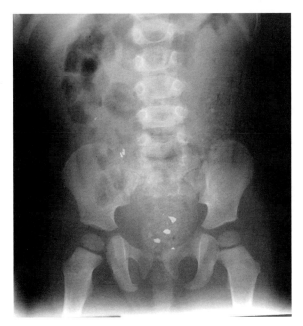

FIG. 18.9. An abdominal radiograph shows radiopaque flecks of material.

to lead. Several nonspecific laboratory findings make lead poisoning likely enough to warrant presumptive chelation therapy until confirmation by lead levels is available: (1) microcytic anemia; (2) elevated erythrocyte protoporphyrin (EP) level; (3) basophilic stippling of peripheral erythrocytes; (4) elevated urinary coproporphyrins; (5) glycosuria; (6) aminoaciduria; (7) radiopaque flecks on abdominal radiographs (Fig. 18.9); and (8) dense metaphyseal bands on radiographs (lead lines) of knees and wrists (Fig. 18.10).

Management

Asymptomatic children found to have lead levels of 45 to 69 μg/dL should have urgent referral and treatment for 5

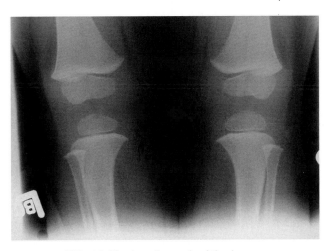

FIG. 18.10. A radiograph of the knees.

days with edetate calcium disodium or succinger acid alone (Table 18.11). If the lead level is greater than 69 μg/dL, dimercaprol plus edetate calcium disodium are used for at least the first 2 days. Supportive care includes adequate hydration to promote good urine output. Symptomatic children without frank encephalopathy should receive chelation therapy with a combination of edetate calcium disodium and dimercaprol for 5 days. Supportive care includes close monitoring for signs of encephalopathy and, again, maintenance of urine flow. Patients with encephalopathy require combination chelation therapy with edetate calcium disodium and dimercaprol, as well as intensive supportive care. Fluid therapy is critical and must be individualized. A reasonable goal is to supply basal water requirements, maintaining urine production at 0.35 to 0.5 mL/kcal per 24 hours.

Organophosphates

Clinical Findings

The symptoms of acute poisoning usually develop during the first 12 hours of contact and include CNS manifestations (dizziness, headache, ataxia, convulsions, and coma); nicotinic signs (sweating, muscle twitching, tremors, weakness, and paralysis); and muscarinic disturbances [SLUDGE (*s*alivation, *l*acrimation, *u*rination, *d*efecation, *g*astrointestinal cramping, and *e*mesis)]. In addition, there may be miosis, bradycardia, bronchorrhea, and wheezing; in severe cases, pulmonary edema develops. Severe intoxications may also cause a toxic psychosis that resembles alcoholism. A depression of plasma or red blood cell cholinesterase activity provides the best laboratory marker of excessive absorption of organophosphates, although it is rarely available on a stat basis; treatment is not to be delayed until confirmation of plasma cholinesterase is obtained.

Management

After decontamination, antidotal therapy begins with the administration of atropine sulfate given in a dose of 0.05 to 0.1 mg/kg to children and 2 to 5 mg for adolescents and adults. This dose should be repeated every 10 to 30 minutes or as needed to obtain and maintain full atropinization, as indicated by clearing of bronchial secretions and pulmonary rales. After atropinization has been instituted, severe poisonings should be treated with the addition of pralidoxime. This drug is particularly useful in poisonings characterized by profound weakness and muscle twitching. A dose of 25 to 50 mg/kg should be administered in 250 mL saline by infusion over approximately 30 minutes; adults may receive 1 to 2 g intravenously. This may be repeated at 1-hour intervals if muscle weakness is not relieved and then at 6- to 8-hour intervals for 24 to 48 hours.

TABLE 18.11. *Guidelines for chelation therapy of lead poisoning*

Condition, BPb (μg/dL)	Regimen	Comment
Encephalopathy	450 mg/m² BAL per day %; 1,500 mg/m² CaNa₂EDTA per day[a]	75 mg/m² IM q 4 hr for 5 days; continuous infusion, or 2–4 divided IV doses, for 5 days (start 4 hr after BAL)
Symptomatic, BPb >70	300–450 mg/m² BAL per day %; 1,000–1,500 mg/m² CaNa₂EDTA[a]	50–75 mg/m² q 4 hr for 3–5 days continuous infusion or 2–4 divided doses IV for 5 days (start 4 hr after BAL)
Asymptomatic, BPb 45–69	700–1,050 mg/m² succimer per day or 1,000 mg/m² CaNa₂EDTA per day[a]	350 mg/m² t.i.d. for 5 days, then b.i.d. for 14 days Continuous infusion, or 2–4 divided doses IV for 5 days

BPb, whole blood lead concentration (μg/dL); BAL, dimercaprol; CaNa₂EDTA, edetate calcium disodium; q, every; IM, intramuscularly; IV, intravenously; t.i.d., three times daily; b.i.d., twice daily.

[a] Doses expressed in milligrams per kilograms; BAL, 450 mg/m² (24 mg/kg); 300 mg/m² (18 mg/kg); CaNa₂EDTA, 1,000 mg/m² (25–50 mg/kg), 1,500 mg/m² (50–75 mg/kg); succimer, 350 mg/m² (10 mg/kg).

Modified from CDC, 1991; AAP, 1995; Henretig, 1998.

Phenothiazines

Clinical Findings

In mild intoxication, CNS signs such as sedation, ataxia, and slurred speech occur. The anticholinergic effects of these drugs may cause constipation, urinary retention, and blurred vision. Hypothermia or hyperthermia occurs in as many as 30% of patients. Orthostatic hypotension may also be noted. In moderate intoxications, the patients may have significant depression in level of consciousness. Dose-dependent extrapyramidal effects become notable at this level of intoxication with muscle stiffness or cogwheel rigidity seen on passive movement of the neck, biceps, or quadriceps. Anticholinergic manifestations are severe and include acute urinary retention and paralytic ileus; hypotension may be profound. Cardiac conduction disturbances may appear and are often heralded by a prolonged QT interval. In severe overdoses, patients are unarousable. Deep tendon reflexes may be hyperactive. Dystonic reactions may occur, involving the head and neck and the cranial nerves. Arrhythmias and shock may result in death. Dystonic reactions may also occur independent of the ingested dose (Figs. 14.1 and 18.11).

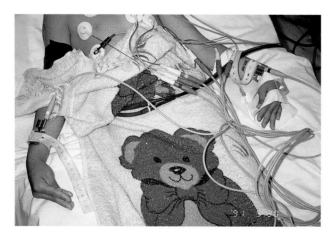

FIG. 18.11. This young child is experiencing a dystonic reaction to a phenothiazine ingestion.

Management

Patients with mild overdoses need no treatment. Those with moderate or severe manifestations require prompt evaluation of vital signs, GI decontamination (if ingestion was within 4-6 hours of ED arrival vascular access and cardiac monitoring or a pressor such as norepinephrine may be used to correct the hypotension). In those rare instances of hypertension, the use of nitroprusside is indicated. Severe arrhythmias should be treated aggressively, as detailed later in the section on tricyclic antidepressants. Dystonic reactions are effectively controlled by the intramuscular or intravenous administration of diphenhydramine in a 1- to 2-mg/kg dose.

Plants/Mushrooms

Plants are among the more commonly reported accidental ingestions in children (Tables 18.12 and 18.13). Charcoal plays a useful role for all toxic plants. Mushrooms can be characterized based on the time interval between ingestion and symptom onset: immediate or delayed. Onset of symptoms within 6 hours of ingestion usually confers a benign prognosis. Most mushrooms have GI effects. In addition, each of five classes of mushrooms possesses unique toxicologic features. Some early-onset mushrooms cause muscarinic effects, usually within 15 minutes, such as sweating, salivation, colic, and pulmonary edema. This syndrome responds to atropine therapy. Other early-onset mushrooms cause anticholinergic effects, including drowsiness, followed by mania and hallucinations. Another subgroup of early-onset mushrooms produces a severe gastroenteritis syndrome. Hallucinogenic mushrooms such as psilocybin make up another class of mushrooms with early-onset symptoms. Finally, some mushrooms precipitate an Antabuse reaction if they are coingested with alcohol. Management for all these agents consists of supportive care and careful monitoring of fluid status.

With the second set of mushrooms, particularly *Amanita phalloides*, after a latent period of many hours, GI upset appears first. Then, approximately 24 hours after ingestion, hepatic dysfunction occurs, which may result in fulminant

TABLE 18.12. *Common nontoxic plants*

Abelia	California holly	Eugenia	Prayer plant
African daisy	California poppy	Gardenia	Purple passion
African palm	Camelia	Grape ivy	Pyracantha
African violet	Christmas cactus	Hedge apples	Rose
Airplane plant	Coleus	Hens and chicks	Sansevieria
Aluminum plant	Corn plant	Honeysuckle	Schefflera
Aralia	Crab apples	Hoya	Sensitive plant
Asparagus fern (may cause	Creeping Charlie	Impatiens	Spider plant
dermatitis)	Creeping Jennie,	Jade plant	Swedish ivy
Aspidistra (cast iron plant)	moneywort, lysima	Kalanchoe	Umbrella
Aster	Croton (house variety)	Lily (day, Easter, or tiger)	Violets
Baby's tears	Dahlia	Lipstick plant	Wandering Jew
Bachelor buttons	Daisies	Magnolia	Weeping fig
Begonia	Dandelion	Marigold	Weeping willow
Bird's nest fern	Dogwood	Monkey plant	Wild onion
Blood leaf plant	Donkey tail	Mother-in-law tongue	Zebra plant
Boston ferns	Dracaena	Norfolk Island pine	
Bougainvillea	Easter lily	Peperomia	
Cactus, certain varieties	Echeveria	Petunia	

hepatic failure. Treatment of the gastroenteric phase includes fluid and electrolyte replacement. If renal failure develops, dialysis may be necessary. Hepatic damage after *A. phalloides* ingestion may be attenuated by the early use of repetitive activated charcos.

Tricyclic and Other Antidepressants

Clinical Findings

The ingestion of 10 to 20 mg/kg of most tricyclic antidepressants represents a moderate to serious exposure, with coma and cardiovascular symptoms expected. The ingestion of 35 to 50 mg/kg may result in death. Anticholinergic activity causes altered sensorium and sinus tachycardia. α-Adrenergic blockade may lead to hypotension. However, the more severe cardiovascular effects are primarily caused by the membrane-depressant or quinidine-like effects that depress myocardial conduction and may lead to multiple focal premature ventricular contractions

and ventricular tachycardia (Fig. 18.12). It has been shown that a QRS interval more than 0.1 second is associated with a significant morbidity and mortality in these patients; this delay in conduction may progress to complete heart block and cardiac standstill and/or the previously mentioned ventricular arrhythmias. Neurologic findings

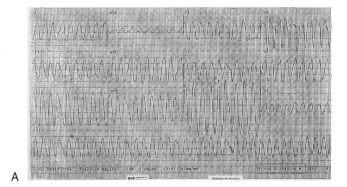

A

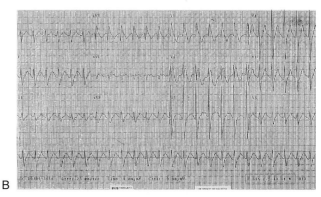

B

FIG. 18.12. This 2-year-old girl ingested imipramine that had been prescribed for her older brother with enuresis. She presented to the emergency department with ventricular tachycardia **(A)**, but her blood pressure was adequate. After she received sodium bicarbonate and lidocaine, her heart returned to a normal sinus rhythm **(B)**. (Courtesy of Dr. Susan Torrey.)

TABLE 18.13. *Common plant toxidromes*

Gastrointestinal irritants	Atropinic effects
Philodendron	Jimsonweed (thorn apple)
Diffenbachia	Deadly nightshade
Pokeweed	Epileptogenice effects
Wisteria	Water hemlock
Spurge laurel	Cyanogenic effects
Buttercup	*Prunus* species (chokecherry,
Daffodil	wild black cherry, plum,
Rosary pea	peach, apricot, bitter
Castor bean	almond)
Digitalis effects	Pear (seeds)
Lily of the valley	Apple (seeds)
Foxglove	Crabapple (seeds)
Oleander	Hydrangea
Yew	Elderberry
Nicotinic effects	
Wild tobacco	
Golden chain tree	
Poison hemlock	

include lethargy, disorientation, ataxia, hallucinations, and, with severe overdoses, coma and seizures. Fever is commonly present initially, but hypothermia may occur later. Additional anticholinergic symptomatology includes decreased GI motility, which delays gastric emptying time, and urinary retention. Muscle twitching has been observed and may be associated with increased deep tendon reflexes. Although the pupils may be dilated, they usually respond to light.

Management

Severe tricyclic antidepressant overdoses require gastric decontamination. Lavage can be considered even for those patients who present as late as 4 to 12 hours after ingestion. Certainly, the administration of activated charcoal should be performed. Significant conduction delays or arrhythmias resulting from tricyclic antidepressants may benefit from alkalinization of the blood. A sodium bicarbonate bolus of 1 to 2 mEq/kg can be given during continuous electrocardiographic monitoring. Bicarbonate infusion can then be used to keep the serum pH at 7.45 to 7.55. If arrhythmias persist, appropriate antiarrhythmic therapy should be instituted, perhaps using lidocaine. Quinidine or procainamide should be avoided because each may increase heart block in this situation. Physostigmine is currently considered to be contraindicated. In the presence of hypotension, many clinicians have advocated the use of norepinephrine infusions (0.1 to 0.3 μg/kg per minute).

Other Antidepressants

Selective serotonin reuptake inhibitors most commonly produce CNS depression in overdose. Seizures may occur after large ingestions. However, life-threatening events from isolated, acute overdoses of these compounds rarely occur. The serotonin syndrome, manifested by muscular rigidity, myoclonus, flushing, and autonomic instability, more typically occurs as the result of drug interactions and is potentially lethal. Amoxapine has anticholinergic activity but is best known for its convulsant properties and the tendency for victims to present with status epilepticus. The α-adrenergic antagonism of trazodone may lead to hypotension.

There are three important clinical pictures of monoamine oxidase inhibitor toxicity. First, patients who take them appropriately and then ingest foods or drugs that contain biogenic amines (e.g., tyramine in wines, cheese, or soy sauce and decongestants) may develop severe hypertension with headache, seizures, or stroke. The second syndrome appears when those who take the drug therapeutically are given particular sympathomimetic or serotonergic agents that cause the serotonin syndrome. Important examples of such drugs include common agents in over-the-counter cough and cold preparations such as dextromethorphan, analgesics such as meperidine, and psychotropic medications such as clomipramine and fluoxetine or other selective serotonin reuptake inhibitors. In these patients,

this drug combination may quickly lead to hyperpyrexia, skeletal muscle rigidity, cardiac arrhythmias, and death. This is one of the few fatal drug interactions known. Finally, those with acute monoamine oxidase inhibitor overdoses develop a clinical syndrome that includes blood pressure instability, hyperpyrexia, skeletal muscle rigidity, seizures, and death.

Because of the toxicity of these agents and the frequent delay in their onset of activity (as long as 24 hours), all patients with a history of monoamine oxidase inhibitor ingestion, regardless of symptoms, should be admitted to the hospital for 24 hours. Management of the patient with monoamine oxidase inhibitor toxicity is largely dictated by the specific toxic manifestations. In those with hypertensive reactions, treatment consists of the immediate administration of an antihypertensive. The ideal agent may be nitroprusside because its brief duration of action permits titration of effect. In the treatment of hyperpyrexia, cooling measures are promptly instituted. Because hyperpyrexia is often accompanied by skeletal muscle rigidity and rhabdomyolysis, serum creatine kinase should be measured and close attention should be paid to the urine for any signs of myoglobinuria. Benzodiazepines are often helpful in this situation and neuromuscular blockade may be beneficial in patients who have severe muscle rigidity with hyperthermia. In the patient with acute overdose, treatment is directed to hemodynamic stability. Because blood pressure changes occur quickly and consist of hypotension and hypertension, hypertension should be treated with short-acting agents and hypotension with fluid and vasopressor support. Intensive care unit admission is mandatory for these patients because of their clinical instability.

Drugs Dangerous in Small Doses

Some drugs cause dangerous toxicity in young children with just one or two doses (Table 18.14). A systematic approach to these patients includes a careful history, an examination with attention to the presence of toxidromes (Table 18.3), and a guided laboratory assessment. An algorithmic approach to this situation is provided in Figure 18.13.

Drugs of Abuse

Table 18.15 provides a summary of the common drugs of abuse, their typical routes of administration, associated symptoms, toxic levels, and duration of action.

γ-Hydroxybutyrate and γ-Hydroxybutyrolactone

The related agents, γ-hydroxybutyrate and γ-hydroxybutyrolactone, have become popular substances of abuse among teenagers and young adults. γ-Hydroxybutyrate and γ-hydroxybutyrolactone are CNS depressants that cause rapid onset of deep sleep that can progress to coma and respiratory depression. Patients who have overdosed may have transient seizure activity and are often hypothermic and bradycardic. The coma is usually relatively short in dura-

TABLE 18.14. *Medications dangerous to toddlers in one to two doses*[a]

Agent	Minimal potential fatal dose (mg/kg)[b]	Maximal dose size	Potential fatal dose	Major toxicity
Benzocaine	<20	10% gel, 20% spray	~2 mL Baby Oragel	Methemoglobinemia, seizures
Beta-Blockers (propranolol)	Unclear	160 mg	1–2 tablets	Bradycardia, hypotension, seizures, hypoglycemia
Calcium antagonists (verapamil)	<40	240 mg	1–2 tablets	Bradycardia, hypotension
Camphor	<100	1 g/5 mL	1 tsp camphorated oil, 2 tsp Campho-phenique, 5 tsp Vicks Vaporub	Seizures, CNS depression
Chloroquine	<30	500 mg	1 tablet	Seizures, arrhythmia
Clonidine	Unclear	0.3 mg tablet, 7.5 mg patch	1 tablet, 1 patch	Bradycardia, CNS depression
Diphenoxylate (Lomotil)	<1.2	2.5 mg/tablet or tsp	2 tablets/tsp	CNS and respiratory depression
Hypoglycemics, oral (glyburide)	~1	5 mg	2 tablets	Hypoglycemia
Lindane	~6	1% lotion	2 tsp	Seizures, CNS depression
Methyl salicylate	~200	1.4 g/mL	1/2 tsp oil of wintergreen, 2 tsp Icy Hot Balm	Seizures, cardiovascular collapse
Phenothiazines (chlorpromazine)	~20	200 mg	1 tablet	Seizures, arrhythmia
Quinidine	~50	300 mg	2 tablets	Seizures, arrhythmia
Quinine	~80	650 mg	2 tablets	Seizures, arrhythmia
Theophylline	~50	500 mg	1 tablet	Seizures, arrhythmia
TCAs (imipramine)	~20	150 mg	1–2 tablets	Seizures, arrhythmia, hypotension

[a] A long list of commonly encountered, highly toxic, nonpharmacologic agents can be severely poisonous in one to two doses. These are not included here.

[b] For the purposes of this table, a dose refers to a single pill or roughly a 5-cc swallow. Calculations are based on a previously healthy toddler of 10-kg body weight.

CNS, central nervous system; TCAs, tricyclic antidepressants.

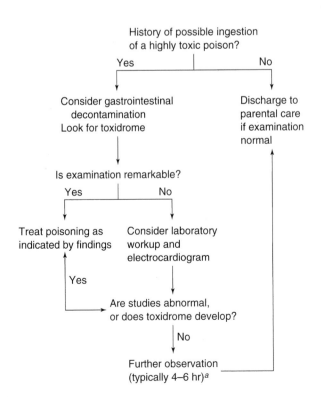

FIG. 18.13. Algorithmic approach to a toddler who has ingested one to two doses (one to two pills or 5 to 10 cc swallow) of a drug. Medications notorious for their ability to have a delayed onset in toxicity, beyond 4 to 6 hours, include oral hypoglycemic agents, sustained-release preparations, monoamine oxidase inhibitors, drugs taken concomitantly with anticholinergic agents, and acetaminophen.

TABLE 18.15. *Drug abuse: summary of toxicity*

Drug of abuse	Symptoms and signs of drug abuse	Diagnosis	Therapeutic dose	Toxic dose	Toxic serum level	Half-life
Cannabis group (marijuana, hashish, Δ9-THC, hash oil)	Pupils unchanged; conjunctive injected; BP decreased on standing; increased heart rate; increased appetite, euphoria, anxiety; sensorium often clear; dreamy; fantasy state; time–space distortions; hallucinations rare. Significant airway obstruction with heavy smoking, decreased forced expiratory volume and decreased vital capacity. Major psychiatric toxic effects: panic reaction most common, psychotic reactions (especially in patients with underlying psychopathology), toxic delirium (disorientation, confusion, memory impairment) in heavy users	Blood, urine levels		20 mg Δ9-THC or 1 g cigarette of 2% Δ9-THC produces effects on mood, memory, motor coordination, cognitive ability sensorium, time sense		*1st phase:* minutes, → distribution in lipid-rich tissues; *2nd phase:* 1½ days, until mobilized from lipid-rich tissue
Hallucinogens	Pupils dilated (normal or small with PCP), elevated BP, increased heart rate, hyperactive tendon reflexes, increased temperature, flushed face, euphoria, anxiety or panic, paranoid thought disorder, inappropriate affect, time and visual distortions, visual hallucinations, depersonalization					
LSD	Psychosis with hyperalertness, changes in body image, sense of profound significance, delusions; hallucinations (also with amphetamines), visual perceptual distortions caused by peripheral effects of LSD on visual system.	Blood, urine levels		20–25 μg produce CNS effects; 0.5–2 μg/kg produce somatic symptoms; between 1 and 16 μg/kg intensity of pathophysiologic effects proportional to dose	Variable	3 hr
PCP	Cyclic coma, extreme hyperactivity violent outbursts, bizarre behavior, amnesia, analgesia, nystagmus, gait ataxia, muscle rigidity. Dystonic reactions, grand mal seizures, tardive dyskinesia, athetosis, bronchospasm, urinary retention, diaphoresis, hypoglycemia. Increased uric	Blood, gastric contents, urine (but level does not correlate with toxicity)		1 cigarette (PCP) = 1–100 mg. Psychosis may last several weeks after 1 dose. Fatal dose = 1 mg/kg; <5 mg/kg = hyperactivty; 5–10 mg = stupor, coma; >10 mg = respiratory depression, convulsions	Individual variability (~0.1 μg/mL)	1–3 days

acid, increased creatine phosphokinase, increased creatine, increased SGOT/SGPT heralds onset of rhabdomyolysis (risk of renal failure)

Drug	Symptoms/signs	Detection	Dose	Toxic/fatal dose	Serum concentration	Half-life
CNS stimulants Amphetamine	Pupils dilated and reactive. Increased BP, pulse, temperature, cardiac arrhythmias; dry mouth; sweating; tremors; sensorium hyperacute or confused; paranoid ideation; impulsivity; hyperactivity; stereotypy; convulsions; exhaustion	Blood level, urine test	5 mg t.i.d.	1. variable; 2. rare <15 mg; 3. severe reactions have occurred at 30 mg; 4. 400–500 mg not uniformly fatal; 5. tolerance is striking; chronic user may take 1,700 mg/d without ill effects	Variable	3 hr
Cocaine	Excitement, restlessness, euphoria, garrulousness; increased motor activity, physical endurance because of decreased sense of fatigue; increased tremors, convulsive movements; increased respiration, pulse, BP, temperature, chills	Urine, serum	Anesthesia; 1 mL of 5% solution for surface anesthesia (≤50 mg)	Fatal dose may be as low as 30 mg; ingested cocaine less toxic than by other routes		1 hr (after oral or nasal route)
CNS sedatives (barbiturates, chlordiazepoxide, diazepam, flurazepam, glutethimide, meprobamate, methaqualone)	Pupils normal or small (dilated with glutethimide); decreased BP, respirations depressed; drowsy, coma, lateral nystagmus, confusion, ataxia, slurred speech, delirium; convulsions or hyperirritability with methaqualone overdose; serious poisoning rare with benzodiazepines alone	Serum level				
Barbiturates (secobarbital, Seconal)	As above	Serum level	30–50 mg, 3–4/d	100 mg/dose	30 µg/mL	19–34 hr
Chlordiazepoxide (Librium)	As above	Serum level	5–20 mg, 3–4 d	25 mg	8 µg/mL	8–25 hr
Diazepam (Valium)	As above	Serum, urine	2–10 mg, 4/d	≥15 mg		20–90 hr
Flurazepam (Dalmane)	As above	Serum, urine	15–30 mg		0.12 µg/mL (fatal)	47–100 hr
Glutethimide (Doriden)	As above	Serum level	125–250 mg, 1–3 d	>500 mg (acute intoxication, 3g)	2 mg/100 mL (but even below, full ICU support may be required)	5–22 hr
Meprobamate	As above	Serum level	400 mg, 4/d	>800 mg	150 µg/mL	6–17 hr
Methaqualone (Parest, Somnafae)	As above	Serum level	100 mg, 4/d	200–400 mg	10 µg/mL	20–60 hr

continued

TABLE 18.15. *Continued*

Drug of abuse	Symptoms and signs of drug abuse	Diagnosis	Therapeutic dose	Toxic dose	Toxic Serum Level	Half-life
Narcotics	Pupils constricted (may be dilated with meperidine or extreme hypoxia); respiration depressed to absent with cyanosis; decreased BP, sometimes shock; temperature reduced; reflexes diminished to absent, stupor or coma; pulmonary edema; constipation; convulsions with propoxyphene or meperidine; arrhythmia with propoxyphene	Serum, urine				
Heroin	As above	Serum	3 mg[a]			1–12 hr[c]
Morphine	As above	Serum	10 mg[a]	60 mg = toxic[b]; 200 mg = fatal dose[b]		3 hr[c]
Codeine	As above	Serum	120 mg[a]	800 mg = fatal dose[b]	1.1 μg/mL	2 hr[c]
Methadone	As above	Serum	7.5–10 mg[a]	100 mg = fatal dose[b]	1.6 μg/mL (fatal)	18–97 hr[c]
Propoxyphene	As above	Serum	65 mg every 4 hr[a]	500 mg = fatal dose[b]	2 μg/mL (fatal)	3–12 hr
Anticholinergics (atropine, belladonna, henbane, scopolamine, trihexphenidyl, tricyclic antidepressants, benzotropine mesylate)	Pupils dilated and fixed, heart rate increased, temperature increased; BP increased; drowsy, coma, flushed, dry skin and mucous membranes, erythematous skin, amnesia, disoriented, visual hallucinations, body image alterations	Urine test				
Atropine	As above		0.5–1 mg	5 mg		24 hr
Belladonna	As above		0.6–1 mg	5 mg		24 hr
Scopolamine	As above		0.6 mg	5 mg		24 hr
Imipramine (Tofranil)	As above		100–200 mg/d	500 mg		8–16 hr
Amitriptyline (Elavil)	As above		75–200 mg	>500 mg	5 μg/mL	32–40 hr
Desipramine	As above			1 g	10 μg/mL	12–54 hr

[a] Dose is amount given subcutaneously that produces same analgesic effect as 10 mg morphine subcutaneously.

[b] Higher doses given for addicts.

[c] Duration is for subcutaneous dose. Intravenous dose peak is more pronounced and overall effects have shorter duration.

BP, blood pressure; PCP, phencyclidine; LSD, lysergic acid diethylamide; CNS, central nervous system; SGOT, serum glutamic-oxaloacetic transaminase; SGPT, serum glutamic-pyruvic transaminase; t.i.d., three times daily; ICU, intensive care unit.

Modified from Dreisbach RH. *Handbook of poisoning.* Los Altos, CA: Lange Medical Publications, 1980.

tion, approximately 1 to 2 hours. During emergence, transient delirium and vomiting are often observed. Depressed respiratory effort and airway-protective reflexes are common in the more severe cases, although aspiration pneumonia as a complication has been rare. Many patients are surprisingly responsive to stimulus, and attempts at laryngoscopy to effect endotracheal intubation in a seemingly deeply comatose patient may result in an angry, combative patient who sits up and swears at the endoscopist. Most patients with acute overdose can be managed with the provision of ambient oxygen, suctioning, and airway and anti-aspiration positioning. A nasal trumpet is helpful in some cases, and endotracheal intubation may be required occasionally, although it may necessitate rapid sequence induction for the reasons previously noted. Atropine has been used for severe bradycardia with success. Blood pressure support is rarely necessary.

Central Anticholinergics

The management of a patient with a known central anticholinergic syndrome is a challenge, particularly because one must also be prepared for the other distinct toxicities of the ingested drug or plant (Table 18.16). Also, most plants and many drugs are not detected on a toxin screen, so the diagnosis must rely on history and clinical suspicion. GI decontamination is essential after anticholinergic ingestion. Unlike most toxic ingestions, there is clear efficacy to decontamination 12 to 24 hours after ingestion because of the likelihood of drug persistence in the gut lumen for an extended time. Activated charcoal with a cathartic is added to enhance fecal expulsion of the drug-charcoal complex in the face of diminished gut motility. Based on presenting signs and symptoms, the patient may require sedation and monitoring in an intensive care unit setting to provide ventilatory support for coma, anticonvulsants for seizures, and antiarrhythmic drugs for cardiac arrhythmias. Adequate sedation may be achieved with titrated doses of benzodiazepines. Physostigmines are reserved for those who have normal electrocardiograms and mental status dysfunction confined to hallucinations or severe agitation. The pediatric dose is 0.5 mg administered slowly intravenously, with repeat every 10 minutes to a maximum of 2 mg. The muscarinic toxicity of physostigmine may be treated with intravenous atropine at one-half of the physostigmine dose given; physostigmine-related seizures may be treated with benzodiazepines.

SUGGESTED READINGS

American Academy of Clinical Toxicology, European Association of Poisons Centres and Clinical Toxicologists. Position statement: single-dose activated charcoal. *J Toxicol Clin Toxicol* 1997;35:721–741.

American Academy of Clinical Toxicology, European Association of Poisons Centres and Clinical Toxicologists. Position statement: whole bowel irrigation. *J Toxicol Clin Toxicol* 1997;35:753–762.

American Academy of Pediatrics, Committee on Drugs. Treatment guidelines for lead exposure in children. *Pediatrics* 1995;96:155–160.

Anker AL, Smilkstein MJ. Acetaminophen: concepts and controversies. *Emerg Med Clin North Am* 1994;12:335–349.

Bates BA, Shannon MW, Woolf AD. Ethanol-related visits by adolescents to a pediatric emergency department. *Pediatr Emerg Care* 1995;11: 89–92.

Furbee B, Wermuth M. Life-threatening plant poisoning. *Crit Care Clin* 1997;13:849–888.

Henretig FM, Slap GB. A guide to acute medical management of intoxication in adolescents. *Am Acad Pediatr Adolesc Health Update* 1994;6:1–7.

Henretig FM. Special considerations in the poisoned pediatric patient. *Emerg Med Clin North Am* 1994;12:549–567.

Koren G. Medications which can kill a toddler with one tablet or teaspoonful. *Clin Toxicol* 1993;31:407–413.

Lewander WJ, Gaudreault P, Einhorn A, et al. Acute pediatric digoxin ingestion—a ten-year experience. *Am J Dis Child* 1986;140:770–773.

Li J, Stokes SA, Woeckener A. A tale of novel intoxication: a review of the effects of gamma-hydroxybutyric acid with recommendations for management. *Ann Emerg Med* 1998;31:729–736.

Liebelt EL, Francis PD, Woolf AD. ECG lead aVR versus QRS interval in predicting seizures and arrhythmias in acute tricyclic antidepressant toxicity. *Ann Emerg Med* 1995;26:195–201.

Liebelt EL, Shannon MW. Small doses, big problems. *Pediatr Emerg Care* 1993;9:292–297.

Liebelt EL. Toxicology reviews: targeted management strategies for cardiovascular toxicity from tricyclic antidepressant overdose: the pivotal role for alkalinization and sodium loading. *Pediatr Emerg Care* 1998; 14:293–298.

Liu JJ, Daya MR, Carrasquillo O, et al. Prognostic factors in patients with methanol poisoning. *J Toxicol Clin Toxicol* 1998;36:175–181.

Mills KC. Serotonin syndrome: a clinical update. *Crit Care Clin* 1997; 13:763–783.

Mueller PD, Benowitz NL, Olson KR. Cocaine. *Emerg Med Clin North Am* 1990;8:481–494.

O'Malley M. Clinical evaluation of pesticide exposure and poisonings. *Lancet* 1997;349:1161–1166.

TABLE 18.16. *Drugs and chemicals that may produce the central anticholinergic syndrome*

Antidepressants
   Amitriptyline (Elavil), imipramine (Tofranil), doxepin (Sinequan, Adopin)
Antihistamines
   Chlorpheniramine (Ornade, Teldrin), diphenhydramine (Benadryl), orphenadrine (Norflex)
Ophthalmologic preparations
   Cyclopentolate (Cyclogel), tropicamide (Mydriacyl)
Antispasmodic agents
   Propantheline (Probanthine), clidinium bromide (Librax)
Antiparkinson agents
   Trihexyphenidyl (Artane), benztropine (Cogentin), procyclidine (Kemadrin)
Proprietary drugs
   Sleep-Eze (scopolamine, methapyrilene), Sominex (scopolamine, methapyrilene), Asthmador (belladonna alkaloids), Excedrin P.M. (methapyrilene)
Belladonna alkaloids
   Atropine, homatropine, hyoscine, hyoscyamus, scopolamine
Toxic plants
   Mushroom (*Amanita muscaria*), bittersweet (*Solanum dulcamara*), jimsonweed (*Datura stramonium*), potato leaves and sprouts (*Solanum tuberosum*), deadly nightshade (*Atropa belladonna*)

Orlowski FP, Paganini EP, Pippenger CE. Treatment of a potentially lethal dose isoniazid ingestion. *Ann Emerg Med* 1988;17:73–76.

Perry H, Shannon M. Emergency department gastrointestinal decontamination. *Pediatr Ann* 1996;25:19–26.

Perry HE, Shannon MW. Diagnosis and management of opioid- and benzodiazepine-induced comatose overdose in children. *Curr Opin Pediatr* 1996;8:243–247.

Shannon M. Toxicology reviews: fomepizole—a new antidote. *Pediatr Emerg Care* 1998;14:170–172.

Shannon M. Toxicology reviews: physostigmine. *Pediatr Emerg Care* 1998;14:224–226.

Victoria MS, Nangia BS. Hydrocarbon poisoning: a review. *Pediatr Emerg Care* 1987;3:184–186.

Wiley JF II. Difficult diagnoses in toxicology: poisons not detected by the comprehensive drug screen. *Pediatr Clin North Am* 1991;38:725–737.

Woodward GA, Baldassano RN. Topical diphenhydramine toxicity in a five year old with varicella. *Pediatr Emerg Care* 1988;4:18–20.

Woolf AD, Shannon MW. Clinical toxicology for the pediatrician. *Pediatr Clin North Am* 1995;42:317–333.

Yip L, Dart RC, Hurlbut KM. Intravenous administration of oral *N*-acetylcysteine. *Crit Care Med* 1998;26:40–43.

SECTION II

Trauma

CHAPTER 19

Trauma: Abdomen

Editor: Gary R. Fleisher

INITIAL MANAGEMENT PRINCIPLES

Basic Principles of Management

In patients with clearly significant injuries, airway management and cervical spine stabilization are priorities (Fig. 19.1). Any child with significant injuries should receive supplemental oxygen, especially if signs of shock are present. Intravenous or intraosseous access should be obtained. Aggressive fluid resuscitation must be pursued. A nasogastric or orogastric (when injuries to the midface are present) tube is indicated to relieve gastric distention (Fig. 19.2). As the initial evaluation proceeds, the priorities of management depend on the extent of multisystem injuries and the stability of the patient (Fig. 19.3). Patients who are unstable as a result of ongoing blood loss or an expanding intracranial hemorrhage require intervention early in the evaluation phase.

The Unstable Patient

Immediate life-threatening injuries, such as airway obstruction, tension pneumothorax, pericardial tamponade, and obvious sources of external blood loss, must be treated promptly. The role of emergency department thoracotomy is controversial in children; its use should be confined to situations in which control of intrathoracic bleeding is needed (e.g., with lung or heart lacerations) or in situations in which previously detected vital signs are lost. If emergent thoracotomy is performed in the latter instance for presumptive intraabdominal hemorrhage, the aorta is cross-clamped at a level just above the diaphragm.

If significant head trauma has occurred, a determination must be made with regard to the need for immediate neurosurgical intervention. A rapidly performed computed tomography (CT) scan of the head is usually sufficient to determine the presence of a hematoma, which can be drained by the neurosurgeon. If hemodynamic instability or the need for immediate craniotomy exists and does not allow CT evaluation of the abdomen (Table 19.1), a diagnostic peritoneal lavage (DPL) should be performed in either the emergency department or operating suite. If the DPL is positive (Table 19.1), laparotomy and craniotomy proceed simultaneously. Finally, if neither thoracotomy nor craniotomy is indicated, emergent laparotomy is performed when pneumoperitoneum is noted on a plain radiograph or when the patient remains hemodynamically unstable in the face of historical or physical evidence of abdominal trauma (Fig. 19.3).

The Stable Patient

Commonly, the injured child can be stabilized with proper airway and cervical spine management and with intravenous fluid therapy and blood transfusion. A complete secondary survey should then be performed. Based on history and careful and serial abdominal examinations, CT is indicated when intraabdominal injuries are suspected (Table 19.2). Children who have had even minor injuries should be examined serially and monitored in the emergency department. At times, an abdominal CT scan is merited based solely on severe force inherent in a particular mechanism of injury, despite an unremarkable physical examination.

Diagnostic Imaging

Radiographic evaluation of children with abdominal trauma includes plain radiographs, contrast studies, radionuclide scans, ultrasonography, and CT. The stable child with abdominal trauma is best evaluated with abdominal CT using intravenous contrast. If a nasogastric or orogastric tube is in place, it should be withdrawn temporarily into the esophagus to avoid an artifact from its radiopaque marker. Abdominal CT has its lowest sensitivity for small gastrointestinal perforations and pancreatic injury. Although abdominal CT is considered the most sensitive diagnostic tool, abdominal ultrasonography may provide important data early in the course of the management of a child with suspected intraabdominal injuries. Data from the adult literature show that the

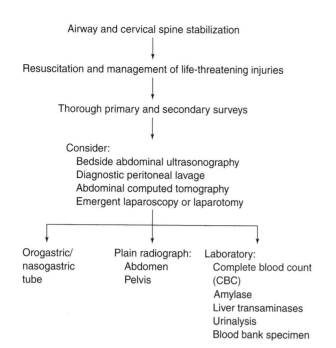

Airway and cervical spine stabilization

↓

Resuscitation and management of life-threatening injuries

↓

Thorough primary and secondary surveys

↓

Consider:
    Bedside abdominal ultrasonography
    Diagnostic peritoneal lavage
    Abdominal computed tomography
    Emergent laparoscopy or laparotomy

Orogastric/
nasogastric
tube

Plain radiograph:
    Abdomen
    Pelvis

Laboratory:
    Complete blood count
    (CBC)
    Amylase
    Liver transaminases
    Urinalysis
    Blood bank specimen

FIG. 19.1. Initial evaluation and treatment of the child with abdominal trauma.

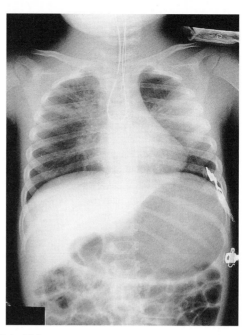

FIG. 19.2. This young boy was struck by a car while crossing a street and subsequently died from massive injury to the brain. He presented with a distended abdomen that was not successfully treated during the first few minutes of the resuscitation due to improper placement of a gastric tube. Also, note the bilateral pulmonary contusions, more prominent on the left, as well as the generalized ileus.

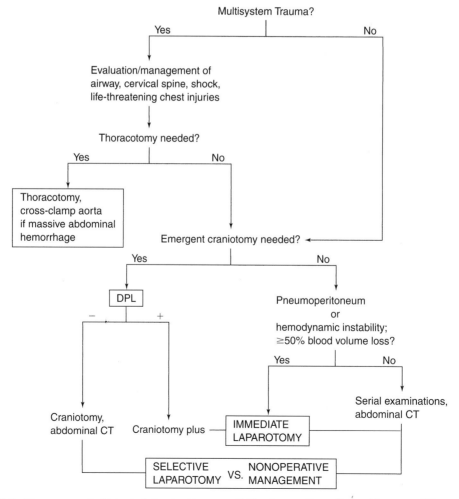

Multisystem Trauma?

Yes — Evaluation/management of airway, cervical spine, shock, life-threatening chest injuries

Thoracotomy needed?

Yes — Thoracotomy, cross-clamp aorta if massive abdominal hemorrhage

No — Emergent craniotomy needed?

No (Multisystem Trauma?) → Emergent craniotomy needed?

Yes — DPL
    − → Craniotomy, abdominal CT
    + → Craniotomy plus

No — Pneumoperitoneum or hemodynamic instability; ≥50% blood volume loss?
    Yes → IMMEDIATE LAPAROTOMY
    No → Serial examinations, abdominal CT

SELECTIVE LAPAROTOMY VS. NONOPERATIVE MANAGEMENT

FIG. 19.3. Management of blunt abdominal trauma. *DPL,* diagnostic peritoneal lavage; *CT,* computed tomography (See Table 19.2).

TABLE 19.1. *Positive diagnostic peritoneal lavage criteria*

1. >5 mL of gross blood
2. Obvious enteric contents (e.g., bile)
3. Peritoneal lavage fluid exiting from chest tube, urinary bladder catheter
4. Positive laboratory analysis of peritoneal lavage fluid
   a. >100,000 RBC/mm^3
   b. >500 WBC/mm^3
5. Elevated amylase in effluent

RBC, red blood cells; WBC, white blood cells.

TABLE 19.2. *Indications for abdominal computed tomography scan in the pediatric trauma patient*

1. Mechanism of injury suggesting major abdominal trauma
2. Slowly decreasing hematocrit
3. Unexplained fluid or blood requirements
4. Neurologic injury precluding accurate abdominal examination
5. Hematuria
6. Acute "need to know" (e.g., before general anesthesia)

TABLE 19.3. *Indications for immediate laparotomy for children with abdominal trauma*

Multisystem injuries with indications for craniotomy in the presence of a positive diagnostic peritoneal lavage, free peritoneal fluid on ultrasonography, or strong historical, physical, or radiographic evidence of abdominal injury
Persistent and significant hemodynamic instability with evidence of abdominal injury in the absence of extraabdominal injury
Penetrating wounds to the abdomen
Pneumoperitoneum
Significant abdominal distention associated with hypotension

sensitivity for the detection of intraperitoneal fluid ranges from 85% to 98%.

Diagnostic Peritoneal Lavage

DPL is occasionally a helpful adjunct to the management of children with abdominal trauma. The disadvantages of DPL include the introduction of air and fluid into the abdomen (subsequent radiographic evaluations are less helpful) and peritoneal irritation caused by the procedure (subsequent physical examinations are less reliable). It is rarely necessary to perform laparotomy on children with free intraperitoneal blood; thus, DPL, which effectively detects small volumes of blood, is often too sensitive in children. The primary indication for DPL in children is an urgent need to know with regard to the status of the peritoneal cavity, such as in the child who is hemodynamically unstable or requires immediate craniotomy, which cannot be delayed for abdominal CT.

Emergent Versus Selective Laparotomy

The indications for immediate laparotomy are limited in blunt abdominal trauma (Table 19.3). In most cases of childhood trauma (Fig. 19.3), emergency laparotomy is not necessary and further diagnostic studies direct either elective (selective) laparotomy or observation and monitoring. The indications for emergent laparotomy in children with penetrating trauma are illustrated in Figure 19.4. Any gunshot wound to the abdomen mandates immediate exploration. Other types of penetrating wounds in the presence of unexplained hemodynamic compromise, evisceration, pneumoperitoneum, or any evidence of violation of the peritoneum require prompt laparotomy.

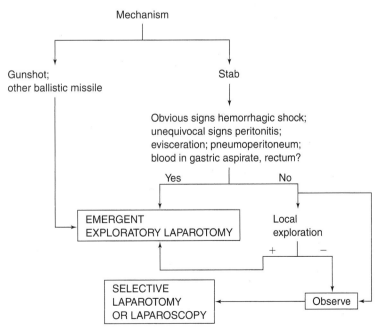

FIG. 19.4. Management of penetrating abdominal trauma.

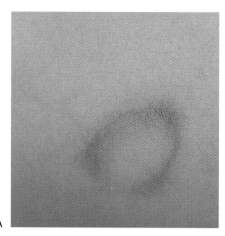
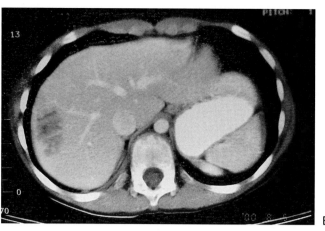

FIG. 19.5. This 10-year-old boy fell while riding his bicycle, landing on top of the handlebars. Although he sustained only a small cutaneous bruise **(A)**, one must be concerned about an impact that is very focused in nature. In fact, the computed tomography scan **(B)** showed a significant hepatic contusion.

BLUNT ABDOMINAL TRAUMA

Abdominal Wall Contusions

Many children have minor trauma to their abdomens in the course of play and as a result of minor accidental events. Balls, bats, swings, toys, and rough play may cause contusions of the abdominal wall. Children without signs of intraabdominal pathology can be sent home. Those with a troubling history or any worrisome signs should receive a diagnostic evaluation and be observed in consultation with a surgeon (Figs. 19.5, 19.6, and 19.7).

Solid Organ Injuries

Patients who have splenic injuries (Fig. 19.8) may present with either diffuse abdominal pain or localized tenderness. Subphrenic blood may cause referred left shoulder pain. Percussion and palpation tenderness is usually of greatest magnitude in the left upper quadrant of the abdomen. Abdominal radiographs occasionally reveal a medially displaced gastric bubble. CT will identify the extent of injury. The safety of nonoperative management of most childhood splenic injuries has been well documented, and postsplenectomy sepsis has decreased.

Blunt liver trauma is the most common fatal abdominal injury. Mechanisms of injury are those common to splenic trauma. Diffuse abdominal tenderness may be a result of hemoperitoneum, but maximal tenderness is elicited in the right upper quadrant of the abdomen. As with trauma to the spleen, nonoperative management of blunt hepatic injuries has become more common and is now the rule rather than the exception.

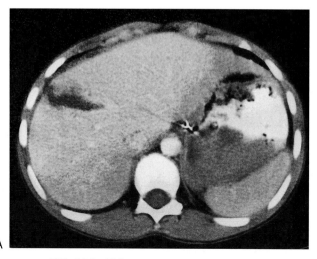
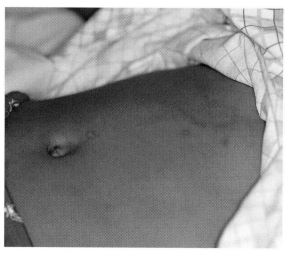

FIG. 19.6. This case serves as a reminder that blunt trauma may cause significant visceral injury such as a laceration of the liver **(A)**, despite minimal cutaneous signs **(B)**.

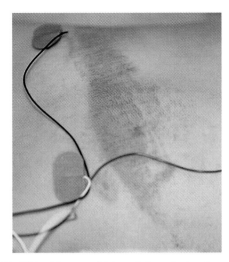

FIG. 19.7. This 10-year-old boy fell and struck a concrete curb, causing an obvious bruise. Despite a somewhat extensive surface wound, he sustained only a minimal hepatic contusion. Thus, a prominent cutaneous finding does not necessarily correlate with the extent of injury, if any, within the abdominal cavity.

Pancreatic Injuries

Blunt abdominal injuries, particularly from bicycle handlebars, are the most common cause of pancreatic pseudocyst formation in children, although this injury is uncommon. The pancreas is relatively well protected, and associated trauma such as hepatic and intestinal injuries commonly are present when injury to the pancreas has occurred. The classic triad of epigastric pain, a palpable abdominal mass, and hyperamylasemia is detected only rarely in children and may develop slowly. Severe injury of the pancreas is rare, but blood loss and leakage of enzyme-laden secretions may result in hypovolemia and peritonitis. Diagnosis depends on a high index of suspicion, consideration of the mechanism of injury, physical examination, serum amylase determination, and diagnostic imaging. Of note, the absence of hyperamylasemia does not preclude pancreatic trauma because elevated serum amylase does not occur

in cases of blunt injury without pancreatic involvement. Similarly, abdominal ultrasonography and contrast CT are useful, but acute pancreatic injuries may not be apparent on the initial scans. Nasogastric decompression and bowel rest are indicated when pancreatic injury is suspected. Nonoperative therapy is normally used initially for children with an isolated pancreatic pseudocyst caused by blunt trauma.

Hollow Abdominal Viscera Injuries

Intestinal perforation caused by blunt abdominal trauma is rare in the pediatric age group, but the most common causes of these injuries are automobile–pedestrian trauma, automobile lap belt injuries, and child abuse. Hollow viscera injury may be difficult to diagnose because physical findings may be minimal and/or nonspecific for the first few hours and abdominal CT is not particularly sensitive. However, succus entericus, bile, and activated pancreatic enzymes are extremely irritating to the peritoneum over time; the development of fever or worsening peritonitis on serial physical examinations should alert the examining physician to the possibility of bowel perforation. Plain radiographs of the abdomen demonstrate free intraabdominal air in only 30% to 50% of cases. Similarly, pneumoperitoneum or leakage of gastrointestinal contrast is only rarely seen on the CT scan. DPL may demonstrate bile or amylase in the effluent and is sensitive for bowel perforations. Most perforations or transections of bowel are discovered at laparotomy, which the surgeon has chosen to perform because of advancing peritonitis or unexplained persistent fever. Management depends on the site and extent of structural injury.

Lap/Shoulder Belt and Air Bag Injuries

Children who are too large for child safety seats but too small for adult seat belts are at increased risk of injuries. In particular, children restrained only by lap belts (Fig. 19.9) in

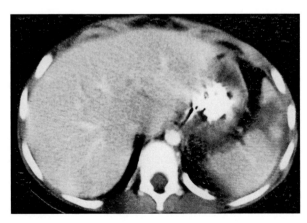

FIG. 19.8. This computed tomography scan shows a major splenic laceration that followed an impact that involved a low level of force but a high degree of focus.

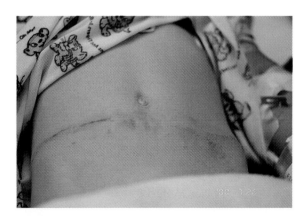

FIG. 19.9. This 5-year-old girl, a victim of a motor vehicle collision, was wearing a lap belt but not a shoulder strap. She presented with a typical lap belt mark and hematuria. After a thorough evaluation, she was diagnosed with a mild renal contusion but not a vertebral (Chance) fracture or a visceral perforation.

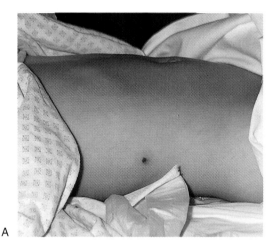
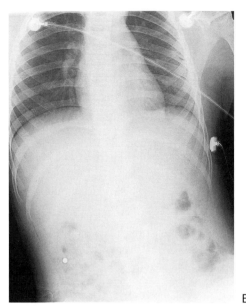

A   B

FIG. 19.10. The brother of this 5-year-old girl unintentionally shot her in the kitchen of their home with a pellet gun. Unfortunately, these toys have sufficient power to cause severe injuries. Despite the seemingly innocuous entry wound **(A)**, the radiograph reveals the projectile within the abdominal cavity **(B)**.

motor vehicles involved in rapid deceleration crashes are at risk of sustaining Chance fractures (compression or flexion–distraction fractures of the lumbar spine) in association with intraabdominal injuries (the lap belt complex). As many as one-half of the children with Chance fractures have intraabdominal injuries; therefore, a high index of suspicion must be maintained to detect such injuries. The hallmark indicator of the lap belt complex is abdominal or flank ecchymosis in the pattern of a strap or belt. A normal abdominal CT does not rule out ruptured viscous, and laparoscopy or laparotomy should be considered for children in whom the lap belt complex is suspected. Carotid injuries caused by high-riding shoulder restraints in motor vehicle collisions are much less common.

Late Presentations of Blunt Intraabdominal Trauma

Some children with abdominal trauma do not have evidence of intraabdominal pathology on the initial evaluation but may return days or weeks later with abdominal distention and/or pain, persistent emesis, or hematochezia. In particular, three injuries are characterized by late presentations: (1) pancreatic pseudocyst (previously discussed), (2) duodenal hematoma, and (3) hematobilia.

Intramural duodenal hematoma is an uncommon injury that results from a direct blow to the epigastrium (blunt force delivered by a small-diameter instrument such as a broom handle or the toe of a boot) or from rapid deceleration and may cause partial or complete gastric outlet obstruction. Bleeding into the wall of the duodenum causes compression

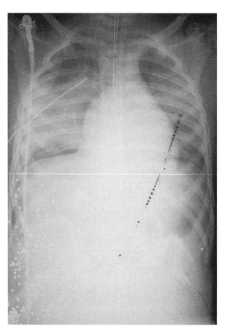

FIG. 19.11. This radiograph demonstrates a penetrating injury (shotgun pellets) to the chest and abdomen of a 6-year-old boy. The child went into a cardiac arrest on arrival but was rapidly resuscitated and taken to the operating room. To control his intraabdominal bleeding, the surgeon performed a right hepatic lobectomy and a right nephrectomy. The patient recovered fully, with the exception of a hemiparesis secondary to a spinal cord contusion caused by the force of the blast.

and therefore symptoms of intestinal obstruction, including pain, bilious vomiting, and gastric distention. Diagnosis is made by ultrasonography or a contrast upper gastrointestinal study, revealing the coiled spring sign. Nonoperative management includes nasogastric decompression and parenteral nutrition for as long as 3 weeks.

Rupture of the gallbladder is rare and is almost always associated with severe blunt trauma to the liver. Likewise, hematobilia is associated with hepatic trauma and is a result of pressure necrosis from an intrahepatic hematoma or direct injury to the biliary tree. Children with hematobilia present several days after a blunt abdominal trauma with abdominal pain and upper gastrointestinal bleeding. Cholangiography confirms the diagnosis. Embolization is used to achieve hemostasis, but hepatic resection is necessary when this treatment fails.

Penetrating Abdominal Trauma

Gunshot Wounds

Gunshots often injure hollow viscera and large vessels, and solid organs such as the liver and spleen may demonstrate burst injuries (Figs. 19.10 and 19.11). Therefore, laparotomy is mandated in all gunshot wounds to the abdomen.

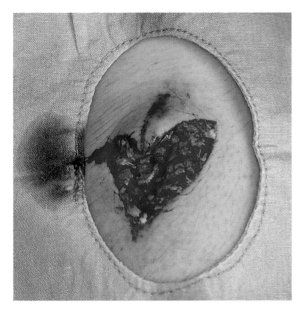

FIG. 19.12. This child fell while climbing over a picket fence, sustaining a "stab" to his anterior abdomen. Careful local exploration by the emergency physician identified the depth of the wound and excluded penetration of the peritoneum.

Stab Wounds

The extent of the injury from stabs depends on the type, size, and length of the weapon and on the trajectory. Major vascular injuries pose the greatest threat; commonly injured vessels include the intraabdominal aorta, the inferior vena cava, the portal vein, and the hepatic veins. Anterior stab wounds are explored via laparotomy if hemodynamic instability or signs of peritonitis are present, if blood is noted in the gastric aspirate or on rectal examination, or if pneumoperitoneum or evisceration is noted (Fig. 19.4). Local exploration is needed to rule out penetration of the peritoneum even in minor stab wounds (Fig. 19.12).

Stab wounds to the flank or back are less readily and less quickly diagnosed than anterior wounds; the retroperitoneal structures are more protected by paraspinal musculature, and bleeding is often tamponaded in this area. Dorsal stab wounds are sometimes managed nonoperatively unless hemodynamic instability or signs of peritonitis are present, although selective laparotomy is a common surgical strategy.

SUGGESTED READINGS

Akgur FM, Aktug T, Olguner M, et al. Prospective study investigating routine usage of ultrasonography as the initial diagnostic modality for the evaluation of children sustaining blunt abdominal trauma. *J Trauma* 1997;42:626–628.

Arkovitz MS, Johnson N, Garcia VF. Pancreatic trauma in children: mechanisms of injury. *J Trauma* 1997;42:49–53.

Bensard DD, Beaver BL, Besner GE, et al. Small bowel injury after blunt abdominal trauma: is diagnostic delay important? *J Trauma* 1996;41: 476–483.

Boyle EM, Maier RV, Salazar JD, et al. Diagnosis of injuries after stab wounds to the back and flank. *J Trauma* 1997;42:260–265.

Branney SW, Moore EE, Cantrill SV, et al. Ultrasound based key clinical pathway reduces the use of hospital resources for the evaluation of blunt abdominal trauma. *J Trauma* 1997;42:1086–1090.

Carillo EH, Bergamini TM, Miller FB, et al. Abdominal vascular injuries. *J Trauma* 1997;43:164–171.

Galat J, Grisoni E, Gauderer M. Pediatric blunt liver injury: establishment of criteria for appropriate management. *J Pediatr Surg* 1990;11: 1162–1165.

Jaffe D, Wesson D. Emergency management of blunt trauma in children. *N Engl J Med* 1991;324:1477–1482.

Keller MS, Stafford PW, Vane DW. Conservative management of pancreatic trauma in children. *J Trauma* 1997;42:1097–1100.

McKenney MG, Martin L, Lentz K, et al. 1,000 consecutive ultrasounds for blunt abdominal trauma. *J Trauma* 1996;40:607–612.

Newman KD, Bowman LM, Eichelberger MR, et al. The lap belt complex: intestinal and lumbar spine injury in children. *J Trauma* 1990;30: 1133–1140.

Patton JH, Syden SP, Croce MA, et al. Pancreatic trauma: a simplified management guideline. *J Trauma* 1997;43:234–241.

Saladino R, Lund D, Fleisher G. The spectrum of live and spleen injuries in childhood: failure of the pediatric trauma score and clinical signs to predict isolated injuries. *Ann Emerg Med* 1991;6:636–640.

Zantut LF, Ivatury RR, Smith RS, et al. Diagnostic and therapeutic laparoscopy for penetrating abdominal trauma: a multicenter experience. *J Trauma* 1997;42:825–831.

CHAPTER 20

Trauma: Burns

Editor: Stephen Ludwig

A first-degree burn is characterized by redness and a mild inflammatory response confined to the epidermis, without significant edema or vesiculation. First-degree burns are not included in the calculation of body surface area (BSA) used for therapeutic decisions. These minor burns are somewhat painful, healing in 3 to 5 days without scarring.

Most burns treated in emergency departments are partial-thickness or second-degree burns (Fig. 20.1). Superficial second-degree burns involve destruction of the epidermis and less than half of the dermis. Blistering is often present (Fig. 20.2). Increased capillary permeability, resulting from direct thermal injury and local mediator release, results in edema (Fig. 20.3). These injuries are usually painful because intact sensory nerve receptors are exposed. The capillary network in the superficial dermis gives these burns a pink-red color and moist appearance. Healing occurs in approximately 2 weeks, and scarring is usually minimal.

Deep partial-thickness burns involve destruction of epidermis and more than 50% of the dermis. Edema can lessen the exposure of sensory nerve receptors, making some partial-thickness burns less painful and tender. Deep partial-thickness burns have a paler, drier appearance than superficial injuries (Fig. 20.4). They are sometimes difficult to distinguish from areas of full-thickness injury. Thrombosed vessels often give the deep partial-thickness burn a speckled appearance. Burns evaluated immediately may appear to be partial-thickness and subsequently become full-thickness injuries, especially if secondary damage from infection, trauma, or hypoperfusion ensues. Deep partial-thickness burns can take many weeks to heal completely. Unacceptable scarring is not uncommon. Skin grafting is often necessary to optimize cosmetic results.

Full-thickness or third-degree burns involve destruction of the epidermis and all the dermis. They usually have a pale or charred color and a leathery appearance (Fig. 20.5). Destruction of the cutaneous nerves in the dermis makes them nontender, although surrounding areas of partial-thickness burns may cause pain. Full-thickness burns cannot reepithelialize and can only heal from the periphery. Most require skin grafting. Fourth-degree burns are those full-thickness injuries that involve underlying fascia, muscle, or bone.

Major Burns

Evaluation and Management

During the first few seconds after arrival, the physician must determine whether a burned patient requires aggressive therapy for major burns (greater than 15% BSA) (Fig. 20.6). In children with severe injuries, the evaluation and initial management take place simultaneously.

Airway

There are several causes of airway obstruction in the severely burned patient. Most life-threatening burns are the result of house fires. The inhalation of hot gases can burn the upper airway, leading to progressive edema and airway obstruction. Any child with burns of the face, singed facial hairs, or hoarseness is at high risk, but airway burns can occur in the absence of these signs. Edema of the burned airway will worsen over the first 24 to 48 hours. Knowledge of the time course of airway swelling warrants intubation of the trachea for subtle signs of airway compromise that occur shortly after the injury.

Breathing

A rapid assessment of ventilation includes respiratory effort, chest expansion, breath sounds, and color. Pulse oximetry is useful, but patients with significant levels of carboxyhemoglobin will look pink and have normal oxygen saturation as measured by a pulse oximeter. Every severely burned child should receive 100% oxygen. Arterial blood gases with cooximetry should be obtained promptly. Patients whose ventilatory status is questionable should receive careful assisted ventilation. Avoidance of high inflating pressures and application of cricoid pressure can minimize gaseous distention of the stomach and reduce the risk of regurgitation with pulmonary aspiration.

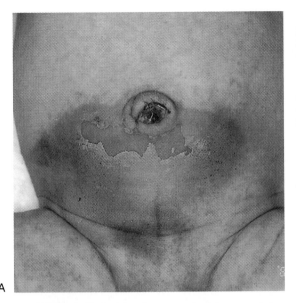

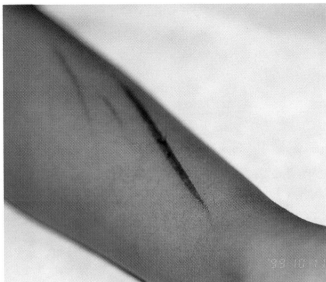

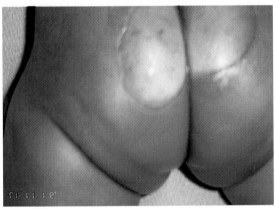

FIG. 20.1. **A:** Second-degree umbilical burn due to silver nitrate. **B:** Second-degree burn of the leg from contact with an iron. **C:** The buttocks of this infant show a second-degree burn as a result of being intentionally immersed in scalding water.

Chest radiographs may be normal initially, even if pulmonary injury has occurred. Smoke is responsible for most of the lower airway abnormalities in burned patients (Fig. 20.7).

Circulation: Burn Shock

The physiology of circulatory impairment in severely burned patients is complex. Burn shock occurs in adults with burns over 30% of BSA but may occur in children with burns over 20% of BSA.

The rapid assessment of circulation includes skin color, capillary refill time, temperature of the peripheral extremities, heart rate, and mental status. Blood pressure is often maintained until decompensation occurs, making it an unreliable measure of early circulatory impairment. Hypertension from increased systemic vascular resistance has been reported immediately after severe burns, particularly in pediatric patients.

Vascular access should be obtained soon after arrival of the severely burned child. Intravenous lines in the upper extremity through intact skin are preferred because they are easier to secure, but access through burned areas may be necessary.

An initial 20-mL/kg bolus of Ringer lactate solution is recommended while assessment of the extent of the burns takes place. A urinary catheter should be placed, and urine output monitored to assess the adequacy of fluid therapy. Major burns cause decreased splanchnic blood flow and ileus. After ensuring that the airway is protected with an endotracheal tube or an adequate gag reflex, the clinician

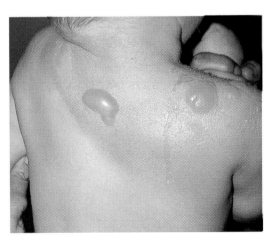

FIG. 20.2. Second-degree sunburn.

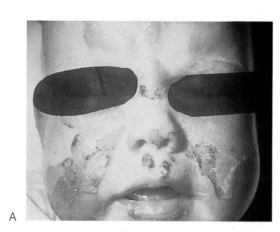

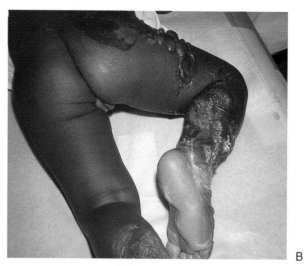

FIG. 20.3. Direct thermal injury burns. **A:** Splatter burn. **B:** Bathtub burn.

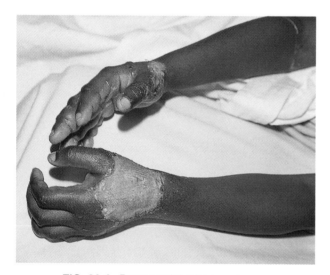

FIG. 20.4. Deep partial-thickness burns.

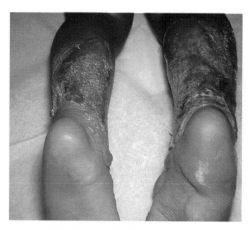

FIG. 20.5. Full-thickness burns.

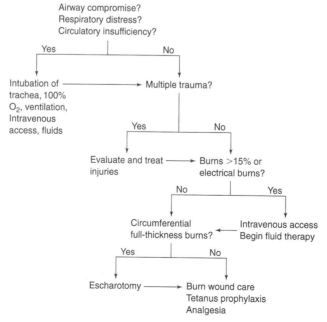

FIG. 20.6. Diagnostic approach to the burn patient.

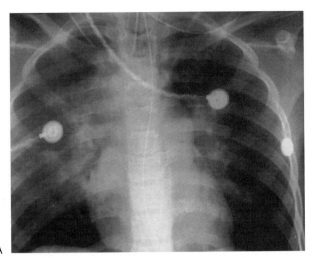
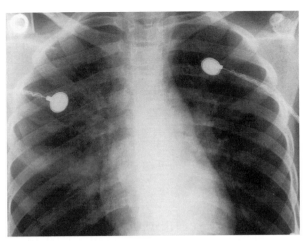

FIG. 20.7. Smoke inhalation in a 9-year-old girl. **A:** There is bilateral central alveolar process with acute smoke inhalation. **B:** A day later, the patient has been extubated, and there is marked improvement in the appearance of pulmonary edema.

should place a nasogastric tube. Hypothermia can occur rapidly in small children, especially in those whose skin injury impairs normal thermoregulation. Core temperature should be monitored and the child kept covered, except as necessary for examination and burn assessment. Tetanus toxoid is indicated if the child has not been immunized in the preceding 5 years; unimmunized patients require tetanus immunoglobulin as well.

Major burns are three-dimensional injuries. To estimate the size of a burn, one must assess the surface area and depth of burned skin. Decisions about fluid therapy, referral, disposition, and prognosis are based on the size of the burn. After stabilization of vital functions in the primary survey, a systematic evaluation of the surface area and depth of burns follows. The rule of nines used to estimate BSA in adults cannot be applied to children with their different body proportions. Young children have relatively larger heads and smaller extremities. Areas of partial- and full-thickness injury should be recorded on an anatomic chart and then total percentage BSA computed using age-appropriate proportions.

Fluid Therapy

Prompt treatment of the hypovolemia that occurs early in children with severe thermal injuries is of prime importance. The fluid status of burned children is a dynamic process that requires careful reevaluation and therapeutic adjustments.

Several formulas for calculation of fluid therapy exist (Table 20.1). The Parkland formula recommends 4 mL/kg per percentage of BSA of crystalloid over the first 24 hours, half during the first 8 hours and half over the next 16 hours. This formula underestimates the needs of young children. Adding maintenance requirements to this volume more accurately supplies the requirements of burn victims younger

than 5 years of age. The Carvajal formula uses BSA rather than weight to calculate fluid therapy. Carvajal recommends 5,000 mL/m^2 per percentage of BSA, half in the first 8 hours and half over the next 16 hours, plus 2,000 mL/m^2 per day as maintenance. Formulas for fluid therapy in burn patients must be used carefully in small children. The calculated volume requirements are useful to the clinician in providing an initial rate of fluid infusion. Adjustments of infusion rates are the rule, not the exception. Many pediatric burn centers prefer to follow urine output rather than central venous pressure to assess the adequacy of fluid therapy. Children should produce at least 1 mL/kg per hour of urine. Oliguria, as determined by this measure, is almost always the result of inadequate fluid administration. Intrinsic renal disease is sometimes noted after electrical injuries because of myoglobinuria. Hyperglycemia may cause an osmotic diuresis and complicate care of the burned patient. Before infusions are decreased in response to excessive urine output, blood sugar should be measured.

Pain Management

Reducing pain is an important consideration in the management of children with burns. Pain is a subjective experience influenced by the preceding events. Children rescued from

TABLE 20.1. *Fluid resuscitation formulas*

Parkland: 4 mL/kg per percentage of BSA second- and third-degree burns, half in the first 8 hr, half in the next 16 hr; add maintenance in children < 5 yr old

Carvajal: 5,000 ml/m^2 per percentage of BSA second- and third-degree burns, half in the first 8 hr, half in the next 16 hr; add 2,000 mL/m^2/d maintenance

BSA, body surface area.

house fires, separated from their parents, transported in ambulances, and brought to emergency departments are usually extremely anxious. Calm, developmentally appropriate verbal reassurance, even to preverbal children, can reduce anxiety and dramatically reduce the perception of pain.

Disposition

Guidelines for admission must be individualized when treating burned children. Hospitals, physicians, and parents have varying capabilities for managing pediatric burn patients. In general, children with burns of lower percentages of BSA than adults require admission, especially patients younger than 2 years old.

Children with partial-thickness burns of more than 10% of BSA should be considered for admission to a hospital. Partial-thickness injury of more than 20% of BSA warrants admission to a children's hospital or burn center. Full-thickness burns over 2% of BSA require inpatient treatment. Burns in some locations present a higher risk of disability or poor cosmetic outcome and should be considered for treatment in the hospital. These include over 1% burns of the face, perineum, hands, feet, circumferential burns, or burns overlying joints (Fig. 20.8). Children with inhalation injury or associated trauma require admission with burns involving lower percentages of BSA. Any time that the physician suspects that the burns cannot be adequately cared for in the home, admission to the hospital is warranted.

Outpatient Management of Burns

A small minority of all burns in children require therapy in the hospital. After a careful assessment has led to a decision to manage a burned patient on an outpatient basis, preparations for treatment at home should begin.

A first-degree burn usually requires no therapy. Moisturizers and acetaminophen or ibuprofen can be given as needed. Partial-thickness burns are first cleansed with mild soap and water, one-fourth strength povidone-iodine

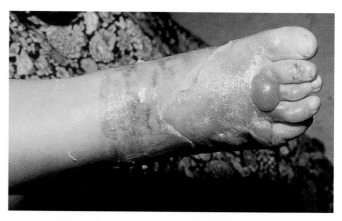

FIG. 20.9. Large bullae likely to be ruptured.

solution, or saline alone. Devitalized tissue can usually be removed by wiping with gauze. Large bullae that are likely to rupture because of their location can be debrided (Fig. 20.9). Clean partial-thickness burns of less than 2% BSA can be dressed with petrolatum gauze. Topical antibiotics are recommended for larger or more contaminated burns. Silver sulfadiazine cream (Silvadene) or bacitracin is the topical antibacterial agent of choice at most burn centers. A $\frac{1}{4}$- to $\frac{1}{2}$-in. layer of silver sulfadiazine is applied to the burn with a sterile tongue blade or gloved hand. Silver sulfadiazine is soothing to the burn and has few side effects. Mild bleaching of the skin may occur. Bacitracin is often chosen for burns of the face. Approximately 5% of children are allergic to sulfa and can be treated with bacitracin or povidone-iodine ointment. Leukopenia has also been reported in patients treated with silver sulfadiazine.

A loose gauze dressing should be placed over the burn and secured with tape. Burns of the face can be treated with an open technique. Dressings should be changed twice each day. The parent should rinse off residual antibacterial cream with warm water and inspect the wound. Signs of infection, such as redness and tenderness around the margin of the burn, warrant immediate evaluation by a physician. A greenish material formed by serous drainage from the burn mixing with the silver sulfadiazine cream is often mistaken for purulence. If the burn is healing well, the parent should reapply the antibiotic cream and dress the wound as demonstrated by the physician or nurse in the emergency department. Burns should be examined by a physician every 2 or 3 days until healing is well under way. Large burns or burns of the hands, feet, perineum, or overlying joints that are managed on an outpatient basis should be referred for follow-up to a burn specialist and evaluated more frequently. Prophylactic antibiotics are not recommended.

Electrical Burns

Burns that result when electrical current passes through the body have unique characteristics. Each year, there are more

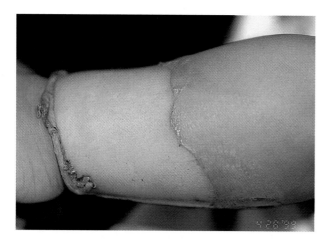

FIG. 20.8. This circumferential burn carries a high risk of leading to complications and disability.

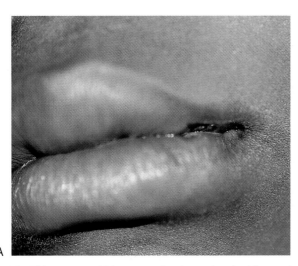

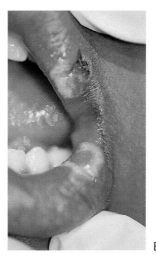

FIG. 20.10. This 5-year-old boy sustained an electrical burn when he bit an electrical cord **(A, B)**. On follow-up after 5 days, only minimal improvement occurred, as is typical for electrical burns.

than 4,000 emergency department visits caused by electrical injuries, mostly in children. Electrical burns account for 3% of burn center admissions and are increasing in number. Most injuries occur in young children from contact with low-voltage (less than 120 V) alternating household current, often from mouthing plugs or extension cords. Severe high-voltage (greater than 500 V) injuries are seen most often in adolescent males as a consequence of risk-taking behaviors.

The initial approach to victims of electrical burns is similar to that for other severely burned children. The potential for arrhythmias requires close cardiac monitoring. Electrical burns are usually more severe than they appear. Significant deep and internal injuries may occur in patients with relatively small entrance and exit wounds. Fluid requirements are higher than predicted by formulas based on estimates of percentage of BSA because a larger portion of the injury is

internal. Destruction of muscle often causes myoglobinuria. Renal failure usually can be prevented with forced diuresis and alkalinization. Electrical injury and edema within fascial compartments can cause a compartment syndrome with vascular insufficiency. Severe electrical injuries require extensive evaluation for internal injuries, which should be done at a children's hospital or regional burn center.

A common electrical injury occurs to the lips and mouths of toddlers (Figs. 20.10 and 20.11) who suck on plugs or extension cords. Deep burns at the corner of the mouth require specialized attention to prevent severe scarring and contracture. Bleeding from the labial artery 1 to 2 weeks after injury, when the eschar separates, can result in significant blood loss. In previous years, these children were hospitalized for 2 weeks, but most burn specialists now manage these children as outpatients. Electrical burns may also occur when a child places a key in an outlet (Fig. 20.12) or

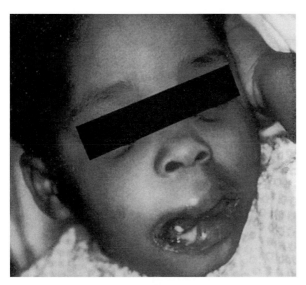

FIG. 20.11. Patient with electrical burns to the corner of the mouth after biting on an electrical cord.

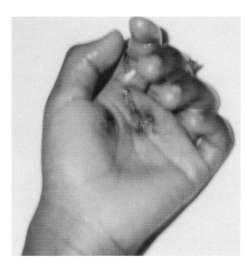

FIG. 20.12. Electrical hand burn.

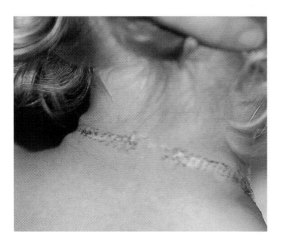

FIG. 20.13. Electrical neck burn.

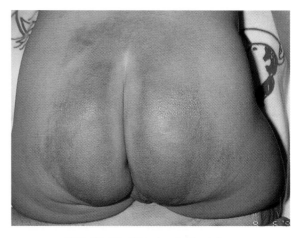

FIG. 20.15. Chlorine buttock burn.

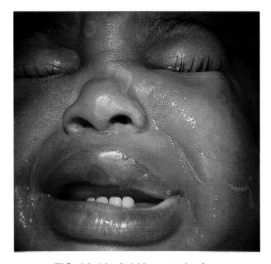

FIG. 20.14. Acid burn to the face.

may be caused by other types of contact with live current (Fig. 20.13).

Chemical Burns

More than 25,000 different caustic products can cause burns. Most are either acidic or alkaline. Acids (Figs. 20.14 and 20.1a) cause coagulation of tissue proteins, which limit the depth of penetration (Fig. 20.15). Alkali results in liquefaction and deeper injury. Caustic chemicals on the skin cause a prolonged period of burning compared with most thermal burns. Edema of the underlying tissue can make full-thickness injuries appear deceptively superficial. Treatment of caustic burns, whether acid or base, involves copious irrigation to dilute the chemical and stop the burning.

SUGGESTED READINGS

Carvajal HF. Fluid resuscitation of pediatric burn victims: a critical appraisal. *Pediatr Nephrol* 1994;8:357–366.

Mozingo DW, Smith AA, McManus WF, et al. Chemical burns. *J Trauma* 1988;28:642–647.

Walker AR. Emergency department management of house fire burns and carbon monoxide poisoning in children. *Curr Opin Pediatr* 1996;8:239–242.

CHAPTER 21

Trauma: Chest

Editor: Marc N. Baskin

Although thoracic trauma in the pediatric population is relatively uncommon, injuries to vital thoracic organs can produce profound physiologic disturbances and many patients die at the scene, never reaching a hospital. In patients who reach the hospital, most thoracic injuries do not require operative intervention other than tube thoracostomy.

INITIAL MANAGEMENT

The first priority in any trauma patient is establishing a secure, patent airway. Indications for endotracheal intubation in the thoracic trauma patient include depressed neurologic status, inadequate oxygenation or ventilation, compromised circulatory status, and an unstable airway.

After the airway is secured, breathing is assessed. Inspection (symmetry, adequate chest rise, neck veins, displaced trachea) and auscultation (equal breath sounds, heart tones) of the chest provide information about ventilation. An oxygen saturation by oximetry provides information on oxygenation.

If a patient has an abnormal examination but appears to be oxygenating and ventilating well and is not in shock, chest radiography is indicated. If, after endotracheal intubation, breath sounds are absent on one side and the trachea is shifted to the opposite side, then the patient requires immediate needle decompression and subsequent tube thoracostomy. Only after the patient is stabilized should a chest radiograph be obtained.

The patient's circulatory status is evaluated after airway and breathing have been stabilized. Pericardial tamponade, tension pneumothorax, or hemothorax should be considered in any shocky patient, especially when sources of blood loss have been excluded and volume resuscitation has not improved the patient's status. Physical examination may reveal muffled heart or breath sounds with decreased or absent pulses.

Once immediate life-threatening injuries such as airway obstruction, tension pneumothorax, hemothorax, and pericardial tamponade are treated, a chest radiograph and thoracic computed tomography (CT) scan should be obtained to assess other potentially life-threatening injuries. Thoracic injuries requiring operative intervention are described in Table 21.1 and Figure 21.1. Thoracic CT is superior to routine chest radiograph in identifying pulmonary contusions, pneumothoraces, and hemothoraces.

CHEST WALL INJURIES

The elasticity and flexibility of a child's thoracic cage make chest wall injuries less common than internal organ injuries, such as a pulmonary contusion. When chest wall injuries occur, the patient is at increased risk of intrathoracic injuries.

Rib Fractures

Rib fractures may occur from either a direct blow to the rib or compression of the chest in an anteroposterior direction. With a direct blow, the rib will fracture inward and may puncture the pleural cavity, causing pneumothorax. Hemothorax is caused by a rib lacerating an intercostal artery, an internal mammary artery, or the lung parenchyma.

Because of the relatively protected nature of the first rib and the amount of force required to fracture it, first rib fractures should be approached with a high index of suspicion for other serious injuries, such as vascular disruption. Patients with vascular injuries are usually symptomatic, usually having hypotension, radial pulse differences, or blood pressure discrepancies between the upper and lower extremities.

Physical examination may reveal point tenderness and, if the pleura has been involved, crepitus. If the patient has any respiratory or circulatory compromise, a tube thoracotomy is indicated for pneumothorax or hemothorax. The tube should be placed at a site separate from the area of the fracture. If the patient is stable, then relief of pain, monitoring the respiratory status, and further evaluation (chest radiography, thoracic CT) for underlying injury is indicated.

TABLE 21.1. *Thoracic trauma injuries requiring operative intervention*

Injury	Signs and symptoms
Tracheal/bronchial rupture	Active chest tube air leak
Lung parenchyma, internal mammary artery laceration, intercostal artery laceration	Chest tube bleeding greater than 2–3 mL/kg/hr or hypotension unresponsive to transfusions
Esophageal disruption	Abnormal esophagogram (leak) or esophagoscopy; gastric contents in the chest tube
Diaphragmatic hernia	Abnormal gas pattern in the hemithorax
	Displaced nasogastric tube in the hemithorax
Pericardial tamponade	Positve pericardiocentesis
Great vessel laceration	Widened mediastinum; tracheal or nasogastric tube deviation; blurred aortic knob; abnormal aortogram (gold standard)

Patients with multiple rib fractures should be admitted to the hospital for pain control, pulmonary physiotherapy, and observation for worsening respiratory status.

Sternal Fractures and Sternoclavicular Joint Injuries

Sternal fractures are uncommon in children and require a thorough evaluation for other thoracic injuries because of the significant force required to fracture this bone (Fig. 21.2). Sternal fractures are rarely associated with cardiac or vascular injuries.

Direct trauma to the sternum may also cause injury to the sternoclavicular joint. Before the age of 18, injury to the sternoclavicular joint causes physeal separations because the epiphysis of the medial clavicle begins to ossify between 13 and 19 years of age and fuses between 22 and 25 years of age. If the separation is posterior, the aorta or trachea may be injured and the patient may complain of choking or difficulty breathing. Plain radiographs may be normal, and CT is usually necessary to delineate the lesion (Fig. 21.3).

Flail Chest

Fracturing two or more ribs on the same side may result in that particular chest wall segment losing continuity with the thoracic cage. This condition is called a flail chest. Direct

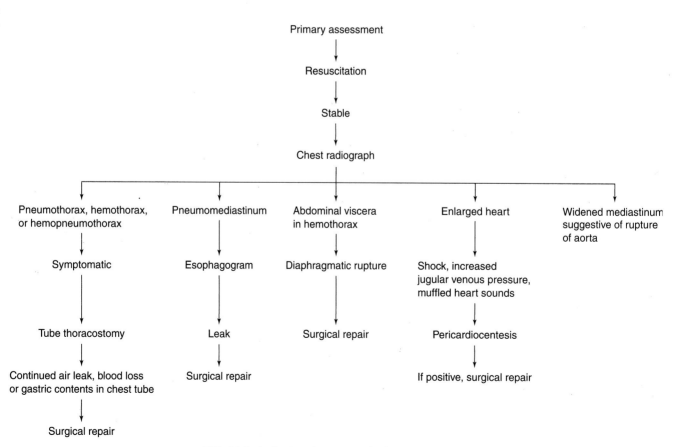

FIG. 21.1. Indicators for surgery in thoracic trauma.

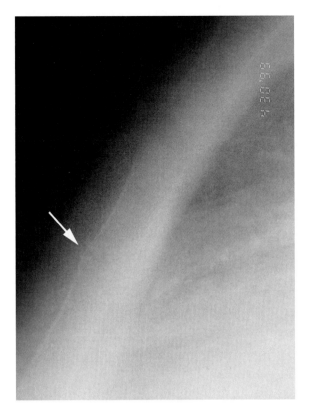

FIG. 21.2. This 17-year-old boy had chest pain after a motor vehicle crash with airbag deployment. His routine posteroanterior and lateral chest radiographs were normal, but this lateral sternal view was obtained because of sternal tenderness. The irregular lucent area is a sternal fracture (arrow).

impact to the rib, as in a crush injury, is the most common mechanism. Flail chest is uncommon in children because of the compliance of the pediatric chest wall. When a flail chest occurs, it is usually associated with an intrathoracic injury, most often pulmonary contusion. The paradoxical movement of the chest impairs the normal inspiratory-expiratory function of the lung. Any patient with respiratory distress should be intubated and placed on positive-pressure ventilation.

PULMONARY CONTUSIONS AND LACERATIONS

Pulmonary contusion is the most common thoracic injury in children and occurs when a blunt force is applied to the lung parenchyma. As in any contusion, the capillary network becomes damaged, leaking fluid into the surrounding tissues. A ventilation-perfusion mismatch occurs because of the extravasation of fluid, interfering with oxygenation. A pulmonary contusion may initially be invisible on a chest radiograph (Fig. 21.4). Chest CT is more sensitive for detecting pulmonary contusion.

Mild contusions require close observation in the hospital for worsening respiratory status and supportive care. Patients with more severe pulmonary contusions may be tachypneic and have an oxygen requirement secondary to shunting within the lung. If the patient can no longer maintain oxygenation, endotracheal intubation and mechanical ventilation with positive pressure are the preferred treatment. Fluid restriction is helpful to avoid exacerbation of pulmonary edema.

Pulmonary lacerations occur more often in penetrating trauma, but rib fractures secondary to blunt trauma may also puncture the lung. Large lacerations may cause hemoptysis. Chest radiographs show pneumothorax or hemothorax.

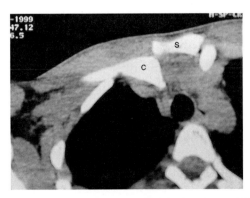

FIG. 21.3. This adolescent was struck in the chest while playing hockey. This computed tomography scan shows his clavicle (c) displaced posteriorly compared with his sternum (s).

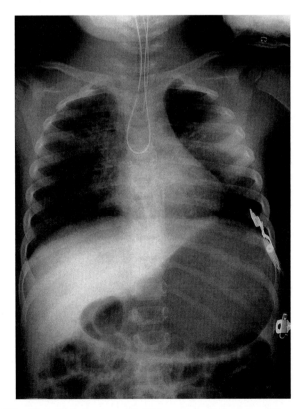

FIG. 21.4. This 3-year-old child was struck by a car. The radiograph shows the pulmonary contusion, looking much like pneumonia. Note the malpositioned nasogastric tube and the resultant distended abdomen.

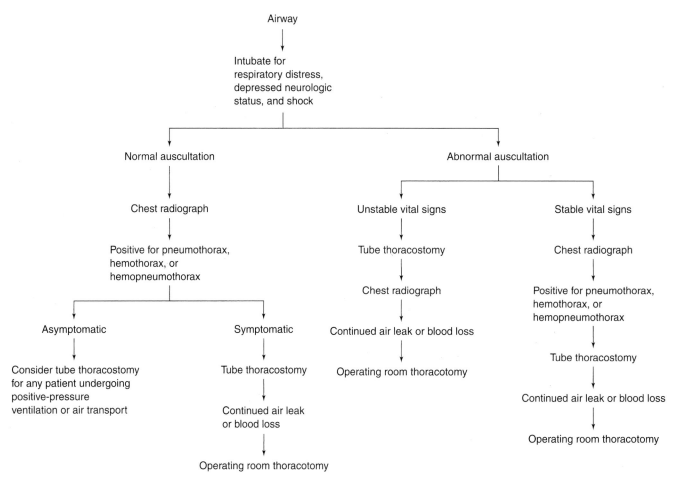

FIG. 21.5. Algorithm for the management of intrapleural injuries.

INTRAPLEURAL INJURIES

Most intrapleural injuries do not need surgical intervention and can be managed either by hospital observation or tube thoracostomy (Fig. 21.5).

PNEUMOTHORAX

Management of pneumothorax and tension pneumothorax is discussed in Chapter 4 (Cardiothoracic Emergencies).

HEMOTHORAX

In blunt thoracic trauma, the most common cause of hemothorax is injury to the intercostal or internal mammary arteries from rib fractures, whereas injuries to the lung or great vessels causing hemothorax are much less common but more serious. Hemothorax is much more common in penetrating than in blunt thoracic trauma.

Patients may present in respiratory distress or in profound shock secondary to massive blood loss. Decreased breath sounds are noted on the affected side. Thirty to 40% of the patient's blood volume may be rapidly lost into the pleural cavity with major vessel lacerations. Bleeding from the intercostal or internal mammary arteries stops secondary to low systemic pressures. If the patient is stable, a chest radiograph should be obtained to confirm the diagnosis (Fig. 21.6). Patients should be typed and cross-matched for packed red blood cells and adequately volume resuscitated, preferably with two large intravenous lines in place. O negative blood, if type-specific blood is not available, should be available at the patient's bedside as soon as possible.

Tube thoracotomy is performed to evacuate blood and re-expand the lung in the same manner as for pneumothorax. Blood within the pleural cavity may tamponade a significant bleeding source within the chest and evacuating that blood may cause new bleeding to occur. Patients can exsanguinate rapidly; therefore, intravenous access, adequate volume resuscitation, and blood available for transfusion should be a priority.

CHYLOTHORAX

Chylothorax is rare in thoracic trauma and most commonly occurs secondary to iatrogenic complications. Disruption of

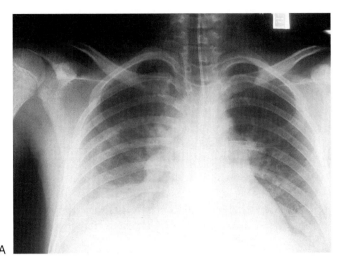
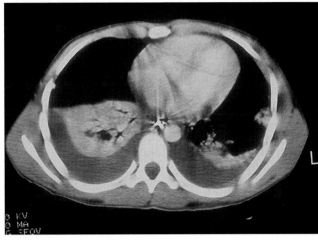

FIG. 21.6. A 15-year-old child involved in an auto–pedestrian accident. Vital signs were stable at the scene, but the child had decreased breath sounds bilaterally. **A:** The chest radiograph shows bilateral hemothorax and pulmonary contusions. **B:** Computed tomography confirmed and better delineated hemothorax and pulmonary contusions.

the thoracic duct will lead to chyle draining into the mediastinum and pleural space. Diagnosis is confirmed when chyle is aspirated from the pleural cavity.

TRACHEOBRONCHIAL INJURIES

This injury is very rare and most commonly caused by acceleration or deceleration forces. Approximately 80% of tracheobronchial injuries occur near the origin of the main stem bronchus. Clinical signs include cyanosis, hemoptysis, tachypnea, and subcutaneous emphysema. Pneumomediastinum and cervical emphysema are seen commonly in airway rupture. If pneumothorax is present with these findings, a bronchial rupture should be suspected. A continued air leak after insertion of a thoracostomy tube should also alert the physician to the possibility of a bronchial tear.

Numerous reports in the literature record a partial tracheal tear becoming complete after endotracheal intubation. Therefore, if the airway is stable, oral tracheal intubation should be performed in the operating room under bronchoscopic guidance. In the stable patient, CT of the chest can also help to confirm the diagnosis and identify other injuries.

ESOPHAGEAL INJURIES

Timely and accurate diagnosis of an esophageal injury is paramount. The complications include mediastinal sepsis and death. The most common cause for esophageal perforation in the pediatric population is iatrogenic, followed by penetrating trauma.

Patients with an esophageal rupture in the cervical region may complain of neck stiffness or neck pain, regurgitate

bloody material, or have cervical subcutaneous emphysema. A lateral neck radiograph may show retroesophageal emphysema. When ruptured in the thoracic region, patients may present with abdominal pain and guarding, chest pain, subcutaneous emphysema, tachycardia, or dyspnea. A chest radiograph may show pneumothorax, pneumomediastinum, or an air-fluid level in the mediastinum.

Patients with suspected esophageal perforation should be adequately volume resuscitated, have a nasogastric tube placed, and receive broad-spectrum antibiotics. The diagnosis can be made by either esophagography, esophagoscopy, or both. Prompt surgical correction is mandatory.

DIAPHRAGMATIC INJURIES

Diaphragmatic injuries are more common in blunt trauma. Even though penetrating thoracoabdominal trauma is uncommon in children, a diaphragmatic injury should be suspected in any thoracic or abdominal penetrating injury. The level of the diaphragm fluctuates greatly with respirations, and injuries of the diaphragm have been reported with penetrating wounds as high as the third and as low as the twelfth rib.

Patients may present in respiratory distress and have a scaphoid abdomen, although they are more likely to be symptomatic from associated injuries than from the diaphragmatic rupture. A nasogastric tube may be difficult to pass in patients with a diaphragmatic injury and gastric herniation. The diagnosis is usually made on initial review of the chest radiograph, but the initial film is occasionally normal (Fig. 21.7). Chest and abdominal CT with contrast or upper and lower gastrointestinal tract series can help to confirm the diagnosis.

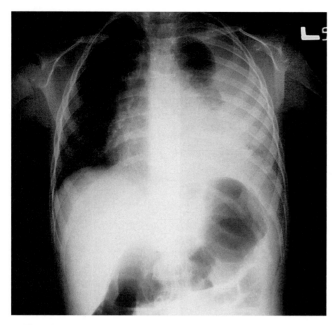

FIG. 21.7. Traumatic diaphragmatic hernia. This 5-year-old boy was on a snowmobile when it crashed into a tree. He was tachypneic, but his breath sounds were reportedly normal. The chest radiograph shows a left-sided diaphragmatic hernia.

TRAUMATIC ASPHYXIA

Traumatic asphyxia results from direct compression of the chest or abdomen. The most common mechanism is a child being run over by a motor vehicle or pinned underneath a heavy object. Patients with traumatic asphyxia usually present with the clinical picture of subconjunctival and upper body petechial hemorrhages, cyanosis, periorbital edema, respiratory distress, altered mental status, and associated injuries. The clinical manifestations occur because the increase in pressure dilates the capillary and venous systems. Areas drained by the superior vena cava are particularly affected.

The primary goal of treatment is to stabilize the patient and identify associated injuries. Pulmonary contusions and hepatic injuries are commonly seen with traumatic asphyxia, and CT is helpful in identifying head, chest, and abdominal injuries.

AORTIC AND OTHER VASCULAR INJURIES

Traumatic rupture of the thoracic aorta (TRA) is uncommon in children but carries a high mortality rate (75% to 95%). TRA is associated with sudden deceleration forces, commonly from automobile accidents, causing a sheering stress. The aortic arch remains fixed, but the descending aorta is mobile. With deceleration, bending or sheering takes place at the level of the ligamentum arteriosum, which is the most common site of aortic tears in adults and children.

Children are usually symptomatic from associated injuries, and TRA can easily be missed. Clinical signs may include difference in pulses between the arms or arms and legs,

thoracic ecchymosis, paraplegia, and anuria. Patients with paraplegia and back pain may be initially diagnosed with a spinal cord injury. Unfortunately, 50% of patients may have no signs pertaining directly to TRA. More than 90% of patients have an abnormal chest radiograph. A widened mediastinum, loss of the aortic knob, left-sided pleural cap, tracheal deviation, and nasogastric tube deviation may all be seen on a chest radiograph (Fig. 21.8).

The preferred method for diagnosing TRA is aortography. Thoracic CT is only 60% accurate but is helpful in diagnosing associated injuries. If the patient is stable and TRA is suspected, aortography should be performed. If the patient is unstable, transesophageal echocardiography can be performed while the patient's other life-threatening injuries are being treated.

PERICARDIAL TAMPONADE

Pericardial tamponade occurs when the myocardium is injured and blood accumulates in the pericardial sac. Because of the nondistendible pericardium, pressure is exerted on the heart. Cardiac output decreases secondary to a decrease in venous return. As the pressure within the pericardial sac increases, the systolic blood pressure decreases, causing a narrowing of the pulse pressure and subsequent hypotension and cardiogenic shock.

Pericardial tamponade is difficult to diagnose because of associated injuries obscuring the signs and symptoms. Patients may present with distant heart sounds, low blood pressure, poor perfusion, a narrow pulse pressure, or electro-

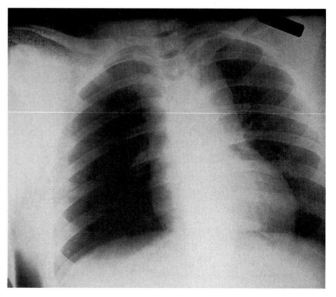

FIG. 21.8. This 12-year-old girl was an unrestrained passenger involved in a motor vehicle accident. The patient was hypotensive at the scene and could not move her legs. In the emergency department, she had no motor or sensory function to her lower extremities and was anuric. The chest radiograph showed a widened mediastinum from traumatic rupture of the aorta.

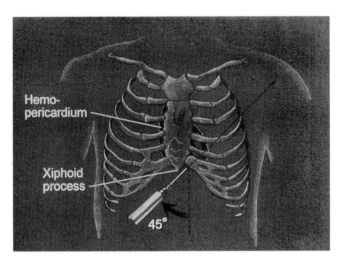

FIG. 21.9. Pericardiocentesis is performed by inserting a 20-gauge spinal needle below the xiphoid process at a 45-degree angle toward the left shoulder.

mechanical dissociation. A chest radiograph may show an enlarged heart and an electrocardiogram may show low-voltage QRS waves. In the stable patient, an echocardiogram can demonstrate fluid within the pericardial sac.

In the unstable patient in whom pericardial tamponade is suspected, treatment includes control of the airway, intravascular volume resuscitation, and pericardiocentesis (Fig. 21.9). Pericardiocentesis is performed by inserting a 20-gauge spinal needle below the xiphoid process at a 45-degree angle toward the left shoulder. If time permits, an electrocardiographic monitor can be attached to the spinal needle. If the needle touches the heart, a current will be noted on the monitor. Blood aspirated from the pericardial sac can be differentiated from intracardiac blood because pericardial blood is defibrinated and does not clot. A catheter should be placed in the pericardial sac over a wire guide for continual drainage of blood until surgical correction can be performed.

BLUNT CARDIAC INJURIES

Myocardial contusion, ventricular or atrial rupture, and valvular disruption are all considered blunt cardiac injury (BCI). Myocardial contusion is the most common and ventricular rupture is the most lethal of injuries. Complications of BCI include arrhythmias, congestive heart failure, and shock.

Cardiac rupture is the most common cause of death in BCI. The right ventricle is the chamber most commonly ruptured because of its location directly beneath the sternum. Patients with valvar injury may present in congestive heart failure with a new regurgitation murmur.

Unlike adults, pediatric patients with BCI often have no chest pain or external evidence of injury. BCI should be considered in any patient with thoracic trauma who develops a cardiac arrhythmia or a new murmur or who is in congestive heart failure.

Patients with suspected BCI can be monitored in the emergency department or hospital and, if no arrhythmias develop on the electrocardiogram, can be safely sent home. Creatine phosphokinase-MB ratios have a high false-positive rate and are not a helpful screening tool. Transesophageal echocardiography should be performed in thoracic trauma patients with an abnormal electrocardiogram or arrhythmia or a new heart murmur.

PENETRATING THORACIC TRAUMA

Penetrating thoracic trauma is less common than blunt thoracic trauma and is usually caused by gunshot or stab wounds. The most common penetrating thoracic injuries are hemothorax and pneumothorax. Intraabdominal injuries should always be suspected because of the close proximity of abdominal contents to the thoracic cavity.

Evaluation and treatment include airway stabilization, fluid resuscitation, and management of the chest wound. Radiopaque markers (paper clips) may be placed by the entry and exit sites to help to determine the course of the missile. Pericardial tamponade should be considered in any unstable patient. In the stable patient, echocardiography is helpful in evaluating the heart and pericardial sac.

SUGGESTED READINGS

Brandt M, Luks F, Spigland N. Diaphragmatic injury in children. *J Trauma* 1992;32:298–301.

Cooper A. Thoracic injuries. *Semin Pediatr Surg* 1995;4:109–116.

Dowd M, Krug S. Pediatric blunt cardiac injury: epidemiology, clinical features, and diagnosis. *J Trauma* 1996;40:61–67.

Gaebler C, Mueller M, Schramm W, et al. Tracheobronchial ruptures in children. *Am J Emerg Med* 1996;14:279–285.

Garcia V, Gotschall M, Eichelberger M, et al. Rib fractures in children: a marker of severe trauma. *J Trauma* 1990;30:695–700.

Peterson R, Tiwary A, Kissoon N, et al. Pediatric penetrating thoracic trauma: a five-year experience. *Pediatr Emerg Care* 1994;10:129–131.

Trupka A, Waydhas C, Hallfeldt KJ. Value of thoracic computed tomography in the first assessment of severely injured patients with blunt chest trauma: results of a prospective study. *J Trauma* 1997;43;405–412.

CHAPTER 22

Trauma: Extremities

Editor: Marc N. Baskin

FRACTURES UNIQUE TO CHILDREN

The anatomic and physiologic differences between adults and children are reflected in a number of fractures and injuries unique to the pediatric age group, including physeal fractures, torus fractures, greenstick fractures, bowing deformities, and avulsion fractures.

OPEN FRACTURES

The incidence of complications is higher with open fractures. Any patient who has a laceration over the site of a fracture must be considered to have an open fracture until proven otherwise (Fig. 22.1). The incidence of infection is increased with open fractures. Initial management should include cleansing the wound, applying a sterile dressing, and administering antibiotics if indicated. Open fractures are orthopedic emergencies possibly requiring surgical debridement and irrigation. The patient should be given nothing by mouth, and an urgent orthopedic consultation should be obtained.

COMPARTMENT SYNDROME

Compartment syndrome refers to vascular insufficiency caused by elevated tissue pressures. It usually occurs after an injury causes hemorrhage or edema within an enclosed fascial compartment. When compartment pressures approach the perfusion pressure of muscle, arterial inflow is reduced. Ischemia of muscle leads to further swelling and can lead to complete cessation of tissue perfusion. Muscle necrosis is irreversible after 6 to 8 hours of tissue anoxia. The emergency physician must identify patients at risk of compartment syndromes and consult with an orthopedist who can monitor tissue pressures and treat compartment syndromes before irreversible injuries occur.

Some pediatric injuries are associated with compartment syndromes. Displaced supracondylar fractures may cause an ischemic deep flexor (anterior) compartment that may lead to a Volkmann contracture if not managed correctly. Diaphyseal tibial/fibular fractures can cause ischemic anterior tibial and peroneal compartments. Less commonly, radial/ulnar and femoral fractures can cause a compartment syndrome. Compartment syndromes may result from crush injuries and other soft-tissue trauma that does not necessarily involve a fracture.

Compartment syndromes are diagnosed clinically by assessing the "five Ps": pain (particularly with passive extension), paresthesia, pallor, paralysis, and pulselessness. All five need not be present for a compartment syndrome to exist. The involved compartment may feel hard and tense.

Treatment of a compartment syndrome should begin when it is suspected. All circumferential bandages should be removed. If symptoms persist, orthopedic consultation should be obtained to measure compartment pressures. Fasciotomy is indicated if compartment pressures remain high.

INJURIES OF THE UPPER EXTREMITIES

Injuries of the Shoulder Region

Sternoclavicular Injuries

The medial clavicular epiphysis is the last one in the body to close. Apparent dislocations of the sternoclavicular joint are invariably epiphyseal separations in children and young adults. Physeal (growth plate) separations of the medial clavicle are caused by indirect trauma that forces the shoulder medially and separates the growth plate or direct trauma to the mid chest, causing posterior displacement. Most separations are anterior, and the patient has swelling and tenderness over the sternoclavicular joint. If the displacement is posterior, the aorta or trachea may be injured and the child may complain of dysphagia or dyspnea, as discussed in Chapter 21 (Trauma: Chest). Plain radiographs may not show the lesion and computed tomography is usually necessary (Fig. 21.3).

Clavicular Fractures

The clavicle may be the most commonly fractured bone in children. More than half of all clavicular fractures occur in children younger than 10 years of age. In pretoddlers

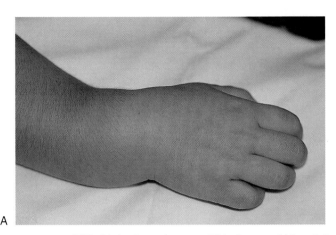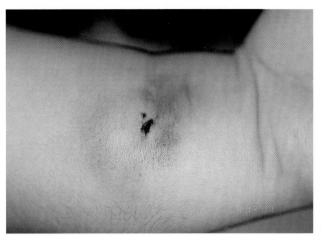

A   B

FIG. 22.1. Open fracture. This 8-year-old boy fell on his hand and was referred to the emergency department with a deformed forearm **(A)** due to a distal radial/ulnar fracture. After removal from his splint, a small ecchymosis and laceration were noted over the ventral aspect of his forearm **(B)**.

(excluding the newborn period), such fractures are uncommon and should provoke consideration of intentional trauma.

Fractures of the clavicular shaft result from direct trauma or from indirect forces (e.g., a fall onto an outstretched hand). Many are greenstick injuries because the thick periosteum enveloping the clavicle prevents significant displacement or angulation (Fig. 22.2). The child complains of shoulder pain and is cradling the injured arm with the opposite one. Occasionally, the initial injury is unnoticed and comes to attention only when a lump appears as a callus forms. Radiographs are confirmatory, although visualization of nondisplaced fractures may require several views. Despite the proximity of the brachial plexus and subclavian vessels, neurovascular injury is rare.

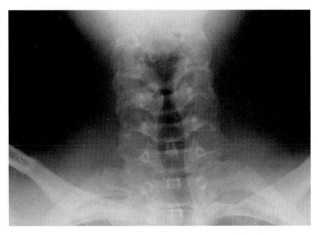

FIG. 22.2. Clavicular fracture. The 14-year-old patient fell off his bike, landing on his left shoulder and complained of left neck pain. His cervical spine and neck examination was normal, but he was tender over his clavicle. Radiographs confirmed the diagnosis of minimally displaced midshaft clavicular fracture.

Laterally, the clavicle is anchored by the coracoclavicular and acromioclavicular ligaments. Once again, fracture through the physis rather than dislocation is the rule. Typically, the proximal fracture fragment is displaced superiorly and the radiographic appearance suggests acromioclavicular separation (Fig. 22.3). Most distal clavicular fractures heal uneventfully with no loss of joint stability.

Only rarely is orthopedic consultation necessary for a clavicular injury. Exceptions include significantly displaced midshaft fractures for which closed reduction is occasionally desirable, posteriorly and significantly anteriorly displaced medial fractures, and grossly unstable distal injuries. Immobilization in a sling and swathe for 3 weeks followed by 3 weeks of restriction from sporting activities is adequate treatment. Nonunion is extremely unusual. Inform parents that a lump will appear as a callus forms and may persist for as long as a year.

Scapular Fractures

Fractures of the scapula are unusual in children and adolescents. The usual mechanism is a severe direct blow (e.g., a motor vehicle crash). The same force that produces the scapular fracture may result in more concerning and potentially life-threatening injuries to the chest, neck, or head (Fig. 22.4). A sling and swathe are usually the only treatment necessary.

Shoulder Dislocations

Dislocations of the shoulder are unusual before physeal closure. Injuries that in an adult would cause dislocation result in fractures in children. Most dislocations that do occur are anterior. Findings on physical examination include swelling with loss of the usual rounded contour of the shoulder (Fig. 22.5). Palpation generally reveals the displacement of the humeral head anterior to the glenoid fossa. Signs of axillary

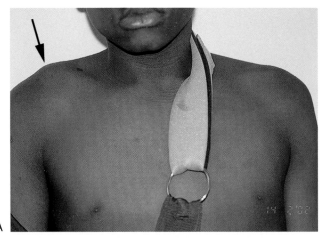

A

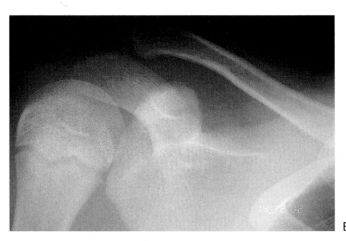

B

FIG. 22.3. Distal clavicle physeal fracture. **A:** This 12-year-old boy fell on his right shoulder. Swelling over his acromioclavicular joint is visible (*arrow*). **B:** The radiograph shows the distal clavicle displaced superiorly from the acromion.

nerve injury may be present. Radiographic studies should include an axillary (Y) view in addition to the customary views of the shoulder. Closed reduction of anterior dislocations can be accomplished by any of a number of techniques. Postreduction radiographs should be performed to ensure that no fracture has occurred with the dislocation. Given their rarity, posterior dislocations merit orthopedic consultation before reduction. Anterior dislocations should be immobilized in a sling and swathe for several weeks and referred to an orthopedist because the rate of recurrent dislocation is high.

Fractures of the Humerus

Proximal Humeral Fractures

Approximately 80% of the growth of the humerus occurs at the proximal humeral physis. As a result, the potential for healing of fractures that involve the proximal humeral shaft and physis is remarkable. Before adolescence, most

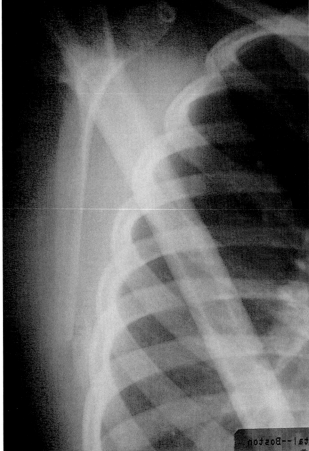

FIG. 22.4. Displaced fracture at the inferior border of the scapula.

FIG. 22.5. An older adolescent patient with a left anterior glenohumeral joint dislocation. Notice the sharp contour of the shoulder, the fullness below the glenoid fossa, and the prominent acromion.

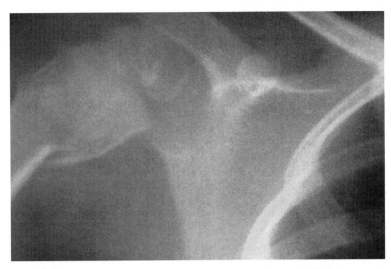

FIG. 22.6. Impacted proximal right humeral fracture with approximately 25 degrees of angulation in a 3-year-old child. Full remodeling can be anticipated.

proximal humeral fractures are metaphyseal (Fig. 22.6). With the onset of adolescence, rapid growth makes the physeal region relatively weak and thus vulnerable to injury. The incidence of proximal humeral fractures is highest in this age group; most are Salter–Harris type II injuries.

Care must be taken not to confuse the normal variations in the epiphyseal line with a fracture; comparison views can be useful. Before adolescence, angulation of as much as 50 or even 70 degrees is satisfactory. Recommendations regarding the degree of deformity acceptable in adolescents vary somewhat; 20 to 50 degrees of angulation and 50% apposition are generally tolerable. A sling and swathe for several weeks are usually the only treatment necessary. Orthopedic follow-up is recommended.

Humeral Shaft Fractures

Fractures of the humeral shaft are much less common than those involving either the proximal or distal segments. The pattern of fracture reflects the mechanism of injury; transverse fractures result from direct blows, whereas spiral fractures are caused by indirect twisting, as with a fall. When a child younger than 3 years of age sustains a spiral fracture of the humerus, the possibility of child abuse must be considered seriously. A prominent vascular groove in the distal humerus is a normal finding that should not be confused with a fracture.

Evidence of radial nerve injury must always be sought. Findings suggestive of radial nerve damage include loss of strength in the extensors of the wrist and fingers and loss of sensation on the dorsal web space between the thumb and index finger. With fracture management, nearly all cases of radial nerve palsy resolve.

The thick periosteal sleeve of the humeral shaft limits fracture displacement and promotes rapid healing. A sling and swathe are all that is needed for incomplete fractures.

For complete or minimally displaced fractures, application of a sugar-tong splint of the upper arm and a sling to support the forearm is recommended. Immediate orthopedic consultation is suggested for any completely displaced fracture, any fracture angulated more than 20 degrees in children and 10 degrees in adolescents, and any fracture with evidence of radial nerve injury. All humeral fractures should be referred for orthopedic follow-up within 5 days.

Injuries of the Elbow

Supracondylar Fractures

Supracondylar fractures account for more than 50% of elbow fractures in the pediatric age group. Most are sustained by children 3 to 10 years of age. A fall on an outstretched arm with hyperextension of the elbow is the most common mechanism. Accordingly, posterior displacement of the distal fracture fragment nearly always occurs (Fig. 22.7). With nondisplaced fractures and only mild soft-tissue swelling, recognition can be difficult. A suggestive history coupled with localized tenderness should prompt a radiographic examination. The radiographic findings also may be subtle. Close attention to the fat pads and the anterior humeral line facilitates diagnosis (Figs. 22.8 and 22.9).

The complications associated with supracondylar fractures range from immediate neurovascular compromise to long-term deformities and range-of-motion abnormalities. For the emergency physician, the first priorities are neurovascular assessment and fracture stabilization. Absence of a pulse by itself is not extremely worrisome. In most instances, vasospasm or arterial compression has occurred and arterial flow will resume with fracture reduction. Conversely, significant muscle ischemia can be present even when pulses and capillary refill appear normal. Forearm pain, pain with passive extension of the fingers, paralysis of finger extension,

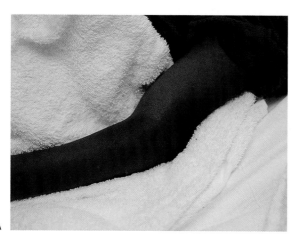
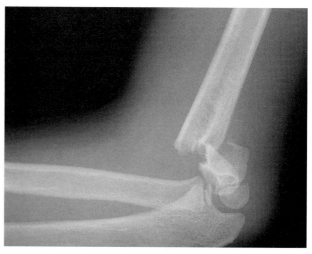

A   B

FIG. 22.7. Supracondylar fracture. **A:** This 5-year-old girl fell on her fully extended left hand. Her elbow is displaced in the posterior direction similar to an older patient with a dislocated elbow. **B:** The radiograph shows a displaced supracondylar fracture. (Courtesy of Dr. Andrew Capraro.)

and paresthesia are each worrisome and should be considered evidence of an impending compartment syndrome.

Minimally displaced or nondisplaced supracondylar fractures may be immobilized in a well-padded long-arm posterior splint with the elbow at 90 degrees and the forearm in pronation or neutral rotation. Orthopedic referral for casting is suggested when the swelling subsides. Immobilization for a total of 3 weeks is adequate in most cases. All nonminimally displaced supracondylar fractures require immediate orthopedic referral.

Lateral Condylar Fractures

Fractures of the lateral condyle are prone to poor functional outcome if misdiagnosed or mismanaged. Unlike supracondylar fractures, lateral condyle injuries involve the articular surface; they are true Salter–Harris type IV injuries. The fracture fragment can be partially or totally avulsed from the distal humerus (Fig. 22.10). Clinically, swelling and tenderness localized over the lateral aspect of the elbow suggest a lateral condylar fracture.

For minimally displaced and nondisplaced injuries, immobilization in a posterior splint with the elbow flexed to 90

FIG. 22.8. Normal lateral radiograph of the elbow of a 2-year-old child. The anterior fat pad is readily seen (*arrow*); the posterior fat pad is not visible. A line drawn along the anterior cortex of the humerus intersects the capitellum in its middle third (*solid line*). A line drawn along the axis of the radius also passes through the center of the capitellum (*dashed line*).

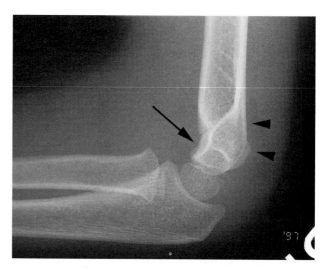

FIG. 22.9. Undisplaced supracondylar fracture. This 4-year-old girl fell on her right arm and was diagnosed with a nurse-maid's elbow. Close review of the radiograph shows the presence of a posterior fat pad (*arrowheads*) that is due to an effusion and suggests a high likelihood of a fracture. In addition, a subtle cortical defect is visible (*arrow*) on the anterior surface of the distal humeral metaphysis.

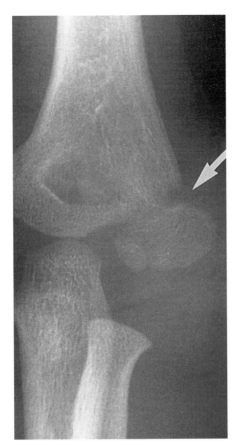

FIG. 22.10. Lateral condylar fracture in a 2-year-old girl (*arrow*).

than 2 years of age. Recognition is both difficult and important because in children younger than 2 years of age, this injury is often the result of child abuse. The proposed mechanism in abused children is forceful twisting of the arm that shears off the distal epiphysis.

Elbow swelling without significant deformity is common. Radiographic diagnosis can be difficult, particularly in infants in whom the capitellum has not yet begun to ossify. Posteromedial displacement of the ulna and radius in relation to the humerus is the most important finding, and recognition may necessitate comparison views. Given the difficulty in recognition and the frequent need for reduction and pinning, all suspected epiphyseal separations of the distal humerus merit immediate orthopedic referral.

Radial Head and Neck Fractures

Falls on an outstretched arm account for most fractures of the radial head and neck. Pain may be referred to the wrist and thus distract from the true injury (Fig. 22.11). The physical examination typically reveals localized tenderness and swelling. The child will have pain with any pronation or supination of the wrist. The incidence of complications, especially loss of motion of the radial head, is significant, and orthopedic referral is recommended for all these fractures. Immobilization with the elbow in 90 degrees of flexion and the forearm in neutral rotation is acceptable emergency management for minimally displaced or nondisplaced fractures. Angulation greater than 15 degrees is an indication for immediate orthopedic consultation.

Elbow Dislocations

Because the ligaments and tendons are relatively stronger than the neighboring bones (particularly the physeal plates) in children, injuries that would lead to dislocations in adults almost invariably result in fractures in the younger age group. In dislocations, the radius and ulna are displaced posteriorly and the anterior capsule is torn. Fractures are commonly associated with the dislocation.

Major neurovascular compromise often accompanies elbow dislocations. The risk of compartment syndrome with

degrees and the forearm in pronation (some authorities suggest supination instead) is satisfactory emergency management. Lateral condylar fractures are prone to displace despite immobilization, and orthopedic follow-up within 3 to 4 days is essential. All fractures displaced more than 2 mm require reduction and often pinning.

Medial Epicondylar Fractures

Fractures of the medial epicondyle occur as the result of falls directly onto the elbow and falls onto an outstretched arm. The flexor muscles of the forearm may avulse the medial epicondyle from the humerus. Medial epicondyle injuries are particularly common with elbow dislocations. The elbow is swollen with tenderness localized to the medial aspect of the elbow. Paresis of the ulnar nerve can occur. Comparison views may be needed on occasion. Open reduction is almost invariably necessary for displaced fractures. Nondisplaced fractures can be placed in a posterior splint with the forearm in pronation for orthopedic follow-up.

Distal Humeral Physeal Fractures

Fractures of the entire distal humeral physis are relatively uncommon. Most such injuries take place in children younger

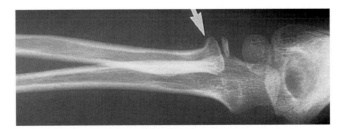

FIG. 22.11. Buckle fracture of the radial neck in a 9-year-old girl. Wrist pain was the chief complaint. The treating physician failed to identify the proximal radial fracture, which was, however, noticed by the radiologist.

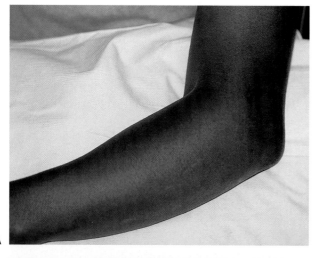

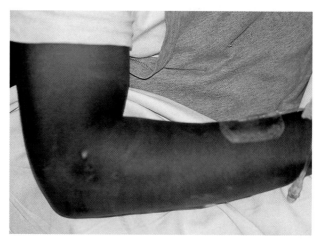

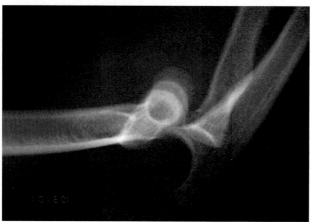

FIG. 22.12. Elbow dislocation. This adolescent football player had his elbow hyperextended when tackling another player. Note the sharp contour due to the prominent olecranon displaced posteriorly on the injured side **(A)** compared with the uninjured elbow **(B)**. **(C)** The radiograph shows the dislocation without an associated fracture.

dislocations of the elbow is such that some authors recommend hospitalization for close observation even after successful closed reduction. Nerve injury, particularly of the ulnar nerve, is even more common than vascular injury. Early recognition and appropriate treatment nearly always lead to complete recovery of ulnar nerve function. Median nerve entrapment is much rarer, but when it occurs, the degree of nerve damage is such that full recovery cannot be guaranteed.

Clinical findings with dislocation of the elbow include obvious deformity and significant swelling (Fig. 22.12). Immobilization before radiographic studies is recommended to minimize the risk of further neurovascular injury. Although most elbow dislocations can be reduced uneventfully, the risks of entrapping a fracture fragment or a nerve in the joint space during the procedure are such that immediate orthopedic consultation is recommended. After appropriate procedural sedation, the physician should encircle the upper arm with his or her hands and use the thumbs to push the olecranon forward. Whatever technique is used, hyperextension should be avoided at all times. Postreduction films are mandatory because only then will many of the associated fractures be evident. Finally, the arm should be immobilized

in a posterior splint with the elbow at 90 degrees and the forearm in mid pronation.

Radial Head Subluxation

Of all the injuries discussed in this section, by far the most common is radial head subluxation, otherwise known as nursemaid's elbow or pulled elbow. This entity is discussed in Chapter 12 (Musculoskeletal Emergencies).

Fractures of the Forearm and Wrist

Fractures of the Radial and Ulnar Shafts

The usual mechanism of injury with forearm fractures is a fall on an outstretched hand, and greenstick injuries are common. Although it is hard to make any absolute rules, any shaft fracture angulated more than 10 degrees merits immediate orthopedic consultation, at least by telephone. A simple rule is that any forearm that looks crooked should be straightened.

If the fracture is complete, the ends of the bones well opposed, and angulation and rotation minimal, a well-applied sugar-tong splint is adequate initial treatment. Otherwise,

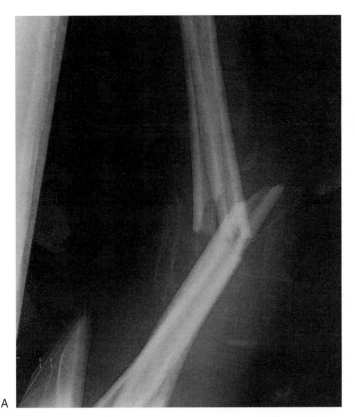

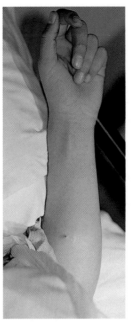

A   B

FIG. 22.13. This 13-year-old patient not only has a sharply angulated midshaft radius and ulnar fracture on the radiograph **(A)**, but a small laceration over the fracture suggesting an open fracture and will require operative management **(B)**. (Courtesy of Dr. Andrew Capraro.)

immediate orthopedic referral is necessary for reduction (Fig. 22.13).

Monteggia and Galeazzi Fracture Dislocations

In general, isolated fractures of the ulna do not occur. Instead, the same force that causes the ulnar fracture leads to a radial injury, often a dislocation of the radial head. The combination of an ulnar fracture and a radial head dislocation is known as a Monteggia fracture. Recognition is most important because failure to reduce the radial head dislocation results in permanent disability. Clues to the diagnosis on physical examination include elbow pain and swelling, which accompany signs of any ulnar fracture.

A line drawn through the axis of the radius should pass through the center of the capitellum on all projections to rule out a radial head dislocation (Figs. 22.8 and 22.14). A true lateral view that includes the elbow should be obtained with all forearm injuries. Even bowing fractures of the ulna, which may require comparison views for recognition, are associated with radial head dislocation. Any suspected Monteggia injury requires immediate orthopedic referral.

The Galeazzi fracture is a radial shaft fracture accompanied by disruption of the distal radioulnar joint. It is rela-

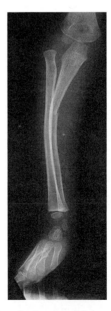

FIG. 22.14. Monteggia fracture/dislocation. A 4-year-old boy fell off his bike. The ulna is fractured and angulated, and a line through the radius clearly does not pass through the center of the capitellum. (Courtesy of Dr. Andrew Capraro.)

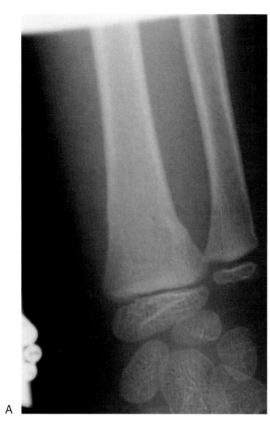
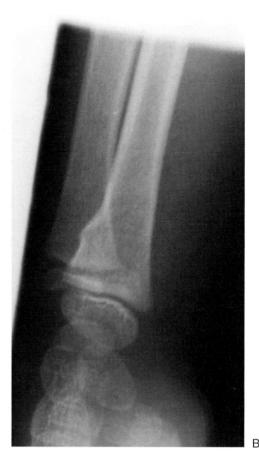

A

B

FIG. 22.15. This buckle fracture of the distal radius is subtle on the anteroposterior view **(A)** but seen more clearly on the lateral view **(B)**.

tively rare. Physical examination reveals prominence of the distal ulna and joint instability. Radiographs are confirmatory. Orthopedic consultation is necessary.

Fractures of the Distal Radius and Ulna

Of all the fractures that occur in childhood and adolescence, those of the distal forearm are by far the most common. Neurovascular complications are rare, and the capacity for remodeling is significant.

Usually, localized swelling and tenderness accompany distal radial fractures. However, wrist pain can be the chief complaint with more proximal injuries (e.g., radial head fractures). Therefore, radiographs should include the whole forearm. Torus fractures are most often overlooked. The fracture may be evident on only one projection and then only as a minor irregularity in the contour of the cortex (Fig. 22.15). When a torus or buckle fracture is identified, a volar splint or, if the swelling is minimal, a short arm cast for 3 to 4 weeks is recommended. Orthopedic referral is optional.

Greenstick and complete fractures are readily recognized. These fractures tend to displace if not properly immobilized. Angulation greater than 10 to 15 degrees is an indication for immediate orthopedic referral. Otherwise, immobilization with either a long arm posterior splint or a well-applied

sugar-tong splint and orthopedic follow-up within 3 to 5 days are adequate emergency management.

Fractures of the Bones of the Wrist and Penetrating Trauma to the Wrist

Adolescents in the later stages of skeletal maturity sustain scaphoid (navicular) fractures. Most injuries of the scaphoid in adolescence are nondisplaced fractures through the distal third of the bone. The rate of nonunion is much lower than in adults, in whom scaphoid fractures generally involve the middle third of the bone and are more often displaced. The patient often has snuffbox tenderness and pain with longitudinal compression of the thumb. Radiographic visualization of a nondisplaced scaphoid fracture may be difficult, even with special views (Fig. 22.16). Should the physical signs suggest a scaphoid fracture, immobilization in a thumb spica splint or cast for 2 weeks is recommended, regardless of the radiographic findings.

The median nerve is very superficial on the ventral side of the wrist and can be transected by even apparently minor lacerations (Fig. 22.17).

Metacarpal Fractures

Perhaps the most commonly encountered metacarpal fracture in pediatrics is one of the distal fifth metacarpal in an adolescent

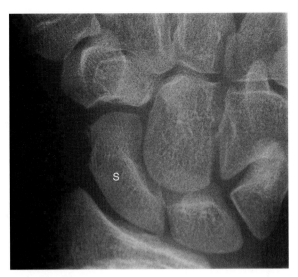

FIG. 22.16. Nondisplaced scaphoid (*S*) fracture. The 15-year-old patient fell on his hand playing soccer. (Courtesy of Dr. David Greenes.)

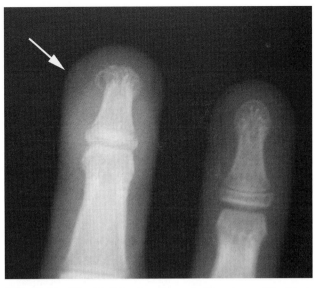

FIG. 22.18. Distal tuft fracture (*arrow*). (Courtesy of Dr. Mark Waltzman.)

who has struck someone or something with a closed fist. Closed reduction is usually performed if the angulation is more than 30 to 40 degrees. Nondisplaced metacarpal shaft fractures, if they are not rotated, may be immobilized in a gutter splint with the wrist neutral and the metacarpal phalangeal joints at 70 degrees and then referred for an orthopedic consultation.

Phalangeal Lacerations, Fractures, Dislocations, and Infections

Distal phalanx fractures typically accompany crush injuries of the fingertips. If only the distal tuft is fractured, anatomic closure of the laceration usually results in adequate realign-

ment of the fracture (Fig. 22.18). Displaced physeal fractures merit immediate referral to an orthopedist. Hyperflexion injuries of the distal phalanx, leading to mallet finger deformities, are also common (Fig. 22.19). Unless recognized and treated, this injury will result in a mallet finger deformity. Recognition of the tendonous disruption is important because proper treatment entails 6 to 8 weeks of continuous splinting of the distal interphalangeal joint only in hyperextension.

Hyperextension can lead to dislocations of the metacarpophalangeal and proximal interphalangeal joints. After a digital block, the joint should be gently hyperextended and the distal bone then pushed back into place (Fig. 22.20). Stability of the collateral ligaments should be carefully

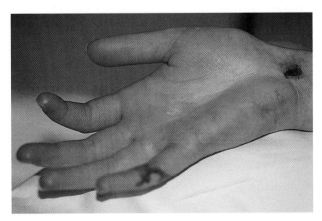

FIG. 22.17. This adolescent cut her wrist on a broken ceramic bowl and complained of numbness of her thumb and index and middle fingers. Although the laceration appeared superficial, she had decreased sensation and abnormal skin perfusion of the thumb and index and middle fingers. Her median nerve transection was repaired in the operating room. (Courtesy of Dr. Mark Waltzman.)

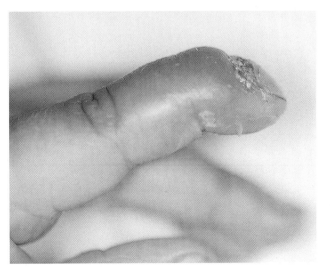

FIG. 22.19. Mallet finger. This child presented with an apparent infection 2 days after his finger was crushed in a door. His examination showed that he could not fully extend his distal phalanx. He had avulsed his extensor tendon from the distal phalanx along with a small piece of bone.

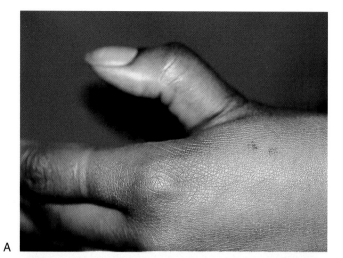

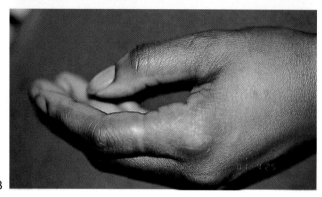

FIG. 22.20. **A:** Metacarpophalangeal joint dislocation prereduction. **B:** Normal thumb position after reduction.

assessed and radiographs, both prereduction and postreduction, should be scrutinized for fractures. Buddy taping for 3 weeks is adequate for routine dislocation.

Superficial infections or lacerations can lead to tenosynovitis, a synovial space infection of the flexor tendon sheath.

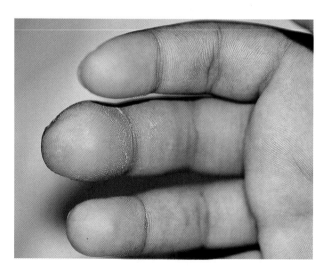

FIG. 22.21. Tenosynovitis. This 13-year-old boy had a painful finger 3 days after a paronychia had been drained. Note the fusiform swelling and erythema of his phalanx.

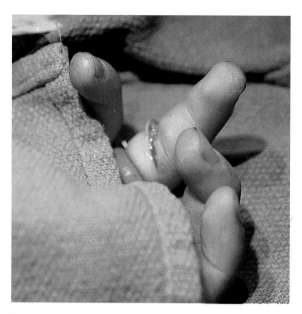

FIG. 22.22. Flexor tendon injury. This patient has his hand in the typical position of a patient with a flexor tendon laceration and was unable to flex the phalanx.

The patients usually have tenderness along the course of the flexor tendon, fusiform swelling of the finger, a flexed posture of the finger, and pain on passive extension (Fig. 22.21). Immediate consultation with a hand surgeon is required as well as parenteral antistaphylococcal antimicrobials.

Apparently superficial finger lacerations can also transect flexor or extensor tendons. These injuries should be recognized before laceration repair by observation and functional testing (Figs. 22.22 and 22.23). Hand surgical consultation should be obtained for all flexor tendon lacerations and are

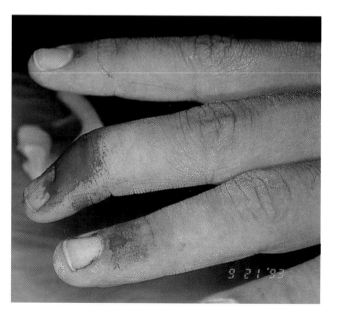

FIG. 22.23. Extensor tendon injury. This patient was asked to straighten his fingers but was unable to extend his middle finger, suggesting an extensor tendon injury.

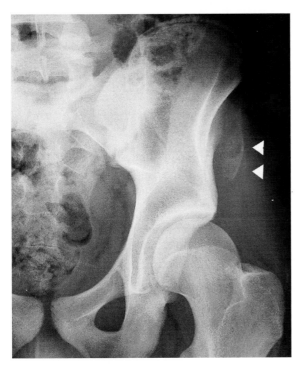

FIG. 22.24. This 14-year-old boy felt a "pop" in his hip while running during a baseball game. The radiograph shows the avulsion fracture (*arrowheads*) of his anterior inferior iliac spine.

usually repaired in the operating room. Some extensor tendon lacerations may be repaired in the emergency department.

FRACTURES OF THE PELVIS

Avulsion Fractures

The muscular attachments to the secondary centers of ossification can be pulled off during active contractions against resistance. Localized tenderness is usually present. The diagnosis is usually readily apparent on plain film radiographs, although bone scintigraphy may be necessary occasionally (Fig. 22.24). Often, crutches with partial or no weight bearing for 4 to 6 weeks with slow resumption of activities are all that is required, even with significantly displaced fractures. With avulsion fractures of the ischial tuberosity of more than 2 cm, some authors recommend open reduction and fixation (Fig. 22.25).

Pelvic Ring Fractures

Single Breaks in the Pelvic Ring

Symphysis pubis diastasis, superior and inferior pubic rami fractures, and straddle fractures are classified as single breaks in the pelvic ring. Although caused by high-energy accidents, they are generally stable fractures. A careful search for accompanying injuries must be made. Fractures of the superior and inferior pubic rami (Fig. 22.26) rarely require any treatment as long as the sacroiliac joints and

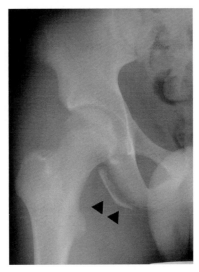

FIG. 22.25. This adolescent soccer player had sudden onset of pain while accelerating during a game. He indicated his buttock as the source of his pain, a rather unusual location, and had increasing hip/buttock pain with palpation of his hamstring muscles in the popliteal space or knee flexion. His radiograph shows an avulsion fracture (*arrowheads*) of his ischial tuberosity (the origin of the hamstrings).

sacrum remain intact. One exception to this rule is a diastasis of the pubic symphysis, associated with disruption of the sacroiliac joint. If significant displacement occurs through the symphysis pubis, closed reduction must be considered.

Double Breaks in the Pelvic Ring

Fractures of the pubic rami or symphysis pubis associated with displaced sacroiliac joint dislocations or sacral fractures result in an unstable hemipelvis. This group of fractures is associated with a high incidence of complications, including life-threatening hemorrhage from pelvic vein disruption. Emergent application of a pneumatic antishock garment in the emergency department with compression of the pelvis may slow bleeding by a tamponade effect. Angiographic

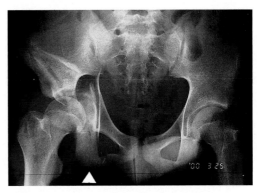

FIG. 22.26. A 13-year-old patient was struck by car. The radiograph shows a fracture of the inferior pubic ramus (*arrowhead*) and mild lateral displacement of the femoral head secondary to hemorrhage within the hip joint.

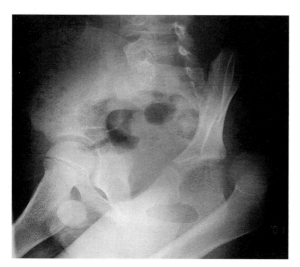

FIG. 22.27. Hip dislocation. This 10-year-old child was "body slammed" during a soccer match. The radiograph shows a left hip dislocation.

embolization should also be considered in the face of persistent bleeding. All unstable pelvic fractures require urgent orthopedic consultation.

INJURIES OF THE LOWER EXTREMITIES

Hip Dislocation

Dislocation of the hip in children and adolescents is uncommon. It probably occurs more often than it is diagnosed, however, because of spontaneous reduction at the time of injury. The injured limb is shortened and externally rotated (Fig. 22.27). A patient presenting with a dislocated hip

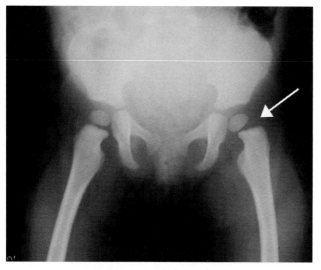

FIG. 22.28. This 14-month-old child was evaluated for hip pain. His radiographs show a displaced proximal femoral physeal fracture (*arrow*) most consistent with child abuse. A skeletal series (not shown) demonstrated old rib and tibial fractures, confirming the diagnosis of child abuse.

should undergo a closed reduction in the emergency department or under general anesthesia within 6 hours of the accident. When closed reduction is unsuccessful or when it is suspected that tissue is trapped in the joint space, open reduction is necessary. Complications of traumatic hip dislocation in children include necrosis of the femoral head, posttraumatic arthritis, and persistent instability of the hip joint.

Proximal Femoral Physeal Fractures

Proximal femoral physeal fractures occur through the proximal femoral growth plate (Fig. 22.28) and may be associated with child abuse. Anatomic reduction is essential. The incidence of osseous necrosis approaches 100% in totally displaced fractures and can lead to long-term disability. In minimally displaced fractures, it may be better to accept mild displacement than to further compromise the vascularity of the femoral head by performing a reduction.

Femoral Neck Fractures

Fractures of the femoral neck are relatively common. Initial treatment is traction and splinting followed by closed or open reduction. Osseous necrosis can occur, especially in displaced fractures.

Intertrochanteric Fractures

Although common in adults, intertrochanteric fractures are uncommon in children and adolescents. Nondisplaced or minimally displaced fractures can be treated in a spica cast for 6 to 8 weeks. The rate of osseous necrosis is approximately 5%.

Fractures of the Shaft of the Femur

Birth to 2 Years of Age

Most femoral fractures in the first 2 years of life result from either a slow twisting motion or a direct blow. A large percentage of femoral fractures in this age group are the result of intentional trauma (Fig. 22.29). Management options include immediate spica casting or a short period of Buck traction followed by spica casting and a full evaluation for child abuse.

2 Years of Age to Adolescence

In this age group, femoral fractures are often the result of high-energy motor vehicle or vehicle–pedestrian accidents. Concomitant injuries are common. Only rarely does an isolated femoral fracture cause hemodynamically significant blood loss. Initial treatment consists of traction or splinting and orthopedic consultation.

Injuries of the Knee

Although relatively uncommon, fractures about the knee arguably rank as the most serious long bone injuries in

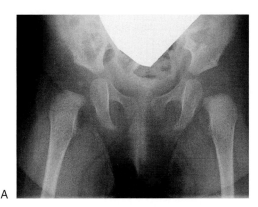
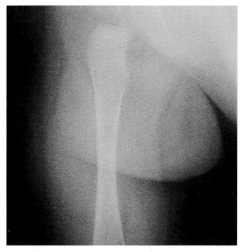

FIG. 22.29. Femur fracture secondary to child abuse. This 3-month-old infant was evaluated for decreased movement of his leg. **A:** Initially hip films were obtained and are normal, but a full femur radiograph **(B)** shows a spiral femur fracture consistent with child abuse.

children and adolescents. The growth centers of the distal femur and proximal tibia together account for two-thirds of lower extremity length. Growth arrest and the resultant limb length discrepancies can occur after physeal injuries about the knee.

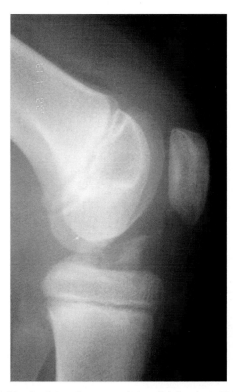

FIG. 22.30. Avulsion fracture of the tibial spine. This gymnast landed directly on her feet without direct trauma and had hemarthrosis. The radiograph shows a complete avulsion fracture of the tibial spine.

Ligamentous Injuries and Avulsion Fractures

Knee injuries in children younger than 14 years tend to result in fractures rather than ligamentous injuries; therefore, radiographs should be ordered routinely for all but the most minor injuries.

Avulsion of the tibial spine is the pediatric equivalent of an anterior cruciate ligament injury in an adult. The most commonly described mode of injury is hyperflexion of the knee. Significant pain and a refusal to bear weight are typical; hemarthrosis is invariably present. Radiographic findings are best seen on lateral views (Fig. 22.30). Immediate management in the emergency department should include splinting in extensions and arthrocentesis when hemarthrosis is causing severe pain.

Another uncommon but severe knee injury observed in adolescents is an avulsion fracture of the tibial tuberosity. This fracture occurs essentially exclusively in boys 12 to 17 years of age. Most such injuries occur during jumping when the quadriceps is strongly contracted and the tibial tubercle is torn from the proximal tibial epiphysis (Fig. 22.31). The severity of the injury dictates whether closed or open management is chosen.

Distal Femoral Physeal Fractures

Fractures of the distal femoral epiphysis are caused by high-energy sports injuries, motor vehicle crashes, and falls from a height. Because the adjacent ligaments are stronger than the physeal plate, stress results in distal femoral epiphysis separation rather than ligament rupture. Stress views after adequate sedation may be required to provide evidence of distal femoral or proximal tibial epiphyseal separation (Fig. 22.32). Such injuries reflect a marked valgus or varus stress. Peroneal nerve damage can accompany severe medial

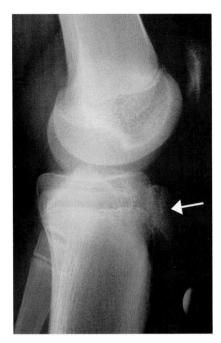

FIG. 22.31. This 15-year-old boy had acute pain as he jumped for a rebound in basketball. The avulsed tibial tubercle is visible (*arrow*).

displacement. Even with adequate reduction, the incidence of premature growth arrest is significant. Both compartment syndrome and direct compression of the neurovascular structures are well-recognized complications. The treatment of these injuries in the emergency department includes splinting in place and prompt orthopedic consultation.

Knee Dislocations

Complete dislocation of the femorotibial joint is extremely uncommon in children because hyperextension is much more likely to cause a distal femoral epiphyseal separation than a dislocation. Given the high likelihood of neurovascular compromise or compartment syndrome, this dislocation is considered a true emergency. Using procedural sedation, axial traction of the tibia with slow flexion of the knee from an extended position may lead to a reduction. After reduction, an arteriogram must be obtained to rule out an intimal tear of the popliteal artery.

Patellar Fractures and Dislocations

Unlike in the adult, the patella in the child is rarely fractured because of the thick covering of cartilage overlying the patella during growth and development.

Diagnosis of a patellar fracture may be difficult. Pain usually prevents active extension of the knee. A congenitally bipartite patella can be easily confused with a fracture. The margins are smooth and rounded. A comparison view of the opposite knee may assist in the diagnosis. Sleeve fractures of the patella, in particular, can easily be misdiagnosed on radiograph (Fig. 22.33).

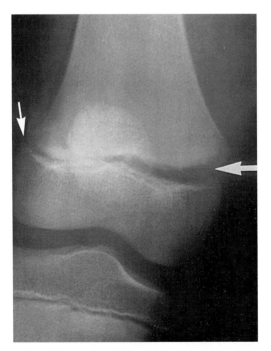

FIG. 22.32. A Salter–Harris type II fracture of the right distal femoral physis in a 9-year-old boy. Widening of the growth plate is seen medially (*large arrow*), and a small metaphyseal fragment has been displaced laterally (*small arrow*). Closed reduction was successful. In an adult, the same mechanism of injury would have resulted in a medial collateral ligament sprain or tear.

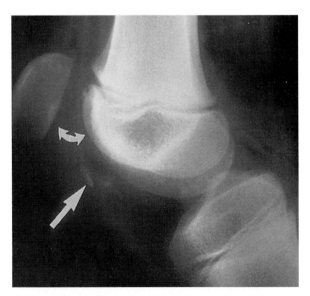

FIG. 22.33. A radiograph demonstrates a sleeve fracture of the patella in a 10-year-old boy. The inferior pole of the patella is displaced anteriorly (*curved arrow*). The bone fragment seen (*large arrow*) was avulsed by and remains attached to the patellar tendon.

Cylindrical cast treatment for 4 to 6 weeks will result in union. Fractures that are displaced more than 3 to 4 mm are best treated with open reduction.

An acute traumatic dislocation of the patella results from a force displacing the patella laterally while the foot is planted. The diagnosis is readily apparent by clinical examination (Fig. 22.34). Reduction of a dislocated patella usually is accomplished easily with extension of the knee and a medial

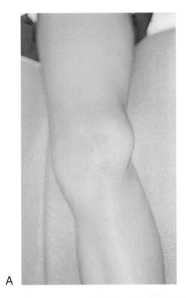

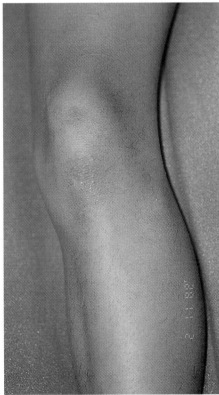

FIG. 22.34. A: This 9-year-old boy was tackled during a soccer match. His patella is displaced laterally. **B:** After closed reduction, the normal patellar profile is restored.

force on the lateral aspect of the patella. After reduction of an acutely dislocated patella, the physician must exclude the presence of an osteochondral fracture of the lateral femoral condyle or the medial patellar facet radiographically.

After closed reduction, immobilization in a posterior splint or a commercially available knee immobilizer until the orthopedic consultation is recommended.

Fractures of the Tibia and Fibula

Proximal Tibial Metaphyseal Fractures

Although usually easy to manage, proximal tibial fractures can lead to two major complications: compartment syndrome and progressive posttraumatic valgus deformity. Progressive valgus deformity can develop after any proximal tibial injury, including greenstick and nondisplaced fractures; therefore, all fractures of the proximal tibial metaphysis should be managed by an orthopedic surgeon.

Tibial and Fibular Shaft Fractures

Fractures of the tibial and fibular shafts are the most common fractures of the lower extremity in children. Most tibial and fibular fractures are stable and in acceptable alignment. If the neurovascular status is normal, no signs of compartment syndrome are present, and the fracture configuration is deemed acceptable, a long leg posterior splint may be applied and orthopedic referral within the next few days arranged. Otherwise, more immediate consultation should be sought. Complications of treatment after tibial and fibular fractures include malunion, limb length inequality, malrotation, and neurovascular deficiency.

Unique childhood fractures such as bowing deformities can occur with fibular trauma (Fig. 22.35).

Toddler's Fractures

Occasionally, the emergency department physician is asked to evaluate a young child with a limp or a refusal to walk. One possibility that should always be considered is a toddler's fracture. Originally, the term toddler's fracture referred to an oblique nondisplaced fracture of the distal tibia in children 9 to 36 months of age. The term is now used more loosely.

In most cases, the history is that of a minor accident. No history of injury may be recalled in some instances. The physical findings are often subtle. The degree of swelling is minimal; warmth and tenderness are more occasionally detected. Gentle twisting of the lower leg may elicit pain.

Like the physical findings, the radiographic abnormalities often are subtle. The anteroposterior or lateral views may reveal a spiral or oblique fracture (Fig. 22.36). If a toddler's fracture is suspected clinically but the routine radiographic views are normal, an internal oblique projection should be ordered. Consideration should also be given to the possibility of a fracture elsewhere in the limb. If no fracture is visualized on routine radiographs, a bone scan or a repeat set of plain films after 10 days to assess for subperiosteal new bone

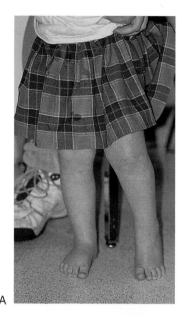

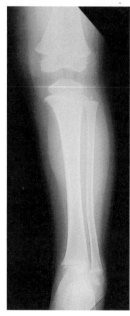

FIG. 22.35. A: This 2-year-old girl fell 4 ft and had a normal examination except that she would not bear weight on her left leg. **B:** The radiograph shows a bowing deformity of the fibula.

formation may be considered. Immobilization provides symptomatic relief and promotes healing.

Injuries of the Ankle and Foot

Ankle Sprains

Adolescents often present to the emergency department complaining of ankle injuries. The differential diagnosis includes ligamentous injuries; nondisplaced Salter–Harris type I fractures; osteochondral fractures of the tibia, fibula, or talus; and

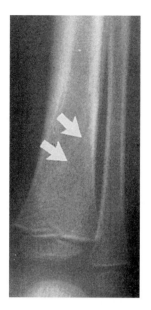

FIG. 22.36. Toddler's fracture of the distal tibia (*arrows*). Not until 2 weeks after the onset of symptoms could the fracture line be demonstrated radiographically.

avulsion injuries. Before growth plate fusion, physeal injuries are much more likely than ligamentous injuries. The most common mechanism is inversion of the foot while it is held in plantar flexion. The anterior talofibular ligament is most commonly injured. Injury to this ligament should be suspected when palpation just anterior to the distal fibula elicits an area of maximal tenderness. Other than with minor injuries, a three-view radiographic examination should be performed.

Controversy exists regarding the appropriate care of ligamentous injuries. If the ligaments are stretched but not torn, the sprain can be treated with an elastic wrap or air splint followed by ice, elevation, and compression for 72 hours. Crutches may be used until the patient is able to walk without a limp. If the ligaments are partially or completely torn, the injury should be immobilized in either a cast or a posterior splint. Ambulation in a cast for 3 weeks aids in initial scar formation and healing. This conservative approach with more severe sprains may help to prevent recurrent ankle sprains in active adolescents.

Distal Tibial and Fibular Fractures

Of the fractures of the distal fibula, a Salter–Harris type I injury is the most common. Tenderness and swelling are present over the growth plate on physical examination. Often the only radiographic finding is soft-tissue swelling overlying the distal fibula (Fig. 22.37). When suspicions of a Salter–Harris type I injury are high, a short leg cast may be applied at the time of initial evaluation. When the diagnosis is less certain, immobilization with a repeat examination in a week is recommended. If tenderness persists, a presumptive diagnosis of a type I fracture should be made and a walking cast applied. After 10 days, repeat radiographs may reveal

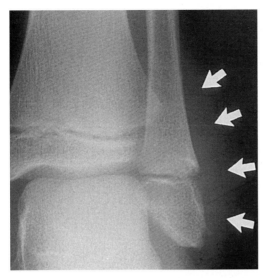

FIG. 22.37. A radiograph of the left ankle of a 10-year-old boy notable only for soft-tissue swelling localized to the distal fibula (*arrows*). If the patient is tender over the growth plate, the presumptive diagnosis is a Salter–Harris type I injury.

periosteal changes confirming the presence of a fracture. In most cases, a total of 3 weeks of immobilization is adequate.

The Tillaux fracture is a Salter–Harris type III injury of the ankle joint that occurs as the medial distal tibial physis begins to close in adolescents. During external rotation of the foot, the anterior tibiofibular ligament avulses the lateral epiphysis from the medial malleolus. When displacement occurs, open reduction with internal fixation is required to ensure restoration of joint anatomy (Fig. 22.38).

The triplane fracture is a complex ankle injury that is a combination of a Salter—Harris type II fracture and a Tillaux fracture. The resultant type IV injury may appear innocuous on the anteroposterior and lateral radiographs, but the degree of growth plate damage is generally significant. Suspected triplane fractures should be evaluated by computed tomography scan to delineate the amount of displacement at the physis and the articular surface.

Nondisplaced physeal and ankle fractures may be treated with a bulky posterior splint, crutches, and a referral to the orthopedist. Immediate orthopedic referral is otherwise necessary.

Hindfoot and Midfoot Fractures and Injuries

Fractures of the talus and the calcaneus are uncommon. When they do occur, they are usually obvious because of swelling and pain. Pain with dorsiflexion may indicate a talar neck fracture. Because calcaneal fractures generally occur as the result of a fall from a height, associated compression fractures of the spine can occur and must be considered. Often, a bulky posterior splint, crutches, and no weight bearing will suffice until an orthopedic consultation can be obtained.

Although uncommon, the Achilles tendon can rupture when the gastrocnemius and soleus muscles contract against force (e.g., pushing off or landing after a jump). The injury may not be very painful, but the patient may report hearing a pop (Fig. 22.39). The injury should be immobilized and operative repair scheduled.

Metatarsal and Foot Injuries

Metatarsal and phalangeal fractures are common in children. Two fractures that occur commonly at the base of the fifth metatarsal bear mentioning. The Jones fracture is a fracture at the diaphyseal-metaphyseal junction at the base of the

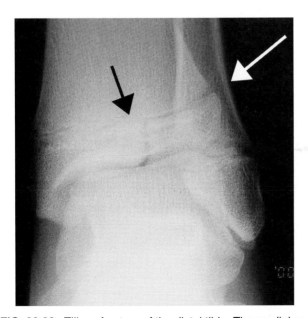

FIG. 22.38. Tillaux fracture of the distal tibia. The medial aspect of the epiphysis is closing. The fracture line runs vertically through the epiphysis (*small arrow*) and then laterally along the open and slightly widened physis (*large arrow*).

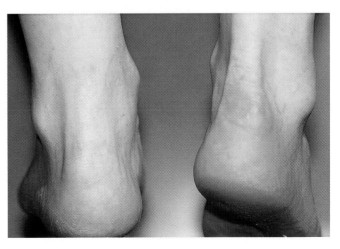

FIG. 22.39. The patient's ruptured left Achilles tendon appears thickened and less distinct than the normal right side, and the patient is unable to plantarflex the left foot.

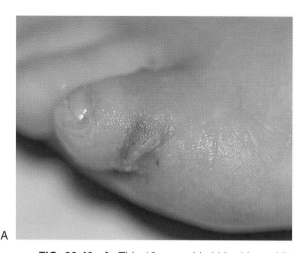

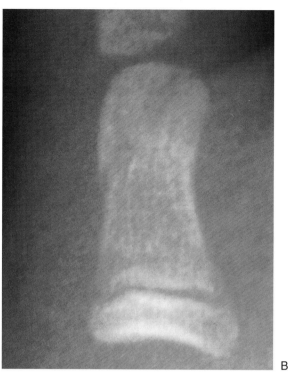

A

B

FIG. 22.40. A: This 12-year-old girl had been bitten by her dog and later hospitalized for cellulitis that improved on intravenous antimicrobials. B: When the infection recurred, a radiograph was obtained that showed a fracture from the initial dog bite. The patient was treated for osteomyelitis, and the infection resolved.

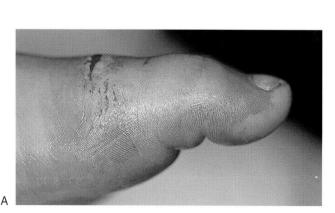

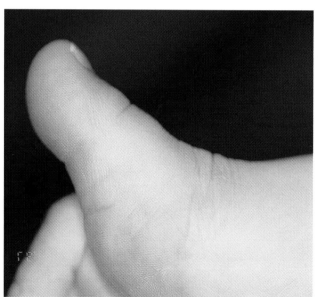

A

B

FIG. 22.41. A: This patient has a slight "droop" of the toe on the affected side, even when asked to extend the toe after digital nerve block. B: Full extension on the unaffected side. His extensor tendon laceration required operative repair.

fifth metatarsal. Although more common in adults, reports in adolescents can be found. This fracture has a high incidence of delayed or nonunion and should be splinted and referred to an orthopedist. An avulsion fracture of the base of the fifth metatarsal at the site of attachment of the peroneus brevis is relatively common in children. This fracture occurs more proximally than the Jones fracture and has a better prognosis. The usual treatment is 3 to 6 weeks of immobilization in a weight-bearing cast.

The care of most metatarsal and phalangeal injuries is relatively straightforward. If the fracture is nondisplaced or minimally displaced, a bulky splint can be applied and crutches prescribed. Intraarticular fractures of the big toe and significantly displaced fractures of the other toes often require pinning. Buddy taping and hard-soled shoes provide adequate stabilization for most other phalangeal fractures.

Bites to the phalanges should always be evaluated for possible bone involvement (Fig. 22.40).

Lacerations of the foot phalanges need a complete examination for tendon laceration just like the hand phalanges (Fig. 22.41).

SUGGESTED READINGS

Anderson WA. The significance of femoral fractures in children. *Ann Emerg Med* 1982;11:174–177.

Boyd KT, Peirce NS, Batt ME. Common hip injuries in sport. *Sports Med* 1997;24:273–288.

Innis PC. Office evaluation and treatment of finger and hand injuries in children. *Curr Opinion Pediatr* 1995;7:83–87.

Kao SC, Smith WL. Skeletal injuries in the pediatric patient. *Radiol Clin North Am* 1997;35:727–746.

Mastey RD, Weiss AP, Akelman E. Primary care of hand and wrist athletic injuries. *Clin Sports Med* 1997;16:705–724.

Micheli LJ. Sports injuries in children and adolescents. *Clin Sports Med* 1995;14:727–745.

Rockwood CA Jr, Wilkins KE, King RE. *Fractures in children*, 3rd ed. Philadelphia: JB Lippincott, 1991.

Swischuk LE. *Emergency radiology of the acutely ill or injured child*, 3rd ed. Baltimore: Williams & Wilkins, 1994.

CHAPTER 23

Trauma: Genitourinary

Editor: Gary R. Fleisher

The clinical approach to the injured child should strictly follow Advanced Trauma Life Support guidelines. Figure 23.1 provides an algorithm for diagnostic evaluation of the pediatric patient with genitourinary trauma.

KIDNEY

Clinical Presentation

Children who sustain significant blunt renal injuries usually present with localized signs such as flank tenderness, flank hematoma, or a palpable flank mass. Generalized abdominal tenderness, rigidity of the abdominal wall, paralytic ileus, and hypovolemic shock may all be part of the clinical picture. Penetrating injuries to the chest, abdomen, flank, and lumbar regions suggest the possibility of renal injury (Fig. 19.11). Although controversy exists about the correlation between the degree of hematuria and the severity of the injury, the presence of any degree of hematuria should be regarded as a potential indication of underlying renal injury or anomaly. Conversely, hematuria may be absent in as many as 50% of patients with vascular pedicle injuries and in 29% of patients with penetrating injuries.

Radiographic evaluation of the genitourinary tract is necessary in patients with gross hematuria or microscopic hematuria associated with a major mechanism, clinical findings indicative of renal injury, or other significant injuries (Fig. 23.1). Hematuria of more than 20 red blood cells per high-power field in patients without associated clinical findings has been recommended as a threshold for radiographic workup. Microscopic hematuria with shock is one of the clinical criteria used to guide radiographic evaluation in the adult population.

Initial evaluation of suspected pediatric renal trauma should include radiographs of the chest, abdomen, and pelvis. Plain films may show obliterated renal and psoas shadows, scoliosis with the concavity toward the injured site, intraabdominal mass effect or a coincident rib, spinous process, or pelvic fracture. Traditionally, intravenous pyelography has been the cornerstone of evaluation in renal trauma (Figs. 23.2

and 23.3). Intravenous pyelography is available in most institutions and provides information about both kidneys. It can be obtained on an unstable patient urgently in the emergency department or in the operating room before surgery. A scout radiograph should be made before the contrast study. More recently, contrast-enhanced computed tomography (CT) has become the preferred study for evaluation of major abdominal injury, including renal injury (Fig. 23.4). A CT scan has particular advantages over intravenous pyelography, the most important of which is the detection of associated injuries. In addition, CT provides three-dimensional views and imaging independent of the vascularity of the kidney.

Management

The principle underlying the management of pediatric renal trauma is preservation of renal tissue and function with minimal morbidity and mortality. After the patient's general condition has been assessed and the presence of associated injuries established, treatment of renal trauma should proceed based on staging of the traumatic lesion. In cases of blunt trauma, minor injuries, such as contusions and lacerations without urinary extravasation (grades I, II, and III), are treated conservatively. Management of the remaining patients (grades IV and V) evokes significant controversy and should be guided by an appropriate surgeon.

URETER

Ureteral injuries can be caused by blunt, penetrating, or iatrogenic trauma. Blunt trauma usually involves the ureteropelvic junction. Trauma to the ureter should be suspected in patients presenting with fracture of the transverse process of a lumbar vertebra. The physical examination may be unremarkable. However, an enlarging flank mass in the absence of signs of retroperitoneal bleeding suggests urinary extravasation. Hematuria is an unreliable sign. When the diagnosis has been delayed, ureteral injury may be manifested by fever, chills, lethargy, leukocytosis, pyuria, bacteriuria,

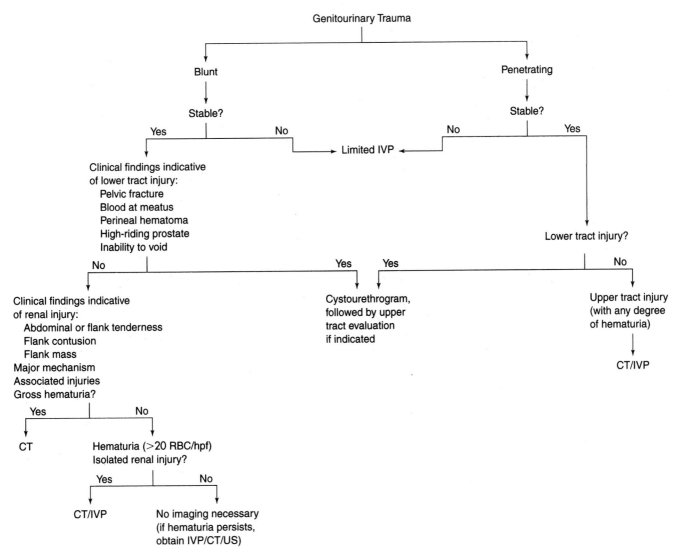

FIG. 23.1. Algorithm for evaluation of the pediatric patient with genitourinary trauma. *IVP,* intravenous pyelography; *CT,* computed tomography; *RBC,* red blood cells; *hpf,* high-power field; *US,* ultrasonography.

flank mass or pain, fistulae, and ureteral strictures. The management of complete transection of the ureter depends on the level of the injury.

BLADDER

Bladder injuries may occur after blunt or penetrating trauma. Approximately 80% of bladder injuries are associated with pelvic fractures and penetration of the bladder by a bony fragment. Hematuria and dysuria are symptoms commonly seen at presentation. Virtually all patients with rupture of the bladder have hematuria. Microscopic hematuria is associated with less severe injuries such as contusions. Inability to void may be associated with large tears. Patients with intraperitoneal ruptures may develop a palpable fluid wave

from extravasation of urine into the peritoneal cavity and peritoneal irritation.

Diagnostic evaluation is indicated in patients who sustain pelvic or lower abdominal trauma with hematuria and inability to void. Evaluation begins with a radiograph to exclude a pelvic fracture. If no pelvic fracture, no blood at the meatus, and no dislocation of the prostate on rectal examination are present, the urethra can be catheterized gently and retrograde cystography can be performed. Cystography of a contused bladder may show a teardrop shape or elevation of the bladder out of the pelvis. No evidence of extravasation of contrast material will be apparent. Extraperitoneal perforation is demonstrated by the presence of extravasated medium in the area of the pubic symphysis and pelvic outlet. In cases of intraperitoneal rupture, contrast may outline intraabdominal

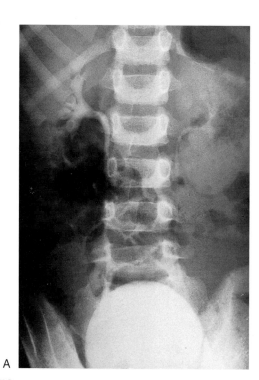

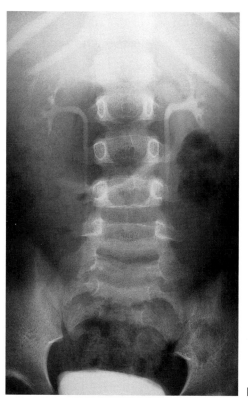

FIG. 23.2. A: Intravenous pyelography in this child reveals a contusion on the left kidney, manifested by decreased concentration of contrast material. **B:** One month later, a repeat study shows a return of normal anatomy and function.

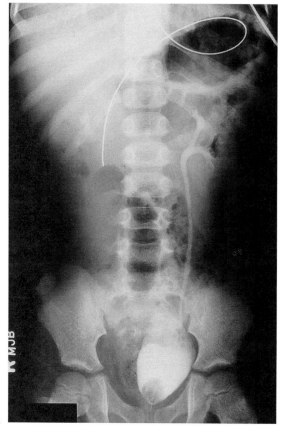

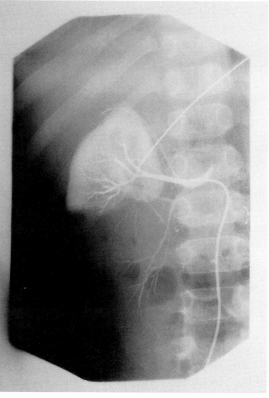

FIG. 23.3. A: Intravenous pyelography demonstrates a renal fracture, with nonvisualization of the lower pole of the right kidney. **B:** An arteriogram confirms the diagnosis.

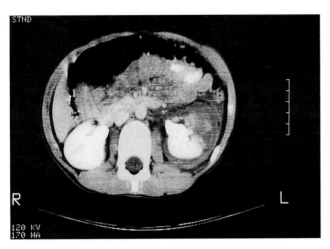

FIG. 23.4. Computed tomography of the abdomen shows a renal fracture and a moderate subcapsular hematoma.

organs or paracolic gutters. Contrast-enhanced CT scan and CT cystography can also be used in the evaluation of bladder injuries.

Conservative management with or without urethral catheter drainage is the standard of care in patients with contusion. Extraperitoneal vesical rupture can be managed by urethral catheter or suprapubic drainage for 7 to 10 days. Treatment of large extraperitoneal tears or intraperitoneal tears involves transperitoneal exploration and repair with placement of a suprapubic cystostomy tube.

URETHRA

Urethral injuries occur primarily in males. In boys, the urogenital diaphragm divides the urethra into anterior (pendulous and bulbous) and posterior (membranous and prostatic) portions. Anterior and posterior urethral injuries (Fig. 23.5) differ from each other by mechanism of injury, clinical presentation, and treatment. Anterior urethral injuries result from direct trauma and are often isolated and associated with a low mortality rate. The pendulous urethra may be damaged by blunt or penetrating forces. Bulbar injuries are commonly caused by a straddle mechanism, as the urethra is compressed between the symphysis pubis and a solid object. Blood at the meatus has been reported in as many as 90% of patients sustaining anterior urethral injuries. Other findings include hematuria, inability or difficulty voiding, and periurethral or perineal edema and ecchymosis. Perineal ecchymosis in the shape of a butterfly is typical for these injuries. Blind placement of a urethral catheter may convert a partial tear into a complete transection and therefore should be discouraged.

Anterior urethral injuries can be managed by 7 to 10 days of urethral catheterization and antibacterial therapy. More severe injuries require urinary diversion by suprapubic cystostomy. Penetrating wounds demand surgical repair with exploration, debridement of devitalized tissue, and copious irrigation. Initial management of posterior urethral injuries remains controversial. Therapeutic options vary from immediate exploration with primary repair to placement of a

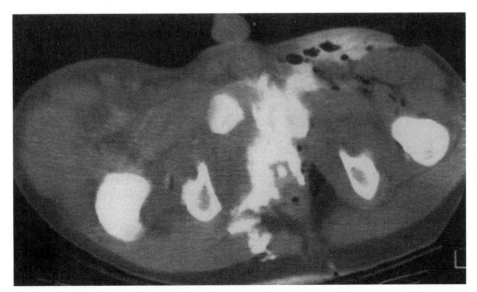

FIG. 23.5. This patient sustained a pelvic fracture complicated by a disruption of the posterior urethra. Computed tomography shows extravasation of contrast from the urethra into the surrounding tissues.

suprapubic tube with delayed urethroplasty. Urethral rupture may also be treated by realigning the urethra over an indwelling urethral catheter. Primary repair or operative realignment should be reserved for urethral injuries associated with rectal laceration, a high-riding bladder, or injury to the bladder neck.

Trauma to the urethra in girls is rare because the female urethra is relatively mobile and short. Injuries may occur after surgical procedures or instrumentation. Most serious injuries involve the vesicourethral junction and result from blunt abdominal trauma in motor vehicle accidents. The lesion generally occurs in association with pelvic fractures. The injury often extends to the vagina. Urethral injuries in female patients are treated with suprapubic drainage and elective repair.

SCROTUM

Scrotal trauma may occur as a result of straddle injuries or bicycle accidents or during sporting events. The patient may present with scrotal tenderness, edema, and ecchymosis. Potential injuries include skin or dartos ecchymoses and lacerations, intrascrotal hematomas, testicular hematomas, testicular dislocation, and testicular rupture. In addition, a testicle may twist after trauma. When inspection of the scrotum and its contents is obscured by local swelling and pain, ultrasonography is helpful to define the extent of the injury. An intratesticular hematoma may show as an echogenic or hypoechoic testicular mass. A hematocele produces a complex extratesticular fluid collection. Sonographic findings of rupture include presence of hematocele, mixed parenchymal echogenicity, intraparenchymal hemorrhage, and disruption of the tunica albuginea or parenchyma.

Patients without evidence of injury to the testes who sustain intrascrotal hematomas, skin ecchymosis, or skin and dartos injury only can be managed conservatively. Treatment consists of ice packs and scrotal support. Minor testicular injuries such as contusions or hematomas can also be treated conservatively. Large testicular hematomas may require surgical management. Testicular dislocation occurs as a result of an upward blow to the scrotum. In most cases, the dislocated testis lies under the abdominal wall. Operative repair is required if closed reduction fails. Testicular rupture with a tear of the tunica albuginea and extravasation of testicular contents into the scrotal sac requires surgical exploration and repair. Other injuries requiring surgical management include tense hematoceles and torsion after trauma. Superficial lacerations of the scrotum can be repaired using absorbable sutures. Local infiltration with lidocaine with epinephrine provides adequate anesthesia.

PENIS

Direct Injury

The most common cause of direct injury to the penis comes from a toilet seat's falling on the penis of a young boy who is learning to stand at the toilet to void. Although the resulting penile edema may be notable, significant injury to the corporal bodies or urethra is rare. The only treatment required is warm soaks and expectant observation. After blunt or sharp trauma, if blood is seen at the urethral meatus, urethral injury must be considered and retrograde urethrography carried out. If a child is seen for a laceration of the shaft of the penis, it is important to be certain that the corporal bodies and urethra have not been injured concurrently. When a question exists, a pediatric urologic consultation, retrograde urethrography, and exploration under anesthetic may be needed. For simple lacerations of the penile skin, repair with chromic catgut suffices.

Zipper Injury

Boys often seem to be in a hurry and sometimes fail to get their penis or foreskin completely back in their pants before they pull up the zipper. This results in the entrapment of penile skin or foreskin in the teeth of the zipper (Fig. 23.6A). The teeth may be so engaged that it is impossible to simply unzip the zipper. The median bar of the zipper may be cut with a pair of wire cutters, which will permit the two halves of the zipper to fall apart, releasing the entrapped skin (Fig.

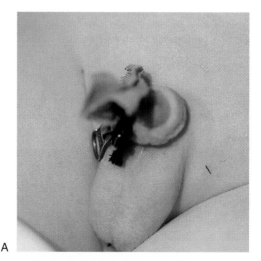

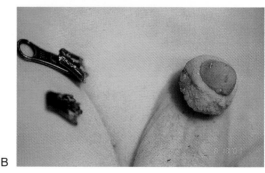

FIG. 23.6. In the act of zippering his pants, this young boy managed to entrap the skin of his penis **(A)**. The emergency physician used a wire cutter to incise the median bar of the zipper, releasing the two sides and freeing the penis **(B)**.

23.6B). Mineral oil has also been used to allow the tissue to slide free of the metal zipper. Infiltration of local anesthesia makes this procedure less traumatic to the child. After the zipper is removed, the penis may become edematous, but generally nothing more than warm soaks is required for further treatment.

Perineum

The mechanism most commonly associated with trauma to the female perineum is a straddle-type injury. These injuries may cause vulvar hematomas, which usually respond to treatment with ice packs and bed rest. Patients experiencing mild urinary retention may be more comfortable voiding in a tub of warm water. Massive or expanding hematomas may require evacuation.

Superficial lacerations of the perineum can be treated conservatively at home with sitz baths. Deep lacerations may extend into the rectum or urethra. Rectal penetration requires a diverting colostomy. Suprapubic cystostomy or primary repair should be performed if the urethra is disrupted.

Vaginal lacerations must always be suspected in patients with severe trauma to the external genitalia or penetration by a foreign object. If a significant vaginal laceration is noted, endoscopy with sedation or general anesthesia is necessary for a full evaluation. The possibility of extension into the urethra, bladder, or rectum must be investigated. The vaginal laceration is debrided and repaired with fine absorbable sutures.

SUGGESTED READINGS

Abou-Jaoude WA, Sugarman JM, Fallat ME, et al. Indicators of genitourinary tract injury or anomaly in cases of pediatric blunt trauma. *J Pediatr Surg* 1996;31:86–90.

Ahmed S, Neel KF. Urethral injury in girls with fractured pelvis following blunt abdominal trauma. *Br J Urol* 1996;78:450–453.

Avanoglu A, Ulman I, Herek O, et al. Posterior urethral injuries in children. *Br J Urol* 1996;77:597–600.

Bass DH, Semple PL, Cywes S. Investigation and management of blunt renal injuries in children: a review of 11 years' experience. *J Pediatr Surg* 1991;26:196–200.

Fleisher GR. Prospective evaluation of selective criteria for imaging among children with suspected blunt renal trauma. *Pediatr Emerg Care* 1989;5:8–11.

Hilton SW, Kaplan GW. Imaging of common problems in pediatric urology. *Urol Clin North Am* 1995;22:13–18.

Kotkin L, Brock JW. Isolated ureteral injury caused by blunt trauma. *Urology* 1996;47:111–113.

Lieu T, Fleisher GR, Mahboubi S, et al. Hematuria and clinical findings as indications for intravenous pyelography in pediatric blunt renal trauma. *Pediatrics* 1988;82:216–222.

Mansi MK, Alkhudair WK. Conservative management with percutaneous intervention of major blunt renal injuries. *Am J Emerg Med* 1997;15:633–637.

McAleer IM, Kaplan GW. Pediatric genitourinary trauma. *Urol Clin North Am* 1995;22:177–188.

Stevenson J, Battistella FD. The one-shot intravenous pyelogram: is it indicated in unstable trauma patients before celiotomy? *J Trauma* 1994;36:828–834.

CHAPTER 24

Trauma: Head and Neck

Editor: Marc N. Baskin

NEUROTRAUMA

Head

Head trauma accounts for approximately 250,000 hospital admissions and nearly five million visits to emergency departments for pediatric patients each year. Brain injury is the leading cause of death and disability among pediatric trauma patients.

Pathophysiology

Discussions of traumatic brain injury typically divide the injury into two main components: primary and secondary. Primary brain injury refers to neural damage that is attributed directly to the traumatic insult itself. Shearing of neuronal axons and contusion or laceration of cerebral tissue all constitute primary brain injury. Secondary brain injury refers to subsequent injury to brain cells not injured by the initial traumatic event. Secondary brain injury has numerous causes, including hypoxia and hypoperfusion resulting from inadequate cerebral blood flow.

Cerebral Herniation

Cerebral herniation refers to the abnormal passage of brain tissue into an anatomic space in which it does not normally reside. Cerebral herniation occurs when the brain tissue is displaced by a large intracranial hematoma and/or massive brain swelling.

In tentorial herniation, as the swelling expands, a portion of the temporal lobe begins to slide through the tentorial notch. As the temporal cortex passes through, it becomes pressed against the brainstem structures and against the third cranial nerve. Classically, the patient first complains of headache, and then a depression in the level of consciousness occurs as the reticular activating system is compressed. The ipsilateral third nerve is compressed next, with resulting pupillary dilation (blown pupil) and eventually loss of third nerve motor function (ptosis and loss of medial gaze). As the process continues and the cerebral peduncle is compressed,

hemiparesis or decerebrate posturing develops. Brainstem control of vital signs is also affected, with the development of bradycardia, hypertension, and irregular respirations (Cushing triad). As herniation and brainstem compression continue to progress, the patient typically loses function of both pupils and develops decerebrate posturing or flaccid paresis bilaterally. Ultimately, respiratory arrest ensues.

Another site of herniation is the foramen magnum, through which the cerebellar tonsils may herniate. As the brainstem and sylvian aqueduct are compressed, ventricular outflow obstruction may occur, with the acute onset of hydrocephalus, which will severely worsen the increased intracranial pressure (ICP), exacerbating the herniation process. Patients with herniation at the foramen magnum may present with symptoms of neck pain, vomiting, depressed mental status, bradycardia, or hypertension. In other cases, the patient may be relatively asymptomatic until sudden cardiorespiratory arrest occurs.

Management and General Principles

Initial Resuscitation

Management of the patient with a head injury focuses on the prevention of secondary brain injury. As with all emergency care, management begins with the ABCs (airway, breathing, and circulation) of resuscitation. Immobilization of the cervical spine with a semirigid cervical collar or with inline manual stabilization must be maintained until the clinician can be certain that no cervical spine injury has occurred.

Unless the ICP is increased, the clinician should aim to achieve normocarbia (Pco_2, 35 to 40 mm Hg) and oxygen saturation of 100%. If the ICP is increased, therapeutic hyperventilation may be indicated.

Endotracheal intubation should be performed for any patients making inadequate or labored respiratory effort or for patients who have a blunted gag reflex, cannot manage their oral secretions, or are comatose. Care must be taken to minimize manipulation of the cervical spine during the process of intubation. In awake patients, rapid sequence intubation with (1) a sedative/anesthetic, (2) a paralytic such as rocuronium, (3) atropine, and (4) lidocaine should be considered.

Brain-specific Therapies

Once the ABCs of resuscitation have been addressed and the patient has been stabilized, attention can be given to the neurologic status. Medical treatment for increased ICP should be undertaken immediately when it is suspected. This treatment includes elevation of the head of the bed to a 30-degree angle, which promotes venous drainage from the head (thereby decreasing the volume of the intracranial vasculature). The head should be maintained in a midline position, which helps to maintain venous outflow through the jugular system as well. Furthermore, sedating medications may be needed to prevent the patient from coughing and choking or from becoming agitated, both of which might be associated with increased intrathoracic pressure and, therefore, impaired venous drainage. Sedation should be used as sparingly as possible, however, so that the neurologic status can be monitored.

Hyperventilation also decreases ICP by decreasing the volume of the intracranial vasculature. The cerebral arteriolar circulation responds to hypocarbia with reflex vasoconstriction. The therapeutic use of hyperventilation requires a delicate balance: too little ventilation leads to vasodilation and increased ICP, but too much ventilation leads to excess vasoconstriction and decreased cerebral blood flow. The optimal balance for therapeutic hyperventilation appears to be achieved at a P_{CO_2} of 30 to 35 mm Hg.

Mannitol can also be given to lower the ICP, at an intravenous dose of 0.5 to 1 g/kg, which increases the serum osmolarity. Because of the lower viscosity of blood, cerebral blood flow is improved. The effect of mannitol on ICP is seen within a few minutes of administration. Clinicians should be cautious about the use of mannitol in any patient with possible hemodynamic compromise because the administration of a diuretic may exacerbate hypovolemia and worsen perfusion.

Although disagreement exists about the optimal use of these maneuvers, stabilization of the patient with impending herniation by using hyperventilation and/or mannitol may allow enough time for the patient to be safely transferred to the radiology suite for an emergency head computed tomography (CT) scan.

Anticonvulsant medications (e.g., benzodiazepines) are indicated for patients who are having ongoing seizure activity. Phenytoin is used as prophylaxis for patients who have intracranial lesions associated with an increased risk of seizure activity, such as cerebral contusion, intraparenchymal hemorrhage, subarachnoid hemorrhage, or subdural hemorrhage.

Disposition

Generally, all patients with intracranial hematomas or brain injuries noted on head CT should be hospitalized, no matter how mild or severe their symptoms. In addition, any patient with an abnormal mental status or neurologic examination should be hospitalized, even if head CT findings are normal. Well-appearing patients with head injuries who either required no head CT scan or who have no intracranial lesions on head CT may be suitable for discharge home with careful instructions. A discussion of the management of these patients follows.

Blunt Trauma: Specific Lesions

Concussion

Concussion is defined by the Centers for Disease Control and Prevention as a head trauma–induced alteration in mental status that may or may not involve loss of consciousness. Common symptoms of concussion include initial loss of consciousness, amnesia, confusion, headache, nausea, vomiting, and dizziness. For the most part, clinicians diagnose concussion in those patients with minor head trauma who have no brain imaging performed or as a diagnosis of exclusion for patients with minor head injury who have no evidence of intracranial pathology on a head CT scan.

In general, patients with concussion can be expected to do well, and no specific therapy is required. These patients may be safely discharged home if no other issues require inpatient care. The American Academy of Neurology has published recommendations for the management of athletes who have sustained a concussion (Table 24.1).

TABLE 24.1. *Recommendations for return to sports activity after concussion*

Grade 1 concussion
  Definition: transient confusion, no loss of consciousness, mental status abnormalities for ≤15 minutes
  Management: return to sports activities same day only if all symptoms resolve within 15 minutes; if a second grade 1 concussion occurs, no sports activity until asymptomatic for 1 week
Grade 2 concussion
  Definition: transient confusion, no loss of consciousness, mental status abnormalities for >15 minutes
  Management: no sports activity until asymptomatic for 1 full week; if a grade 2 concussion occurs on the same day as a previous grade 1 concussion, no sports activity for 2 weeks
Grade 3 concussion
  Definition: concussion involving loss of consciousness
  Management: no sports activity until asymptomatic for 1 week if loss of consciousness was brief (seconds) or for 2 weeks if loss of consciousness was prolonged (minutes or longer)
  Second grade 3 concussion, no sports activity until asymptomatic for 1 month
  Any abnormality on computed tomography or magnetic resonance imaging, no sports activity for remainder of season; patient should be discouraged from any future return to contact sports

Modified from *MMWR, Morb Mortal Wkly Rep*, Centers for Disease Control and Prevention.

Skull Fracture

Infants are clearly at a higher risk of skull fracture than older children, probably because their skulls are thinner. Many skull fractures in infants result from short distance falls; approximately 50% of infants with skull fracture have fallen less than 4 or 5 ft.

Fractures may occur in any bone of the skull, although fractures of the parietal bone constitute approximately 70% of cases. The occipital and temporal bones are the next most commonly involved, with the frontal bone least likely to fracture.

Most cases of skull fracture are associated with soft-tissue swelling or hematoma overlying the fracture site. Skull fracture may occur in the absence of recognized soft-tissue findings as well, perhaps because subtle swelling is missed beneath the patient's hair.

Signs of basilar skull fracture may include hemotympanum, Battle sign (hematoma or discoloration overlying the mastoid bone), "raccoon eyes" (blue or purple discoloration of the periorbital tissue) (Fig. 24.1), or cerebrospinal fluid (CSF) rhinorrhea or otorrhea. Skull fracture may be diagnosed by plain radiographs of the skull or by head CT. A head CT scan is usually preferred for evaluating children with head injuries because it provides information not only about the skull but also about the intracranial contents. Skull radiographs are more sensitive for detecting skull fracture, especially for those horizontal fractures that run parallel to and between adjacent "cuts" on the CT scan.

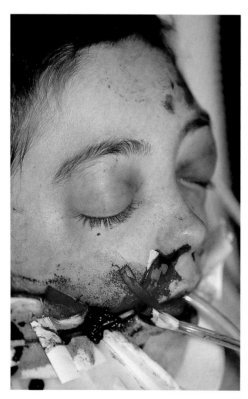

FIG. 24.1. "Raccoon eyes" secondary to severe closed head injury with basilar skull fracture.

Linear Skull Fracture

The main significance of linear skull fractures is that they indicate that the risk of intracranial injury is increased by as much as 10-fold. In cases in which acute linear skull fracture is diagnosed, therefore, a head CT scan is essential to evaluate for possible intracranial injury. In addition, any diagnosis of skull fracture should lead the clinician to consider the possibility of child abuse. If the history provided is not a plausible explanation for the injuries observed, further evaluation for possible child abuse should be initiated.

Many clinicians routinely admit children with skull fracture to the hospital for a period (e.g., 24 hours) of observation to exclude the small possibility of late complications. However, if a child with skull fracture but no intracranial lesions remains well over a short period of observation in the emergency department and child abuse is not suspected, the child may be considered for discharge home. The warning signs of advancing intracranial injury should be carefully reviewed with the family, with advice to return immediately if any of these signs is noticed. The family should also be counseled to expect the possible development of a subgaleal hematoma, which becomes more evident as the clotted blood overlying the fracture site begins to liquefy and which presents as a large boggy swelling of the scalp, usually between 5 and 7 days after the injury. Unless the hematoma develops signs of infection, it will resolve gradually on its own and should not be aspirated.

Linear skull fractures generally heal well, with no specific therapy required. Fewer than 1% of patients will develop a growing skull fracture (i.e., a fracture that fails to heal and becomes wider over time). All patients should have a follow-up examination 1 month after the initial injury.

Depressed Skull Fracture

If no other complicating features exist, isolated skull fractures with minimal depressions can be managed in a fashion similar to that previously described for linear skull fractures. More significant depressions of the skull are more serious. In cases in which injury to underlying brain is noted on head CT, especially if there are seizures or focal neurologic findings referable to the brain injury, prompt surgical elevation of the fracture fragments may be required. Surgical intervention is also usually necessary for compound, or open, depressed skull fractures, for any skull fracture with a 1-cm or greater depression, or for depressions with a depth greater than the thickness of the skull.

Basilar Skull Fracture

Fractures through the skull base are unique in that they may involve disruption of the mastoid air cells or the paranasal sinuses. The most recent studies suggest that the risk of meningitis after basilar skull fracture is between 0.4% and 5%. The highest risk is in patients with evident CSF rhinorrhea or otorrhea. It is therefore recommended by many clinicians that these patients be admitted to the hospital for prophylactic intravenous antibiotics.

Parenchymal Injuries

Cerebral Contusion and Intraparenchymal Hematoma

Cerebral contusion refers to bruising of the cerebral cortex. Focal neurologic deficits associated with dysfunction of the contused tissue should be expected. In addition, cerebral contusion leads to a risk of secondary brain injury because the contusion may exert some mass effect on surrounding tissue, with resulting cerebral dysfunction and risk of further ischemia. Finally, contusions are associated with a risk of late intraparenchymal hematoma.

The severity of the clinical manifestations associated with cerebral contusion can vary widely. Often, there is history of loss of consciousness or some disturbance in mental status. With the increasing use of CT for patients with mild head trauma, an increasing number of contusions are being discovered in patients with no or mild symptoms (headache, nausea and vomiting, lethargy).

Most patients with intraparenchymal hematomas are comatose, and they may have focal neurologic deficits. Rare patients with intraparenchymal hematoma may initially be alert, but they have a high risk of deterioration over the ensuing hours.

Cerebral contusions are generally evident on a head CT scan as hypodense areas of edema, sometimes intermingled with hyperdense areas of hemorrhage (Fig. 24.2). Intraparenchymal hematomas are more uniformly hyperdense, although areas of active bleeding may be isodense.

All patients with acute cerebral contusion and intraparenchymal hematoma should be admitted to the hospital for observation. Management of cerebral contusions focuses on efforts to prevent secondary brain injury, with the recognition that the contused tissue and surrounding areas are at especially high risk of ischemia. For patients in a coma, ICP monitoring is generally indicated, and maneuvers for managing increased ICP may be required. The clinician must be especially alert for the possibility that an initially nonhemorrhagic contusion will undergo late hemorrhage, which would manifest as a sudden increase in ICP and/or deterioration in clinical status.

Diffuse Axonal Injury

Diffuse axonal injury (DAI) is characterized pathologically by injury to the white matter tracts of the brain. In addition, DAI is often associated with other focal lesions or with global brain swelling. DAI results from the application of severe acceleration/deceleration or angular rotational forces to the brain, which lead to shear injuries of the axons and associated vasculature.

The clinical manifestations of DAI can vary greatly, ranging from those patients who have symptoms of concussion to those who present in a coma. Loss of consciousness is

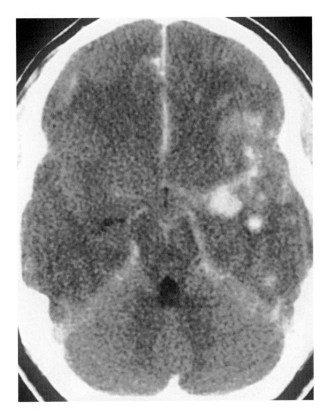

FIG. 24.2. Cerebral contusion. This 16-year-old girl was comatose after being a passenger in a high-speed motor vehicle collision. A head computed tomography scan shows hemorrhagic contusion of the left temporal lobe, subdural hematoma along the tentorial margins, and effacement of the sulci throughout. The patient expired despite intensive medical management for increased intracranial pressure.

common. In one study of patients with DAI, 82% developed a coma.

DAI is evident on CT scan as small, nonexpansive hemorrhagic lesions of the white matter. DAI is often accompanied by cerebral swelling, intraventricular hemorrhage (Fig. 24.3), intraparenchymal hemorrhages, or cerebral contusions.

Patients with a radiographic diagnosis of DAI should be admitted to the hospital for observation. Management of patients with DAI is supportive, with efforts directed mainly at preventing secondary brain injury.

Diffuse Brain Swelling

Diffuse brain swelling (DBS) is a common manifestation of head trauma, especially in pediatric patients. DBS appears to be caused by an increase in intracerebral vascular volume. This may be caused by diffuse vasodilation and a loss of normal autoregulatory reflexes or cerebral edema that is vasogenic (extravasated from injured or inflamed blood vessels), cytotoxic (representing intracellular swelling of injured brain cells), or interstitial (from inadequate drainage of CSF).

Most patients with DBS are comatose on initial evaluation but rarely have only minor neurologic deficits. These

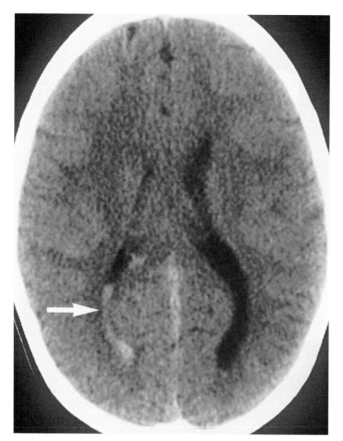

FIG. 24.3. Intraventricular hemorrhage. This head computed tomography (CT) scan was performed on an 8-year-old girl who was involved in a sledding accident. She presented in a coma. There is hemorrhage in the right lateral ventricle (*arrow*). Note the layering of blood inferiorly in this supine patient. Other "cuts" of the CT showed areas of punctate hemorrhage consistent with diffuse axonal injury. The patient made an excellent recovery, with minimal neurologic deficits.

patients often experience neurologic deterioration over the ensuing several hours.

DBS is diagnosed by a head CT scan when evidence exists of smaller ventricles, effacement of the sulci, or obliterated basal cisterns in the absence of other intracranial pathology that may be exerting a significant mass effect (Fig. 24.4). Other accompanying intracranial lesions, such as DAI, subdural hemorrhage, or cerebral contusion, are often diagnosed as well. Patients with DBS need to be admitted to the hospital. Generally, admission to the intensive care unit is required for careful monitoring of hemodynamics, oxygenation and ventilation, and ICP. ICP monitors are indicated for any patient with DBS in a coma.

Epidural Hematoma

Most epidural hematomas (EDHs) result from blunt impact to the cranium, with a skull fracture and an associated laceration to the epidural vessels underlying the fracture. In other cases, there is no fracture, but the deformation of the skull from impact leads to shearing of the epidural arteries or veins. Many patients with EDH have experienced relatively low-energy mechanisms of injury (e.g., approximately half of pediatric cases result from falls of 6 ft or less). Other mechanisms of injury, such as the shaking often implicated in cases of child abuse, are less likely to be associated with EDH because they do not lead to deformation of the skull. As the EDH expands, it begins to occupy an increasingly large intracranial volume. This increasing mass effect leads to an increase in ICP and may result in diffuse secondary brain injury and ultimately lead to cerebral herniation.

Clinical Symptoms and Signs

Pediatric patients with EDH rarely present with the classic deterioration after a "lucid interval." The most common symptoms of EDH in pediatric patients are headache, vomiting, and lethargy. A small number of patients with EDH may not have any symptoms indicative of brain injury. Skull fracture, especially temporal or parietal, may be a particularly important indicator of the risk of EDH, especially in patients with few other symptoms.

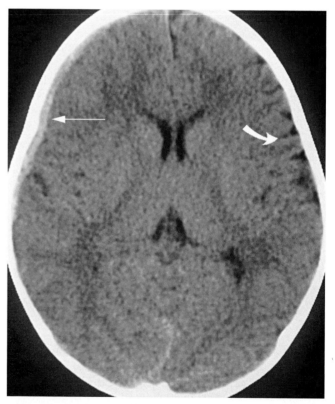

FIG. 24.4. Brain swelling. This 1-year-old boy fell from a second-story window. The neurologic examination was normal. A head computed tomography scan shows a small, right-sided subdural hematoma in the temporal region. Note also the effacement of the sulci on the right (*straight arrow*), which can be compared with the normal sulci on the left (*curved arrow*). There is also a mild shift of the midline toward the left.

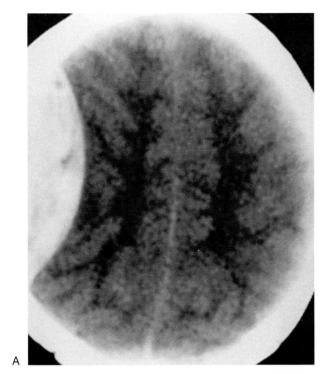
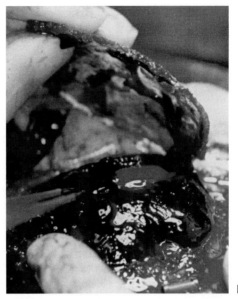

A

B

FIG. 24.5. Epidural hematoma. This 8-year-old boy presented after a sledding accident. He had no loss of consciousness but complained of headache and vomiting. **A:** A head computed tomography scan shows the classic biconvex hyperdensity of an epidural hematoma. He proceeded to the operating room, where a large mass of clotted blood **(B)** was removed.

EDH can be readily diagnosed by noncontrast CT of the head (Fig. 24.5).

Management

The mainstay of treatment of EDH is craniotomy, with drainage of the hematoma and repair of the lacerated epidural vessels. Neurosurgeons have recognized that some patients with EDH may safely be managed with observation, e.g., those with a small EDH (generally less than 30 mL in volume and with a thickness of less than 2 cm), no focal neurologic deficits, and a normal level of consciousness. Mortality rates in EDH range from 0% to 10%. Approximately 85% of surviving children with EDH have a good neurologic outcome.

Subdural Hematoma

Subdural hematomas (SDHs) result from tearing of the bridging veins that traverse the subdural space. Mechanisms of injury that are associated with shear forces, especially acceleration/deceleration, are especially likely to lead to SDHs. In older children and adolescents, SDHs most commonly result from motor vehicle collisions. In infants, SDHs are commonly a result of the shaking impact syndrome of child abuse.

Clinical Manifestations

SDHs are often associated with an initial loss of consciousness and a depressed mental status. Coma and pupillary abnormalities may indicate impending herniation. In less ill patients, headaches, vomiting, lethargy, irritability, visual difficulties, or seizures may be noted. In patients with SDHs involving the posterior fossa, cerebellar signs such as ataxia or nystagmus may be noted. Because CT scanning is being used more routinely in cases of minor head injuries, many cases of asymptomatic SDH are being discovered as well. Although most cases of SDH present within hours after the trauma, occasional cases of chronic SDH are diagnosed days or even weeks later. Chronic traumatic SDH is most commonly seen in infants, usually as a consequence of child abuse. Presenting symptoms in these infants may include a tense fontanelle, macrocephaly, depressed activity, seizures, vomiting, or irritability (Fig. 24.6).

On head CT, acute SDH is seen as a hyperdense, crescentic collection of extraaxial fluid. The density of the subdural fluid collection varies over time. With older chronic hematomas, the collection may be almost isodense with CSF.

Management

In the early 1980s, several researchers were able to show remarkable decreases in mortality from SDH if patients

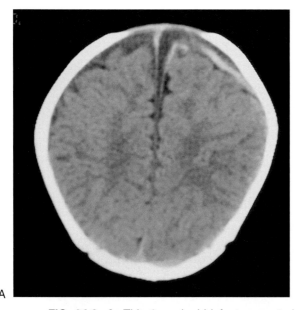
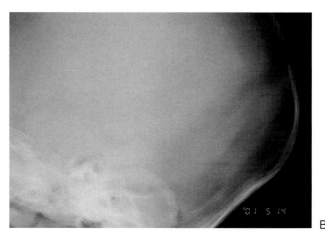

A

B

FIG. 24.6. A: This 6-week-old infant presented after a short seizure. The noncontrast computed tomography scan shows hyperdense blood overlying the left frontal lobe and a small amount of subdural blood over the right frontal lobe. There is no mass effect, and a small amount of blood is seen adjacent to the tentorial membrane. **B:** Skull radiographs show diastatic suture lines suggesting a chronic course. A skeletal survey (not shown) demonstrated old healing fractures consistent with child abuse.

underwent timely surgical drainage. Not surprisingly, this effect was most evident in those patients with large SDHs associated with midline shift and coma.

Many patients with SDH who are not as severely ill can be managed nonoperatively. Some authors have proposed nonoperative management for patients with SDHs who are not comatose, who have small SDHs with no mass effect, and who have patent basal cisterns. Immediate consultation with a neurosurgeon is essential because of the potential for rapid clinical deterioration over the first several hours of observation.

The clinician must recognize the strong association of SDH with child abuse, especially in infants with no clear mechanism of injury reported. If the circumstances of the injury cannot be clearly explained, further evaluation for nonaccidental trauma should be pursued.

In several studies, mortality rates for children with acute SDH range from 10% to 20%. Of those who survive, persistent neurologic sequelae are common.

Subarachnoid Hemorrhage

Subarachnoid hemorrhage (SAH) is a common complication of head trauma, especially in more severely injured patients. SAH results from tearing of the small vessels of the pia mater. Because the cerebral subarachnoid space is large and freely communicates with the basal cisterns and spinal subarachnoid space, SAH rarely accumulates to the extent that it causes a clinically important mass effect. SAH is often seen

in association with other intracranial injuries, and its presence may be most important as a marker for severe primary brain injury rather than as a cause of secondary injury in itself.

Clinical Manifestations

Patients with posttraumatic SAH often have other intracranial hemorrhage or parenchymal injuries as well; therefore, they may present with a wide range of symptoms, from those who have minimal if any symptoms to those who are comatose with signs of impending cerebral herniation. As an isolated intracranial lesion, SAH most commonly causes headache and other signs of meningeal irritation, such as nausea and vomiting, nuchal rigidity, and photophobia. Seizures are reported in 2% to 10% of cases. Subhyaloid or preretinal hemorrhages, located just adjacent to the optic nerve head, may be seen with SAH as well.

SAH can usually be detected on noncontrast head CT as a collection of hyperdense fluid in the CSF spaces, either in the subarachnoid space overlying the cerebral convexity or in the basal cisterns. Subarachnoid blood overlying the cerebral hemisphere can be distinguished from SDH in that the subarachnoid blood may flow into the depths of the brain sulci, fissures, and cisterns, whereas the subdural space does not penetrate to these depths. Head CT imaging has a sensitivity of only approximately 90% for detecting SAH, with a lower sensitivity for patients seen later than 24 hours after the SAH began. However, lumbar puncture is not recommended and may be dangerous in the setting of focal intracranial pathology or brain swelling because it may increase the risk of cerebral herniation.

In all patients with trauma, the clinician should consider the possibility that the trauma was inflicted (see Chapter 26, Child Abuse).

Management

All patients with traumatic SAH should be admitted to the hospital for observation. In most cases, specific therapy directed at the SAH is not required beyond the general principles of management for patients with head injuries. Prophylactic anticonvulsants are often used for patients with SAH. Patients with associated intracranial injuries have the worst outcome. Patients with minor or no symptoms and small SAHs generally do well.

Penetrating Trauma

Penetrating trauma includes injury from sharp objects, such as knives or animal bites, and from missiles, usually bullets. Penetrating head trauma leads to brain injury by several mechanisms. First, there is direct injury along the path of the penetrating object, with laceration or contusion of neural tissue and hemorrhage from injured vessels. Higher velocity injuries (from bullets) also cause significant damage because of the shock waves created by the impact of the penetrating object. These shock waves can cause contusions or vascular injury at sites that had no contact with the penetrating object itself. Because the skull and dura are violated by the penetrating object, there is direct communication of the CSF spaces or brain with the outside world and, consequently, a risk of intracranial infection.

Clinical Manifestations

The local signs of penetrating injury can sometimes be subtle, especially if the penetrated area is covered by hair or a dressing. Without careful exploration, the entrance wound might be mistaken for a superficial scalp laceration. Parenchymal tissue may be visualized in the wound or CSF may be oozing (Fig. 24.7). Signs of neurologic injury are often severe for patients with high-velocity injuries. Patients with progressively enlarging intracranial hematomas or worsening brain swelling may deteriorate quickly over the several hours after presentation.

Management

The initial management of the patient who has sustained penetrating head trauma focuses on the ABCs of resuscitation, as outlined previously. In addition to general trauma management, (1) the clinician should recognize the potential for multiple penetrating wounds or for exit wounds in unpredicted locations because of a complicated migratory path of the penetrating object; (2) patients with penetrating head injuries generally require prophylactic antibiotic therapy (30 mg/kg cefazolin intravenously, to a maximum dose of 2 g is usually appropriate); (3) most patients with penetrating head injuries are started on prophylactic anticonvulsant therapy (usually with fosphenytoin).

Patients with penetrating injuries to the head require immediate head CT to delineate the extent of brain injury and to demonstrate the presence of intracranial foreign material. Most patients with penetrating head injuries need to have angiography performed (either conventional or magnetic resonance angiography) to exclude the possibility of

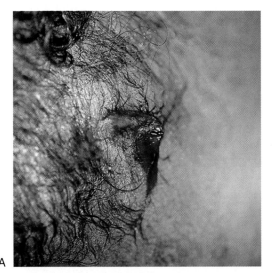
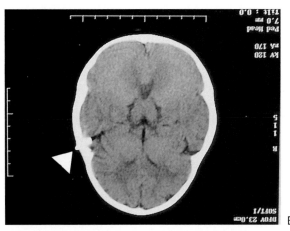

FIG. 24.7. A: This 1-year-old child fell on the floor just after his mother dropped and broke a glass. The glass appears superficial but seemed unusually solidly implanted. **B:** The computed tomography scan shows the piece of glass (*arrowhead*) penetrating through the skull into sylvian fissure. (Courtesy of Dr. Mark Walzman.)

traumatic injuries to the cerebral vasculature. In addition, most patients with penetrating injuries to the head require prompt surgery to debride the infected or contused brain tissue at the entry site.

The prognosis after penetrating head injury depends mostly on the level of neurologic function at the time of presentation. For patients with severe neurologic dysfunction (Glasgow Coma Scale scores in the range of 3 to 5), the likelihood of a good functional outcome is low.

Spinal Cord Trauma

Spinal cord injury is rare in pediatric patients. Nonetheless, when these injuries do occur, they are associated with significant morbidity and mortality, and the consequences of missing early signs of spinal cord injury can be devastating.

Clinical Manifestations

Spinal cord injuries are generally associated with severe mechanisms of injury, such as motor vehicle collisions, falls from significant heights, or child abuse. Patients with injuries to the spinal cord often have evidence of injuries to other organ systems.

Patients with high cervical cord injuries may sometimes have abnormal vital signs, reflecting an interruption of autonomic impulses to the heart and vasculature. These patients demonstrate bradycardia and hypotension, along with peripheral vasodilation, a syndrome known as spinal shock. They may also have abnormal or absent respiratory effort. Because most trauma patients with hypotension are hypovolemic and have a reflex tachycardia, those with bradycardia should be strongly suspected of having spinal shock.

Spinal cord injuries should also be suspected in any traumatized patient who complains of decreased motor strength or in whom focal deficits in strength or tone are noted on examination. In the acute setting, severe spinal cord injuries are usually associated with decreased or absent reflexes. Partial injuries to the spinal cord, conversely, may be associated with initial hypertonia and hyperreflexia. Abnormalities of bladder control and rectal tone may also be noted. Motor deficits correspond to the spinal roots whose neural impulses are compromised by the spinal cord injury. Most typically, all motor impulses that originate from spinal nerve roots at or below the level of the spinal cord injury are affected.

Sensory deficits may be noted as well, and these may range from paresthesias to complete loss of sensation. Often, a well-demarcated sensory "level" of the spinal cord can be identified, below which sensory impulses are absent and above which sensation is intact.

Many injuries to the spinal cord involve solely or predominantly one of the two lateral sides of the cord. Because of the distribution of sensory and motor neurons in the spinal cord, a lesion to the left spinal cord affects left-sided motor strength but right-sided sensation. This classic crossed pattern of sensory and motor deficits is known as the Brown–Séquard syndrome.

Partial injuries to the spinal cord may result in partial deficits. In some cases of ventral cord injury, for instance, only motor deficits may be observed. Cases of hyperextension injury may cause more severe injury to the central or deep regions of the cord (the gray matter) while sparing the more superficial white matter. This leads to a paradoxical pattern of symptoms known as the central cord syndrome, in which the more distal function (served by the white matter) is spared, but the more proximal function (served by gray matter) is compromised. Finally, occasional patients with more minor injuries to the spinal cord report transient symptoms of paresthesias, numbness, or weakness that may have resolved by the time of evaluation.

Management

Care of the patient with spinal cord injury begins with the ABCs of resuscitation. This initial resuscitation must be accomplished with meticulous attention to the stabilization of the spine. For older children and adolescents, a semirigid cervical collar or manual inline stabilization should be used. For infants, a semirigid cervical collar might actually be too large and may lead to distraction or hyperextension, which could be deleterious. For some infants, therefore, it may be preferable to immobilize instead with sandbags on the sides of the head. In addition, the patient should be maintained in a supine position on a backboard so that no undue manipulation of the spine occurs. Because infants have a relatively large occiput, supine positioning on a flat surface may result in flexion of the neck. Proper neutral positioning for these young patients may require that the occiput be allowed to rest at a level slightly lower than the shoulders.

As soon as possible after an injury, the patient's neurologic status should be assessed and recorded so that any early progression of neurologic symptoms can be noted and no undue concerns are raised that the injuries were a result of the emergency care provided. For cooperative patients, the neurologic examination should include a test of motor strength, tone, and deep tendon reflexes in all four extremities. Rectal tone should also be assessed. The sensory examination, assessing for light touch, pain sensation (as from a pinprick), and joint position sense (of fingers and toes) should be assessed as well.

Patients with suspected spinal cord injury should have plain radiographs of the spine to evaluate for fractures or subluxations. However, the absence of abnormalities on radiographic imaging does not eliminate the possibility of spinal cord injury. The syndrome of spinal cord injury without radiographic abnormalities (SCIWORA) is well reported in the literature. Children have an especially high risk of SCIWORA because of the flexibility of the pediatric spinal column, which allows the spinal cord to withstand shear or compressive forces without necessarily causing a fracture.

Magnetic resonance imaging (MRI) has become a mainstay for the diagnostic evaluation of patients with suspected spinal cord injury because it provides good detail of the soft tissue of the spinal cord itself, which cannot be well imaged by plain radiographs or CT.

Specific therapy directed at the spinal cord focuses on the prevention of secondary spinal cord injury. The mainstay of this therapy is careful immobilization. In all cases of spinal cord injury, a neurosurgeon should be consulted immediately. If compressive spinal cord lesions are noted, especially with incomplete but progressing neurologic injury, emergent laminectomy with surgical evacuation of the lesion may be necessary. Displaced fractures or subluxations of the spinal column require immobilization and generally some form of traction (e.g., a halo brace, skull tongs) to reduce them and maintain stability. Patients with SCIWORA usually require long-term immobilization as well because they should be presumed to have some ligamentous instability of the spine, even if the initial radiographic studies show normal alignment.

High-dose corticosteroid therapy is widely used in the setting of spinal cord injury. It is believed that corticosteroid therapy decreases the extent of secondary cord injury by interfering with the lipid peroxidation pathway. The National Acute Spinal Cord Injury Study found that high-dose corticosteroid therapy significantly improved the outcome for those patients treated within 8 hours of injury. Patients with neurologic deficits attributable to spinal cord injury who are seen within 8 hours of injury should receive methylprednisolone at an initial intravenous bolus dose of 30 mg/kg followed by an infusion of methylprednisolone at 5.4 mg/kg per hour for the subsequent 23 hours.

Penetrating Spinal Cord Trauma

Penetrating spinal cord trauma is an especially rare phenomenon in pediatrics and is usually from stabbing or a gunshot wound. When penetrating spinal cord injury is suspected, the principles of management, as outlined previously, should be followed. Plain radiographs demonstrate the presence of many radiopaque foreign bodies; in some cases, CT may be required to demonstrate less radiodense materials. MRI is the best imaging modality for delineating injury to the spinal cord itself.

NECK TRAUMA

Although pediatric neck injuries are uncommon, they can be life threatening and need to be assessed in a timely and orderly manner. It is imperative to appreciate how apparently minor or innocuous neck injuries can progress rapidly to more serious and life-threatening events. Subtle neck injuries can be easily overlooked in a patient with obvious head or chest trauma.

The neck can be divided into three anatomic zones. Zone I encompasses the area between the thoracic inlet and the cricoid, zone II is the area between the cricoid (clavicle or sternal notch) and the angle of the mandible, and zone III is the area above the angle of the mandible. Knowledge of the divisions and structures that they contain is useful in evaluation and management of neck trauma. Lesions in zones I and III are often occult and difficult to diagnose by physical examination alone.

Penetrating Trauma

Penetrating trauma may involve multiple organ systems within the neck. Most penetrating trauma in pediatric patients is the result of a gunshot wound (usually low velocity), knife, other sharp object, or explosion. Unlike higher velocity missiles (military-style weapons), low-velocity missiles (handguns) tend to be redirected when they encounter vascular or other structures. Visceral injuries may be anticipated but not completely predicted by the path of the missile.

Vascular injury is the most common complication of penetrating trauma. Injury to the vessels can be dramatic, with exsanguination, rapidly expanding hematoma causing airway compromise, and acute neurologic deficits from ischemia, or it may be subtle with an initially normal examination. Only one-third of arterial injuries present with neurologic deficits. The symptoms and signs suggestive of vascular and other neck injuries are presented in Table 24.2.

Direct nervous system injury (brachial plexus, spinal cord, cervical nerves, cervical sympathetics) is possible, and symptoms will correspond to the injured structure. When assessing neurologic findings or predicting the location of injury, it is important to remember that spinal cord and vertebral levels are not the same. In the cervical area, the cord level lies one segment higher than the corresponding vertebral level (C4 cord level lies opposite the C3 vertebral body).

Blunt Trauma

Blunt trauma is often the result of a motor vehicle accident, although it can also result from sports, clothesline-type and handlebar injuries, strangulation, hanging, blows from fists or feet, and the battered child syndrome. The airway is often injured with direct blunt trauma as a result of the anterior and relatively fixed position of the larynx and trachea. The presence of dyspnea, stridor, or hemoptysis suggests laryngeal injury.

Cervical Spine Evaluation

Cervical spine injuries are also uncommon in children, occurring in an estimated 1% to 2% of patients with multiple trauma. However, the clinician must assume that all children who sustain multiple trauma, have head or neck injuries, or have an altered level of consciousness have a cervical spine injury until proven otherwise. Goals in the care of these children include effectively stabilizing the primary injury that has occurred and preventing progression to a more severe injury. The devastating nature of a cervical cord injury makes it imperative to not inadvertently miss a potentially unstable cervical spine injury.

TABLE 24.2. *Symptoms and signs of neck injuries*

Laryngotracheal	Digestive	Vascular	Neurologic
Airway obstruction	Crepitus	Vigorous bleeding, internal or external	Altered consciousness
Dyspnea	Retropharyngeal air	Expansile or pulsatile hematoma	Generalized weakness
Stridor	Subcutaneous emphysema	Bruit	Hemiparesis
Retractions	Pneumomediastinum	Absent pulsations (carotid superficial temporal, or ophthalmic artery)	Hemiplegia
Cough	Hematemesis	Unexplained hypotension	Quadriplegia
Aspiration	Chest or neck pain	Hemothorax	Seizures
Pneumomediastinum	Neck tenderness	Cardiac tamponade	Bruit
Pneumothorax	Dysphagia	Hemiplegia	Cervicosensory deficits
Crepitus	Odynophagia	Hemiparesis	Aphasia
Subcutaneous emphysema	Saliva in wound	Aphasia	Horner syndrome (Ipsilateral cervical sympathetics)
Tracheal deviation	Drooling	Monocular blindness	Cranial nerve IX–XII dysfunction
Endobronchial bleeding	Fever	Loss of consciousness	Tongue deviation (hypoglossal)
Hemoptysis	Mediastinitis	Neck asymmetry, swelling or discoloration	Drooping of corner of mouth (mandibular branch of facial nerve)
Epistaxis		Wide mediastinum	Hoarseness (vagus/recurrent laryngeal)
Hematemesis		Cranial nerve abnormality	Immobile vocal cords (vagus/recurrent laryngeal)
Dysphagia		Clavicle/first rib fracture	Trapezius weakness (spinal accessory)
Odynophagia			Brachial palsy (arm paresthesias)
Bubbling, sucking, or hissing wound			Monocular blindness (vertebral artery)
Neck deformity			Diaphragm paralysis (phrenic)
Asymmetry			
Loss of landmarks			
Flat thyroid prominence			
Laryngotracheal tenderness			
Dysphonia			
Aphonia			
Voice changes			
Hoarseness			
Drooling			
Neck pain, tenderness (with coughing or swallowing)			

Hyperextension of the neck to facilitate intubation should be avoided. A vigorous chin lift or jaw thrust may also inadvertently hyperextend the unstable cervical spine. Tracheal intubation in a patient with a potential cervical spine injury ideally requires at least two participants to perform the procedure safely and efficiently. One should maintain inline immobilization (being careful to avoid applying traction of the neck) while another performs the intubation. The hard cervical collar should be opened anteriorly while this process is being performed. It is difficult to intubate a child with an anterior trachea unless the jaw immobilization afforded by the collar is temporarily removed.

Several concepts should be kept in mind concerning cervical immobilization in children. Soft cervical collars offer no protection to an unstable spine and hard (Stifneck, Philadelphia) collars alone still allow a fair amount of movement of the cervical spine. Ideal immobilization involves a hard cervical collar in conjunction with a full spine board and securing straps. The tallest collar that does not hyperextend the neck should be chosen. When a child is immobilized on a spine board, the clinician must consider that the child's head is disproportionately large compared with the adult's.

A child's head reaches 50% of postnatal growth by approximately age 2 years, whereas chest circumference reaches 50% of postnatal growth by approximately age 8 years. This disparate growth of the head and trunk causes the neck to be forced into relative kyphotic position when a child is placed on a hard spine board. This is distinctly different from the adult patient whose neck is in 30 degrees of lordosis, the neutral position, when immobilized on a hard spine board. Suggestions have been made to place a spacing device such as a blanket underneath the torso to allow the neck to rest in a neutral position.

The pediatric cervical spine and its evaluation differ in many ways from the adult cervical spine and its evaluation. The fulcrum of the cervical spine of an infant is at approximately C2-3 and reaches C3-4 by the age of 5 to 6 years. At approximately the age of 8, the fulcrum (C5-6) and other characteristics of the cervical spine approximate that of an adult. The higher fulcrum of a child's spine in combination with relatively weak neck muscles account for young children often having fractures that involve the upper cervical spine, whereas older children and adults have fractures that more often involve the lower cervical spine. Neurologic disability can occur from cervical lesions at all levels, but high cervical cord injuries are more likely to be fatal than are lower cervical cord injuries.

A neurologic history is imperative to assess whether there was any paresthesia, paralysis, or paresis at any time after the injury. These symptoms may have been transient and may not be present at the time of the examination or volunteered by the patient, yet they are important because they may suggest a cervical contusion, concussion, or SCIWORA.

Cervical spine radiographic evaluation is the next step in assessment. Radiographic options include radiographs, CT, and MRI. MRI scans are more appropriate when evaluating the subacute or chronic stages of injury or when looking for an acute problem with cord impingement by blood or soft tissues such as tumors or intervertebral discs. MRI does not image cortical bone well and should not be used to evaluate the cervical spine for fractures; the CT scan demonstrates fractures clearly. A CT scan is often used as a secondary screen when adequate plain radiographs cannot be obtained or to substantiate suspected fractures. A common scenario is the use of CT to supplement viewing the C1-2 region in young, traumatized children. The CT scan images soft tissue well; however, it does not demonstrate the intrathecal, ligamentous disc or vascular detail that can be obtained with an MRI scan.

The plain radiograph remains the preferred initial test for acutely traumatized patients. The perception of unnecessary tests should be balanced against the severity of consequences that may occur with a missed cervical spine injury. If the patient does not have a high-risk mechanism of injury (motor vehicle accident, fall, dive, sports injury), is awake and alert, can have an interactive conversation (not inebriated, no altered level of consciousness, older than 4 to 5 years of age), does not complain of cervical spine pain, has no tenderness on palpation (especially in the midline), has normal neck mobility, has a completely normal neurologic examination without history of abnormal neurologic symptoms or signs at any time after the injury, and has no other painful injuries (which may distract the patient and mask neck pain), the patient probably does not need radiographic evaluation of the cervical spine. The clinician must be sure, however, to never "clear" the cervical spine, regardless of studies performed, in an unconscious patient in the emergency department.

When radiographs are obtained, a normal lateral radiograph does not clear the cervical spine. The sensitivity of a lateral cervical spine radiograph varies between 82% and 98% in the literature. When evaluating a lateral cervical spine radiograph, the clinician must ensure that C1 through C7 are included as well as the C7-T1 junction. Additional films that include an anteroposterior view of C3 through C7 and an anteroposterior open-mouth (odontoid) view of the C1-2 region increase the sensitivity of the initial radiographic evaluation to more than 95%. An adequate open-mouth (odontoid) view is often technically difficult to obtain in young children and those who are intubated. If further information is required, a CT scan of the C1-2 region can be useful to augment or replace the open-mouth view.

The cervical spine has anterior (vertebral bodies, intervertebral discs, ligaments) and posterior (lamina, pedicles, neural foramen, spinous processes, ligaments) components. The initial three-view series evaluates the anterior cervical spine well; however, it is not ideal for evaluating the posterior cervical spine. Oblique (pillar) views are helpful in imaging those posterior elements. In practice, however, oblique films rarely add significant information to the initial radiographic assessment. Flexion and extension films are accomplished in an awake patient by having the patient flex and extend the neck as far as possible without discomfort. Because the end point involves the sensation of pain, flexion/extension films should not be performed in a patient who has preexisting neck pain. These studies can help to evaluate underlying soft-tissue or ligamentous injury that was not evident on the initial films. If a question remains concerning the integrity of the cervical spine after following this radiographic scheme, a CT scan should be considered. MRI should be considered to detect ligamentous, soft-tissue, or subtle cord injuries.

A systematic approach should be used when evaluating radiographs of the cervical spine. The ABC method is a useful approach. Alignment is assessed, keeping in mind that the spinal cord lies between the posterior spinal line and the spinolaminar line. These lordotic curves may not be present in children younger than 6 years of age, those on hard spine boards or in cervical collars, or those with cervical neck muscle spasm.

Soft-tissue evaluation is extremely important. Abnormal soft-tissue spaces may be the only clue to the underlying ligament, cartilage, or bone injury, which may not be obvious on the radiograph. The soft-tissue widening may represent blood or edema, which suggests an underlying injury. The prevertebral space at C3 should be less than one-half to two-thirds of the anteroposterior width of the adjacent vertebral body. This space will double to approximately the width of the adjacent vertebral body below C4 (the level of the glottis) because the usually non–air-filled esophagus is present at this area. Care must be taken when evaluating the prevertebral soft-tissue space because crying, neck flexion, or the expiratory phase of respiration may produce a pseudothickening in the prevertebral space (Fig. 24.8).

Specific Injuries

The Jefferson fracture is a bursting fracture of the ring of C1 as a result of an axial load. The radiographic criterion for diagnosis of a Jefferson fracture is lateral offset of the lateral mass of C1 more than 1 mm from the vertebral body of C2 (Fig. 24.9). Neck rotation may give a false-positive radiograph.

The hangman's fracture is a traumatic spondylolisthesis of C2. This injury occurs as a result of hyperextension, which fractures the posterior elements of C2. Hyperflexion, with

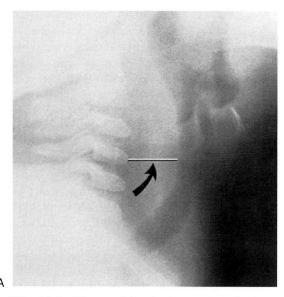

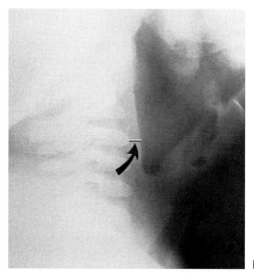

FIG. 24.8. Effects of inspiration and expiration on prevertebral (retropharyngeal) soft tissues. **A:** Increased soft-tissue space with expiration. **B:** Repeat radiograph in the same patient during inspiration demonstrates normal prevertebral (retropharyngeal) soft tissue space.

resultant ligamentous damage, may lead to anterior subluxation of C2 on C3 and subsequent damage of the cervical cord Figure 24.10. The subluxation associated with a hangman's fracture can sometimes be mistaken for the normal or physiologic subluxation that exists in the C2-3 or C3-4 region in approximately 25% of children younger than 8 years of age; it also may be seen up to the age of 16. Distinguishing between a subtle hangman's fracture and pseudosubluxation can be accomplished using the Swischuk "posterior cervical line," as described in Figure 24.11.

Atlantoaxial subluxation is a result of movement between C1 and C2 secondary to transverse ligament rupture or a fractured dens. Ligament instability may be precipitated by tonsillitis, cervical adenitis, arthritis, or connective tissue disorders. Approximately 15% of patients with Down syndrome have radiographically demonstrated atlantoaxial subluxation and therefore should be discouraged from contact sports. A dens fracture is the cause of atlantoaxial subluxation more often than ligamentous disruption in a young child because the weakest part of the musculoskeletal system in a child is the osseus component.

Cervical distraction injuries may result from rapid acceleration- or deceleration-type incidents, such as high-speed motor vehicle or pedestrian accidents. An injury that was

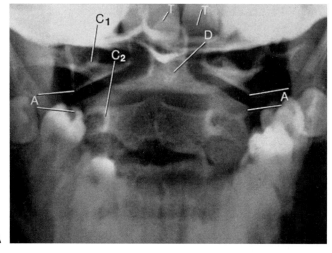

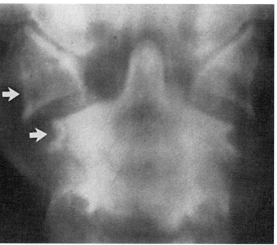

FIG. 24.9. A: Normal anteroposterior (AP) (open-mouth, odontoid) view of C1 and C2. C_1, first cervical vertebra (lateral mass); C_2, second cervical vertebra; *T*, central incisors overlying dens *D*; *A*, normal relationship between lateral mass of C1 and vertebral body of C2. **B:** Jefferson fracture in AP view. Note the lateral offset of C1.

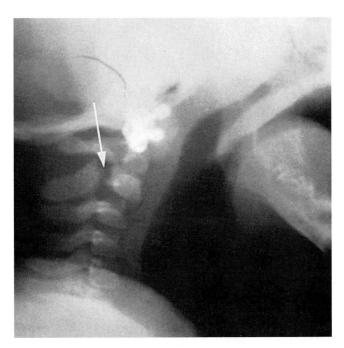

FIG. 24.10. Hangman's fracture. A 7-week-old infant with fracture through the posterior elements of C2 (*arrow*). (From Sumchai A, Sternback G. Hangman's fracture in a 7-week-old infant. *Ann Emerg Med* 1991;20:87, with permission.)

incompatible with long-term survival but for which initial cardiopulmonary resuscitation was successful is shown in Figure 24.12.

Vertebral compression injuries are suggested by isolated anterior wedging or teardrop fractures. The vertebral bodies should be cuboid and consistent between adjacent cervical levels (Fig. 24.13).

The clay shoveler's fracture is a fracture of the inferior aspect of a lower cervical or T1 vertebra spinous process. Today, the usual mechanism for this stable fracture is direct trauma rather than neck flexion during clay mining (Fig. 24.14).

A flexion/rotation stress can lead to anterior subluxation of one vertebral body on another with facet dislocation ("locked" or "jumped" facet). If the anterior displacement is less than 50% of the vertebral body width, it is consistent with a unilateral facet dislocation. More than a 50% anterior subluxation suggests a bilateral facet dislocation. These injuries are often accompanied by widened interspinous and interlaminar spaces, anterior soft-tissue swelling, and a narrowed disc space (Fig. 24.15).

SCIWORA probably accounts for approximately 25% of cervical cord injuries in children younger than 8 years of age. These injuries mainly occur in children younger than 8 years

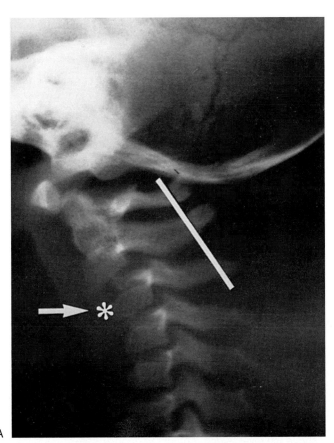

A

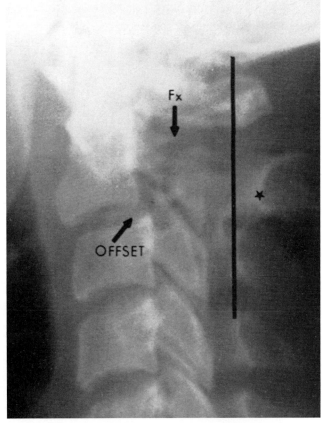

B

FIG. 24.11. A: Pseudosubluxation of C2 on C3 with normal posterior cervical line in a 2-year-old child. Note the apparent widening of prevertebral soft tissue. **B:** Abnormal posterior cervical line with underlying hangman's fracture. Actual offset is 4 mm. (From Swischuk L. *Emergency radiology of the acutely ill or injured child*, 2nd ed. Baltimore: Williams & Wilkins, 1986:562–563, with permission.)

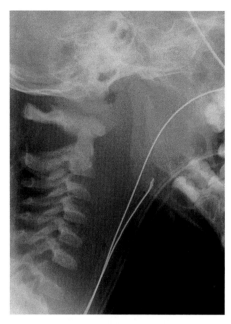

FIG. 24.12. This 3-year-old boy was struck by a car. His radiograph shows C1-2 and C6-7 distraction.

of age who present with or develop symptoms consistent with cervical cord injuries without any radiographic or tomographic evidence of bony abnormality. SCIWORA is not often seen in patients older than 8 years of age because the forces necessary to injure the spinal cord also cause bony abnormalities. Many authors recommend hospitalization and

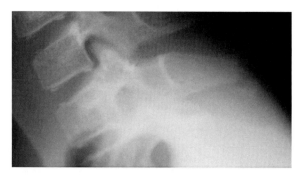

FIG. 24.14. Clay shoveler's fracture. This 12-year-old boy fell on the back of his neck playing basketball and had persistent posterior neck pain for 2 weeks. The coned down view of T1 shows the spinous process fracture.

immobilization for young patients who have a history of transient neurologic symptoms. At the least, neurologic consultation is recommended if the history suggests a SCIWORA-type injury.

Torticollis (wry neck) is a common complaint in the pediatric emergency department. The clinician should always inquire about traumatic causes because an underlying bone injury may be present. Often, however, torticollis is caused by spasm of the sternocleidomastoid muscle. The patient with muscular torticollis has muscle spasm of the sternocleidomastoid on the opposite side that the chin points because the cause of torticollis is muscular spasm. This condition is the

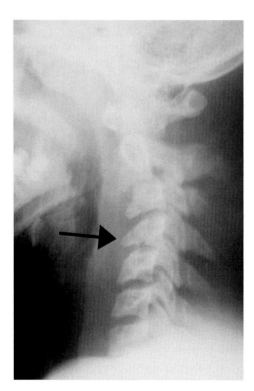

FIG. 24.13. This adolescent swam full speed into the pool wall. He has a crush injury of C4 and C2-3 subluxation (*arrow*).

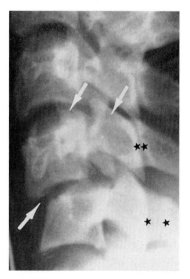

FIG. 24.15. Unilateral facet dislocation. C4 is offset anteriorly on C5 less than 50% of the width of the vertebral body and apophyseal joints. The disc space between C4 and C5 is narrowed. Note that the distance between the posterior cortex of the apophyseal joint facet and the anterior cortex of the spinous process tip is wider below the level of dislocation than above the level (*stars*). Anterior vertebral offset of more than 50% would denote a bilateral facet dislocation. (From Swischuk L. *Emergency radiology of the acutely ill or injured child*, 2nd ed. Baltimore: Williams & Wilkins, 1986:697, with permission.)

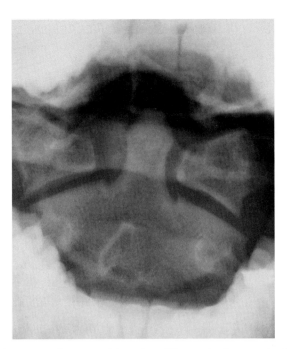

FIG. 24.16. Rotary subluxation. The patient came to the emergency department with persistent "torticollis" for 3 days. The radiograph shows asymmetry between the odontoid and the lateral masses of C1.

opposite of rotary subluxation, in which the patient assumes the typical (cockrobin) position with the muscle spasm of the sternocleidomastoid on the same side that the chin points. Rotary subluxation is a cervical spine injury that may be spontaneous or may follow an upper respiratory infection or minor trauma. These patients rarely present with abnormal neurologic findings. Rotary subluxation should be suspected if, on an open-mouth radiograph, there is asymmetry between the odontoid and lateral masses of C1 or if one of the lateral masses of C1 appears forward and closer to the midline and the opposite lateral mass appears narrow and away from the midline (lateral offset) (Fig. 24.16). A normal film does not rule out rotary subluxation, and a CT scan may be needed for diagnosis. Patients with mild rotary subluxation should be treated with a cervical collar and analgesia for comfort, whereas those with more severe displacement may need immobilization and traction.

EYE TRAUMA

Ruptured Globe

Laceration or puncture of the cornea and/or sclera creates a ruptured globe. This condition can occur after trauma by projectile, sharp implement, or blunt trauma. Immediately on laceration, the iris or choroid (which is the extension of the iris underneath the sclera) plugs the wound. This plug may appear as a dark material on the surface of the sclera or at the cornea–sclera junction. The iris will come forward and plug a corneal wound. Because of this iris or choroid movement,

the pupil may take on a teardrop shape, with the narrowest segment pointing toward the rupture. With small lacerations that are plugged by the iris or choroid, the eyeball may retain a remarkably normal external appearance. Subconjunctival hemorrhage for 360 degrees may obscure an underlying scleral rupture but leave the eye fairly intact. Patients who present after trauma with this finding or with severe 360-degree conjunctival swelling without hemorrhage should be treated as if they had a ruptured globe and referred immediately to an ophthalmologist.

Management

Eyeball rupture is an ominous sign that warrants emergent referral for ophthalmology consultation. Further ocular examination should be stopped immediately. No eyedrops should be instilled. A patch should never be used in this circumstance. A plastic shield should be placed over the eye such that the edges of the shield make contact with the bony prominences above and below the eyeball. If a commercially marketed shield is not available, the clinician should cut off the bottom of a Styrofoam or plastic cup and use it as a shield.

Every attempt should be made to keep the child calm, even if sedation must be used. Crying, screaming, and vomiting can result in extrusion of intraocular contents through the rupture. Although broad-spectrum intravenous antibiotic coverage is desirable, particularly if a delay may occur before the patient sees an ophthalmologist, this treatment must be weighed against the potential aggravation of the child, which might accompany intravenous catheter placement.

Even if a ruptured globe is not seen clearly on examination, any patient who has a high-risk history, severe lid swelling, and extreme resistance to examination should be given an eye shield and referred to an ophthalmologist as if a ruptured globe were confirmed.

Blowout Fracture

Photographs and further discussion of these fractures are found later in this chapter in the otolaryngologic section. Approximately 20% of orbital fractures are associated with eyeball injury. Therefore, ophthalmology consultation for complete dilated retinal examination and slit-lamp biomicroscopy is indicated in virtually every case. Axial (proptosis) or coronal displacement of the eyeball is an ominous finding because it may be a sign of orbital hemorrhage, which can cause compression of the optic nerve, requiring emergency surgical intervention.

Eyelid Lacerations

Although eyelid lacerations are usually easy to detect, one must remember that the underlying eyeball also might have been lacerated. Superficial lacerations of the eyelid may be associated with penetration into the orbit or intracranial cavity, particularly when the injury was caused by a pointed object such as a tree branch or pencil. If possible, the eyelid should be everted to look for a conjunctival wound indicating that the laceration is actually a complete perforation of the eyelid.

Oblique lacerations that extend into the medial canthal area (juncture of the upper and lower lids medially) may involve the proximal portion of the nasolacrimal duct. The involvement of the nasolacrimal duct may not be visible on initial inspection (Fig. 24.17). Lacerations in this area should usually be referred for ophthalmology consultation if any question persists regarding whether the tear drainage system is intact.

Table 24.3 summarizes those findings that, when associated with eyelid lacerations, should prompt ophthalmology consultation for wound closure.

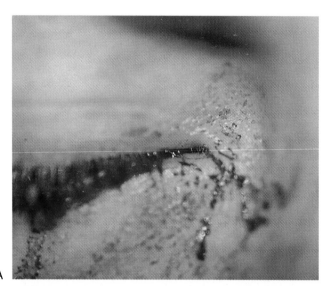

A

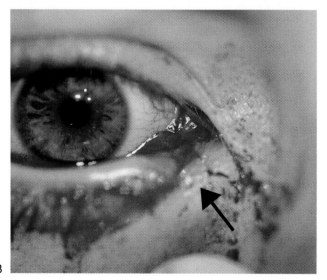

B

FIG. 24.17. Lacrimal duct laceration. A 13-year-old child was struck by a bike handlebar. **A:** On initial inspection, a tiny laceration is visible in the medial canthal area. **B:** With gentle inferior traction, the full-thickness laceration and involvement of the area of the lacrimal duct become visible (*arrow*).

TABLE 24.3. *Eyelid lacerations*

Consult ophthalmologist if laceration associated with
    Full-thickness perforation of lid
    Ptosis
    Involvement of lid margin
    Possible damage to tear drainage system
    Tissue avulsion
    Eyeball injury

Corneal and Conjunctival Injury

The conjunctiva can be abraded or lacerated, although the management of this problem is usually identical with that of corneal abrasion because the tissues heal so rapidly. Bacterial keratitis and corneal ulcers (Fig. 15.9) can develop after corneal lacerations or corneal foreign body removal.

Corneal abrasion can be painful and accompanied by dramatic photophobia and resistance to opening of the eyes. A drop of topical 0.5% proparacaine or 0.5% tetracaine may have both diagnostic and temporary therapeutic usefulness. Any patient who is made more comfortable by the instillation of these drops must have an ocular surface problem (conjunctiva or cornea) as the cause of pain. The child who is crying and refusing to open the eyes may be easy to examine a few minutes after the instillation of a topical anesthetic. Onset of action is approximately 20 seconds, and duration is approximately 20 minutes.

Topical fluorescein is used to stain the affected area. If the staining pattern reveals one or more vertical linear abrasions, the examiner should suspect the presence of a retained foreign body under the upper lid. This foreign body may be viewed by upper lid eversion. The patient should be asked to look down repeatedly throughout this procedure. With the eye in downgaze, a cotton swab should be placed against the midbody of the upper eyelid and gently rotated downward toward the eyelashes so that the skin is rolled with the swab by friction. This procedure causes the eyelashes to turn out toward the examiner so that they may be grasped between the examiner's thumb and forefinger. After the lashes (or margin) are grasped, they should be lifted vertically while the cotton swab is used to apply gentle downward pressure in the opposite direction. The eyelid then flips around the cotton swab. If a foreign body is identified, it can be gently lifted away using a cotton swab or forceps. To revert the eyelid, have the patient look upward or massage the lid down.

Subconjunctival hemorrhage (Fig. 24.18) may result from blunt trauma, conjunctivitis, chemical irritation, and increased intrathoracic pressure (e.g., chest trauma, suffocation). Hypertension, coagulopathy, or anticoagulant medications may result in subconjunctival hemorrhage out of proportion to the injury. After blunt eyeball trauma, a 360-degree subconjunctival hemorrhage may mask an underlying ruptured globe. No treatment is needed for isolated subconjunctival hemorrhages. They may take as long as 2 weeks to resolve, turning yellowish in the process.

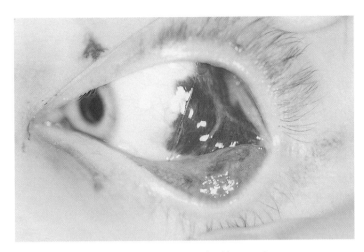

FIG. 24.18. Subconjunctival hemorrhage.

Management

Several studies have suggested that patching may not accelerate healing or decrease symptoms. Although some controversy exists, many physicians apply lubricating antibiotic ointment to the ocular surface, followed by a pressure patch over the closed eyelid. For patients who are in significant pain, a drop of 1% cyclopentolate can be instilled to relieve spasm of the ciliary muscle. Ointments containing steroids or neomycin should not be used. A pressure patch can be created by stacking three patches on top of each other over the closed eyelid before applying tape. The patch should be worn overnight. For conjunctival abrasions and small corneal abrasions not involving the central cornea, the patch may be removed by the patient or parents in 24 hours. If the patient is asymptomatic, no follow-up is required. However, if pain or foreign body sensation continues, the patient should be instructed to seek ophthalmologic care. A topical antibiotic ointment may be prescribed for use after patch removal two to three times daily for approximately 3 days. Larger corneal abrasions and those involving the visual axis should be seen the next day by an ophthalmologist.

Hyphema

The presence of blood between the cornea and iris is a sign of severe ocular trauma. Although the entire anterior chamber may be filled with blood ("eight-ball hyphema") (Fig. 24.19), clots may also be small, requiring careful inspection while the patients is upright for detection (Fig. 24.20). Patients with hyphema enter a vulnerable period 3 to 5 days after injury when spontaneous rebleeding may occur. Patients with hemoglobinopathies are also at particular risk of ocular complications of hyphema. Therefore, all patients who are in a high-risk

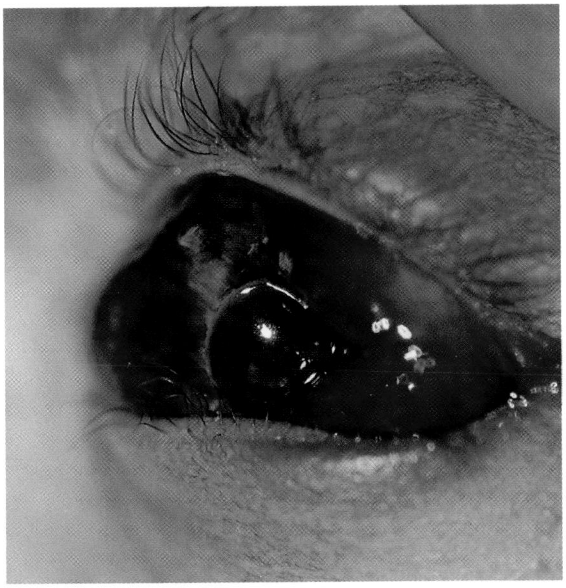

FIG. 24.19. Hyphema, 100%. A 17-year-old boy with Sturge–Weber syndrome has his entire pupil obscured by blood and massive subconjunctival hemorrhage. (Courtesy of Dr. Mark Waltzman.)

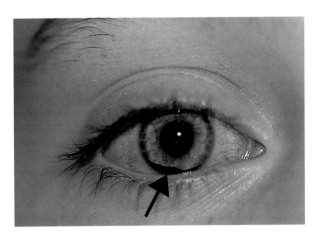

FIG. 24.20. Hyphemas. This 7-year-old girl was struck by a hard rubber ball and presented with blurred vision. The 1-mm hyphema (*arrow*) was only visible when she was upright. (Courtesy of Dr. Andrew Capraro.)

ethnic group should have hemoglobin electrophoresis at presentation unless their status is already known.

Management

All patients who have hyphema must be seen by an ophthalmologist. Although some small hyphemas may be managed in select clinical situations as outpatients with careful daily follow-up, hospital admission is often recommended. The eye should be shielded, not patched, and the patient should be placed on bed rest with the head elevated 45 degrees. This position helps blood within the anterior chamber to settle inferiorly, clearing the visual axis and allowing a better view for the ophthalmologist. Some ophthalmologists may even recommend sedation of an active or distressed child. Oral antifibrinolytics may be used to prevent spontaneous rebleeding. However, these agents should be used only under the supervision and recommendation of an ophthalmology consultant.

Traumatic Iritis

Inflammation within the anterior chamber may not present for 24 to 72 hours after blunt trauma to the eyeball. The patient may complain of eye pain, redness, photophobia, or visual loss. The pupil on the affected side may be constricted. The ocular injection may be confined to a ring of redness surrounding the cornea (ciliary flush). Definitive recognition of traumatic iritis requires slit-lamp microscopy.

Management

Traumatic iritis may be an indicator that other ocular injuries have occurred. Ophthalmology consultation should be obtained in the diagnosis and management of this condition. The ophthalmologist often recommends dilating drops and topical steroids for treatment. Because of the risks associated with the use of topical steroids, they should not be prescribed except in consultation with an ophthalmologist.

Traumatic Visual Loss

Occasionally, the emergency physician is faced with a child who is feigning visual loss after injuries. Functional visual loss can also be idiopathic or associated with stress in the child's life. In the absence of other signs of ocular or head trauma, this diagnosis should be suspected. It then becomes necessary to "trick" the child into demonstrating that he or she can actually see. Patients who are truly acutely blind should demonstrate some degree of anxiety. When asked to write their names on a piece of paper, truly blind patients can do so accurately, unlike children who are functionally blind who assume that they are unable to write. When a mirror is held before a truly blind eye and then tilted in the vertical and horizontal planes, the eye will not follow. However, any eye that truly has enough sight to recognize its own image moves involuntarily with the motion of the mirror.

A rare cause of visual loss after head trauma is transient cortical visual impairment/blindness. As a result of an occipital contusion, a child may experience acute blindness despite an otherwise normal eye examination. This centrally mediated phenomenon may resolve spontaneously. Ophthalmology consultation can help to rule out other causes of the visual loss.

A multitude of intraocular injuries, including traumatic cataract, vitreous hemorrhage, retinal bruising (commotio retinae), retinal detachment, and optic nerve injury, can result in true visual loss or blindness. The pediatric emergency physician must recognize that true intraocular injury has occurred and obtain an ophthalmology consultation.

OTOLARYNGOLOGIC TRAUMA

Ear

Foreign Bodies

Foreign bodies in the ear canal are common in children. Solid objects, such as stones, beads, or paper, are the most commonly encountered foreign bodies, but live insects may also enter the ear canal. Foreign bodies should be removed as soon as possible. Most objects can be gently rolled out of the external meatus with an ear curette or grasped and removed with a forceps. Round or occluding objects may be removed by irrigation of the canal with body-temperature water. Irrigation should not be performed if a tympanic membrane (TM) perforation is suspected or if a ventilating tube is in place. The stream is directed along the side of the foreign body, forcing it to the external meatus. Insects should be killed by filling the ear canal with alcohol or mineral oil before they are removed from the ear canal by the techniques already described. Objects resting against the TM are best removed by irrigation to avoid injury by manipulation. Care must be taken to remove the foreign material without causing pain; if the removal is unsuccessful, a general anesthetic is usually necessary for removal of the object by the otolaryngologist.

Trauma

External Ear Trauma

External ear trauma is common in children because the pinna is in an exposed position on the side of the head. The injury may result in simple ecchymosis or disrupt perichondrial blood vessels with subsequent hematoma formation. Hematomas must be evacuated immediately to prevent cartilage necrosis (Fig. 24.21). The physician needs to consider the possibility of child abuse for any unexplained external ear trauma.

Thermal injury of the external ear commonly occurs because the ear protrudes from the head and is exposed to burns and cold. Burns of the ear should be treated in the same manner as burns of other parts of the body.

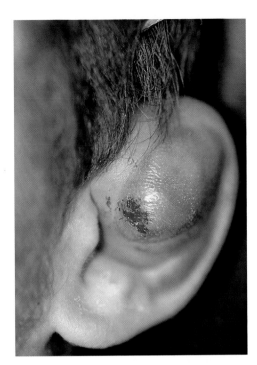

FIG. 24.21. This patient presented 2 days after external ear trauma. The smooth, discolored mass obscuring the normal contour of the pinna is a hematoma.

Middle Ear Trauma

A slap to the side of the head may result in perforation of the TM by sudden compression of the air in the external auditory canal, but traumatic perforation of the drum is usually caused by poking an object into the ear canal. The structures of the middle ear may also be damaged by the penetrating object. The ossicles may be fractured and a perilymph fistula may be created in the footplate of the stapes. This reaction causes immediate vertigo and a sensorineural hearing loss. The facial nerve may be injured, causing facial paralysis. Traumatic perforations of the TM must be examined carefully to be certain that the edges of the perforation do not fold into the middle ear. If they do, skin may grow into the middle ear and a cholesteatoma will develop. Clean perforations with margins that do not fold into the middle ear usually heal spontaneously in 2 to 3 weeks. The perforation should be kept clean and dry. If the ear is draining, topical otic drops (neomycin, polymyxin, and hydrocortisone) should be used for 10 days. Any perforation that does not heal within 3 weeks should be referred to an otolaryngologist for evaluation and repair.

Barotrauma to the ear may occur during an airplane trip or while scuba diving, especially if the child has an acute upper respiratory infection. A direct, open communication between the middle ear and nasopharynx normally permits prompt equalization of changes in ambient pressure. If the eustachian tube is obstructed, however, changes in ambient pressure may not be transmitted to the middle ear, and barotrauma can result. As the child descends in an airplane (or during an underwater dive), the increased ambient pressure is transmitted to the cardiovascular system and, thus, to the vessels of the mucosal lining of the middle ear. The mucosa becomes edematous and the vessels become engorged. If the eustachian tube is obstructed and has not equalized the air pressure, a large differential pressure occurs between the middle ear mucosa and its air-filled cavity. This condition results in a rupture of the blood vessels within the mucosa and bleeding into the middle ear. Rarely, perforation of the TM occurs. These injuries usually resolve spontaneously over several weeks. Antimicrobials may be prescribed to prevent infection of the middle ear fluid/blood. Persistent symptomatic fluid may require myringotomy and ventilation tube placement. Barotrauma with acute sensorineural hearing loss and/or vertigo may indicate the presence of a perilymph fistula.

Inner Ear Trauma

Concussive injuries to the head may cause inner ear trauma by disrupting the intracochlear membranes. Sensorineural hearing loss and/or vertigo may occur as a result of such an injury. Occasionally, the losses from these injuries can improve spontaneously, but most are permanent. Loud blasts from explosions may cause sudden, permanent sensorineural hearing loss.

Cerebrospinal Fluid Otorrhea

CSF otorrhea may occur secondary to a temporal bone fracture that results in a fracture through the inner ear and a ruptured TM. Manipulation or instrumentation of the external auditory canal in the presence of CSF otorrhea is discouraged because it could introduce bacteria and contribute to the development of meningitis.

Facial Nerve Paralysis

Facial nerve paralysis may occur as a result of temporal bone trauma. Patients with traumatic facial nerve paralysis should be referred to the otolaryngologist for possible exploration and nerve repair.

Nose and Paranasal Sinuses

Nasal Trauma

Trauma to the nose most often causes ecchymosis and edema of the overlying skin. However, a direct blow to the nose can fracture the nasal skeleton with resultant deviation and/or depression of the nasal bones and septum. The deformity should be readily apparent by clinical examination, but the postinjury edema may prevent its recognition for several days until the swelling has subsided. A step-off or bony irregularity may often be detected in these patients. Radiographs of the nose are notoriously unreliable in the evaluation of nasal injuries and are not recommended in the routine management of simple nasal fractures. Epistaxis commonly accompanies nasal trauma (see the section on epistaxis in

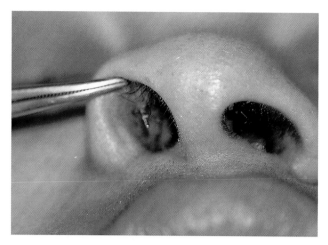

FIG. 24.22. Embedded nasal stud from a nose ring.

Chapter 15, Ophthalmic and Otolaryngologic Emergencies). The presence of any associated ocular injury, such as hyphema, must be detected, and ophthalmologic consultation must be obtained.

The amount of nasal deviation and/or depression should be noted. Because this condition can be masked by postinjury edema, it may be best to examine the child again in 3 to 4 days when the swelling has subsided to allow an accurate determination of nasal deviation and/or depression. If no septal hematoma or associated ocular or intracranial injuries are present, then the deviated nose and septum can be reduced by the otolaryngologist between days 4 and 7 when the swelling has subsided enough to permit an accurate evaluation of the nasal deformity.

One complication of body piercing is embedded jewelry (Fig. 24.22). These can often be removed using a hemostat after application of topical or infiltrative anesthesia.

Septal Hematoma

The presence of a septal hematoma must be recognized as soon as possible after the injury. A septal hematoma appears as a bulging of the nasal septum into one or both sides of the nasal cavity. Accumulation of blood between the septal cartilage and its overlying mucoperichondrium deprives the cartilage of its blood supply. Otolaryngologic consultation should be obtained as quickly as possible if a septal hematoma is suspected. The hematoma is drained as soon as possible, and the mucoperichondrium is packed back against the septal cartilage to restore its blood supply.

Cerebrospinal Fluid Rhinorrhea

A clear, watery rhinorrhea occurring after nasal trauma may be CSF rhinorrhea, which would indicate a skull fracture, usually through the cribriform plate. If the patient leans forward, allowing the nasal drainage to drip onto a piece of paper, a characteristic target pattern will often appear, with a blood stain in the center of the drop and a clear halo of CSF around it. If CSF rhinorrhea is suspected by history or clinical examination, the child should be admitted and restricted to bed rest with his or her head elevated in an attempt to decrease the leak, and a neurosurgical consultation should be obtained.

Sinus Trauma

Fractures of the paranasal sinuses may occur as isolated injuries or in association with trauma to the nose and orbital structures. Fractures of the ethmoid sinus and anterior wall of the maxillary sinus usually occur as a result of blunt trauma to the nose and cheek, respectively (Fig. 24.23). The otolaryngologist and ophthalmologist should assist the emergency physician in evaluating these injuries.

Foreign Bodies

Children with nasal foreign bodies are usually brought to the emergency department with the history of putting an object into the nose, but the presence of a foreign body may often be unsuspected and may be discovered only during evaluation of a child with persistent, unilateral, foul-smelling, purulent rhinorrhea. This mode of presentation for these problems is so common that any child with a foul-smelling unilateral nasal discharge (even without a history of placing an object in the nose) should be evaluated for a nasal foreign body. The foreign body is usually visible on anterior rhinoscopy. However, purulent secretions may have to be suctioned from the nose before the object is seen. Radiographs are of limited value because most of the foreign bodies are radiolucent (e.g., paper, cloth, sponge, food).

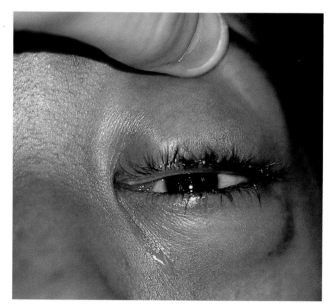

FIG. 24.23. This 15-year-old boy struck his eye on the head of his wrestling opponent. He has local swelling and impaired upward gaze caused by an ethmoid fracture. (Courtesy of Dr. Mark Waltzman.)

If the object is located in the nasal vestibule, the emergency physician may attempt to remove it. The child should be adequately restrained, and the necessary equipment, including a nasal speculum, directed light, suction, small hooks, and forceps, should be available. A few drops of 4% lidocaine can be placed in the nostril to provide topical anesthesia before removing the foreign body.

Pharynx and Esophagus

Trauma

Children may have oropharyngeal lacerations or puncture wounds when they fall with an object, such as a stick, in their mouths. If the injury is restricted to the central portion of the palate, damage to vascular or neural structures of the neck is unlikely. These children are usually safe to send home after confirmation of absence of any retained foreign body. However, trauma to the lateral aspects of the palate or the posterior pharyngeal wall may be associated with vascular injuries of the carotid artery or the jugular vein (Fig. 24.24). Expanding hematoma of the neck or pharynx, continued intraoral bleeding, and diminished pulses in the neck are all signs of serious vascular injury. These children need to be admitted and have urgent angiography or magnetic resonance angiography and possible neck exploration. If a lateral pharyngeal or palatal puncture injury is present without signs of vascular injury, the child should be observed closely in the hospital or at home for signs of neurologic deterioration.

In treating puncture wounds of the pharynx, it is imperative to determine whether the foreign body has been recovered intact or if a portion of the foreign body may have been left in the palatal tissues. Plain radiographs may not be useful in determining whether a foreign body has been left in the wound because most of the objects are radiolucent and/or too

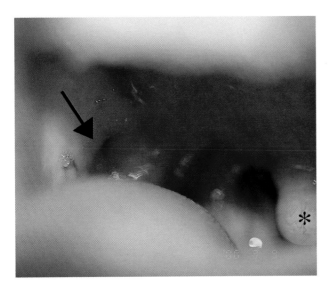

FIG. 24.24. Puncture wound (*arrow*) lateral to tonsillar pillar. Midline uvula (*asterisk*). Computed tomography showed the puncture wound to be adjacent to the carotid artery.

small to be seen. Inspecting the actual object that caused the wound to make sure that it is intact is more important. If a retained portion of the foreign body is suspected, CT scan may be required, followed by exploration of the wound, usually under general anesthesia.

Caustic Injuries

Caustic substances (lye or acid) may be ingested, causing burns anywhere from the lips to the stomach. Burns of the oral mucosa appear as patches of erythema, blebs, or ulcerated areas. Although caustic burns are usually visible in the oral cavity and pharynx, large skip areas may exist. Therefore, the absence of oral or pharyngeal burns does not rule out esophageal injury. If a history of significant caustic ingestion exists, an esophagoscopy should be performed 6 to 12 hours later to establish the presence of esophageal burns, regardless of the condition of the oral cavity and pharynx.

Caustic substances may burn the larynx when ingested and can cause rapidly progressive edema and respiratory distress. Orotracheal intubation for acute airway management should be performed in the emergency department if necessary. A tracheotomy should be performed as soon as possible after the intubation to minimize the possibility of laryngotracheal stenosis.

Foreign Bodies

Objects of all types may lodge in the hypopharynx or esophagus. The most common sites are the cricopharyngeal area, thoracic inlet, arch of the aorta, and gastroesophageal junction. If the child can breath and talk, no attempt should be made to remove the object in the emergency department. If the child is gagging and unable to breathe, the Heimlich maneuver should be used. If this method is not effective, emergency intubation or tracheotomy may be required to bypass the obstructing object. Lateral neck and chest radiographs reveal radiopaque hypopharyngeal and esophageal foreign bodies. Plastic and other nonradiopaque objects cause the same foreign body sensation but are not visible on radiograph. Young children often have dysphagia and drooling because of painful swallowing.

If a child presents to the emergency department with a history of swallowing an object, such as a toy or a fish bone, and complains of a foreign body sensation, a careful examination of the oral cavity and hypopharynx must be performed. If no foreign body is seen, plain radiographs of the neck should be obtained. Barium esophagrams are rarely helpful in pinpointing sharp foreign bodies in the esophagus but may be useful to confirm esophageal obstruction from an impacted foreign body such as a bolus of food. Foreign bodies seen in the oral cavity may be removed by the emergency physician. Consultation with an otolaryngologist (or similarly skilled specialist) should be obtained if a foreign body is detected in the pharynx or esophagus because removal usually requires endoscopic examination under anesthesia. If the physical examination and radiographs fail to detect a foreign body, management is determined by the child's symptoms. If the child is having significant pain, the otolaryngologist should be consulted to perform esophagoscopy in the operating room.

Larynx and Trachea

Trauma

Blunt or penetrating injuries of the larynx can result in mucosal lacerations, laryngeal hematomas, vocal cord paralysis, or fractures of the thyroid and cricoid cartilages. Patients with laryngeal trauma present with varying degrees of neck pain, hoarseness, hemoptysis, and airway obstruction. Physical examination of a child with blunt trauma can reveal anterior neck tenderness, crepitance, and absence of the normal prominence of the thyroid cartilage or Adam's apple. The otolaryngologist may be needed to perform an indirect examination of the larynx. A direct laryngoscopy may be required when the child is in respiratory distress. The otolaryngologist should be prepared to intervene with intubation, tracheostomy, and/or surgical exploration of these laryngeal injuries.

Foreign Bodies

Foreign bodies may become trapped in the laryngeal inlet, causing acute upper airway obstruction. The child usually presents with severe coughing, hoarseness, and significant respiratory distress. If the child is able to phonate, air is moving through his or her larynx, indicating only partial obstruction. Back blows or the Heimlich maneuver should not be

performed in these children because this action may convert a partial obstruction into a complete one. The child should be taken immediately to the operating room where the otolaryngologist (or similarly skilled specialist) can perform direct laryngoscopy and remove the foreign body. In contrast, if the child is unable to speak, becomes cyanotic, or loses consciousness, the foreign body may be causing total obstruction. In this case, back blows and chest thrusts in infants or the Heimlich maneuver in children as per basic life support guidelines may be lifesaving. If a patient has complete obstruction requiring back blows or Heimlich maneuver, postobstructive pulmonary edema may develop. Emergency laryngoscopy, intubation, or tracheostomy is rarely required.

Foreign bodies that pass the larynx to lodge in the trachea or proximal bronchi can present problems in diagnosis and management. A history of coughing or choking on food or a toy is usually obtained. The child is often in no acute distress but may demonstrate a mild cough and/or wheezing. Inspiratory and expiratory stridor are characteristic of tracheal foreign bodies. Unilateral wheezes and decreased breath sounds are often heard with unilateral bronchial obstruction, or the patient may have a completely normal chest examination. Because most of the foreign bodies are radiolucent, they are not identifiable on radiographs. However, a radiographic difference in aeration of the lungs often helps to detect the presence and identify the site of bronchial obstruction. Volume decrease, atelectasis, and infiltrate on the involved side may be seen on plain chest films if the bronchus is completely occluded by the foreign body (Fig. 24.25). Hyperaeration (air

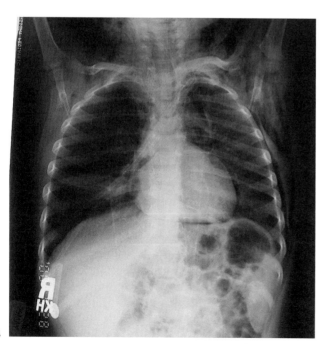
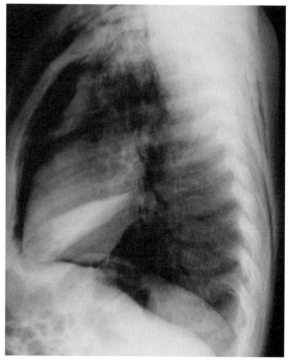

FIG. 24.25. A 19-month-old child with wheezing since choking on walnut toast. **A:** The posteroanterior view shows subcutaneous air, pneumomediastinum, and right middle lobe (RML) collapse. **B:** The lateral view shows marked hyperaeration with flat diaphragms and increased retrosternal space and RML collapse. (Courtesy of Dr. Mark Waltzman.)

trapping) secondary to a ball–valve effect of a foreign body that is partially blocking the bronchus is best seen by comparing inspiration and expiration films. If the child will not cooperate to obtain these views, right and left lateral decubitus films can often demonstrate the same phenomenon. Any radiographic asymmetry signals a possible foreign body and may require endoscopy; however, a normal chest radiograph does not rule out the possibility of a foreign body. If a foreign body is suspected, the child should be admitted and otolaryngologic consultation should be obtained to perform the endoscopy necessary for the prompt and safe removal of the object.

DENTAL TRAUMA

An initial general assessment includes the ABC evaluation. Control of bleeding, assessment of the degree of shock, evaluation of neurologic status, and notation of other injuries must all be done sequentially.

A thorough history and physical examination are paramount to any treatment considerations. The practitioner should always be alert to the possibility of nonaccidental trauma (i.e., child abuse) if the history is not consistent with the observed injury.

Physical Examination

Extraoral Examination

The clinician should note the symmetry of the face. The child should be inspected for any nasal or orbital malalignments. The clinician should carefully note the location and nature of any swollen or depressed structures and should look for lacerations and ecchymoses. The child should be asked to open and close his or her mouth while facing the clinician to see whether the mandible deviates during function. The clinician should inspect for lip competency (the ability of the lips to cover the teeth) because loss of competency may indicate displacement of the teeth from trauma.

The clinician should feel the temporomandibular joints as the child opens and closes his or her mouth. One should palpate to the orbital rim, the zygoma, the mandibular ramus, and then the nose to assess for tenderness, crepitus, or mobility and should note any paresthesia or hypoesthesia of the lips, nose, and cheeks, which may indicate a fracture.

Intraoral Examination

Hematomas or mucosal ecchymoses in the floor of the mouth or vestibular area are highly suggestive of mandibular fractures. Traumatically displaced teeth often produce the complaint that the child's teeth do not fit together when he or she bites on the back teeth. The child should be inspected for any chipped or missing teeth. If a tooth is chipped or missing, the clinician should check for any fragments of teeth or foreign bodies in adjacent soft tissues. If the child's teeth are missing yet no bloody socket is present, the eruption/exfoliation timetables (Tables 24.4 and 24.5) can be helpful in determining whether the loss is normal. Table 24.6 indicates the radiographic view that would be the preferred diagnostic aid for these injuries.

TABLE 24.4. *Eruption schedule for specific teeth*

Primary teeth	Age at eruption (mo)		Age at shedding (yr)	
	Lower	Upper	Lower	Upper
Central incisor	6	$7\frac{1}{2}$	6	$7\frac{1}{2}$
Lateral incisor	7	9	7	8
Cuspid	16	18	$9\frac{1}{2}$	$11\frac{1}{2}$
First molar	12	14	10	$10\frac{1}{2}$
Second molar	20	24	11	$10\frac{1}{2}$
Incisors	Range, ± 2 months			
Molars	Range, ± 4 months		Range, ± 6 months	

Permanent teeth[a]	Age (yr)	
	Lower	Upper
Central incisors	6–7	7–8
Lateral incisors	7–8	8–9
Cuspids	9–10	11–12
First bicuspids	10–12	10–11
Second bicuspids	11–12	10–12
First molars	6–7	6–7
Second molars	11–13	12–13
Third molars	17–21	17–21

[a] The lower teeth erupt before the corresponding upper teeth. The teeth usually erupt earlier in girls than in boys.
Modified from Massler M, Schour I. *Atlas of the mouth and adjacent parts in health and disease.* The Bureau of Public Relations Council on Dental Health, American Dental Association, 1946.

TABLE 24.5. *Sequence of primary tooth exfoliation*

Rank	Mandibular arch	Maxillary arch	Mean age*a* (yr·mo) Boys	Girls
First	Central incisors		6.0	5.7
Second		Central incisors	6.10	6.7
Third	Lateral incisors		7.2	6.10
Fourth		Lateral incisors	7.10	7.5
Fifth	Canines		10.5	9.7
Sixth	First molars		10.8	10.2
Seventh		First molars	10.11	10.6
Eighth		Canines	11.3	10.7
Ninth	Second molars	Second molars	11.9	11.5

a Ages are for the right side of the mouth; however, exfoliation is generally bilaterally symmetric.
From Ripa LW, Lesks GS, Sposanto AL, et al. Chronology and sequence of exfoliation of primary teeth. *J Am Dent Assoc* 1982;105:641, with permission.

Orofacial/Dental Trauma

The emergency physician needs to know which injuries can be managed without dental consultation, which need follow-up care, and which need emergency dental care.

Soft-tissue Lacerations

Management of injuries to the soft tissues of the oral cavity follows the same emergency care principles used for other soft-tissue injuries. Lacerations of the tongue and frenum bleed profusely because of the richness of their vascularity. However, ligating specific vessels is usually unnecessary because the bleeding normally stops with direct pressure and careful suturing. Because they heal well spontaneously, frenum lacerations usually do not require suturing. If the gingiva is fully avulsed, a dental consultation should be considered to reapproximate the gingiva over the exposed tooth (Fig. 24.26).

Injuries to the Teeth

Traumatic dental injuries can be categorized into two groups: (1) injuries to the teeth (hard dental tissues and pulp)

TABLE 24.6. *Radiographic diagnostic aids*

Radiographic view	Diagnostic aid for
Right and left lateral oblique	Fractured body and ramus of mandible
Anteroposterior view of mandible	Fracture of mandibular condyles and symphysis
Towne	Fractured condyles
Waters	Maxillary fractures
Intraoral radiographs	
Panoramic, occlusal, periapical/bite wing	Maxillary and mandibular fractures and related pathology
	Tooth fractures and pathology
	Alveolar fractures and pathology

and (2) injuries to the periodontal structures (periodontal ligaments and alveolar bones).

Injuries to Hard Dental Tissues and Pulp

Uncomplicated tooth fractures are confined to the hard dental tissue (enamel, dentin, cementum). Clinically, there may be a jagged edge of tooth (Fig. 24.27). The fracture line may appear deep, but no sign of bleeding from the central core (pulp) of the tooth is apparent. The child may complain of sensitivity, especially to cold air and fluids. Emergency treatment is aimed at protecting the pulp, even if no frank pulp exposure is noted. The dentist should be called as soon as possible to place a dressing of calcium hydroxide or glass ionomer over the exposed dentin for prevention of (pulpal) necrosis.

A complicated tooth fracture involves the pulp of the tooth. Often, bleeding is noted from the central core of the

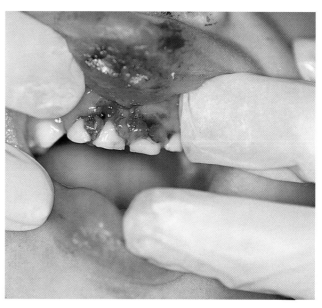

FIG. 24.26. Gingival avulsion.

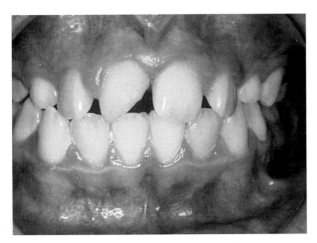

FIG. 24.27. Enamel and dentin fracture of a permanent incisor.

tooth. Prognosis depends on the time interval between the trauma and therapy (less than 24 hours carries the best prognosis). Thus, calling the dental consultant as soon as possible to institute pulpal therapy is important.

In any injury resulting in fragmentation of teeth, the emergency physician should attempt to account for all the fragments. Soft-tissue lacerations, especially of the lower lip and tongue, should be evaluated clinically and, if necessary, radiographically to rule out embedded tooth fragments. Infection and poor wound healing are the sequelae of such an oversight.

Displaced Teeth

The physician may note either an increase or decrease in mobility of the tooth. Periodontal injuries may be subdivided into five clinical types: (1) concussion, (2) subluxation, (3) intrusion, (4) extrusion/lateral luxation, and (5) avulsion.

Avulsion describes a tooth that has been completely displaced from its socket. Radiographs may show the tooth to be intruded, ingested, or aspirated. The best prognosis exists if therapy is instituted within 30 to 60 minutes of the avulsion. The emergency physician or the parent should do the following: (1) find the tooth; (2) determine whether it is a primary tooth by checking the child's age and the table of tooth eruption (if it is a primary tooth, do not reimplant); (3) if it is a permanent tooth, gently rinse the tooth under running water or saline, taking care to hold the crown of the tooth and not the root (do not scrub the crown or root); and (4) insert the tooth into the socket in its normal position (do not be concerned if it extrudes slightly).

A commercial product such as the 3M Save-a-Tooth Emergency Tooth Preserving System (Smart Practice, Phoenix, AZ) containing Hanks solution is available to place the tooth into during transportation to the dental office. If such products are not available, milk is an excellent alternative transport medium. Although saliva or saline are not ideal, they are alternative mediums that are preferred over allowing the root surface to air dry. The patient should go directly to the dentist

for immobilization (splint) and to arrange dental follow-up. Avulsed primary teeth are generally not reimplanted because of the close proximity of the permanent tooth and possible negative effects on development of this tooth.

Orthodontic Trauma

Orthodontic trauma often results from loose wires that are attached to orthodontic brackets or bands. If dental service is unavailable, the physician can bend or cut the wire away from the soft tissues with a hemostat. Softened wax can be molded over the loose wire as a temporary method to allow the traumatized soft tissues to heal. Dental follow-up should be arranged.

Mandibular Fractures/Dislocations

The examination of the mandible and appropriate radiographs (Table 24.6) should confirm the diagnosis of mandibular fracture. Most fractures occur at the neck of the condyles. Pain when opening the mouth often indicates mandibular fracture. If the mandible is fractured, an appropriate consulting service should be called to stabilize the fracture.

Mandibular dislocation occurs when the temporomandibular joint ligaments are stretched to allow the condyle to move to a point anterior to the articular eminence during mouth opening. Treatment consists of gently massaging the muscles of mastication. If this fails, 0.2 mg/kg intravenous diazepam (maximum, 10 mg) can be administered. When relaxation is achieved, gentle downward and backward pressure should be applied by the physician's thumb (wrapped in gauze) on the surfaces of the posterior teeth (Fig. 24.28). The downward pressure moves the dislocated condyle below the

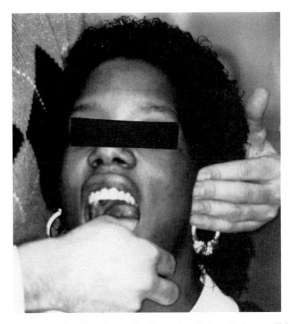

FIG. 24.28. Position for reduction of a dislocated mandible.

articular eminence; subsequent backward pressure on the molars shifts the condyle posteriorly into the mandibular fossa. Figure 24.29 shows the anatomic landmarks and repositioning of the temporomandibular joint.

SUGGESTED READINGS

Andraeson JO, Andraeson FM. *Textbook and color atlas of traumatic injuries to the teeth*, 3rd ed. St. Louis: Mosby, 1994.

Arbour JD, Brunette I, Boisjoly HM. Should we patch corneal erosions? *Arch Ophthalmol* 1997;115:313–317.

Back MR, Baumgartner FJ, Klein SR. Detection and evaluation of aerodigestive tract injuries caused by cervical and transmediastinal gunshot wounds. *J Trauma* 1997;42:680–686.

Baker M. Foreign bodies of the ears and nose in childhood. *Pediatr Emerg Care* 1987;3:67–70.

Balkany T, Rutherford R, Narrod J, et al. The management of neck injuries. In: Zuidema G, Rutherford R, Ballinger W, eds. *The management of trauma*, 4th ed. Philadelphia: WB Saunders, 1985:359–378.

Bezircioglu H, Ersahin Y, Demircivi F, et al. Nonoperative treatment of acute extradural hematomas: analysis of 80 cases. *J Trauma* 1996;41:696–698.

Bracken M, Shepard M, Collins W, et al. Methylprednisolone or naloxone treatment after acute spinal cord injury: 1-year follow-up data. *J Neurosurg* 1992;76:26–31.

Bullock R, Chesnut R, Clifton G, et al. *Guidelines for the management of severe head injury*. New York: Brain Trauma Foundation, 1996.

Cohen A, Hirsch M, Katz M, et al. Traumatic atlanto-occipital dislocation in children: review and report of five cases. *Pediatr Emerg Care* 1991;7:24–27.

Eckstein M. The prehospital and emergency department management of penetrating head injuries. *Neurosurg Clin North Am* 1995;6:741–751.

Ersahin Y, Mutluer S, Mirzai H, et al. Pediatric depressed skull fractures: analysis of 530 cases. *Childs Nerv Syst* 1996;12:323–331.

Gold SM, Gerber ME, Shott SR, et al. Blunt laryngotracheal trauma in children. *Arch Otolaryngol Head Neck Surg* 1997;123:83–87.

Greenes DS, Schutzman SA. Isolated skull fractures in infants: what are their clinical characteristics, and do they require hospitalization? *Ann Emerg Med* 1997;30:253–259.

Grewal H, Rao PM, Mukerji S, et al. Management of penetrating laryngotracheal injuries. *Head Neck* 1995;17:494–502.

Hester TO, Campbell JP. Diagnosis and management of nasal trauma for primary care physicians. *J Kentucky Med Assoc* 1997;95:386–392.

Kadish HA, Corneli HM. Removal of nasal foreign bodies in the pediatric population. *Am J Emerg Med* 1997;15:54–56.

Kriss VM, Kriss TC. SCIWORA (spinal cord injury without radiographic abnormality) in infants and children. *Clin Pediatr* 1996;35:119–124.

Levin AV. Eye emergencies: acute management in the pediatric ambulatory setting. *Pediatr Emerg Care* 1991;7:367–377.

Levin AV. General pediatric ophthalmic procedures. In: Henretig FM, King CK, eds. *Textbook of pediatric emergency procedures*. Philadelphia: Williams & Wilkins, 1997:579–592.

Martin W, Gussack G. Pediatric penetrating head and neck trauma. *Laryngoscope* 1990;100:1288–1291.

Proudfoot J. Pediatric cervical spine injury: navigating the nuances and minimizing complications. *Pediatr Emerg Med Rep* 1996;1:83–94.

Radkowski D, McGill TJ, Healy GB, et al. Penetrating trauma of the oropharynx in children. *Laryngoscope* 1993;103:991–994.

Reilly JS, Cook SP, Stool D, et al. Prevention and management of aerodigestive foreign body injuries in childhood. *Pediatr Clin North Am* 1996;43:1403–1411.

Schutzman S, Barnes P, Mantello M, et al. Epidural hematomas in children. *Ann Emerg Med* 1993;22:535–541.

Shingleton BJ. Eye injuries. *N Engl J Med* 1991;325:408–413.

Shugerman R, Paez A, Grossman D, et al. Epidural hemorrhage: is it abuse? *Pediatrics* 1996;97:664–668.

Woodward GA, Kunkel CN. Cervical spine immobilization and imaging. In: Henretig FM, King C, eds. *Textbook of pediatric emergency procedures*. Baltimore: Williams & Wilkins, 1997:329–341.

CHAPTER 25

Minor Lesions, Soft-tissue Trauma, and Foreign Bodies

Editor: Gary R. Fleisher

MINOR LESIONS

Paronychia

Most paronychiae (Fig. 25.1) arise after minor injuries (a traumatized hangnail, finger sucking, or nail biting) that causes a breakdown in the epidermal barrier. In its initial stage, the infection consists of a superficial cellulitis that remains localized to the cuticle and is termed an eponychia. With progression, pus collects in a single thin-walled pocket under the cuticle, forming a paronychia. Treatment of a simple eponychia involves frequent warm soaks and attention to local hygiene. Incision and drainage are the treatment of choice for a paronychia (see Chapter 27, Selected Procedures). If an onychia (collection of pus under the nail) has formed, removal of the proximal portion of nail overlying the abscess is essential. The role of oral antibiotics after incision and drainage has not been clearly established, but most physicians choose a short course of a β-lactamase stable antibiotic (e.g., dicloxacillin, cephalexin).

Felon

A felon consists of a deep infection of the distal pulp space of a fingertip. Felons are caused by introduction of bacteria into the pulp space usually by punctures (which may be trivial) or splinters. A felon typically presents as an exquisitely tender and throbbing fingertip that is swollen, tense, warm, and erythematous. In some cases, organisms may spread to invade the phalanx, resulting in osteomyelitis. In others, the process may point outward to the center of the touch pad, where the septae are least dense, producing an obvious area of fluctuation. A longitudinal incision over the area of maximal tension or fluctuance is the procedure of choice. Care should be taken not to extend the incision past the distal interphalangeal joint to prevent formation of a flexion contracture. Older techniques, such as the extended fishmouth incision, incision through the touch pad, and the through-and-through incision,

should be abandoned. After drainage, a course of oral antibiotics is indicated.

Subungual Hematoma

A subungual hematoma (Fig. 25.2) is a collection of blood located under a nail that arises after trauma to the nailbed. The typical mechanism is a crush injury. Because this mechanism is a common cause of phalangeal fractures, radiographs are advisable. The patient experiences throbbing pain that worsens with increasing pressure as more blood collects. The underlying nailbed injury may be trivial or may involve a laceration that requires repair. If the subungual hematoma involves more than 50% of a nail surface, is associated with a distal phalanx fracture, or the nail or its margins are disrupted, the presence of a significant nailbed injury should be suspected. Nail trephination provides drainage with attendant relief of pressure and pain and suffices for uncomplicated subungual hematomas. When the hematoma is large, the nail or its margins are disrupted, and/or a phalangeal fracture is present, the nail should be removed and the nailbed repaired. Antimicrobial prophylaxis for these injuries remains a source of controversy but is prescribed by most practitioners for patients with underlying fractures and those with severe soft-tissue injuries.

Ganglion

A ganglion is a cystic outgrowth or protrusion of the synovial lining of a tendon sheath or joint capsule. Common locations of such lesions include the dorsal or volar surface of the wrist (usually on the radial side) (Fig. 25.3), the dorsum of the foot, or near the malleolus of an ankle. The cysts are soft, and slightly fluctuant, and transilluminate. Most are painless or only mildly uncomfortable. However, those on the foot or ankle may cause pain when shoes are worn. Elective surgical excision with obliteration of the base is in-

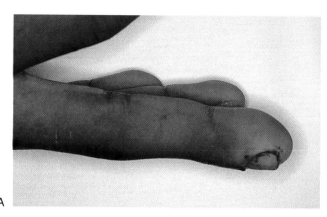
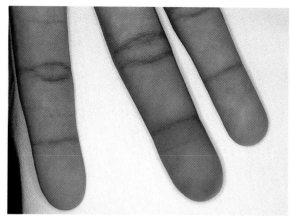

FIG. 25.1. Paronychia of the right middle finger. The infection is clearly localized to the dorsal surface **(A)**, although the pulp is slightly swollen **(B)** due to edema.

dicated only if function is impaired or the lesion is of cosmetic significance. Even then, as many as 20% recur. The old folk remedy of striking the cyst with a large book or against a hard surface should be strongly discouraged because the cystic fluid may be dispersed through the surrounding soft tissue, inciting diffuse scar formation.

Lipoma

Lipomas are benign subcutaneous tumors composed of mature adipose cells. They often present in adolescence as painless and usually solitary nodules. Although they may be located anywhere on the body, preferential sites include the neck, shoulders, back, upper chest, abdomen, and arms. Clinically, lipomas are nontender and have a soft, rubbery consistency, often with lobulations. Overlying skin is normal and easily slides across the mass. Lesions that are cosmetically significant, large, or painful warrant elective surgical excision.

Pyogenic Granuloma

Pyogenic granulomas (also called lobular capillary hemangiomas) are benign vascular lesions most commonly found on exposed skin surfaces such as the face, hands, and forearms. They are composed of granulation tissue with significant vascular overgrowth and are considered the result of an exaggerated vascular growth factor response after local trauma (Fig. 25.4). Lesions are usually solitary and pedunculated, measuring from 0.5 to 2 cm. The color and character of a pyogenic granuloma vary according to its stage of growth. Early on, the lesion appears as a glistening, red, polypoid nodule with a friable surface that bleeds easily. Later (weeks to months), the lesion becomes fibrotic and shrinks, taking on a reddish brown hue. The most common reasons for presenting to the emergency department are bleeding or chronic oozing of an early lesion. Treatment consists of excision followed by silver nitrate cauterization of vessels at the base. Recurrence merits referral to a dermatologist.

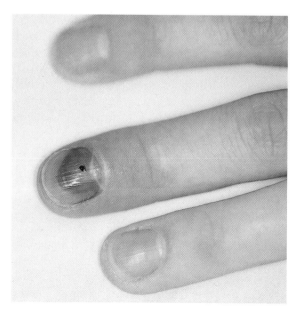

FIG. 25.2. A subungual hematoma that required drainage for relief of pain.

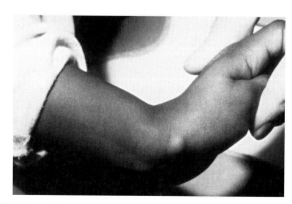

FIG. 25.3. Ganglion cyst of the tendon sheath of the flexor carpi radialis at the wrist.

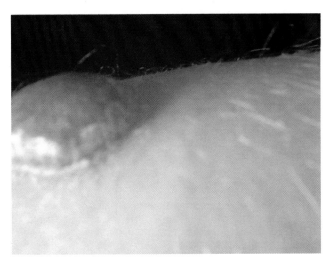

FIG. 25.4. Pyogenic granuloma.

Granuloma Annulare

The lesions of granuloma annulare are composed of infiltrates of lymphocytes and altered collagen within the dermis. They first appear as raised nodules that gradually expand centrifugally to form annular rings ranging from 1 to 5 cm in diameter. They have a firm, fibrous, sometimes lumpy consistency on palpation. Overlying skin is usually normal or slightly hyperpigmented (Fig. 25.5). Although most are asymptomatic, a patient occasionally may report mild pruritus and present with superficial excoriation caused by scratching. The lack of an active microvesicular border, firm consistency on palpation, and the deeper dermal location of these lesions helps to distinguish them from tinea corporis. Lesions are commonly found on the extensor surfaces of the lower legs and the dorsum of the hands and feet and, less often, on the trunk or abdominal wall. Because most lesions undergo resolution within 1 to 2 years, reassurance is usually all that is necessary.

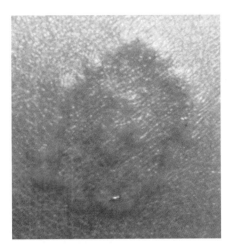

FIG. 25.5. Granuloma annulare. Compared with tinea corporis (See Fig. 6.19), this lesion has central clearing and no microvesicles of the border.

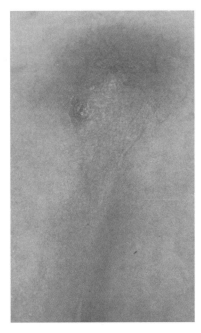

FIG. 25.6. Infected pilonidal cyst.

Pilonidal Sinus

Pilonidal sinuses have a small surface opening to a tract lined by stratified squamous epithelium that extends toward, but not into, the spinal canal. These sinuses and cysts are asymptomatic unless the sinus becomes obstructed and/or infected, usually during adolescence or early adulthood. After infection occurs, an abscess forms and tends to enlarge rapidly (Fig. 25.6). Patients typically complain of low back pain that increases on sitting and local tenderness. On examination, a tender, indurated swelling is noted overlying the sacrococcygeal area with the original sinus at its cephalad end. Treatment consists of incision and drainage with careful probing to break up loculations and extract any hairs present because these act as foreign bodies.

MINOR TRAUMA

Blunt

Blunt forces cause a spectrum of injuries that range from superficial to deep. Internal hemorrhages, visceral disruptions, fractures, and a host of other deep injuries are covered in the chapters on head and neck, thoracic, abdominal, genitourinary, and orthopedic trauma. Superficial wounds proceed from contusions and ecchymoses (Fig. 25.7) at the surface to bleeding beneath fascial planes, leading in some cases to compartment syndrome (Fig. 25.8).

Geometric lesions, especially if multiple, should suggest either child abuse (Chapter 26) or self-inflicted injuries such as cupping (Fig. 6.28). Various cultural practices may produce a similar appearance, particularly "coining," during which parents rub hot coins over the bodies of their

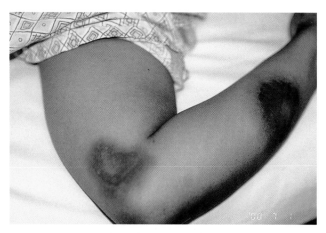

FIG. 25.7. Severe ecchymoses resulted from minor trauma in this child taking anticoagulant medication.

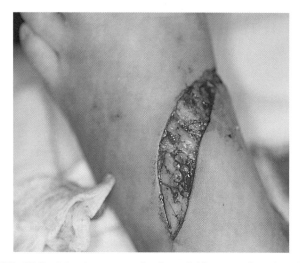

FIG. 25.8. A truck ran over the foot of this young boy. In addition to the obvious laceration, observation reveals a pale blue color resulting from impaired circulation that occurred as a result of increased pressure in all compartments of the foot.

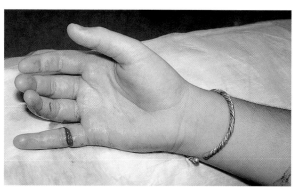

FIG. 25.10. This laceration of the fifth digit appears superficial, but it extended through the extensor tendon and required repair in the operating room. As an aside, this photograph illustrates the point that careful observation is an extremely important tool in the evaluation of children. Although this patient would not cooperate with an evaluation of neurovascular function, the position of her finger at rest proved sufficient for the detection of the severed tendon.

children, reportedly as a treatment for fever (Fig. 25.9 and Fig. 6.29).

Penetrating

As with blunt trauma previous chapters discuss serious injuries that penetrate through the cranium, platysma, pleura, peritoneum, and fascial layers of the extremities. Superficial penetrating forces cause primarily lacerations that vary in size, depth, and complexity (Fig. 25.10).

As described in Chapter 27, physicians may choose to repair lacerations with adhesive strips, tissue glue, or sutures. Each method entails potential complications; occurring most frequently and common to all approaches are infection and dehiscence.

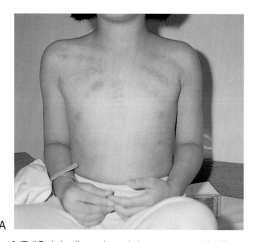

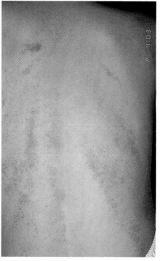

A   B

FIG. 25.9. A,B "Coining" produced these geometrically arranged contusions as a result of friction over the bony prominences in this child, who was referred to the emergency department for suspected child abuse.

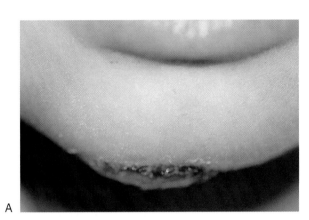
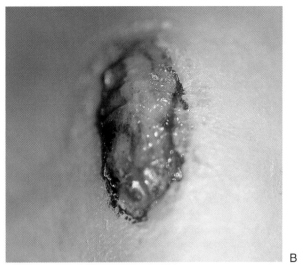

A

B

FIG. 25.11. A,B: Hemorrhage occurred in this incorrectly closed wound and resulted in swelling contained within the pocket formed by the tissue adhesive. In this case, the adhesive was Dermabond and the lesion might be considered a "Dermabondoma." This laceration, as do most wounds of the face and chin, required a meticulous, layered repair, rather than a simple application of tissue adhesive.

Unique to the use of tissue adhesives is hemorrhage and exudation contained within the pocket formed during the repair (Fig. 25.11).

FOREIGN BODIES

Children frequently visit emergency departments for foreign bodies, acquired either unintentionally or as the result of experimentation. Ingestion into the gastrointestinal tract and aspiration into the airways were discussed previously.

Foreign bodies may also become embedded in or just under the skin as well as deeper in the soft tissues or may simply encircle a digit or extremity, which swells to the point that the edema prevents simple removal by traction. A wide variety of objects may be involved, including human hairs, wooden splinters, glass, manufactured objects, rocks, and other debris. Objects that tightly encircle a digit require prompt removal before circulatory compromise ensues (Fig. 25.12). Superficial foreign bodies can usually be removed with a forceps (Fig. 25.13). Deeper objects that have

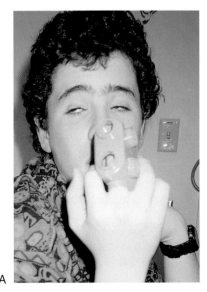
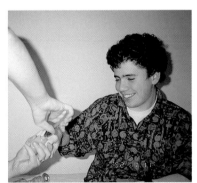

A

B

FIG. 25.12. A: The foreign body around this child's finger was stuck, secondary to swelling. B: The foreign body had to be cut before removal.

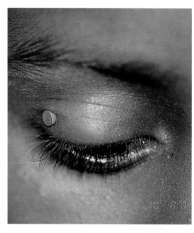

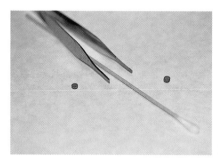

A

B

FIG. 25.13. A, B: Superficial, palpable objects, such as the magnetic metal cylinders adherent to both the inner and outer aspect of this child's upper eyelid, are easily removed. Deeper foreign bodies, particularly sewing needles submerged in the sole of the foot, often require an inordinate amount of time for removal.

a visible fragment or are easily palpated (Fig. 25.14) are generally amenable to removal in the emergency department. Those that are sufficiently remote from the surface as to be neither visible nor palpable (Fig. 25.15) require an inordinate amount of time to locate; thus, the emergency physician may choose to refer the patient to a surgeon for removal in the operating room. The availability of fluoroscopy facilitates the extraction of deeper foreign bodies that are radiopaque. Radiographs should be obtained before and after the removal of subcutaneous radiopaque objects.

Subungual Foreign Body

Foreign bodies such as a wood splinter or metallic shaving may become embedded under the nail and may be the source of pain and/or infection. When a foreign body is only partially embedded, the nail can be trimmed close to the nailbed, and the object's projecting end grasped with splinter forceps

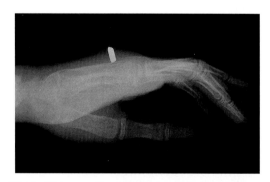

FIG. 25.14. This metallic object (not a bullet, despite the suggestive appearance) penetrated just beyond the dermis and was easily palpable in its superficial location, although not visible, because the family delayed for several weeks before seeking treatment and the wound had closed.

and gently extracted. If a portion remains, or the foreign body is deeply embedded from the outset, the nail can be lifted and the object removed.

Hair Tourniquet

A hair tourniquet injury is an entity unique to pediatrics. It involves strangulation of a digit (or occasionally the penis, less commonly the clitoris) by a hair or fine thread (Fig. 25.16). It is seen most commonly in young infants and can be the cause of unexplained irritability or crying. The mechanism involves entwinement of the hair around an infant's appendage. This may occur during a bath, during subsequent toweling, or as a result of wiggling of the toes in a sock, bootie, or mitten that inadvertently has a hair or loose thread in it. A hair shed from a parent during diapering is the probable source of penile tourniquets. As the hair or thread becomes more tightly entwined, it produces a tourniquet effect, impairing blood flow with resultant ischemic pain and distal swelling. When noted early, the hair is often visible in a crease just proximal to the swollen area. If seen later, the hair may have cut through the skin, making it difficult to visualize. In rare cases, frank ischemic necrosis of the distal digit may be seen on presentation. Removal requires a fine-tipped forceps and the aid of a thin loupe or probe that is inserted proximally under the constricting hair. Usually the hair can be unwound from the digit intact or cut with scissors. When the hair is deeply embedded or there is any question of a remaining constricting band, a nerve block should be performed and a perpendicular incision made over the hair. To avoid damage to neurovascular structures, such an incision should be made on the lateral aspect of a finger or toe at the 3 or 9 o'clock or the 4 or 8 o'clock position along the penile shaft. When the entire hair cannot be removed with certainty, surgical consultation is indicated.

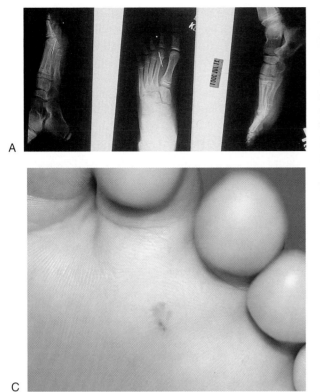

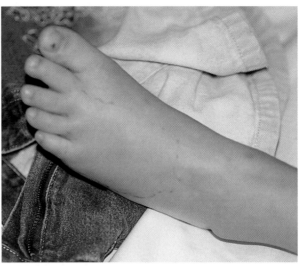

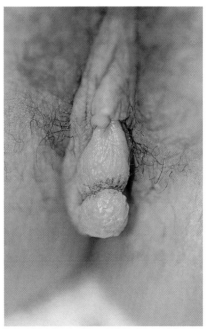

FIG. 25.15. A: A radiograph shows a sewing needle that embedded itself in the deep tissues of the sole of the foot. The child presented with dorsal erythema **(B)**, from a cellulitis, but the finding of a small puncture wound **(C)**, suggested a foreign body despite the absence of any history along this line.

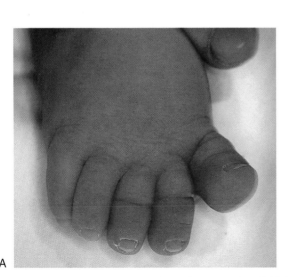

FIG. 25.16. Hair tourniquets encircle the second and third toes of this infant **(A)**. **B:** A patient presented with a hair tourniquet involving the labia minora.

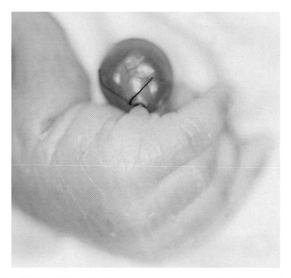

FIG. 25.17. This infant presented at 1 week of age with a swollen, supernumerary digit. The suture ligature had not been tied sufficiently tightly.

In the newborn period, when an infant is born with extra digits, the technique of applying a tourniquet around the supernumerary digit is used therapeutically. The physician ties a suture at the base of the extra digit, causing it to slough off. Occasionally, this procedure can lead to complications, similar to what might be encountered with an incompletely, persistently constricting hair tourniquet (Fig. 25.17).

SUGGESTED READINGS

Hurwitz S. *Clinical pediatric dermatology*, 2nd ed. Philadelphia: WB Saunders, 1993.

Knight PJ, Reiner CB. Superficial lumps in children: what, when, and why? *Pediatrics* 1983;72:147–153.

Mooney MA, Janniger CK. Pyogenic granuloma (review). *Cutis* 1995;55: 133–136.

Prendville JS. Diseases of the dermis and subcutaneous tissues. In: Schachner LA, Hansen RC, eds. *Pediatric dermatology*, 2nd ed. New York: Churchill Livingstone, 1995.

Sebastian MW. Pilonidal cysts and sinuses. In: Sabiston DC Jr, ed. *Textbook of surgery*, 15th ed. Philadelphia: WB Saunders, 1997:1330–1334.

Simon RR, Wolgin M. Subungual hematoma: association with occult laceration. *Am J Emerg Med* 1987;5:302–304.

SECTION III

Psychosocial Emergencies

CHAPTER 26

Child Abuse

Editor: Stephen Ludwig

Child abuse is the single diagnostic term used to describe a range of behaviors from somewhat harsh discipline to intentional, repetitive torture. This phenomenon is complex and results from a combination of individual, familial, and societal factors. The common pathway for all these factors is parental behavior destructive to the process of normal growth, development, and well-being of the child. Abuse may be subdivided into four broad categories: (1) physical abuse, (2) sexual abuse, (3) neglect, and (4) emotional abuse. This chapter covers only the findings of physical and sexual abuse.

PHYSICAL ABUSE

There are four major types of child maltreatment: (1) physical abuse, (2) child neglect, (3) sexual abuse, and (4) emotional abuse. Physical abuse is the infliction of physical injury as a result of punching, beating, kicking, biting, burning, shaking, or otherwise harming a child. The parent or caretaker may not have intended to hurt the child, but rather the injury may have resulted from overdiscipline or physical punishment.

Manifestations

The manifestations of physical abuse may affect any body system. Thus, the emergency physician must be prepared to recognize a variety of signs and symptoms. Abuse may also be seen by physicians in other specialties. National data show neglect to be most common.

Integument

The skin is the most commonly injured body organ. Cutaneous injuries may be divided into nonspecific and specific traumatic lesions, burns, and hair loss. Of the nonspecific traumatic injuries, the bruise or contusion is the most commonly seen. Although bruises are also common in children who are not abused, accidental bruises usually have a different distribution and appearance. Accidental injuries occur most commonly on the extremities and forehead. As bruising

moves (Fig. 26.1) centrally and becomes extensive, the likelihood of abuse rises. The bruise should be dated and compared with the history provided. A prothrombin time, partial thromboplastin time, bleeding time, and platelet count should be obtained if easy bruisability has been offered as a possible explanation.

Other nonspecific cutaneous injuries include lacerations, punctures, and abrasions. The following criteria are important for the evaluation of any nonspecific injury: (1) the history of injury, (2) the child's age and developmental level, (3) the presence of other old or new injuries, (4) the interaction between the parents and child, and (5) the interaction between the parents and the emergency department (ED) staff.

Specific skin injuries are those that clearly reflect the method or object used to inflict the trauma. Loop-shaped marks are readily seen after a beating with an electric cord or wire (Fig. 26.2A–C). Linear marks may be seen from a belt or paddle injury. Rope burns result in circumferential marks on the wrists, ankles, or around the neck when a child has been bound (Fig. 26.2D). Another common specific integument lesion is a handprint on the side of the face or symmetrically on the upper arms (Fig. 26.2E). The lesion produced by a slap leaves ecchymotic areas in the location of the interphalangeal spaces. Human bites appear as circular lesions 1 to 2 in. in diameter (Fig. 26.2F). Forensic dentistry is able to match the skin lesion with the dentition of the alleged perpetrator.

Burns of the skin may be caused by abuse or neglect. Burns account for 5% of cases of physical abuse. In particular, tap water scald burns that occur in an immersion pattern are often the result of intentional trauma. Immersion burns are likely to be inflicted by an abusive parent when they occur on a child who is being toilet trained (Figs. 20.1C and 26.3A). Other indications of abuse are a delay in seeking treatment, a history of the child being unsupervised, and the child being brought to the hospital by the parent who was not present when the burn occurred.

In attempting to match the physical findings of the burn with the available history, several factors must be appreciated. The extent of the burn depends on the temperature of the

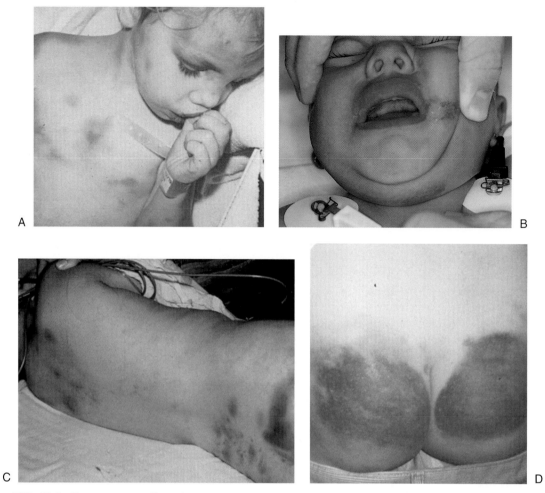

FIG. 26.1. Cutaneous manifestations of child abuse. **A:** Multiple bruises in a central pattern. **B:** Bruises around the face. **C:** Bruises at various stages of healing. **D:** Buttocks bruises as a cause of myoglobinuria.

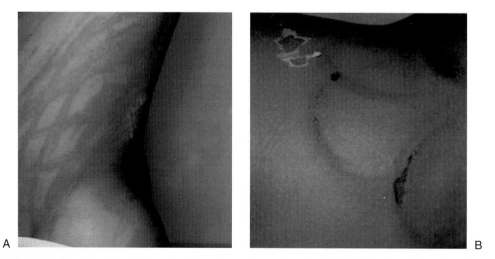

FIG. 26.2. Specific skin injuries. **A:** Linear loop-shaped marks. **B:** Multiple loop-shaped marks.

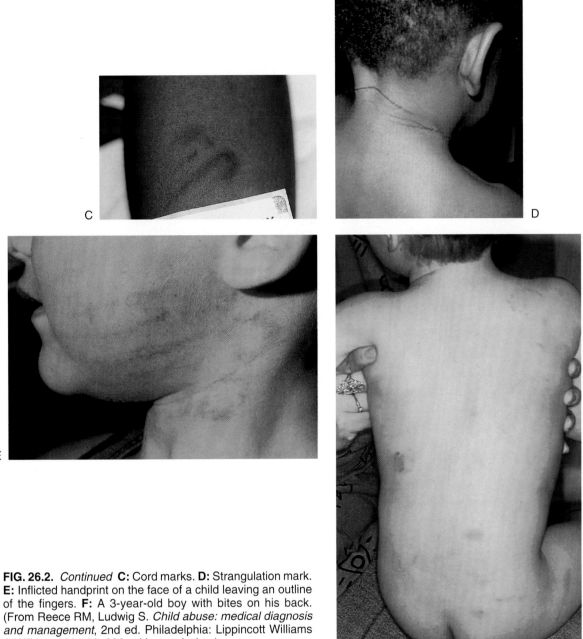

FIG. 26.2. *Continued* **C:** Cord marks. **D:** Strangulation mark. **E:** Inflicted handprint on the face of a child leaving an outline of the fingers. **F:** A 3-year-old boy with bites on his back. (From Reece RM, Ludwig S. *Child abuse: medical diagnosis and management*, 2nd ed. Philadelphia: Lippincott Williams & Wilkins, 2001:28, 396, with permission.)

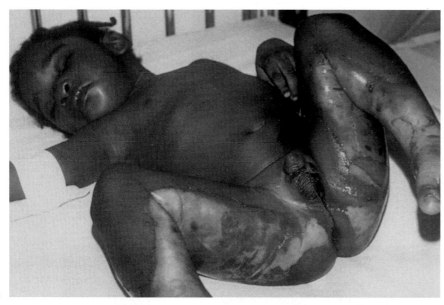

A

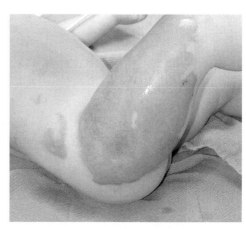

B

FIG. 26.3. Immersion burns. **A:** Hot water burn in an immersion pattern. **B:** Hot liquid spill burns sustained by a 6-month-old child. (From Reece RM, Ludwig S. *Child abuse: medical diagnosis and management*, 2nd ed. Philadelphia: Lippincott Williams & Wilkins, 2001:402, with permission.)

water, duration of exposure, thickness of the skin involved, and presence or absence of clothing. A water temperature of 54°C (130°F) or greater causes a full-thickness burn with less than a 30-second exposure. Because palms and soles are thick, they are often spared. Clothing tends to keep the hot water in contact with the skin and causes more severe burns. Burns presumably caused by falling or thrown fluids should produce a droplet or splash pattern (Fig. 26.3B).

Other burns may occur through contact with a hot solid rather than a hot fluid. Cigarette burns are the most common of this type. If the history given is of a child brushing against a cigarette or of hot ashes falling on the child, the resulting injury should be a nonspecific first- or second-degree burn. When a cigarette is extinguished on the child's skin, the injury is a burn that is 8 to 10 mm in diameter and indurated at its margin. A healed cigarette burn is indistinguishable from any other circular skin lesion such as impetigo, abscess, or vesicles. Burns from radiators, hot plates, cigarette lighters, curling irons, or standard irons imprint the shape of the hot object (See Fig. 20.2 and 26.4). Recently, there have been reports of children burned by microwave ovens.

The final category of integumental injury is injury to the hair. Traction alopecia (Fig. 26.5) is seen when a parent pulls the child by the hair. The scalp is usually clear, differentiating this lesion from tinea capitis, seborrhea, and scalp eczema. Alopecia areata produces a lesion in which the hair is uniformly absent. In the cases of traction or traumatic alopecia, patches of broken hair remain.

Skeletal System

The skeletal system is also commonly traumatized when children are physically abused. As previously mentioned,

matching the history of injury with the physical findings is important. Considering the mobility and strength of the child is also important to identify suspicious injuries. The radiologist needs to review the patient's past radiographs to identify the child with multiple visits to the hospital for fractures. When suspicion of abuse is high, a radiographic skeletal survey should be obtained to ascertain the condition of the entire skeletal system.

Support for the use of radioisotope scans as a more sensitive and immediate way of demonstrating bone injury is increasing. However, radionuclide scans are still second-line studies. Some of the indications for a radiographic skeletal survey or bone scans are listed in the Management section of this chapter. Skeletal surveys are often performed on a young child with an obvious fracture and then reveal multiple old fractures. The skeletal survey is the preferred radiographic study because it provides information on the type, location, and age of fractures as well as the presence or absence of bone diseases.

Bone injuries may be of several types, including simple transverse fractures, impacted fractures, spiral fractures, metaphyseal fractures, or subperiosteal hematomas. Radiographs of some of these injuries are shown in Figure 26.6. To explain a transverse fracture, the history should be that of direct force applied to the bone. Differentiating the true cause of this type of fracture is often difficult. The impacted fracture should have an accompanying history of force along the long axis of the bone, such as the child's falling on his or her outstretched hand. In the case of a spiral fracture, a history of twisting or torque during the traumatic event should be present. Metaphyseal chip fractures occur when the extremity is pulled or yanked; the periosteum is most tightly adherent at the metaphysis, causing

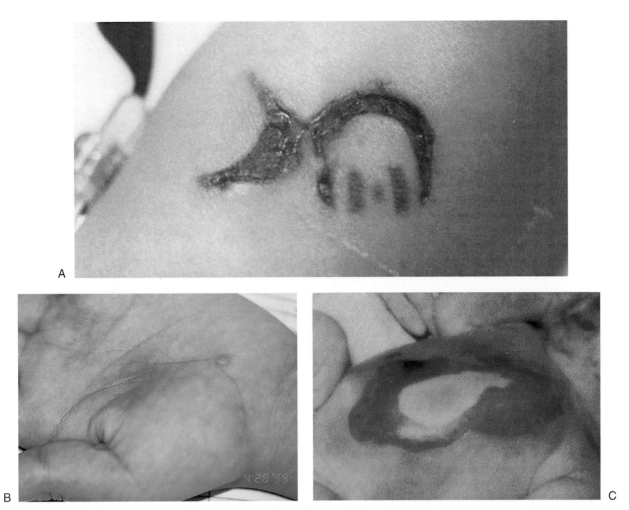

FIG. 26.4. Hot solid burns. **A:** Pattern burn from cigarette lighter. **B:** Coin burn. **C:** Ventral burns. There are full-thickness burns to the left abdomen and thorax and partial-thickness burns to left anterior thigh. Extensive circumferential burns of right foot and left hand are not seen. This infant presumably was placed on her back in the microwave oven. From Reece RM, Ludwig S. *Child abuse: medical diagnosis and management*, 2nd ed. Philadelphia: Lippincott Williams & Wilkins, 2001:455, with permission.)

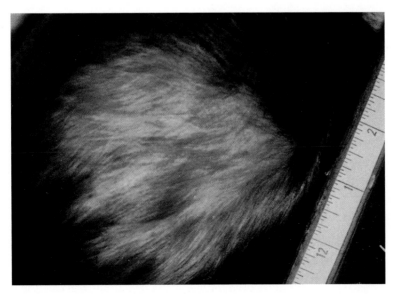

FIG. 26.5. Traumatic alopecia. (From Reece RM, Ludwig S. *Child abuse: medical diagnosis and management*, 2nd ed. Philadelphia: Lippincott Williams & Wilkins, 2001:29, with permission.)

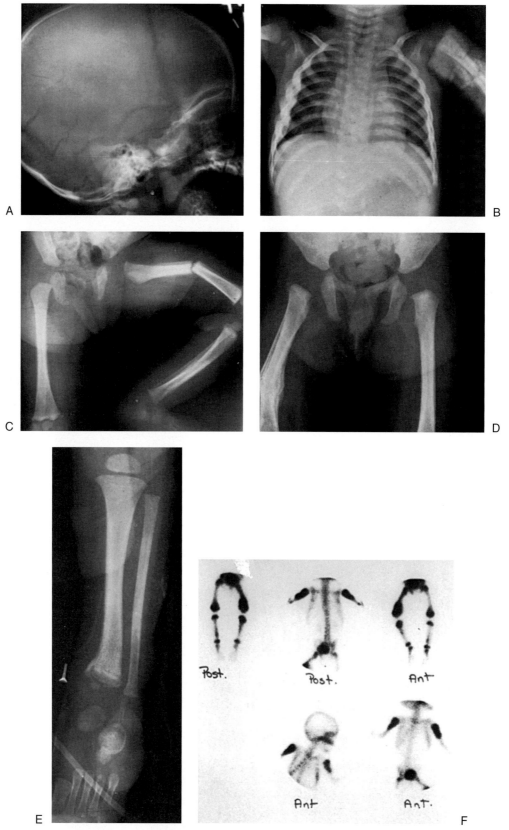

FIG. 26.6. Radiographic findings of child abuse. **A:** Multiple skull fractures in an infant. **B:** Left humeral fracture and multiple old healing rib fractures. **C:** Left femoral fracture and metaphyseal chip avulsion fractures of the right distal femur. **D:** Healing fracture of the right femur with callus formation and new periosteal bone formation. **E:** "Bucket-handle" deformity of healing distal tibial epiphyseal fracture. **F:** Bone scan shows multiple areas of increased uptake caused by trauma. Some of these areas appeared normal on the original radiographs.

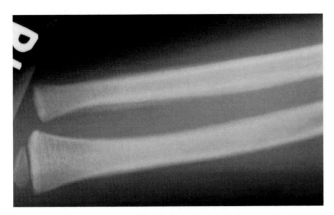

FIG. 26.7. Periosteal elevation not secondary to abuse.

small bone fragments to avulse. Metaphyseal chip fractures are almost exclusively caused by abuse. Subperiosteal hematomas produce a characteristic radiograph. The elevation of the periosteum is seen as a linear opacification running parallel to the bone surface. Subperiosteal hematomas are produced by direct trauma to the bone. However, in as many as 10% of small and premature infants, symmetric periosteal elevation (Fig. 26.7) that is not caused by abuse may occur along the tibia or humerus. The reason for this finding is unknown, but it should not be confused with abuse.

The location of the fracture is important in the identification of abuse. The fracture of a clavicle and the dislocation of a radial head are common noninflicted injuries. However, when the femur of a young child is fractured or when ribs are fractured, the suspicion of abuse increases (Fig. 26.8).

Other uncommon and, therefore, suspicious fractures are located in the vertebrae, sternum, pelvis, or scapulae. Uncommon fractures need to be carefully evaluated unless a clear history of significant trauma, such as an automobile injury, is reported.

The age of a fracture may be estimated from the amount of callus formation and bone remodeling seen on the radiograph

(Fig. 26.9). Table 26.1 lists fracture landmarks by date. Dating of fractures is not an exact science because many confounding variables, such as the child's age, location of the fracture, and nutritional status must be considered. Nonetheless, the child who presents with an acute fracture and has a second fracture with a callus stands out as having sustained more than one episode of trauma. The usual longbone fracture may take 8 to 10 days to form a callus and several months to heal completely. In the acute stages of injury, soft-tissue swelling should be seen for 2 to 5 days. Soft-tissue swelling may be clearly seen on standard radiographs. Skull fractures or fractures of other flat bones cannot be dated in the same way.

When a young child sustains multiple fractures, the differential diagnosis must be widened beyond accidental trauma and abuse to include osteogenesis imperfecta, infantile cortical hyperostosis, scurvy, syphilis, osteoid osteoma, neoplasms, rickets, hypophosphatasia, and osteomyelitis. Table 26.2 details the distinction between child abuse and osteogenesis imperfecta (Fig. 26.10). All the other conditions are much rarer than abuse and can be ruled out by the appearance of the bone on the radiograph and by the levels of calcium, phosphorus, and alkaline phosphatase in the serum.

Central Nervous System

Injuries to the central nervous system are the main cause of child abuse deaths. These injuries may be subdivided into two categories: direct trauma and shaking injuries. Direct trauma is inflicted by striking the child with an object or by dropping or throwing the child against a wall or onto the floor. The extent of the resulting trauma depends on the amount of force used, the surface contacted, and the child's age. The child may be brought to the ED with a small subgaleal hematoma or in coma. Injuries may vary from scalp contusions to intracerebral hematomas.

Shaking injuries characteristically cause serious central nervous system damage without evidence of external trauma

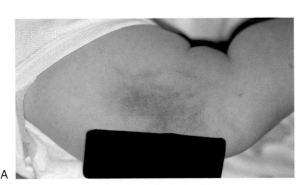

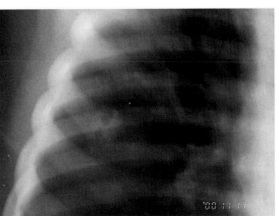

FIG. 26.8. Importance of fracture locations. **A:** Swollen thigh overlying a femoral fracture. **B:** Fourth rib fracture.

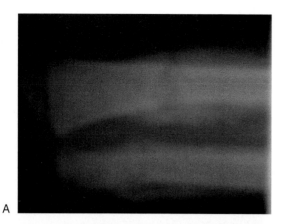

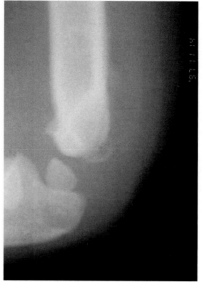

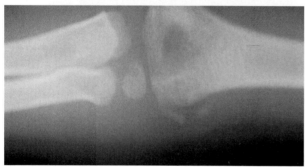

FIG. 26.9. Fractures. **A:** Radial/ulnar fractures. **B:** Humeral fracture. **C:** "Bucket-handle" fracture.

TABLE 26.1. *Dating fractures*

0–10 days
  Soft-tissue edema
  In an adjacent joint fluid
  Visible fracture fragments
  Visible fracture lines
10 days–8 weeks
  Periosteal new bone (layered)
  Callus (first subtle and then heavy)
  Bone resorption along fracture line makes fracture line
    more visible
  Metaphyseal fragments often more visible
≥8 weeks
  Periosteal new bone matures, becomes thicker
  Callus formation becomes denser and smoother
  Metaphyseal fragments are incorporated into a metaphy-
    seal callus and become smoother
  Fracture line less visible and then invisible
  Deformities and cortical bumps persist

TABLE 26.2. *Osteogenesis imperfecta versus child abuse*

Finding	Osteogenesis imperfecta	Child abuse
Incidence	Rare	Common
Positive family history	Common	Common
Blue sclerae	Common	Rare
Abnormal teeth	Common	Rare
Hearing impairment	Common	Uncommon
Osteoporosis	Common	Rare
Abnormal fracture healing	Common	Rare
Wormian bones	Common	Rare
Joint laxity	Common	Rare
Short stature	Common	Occasional
Fracture recurrence in protected environment	Common	Rare
In utero fracture	Occasional	Rare
Biochemical studies	Abnormal	
		Normal

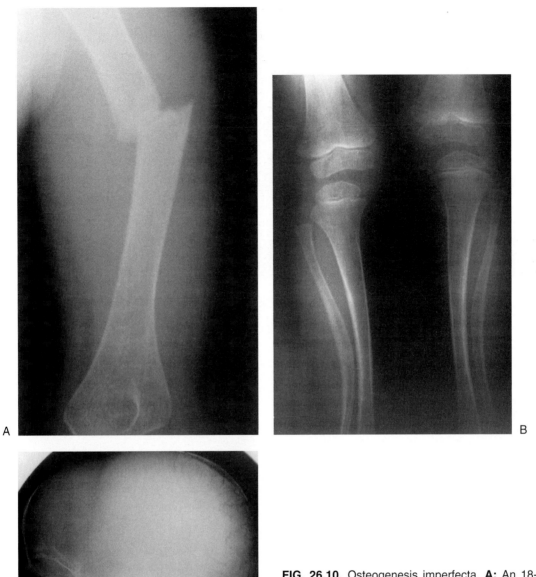

FIG. 26.10. Osteogenesis imperfecta. **A:** An 18-month-old child (osteogenesis imperfecta) with clinically short stature has a transverse fracture of the left humerus. **B:** Symmetric tibial and fibular bowing. The bones are generally demineralized with thin cortices. **C:** The skull shows multiple sutural (wormian bones). (From Reece RM, Ludwig S. *Child abuse: medical diagnosis and management*, 2nd ed. Philadelphia: Lippincott Williams & Wilkins, 2001:150, with permission.)

(Fig. 26.11A). The infant's relatively large head size and weak neck muscles are predisposing factors for whiplash injury. Whether the injury is caused by shaking alone or shaking followed by an impact is controversial. In most fatal cases, minor bruising to the scalp is seen, although such scalp injuries may not be apparent until the scalp is reflected during the autopsy.

The shearing and contusive forces that result from shaking the infant produce this type of injury. Specific lesions that occur include hematomas, subarachnoid hemorrhages, or brain contusions, particularly in the frontal and occipital lobe. The child may present with lethargy and a "septic" appearance, with seizures, or in a coma. The physical examination is otherwise unremarkable except for retinal hemorrhages (Fig. 26.11B–D). Occasionally, bruises on the upper arms or shoulders indicate the sites where the child has been grasped. Lumbar puncture produces grossly bloody or xanthochromic spinal fluid. If computed axial tomography is available, it shows the characteristic findings of occipital contusion and intrahemispheric blood. This form of abusive behavior by the parent is usually triggered by the infant's persistent crying. Occasionally, excessively rough forms of play or misguided resuscitative efforts may result in shaking injuries.

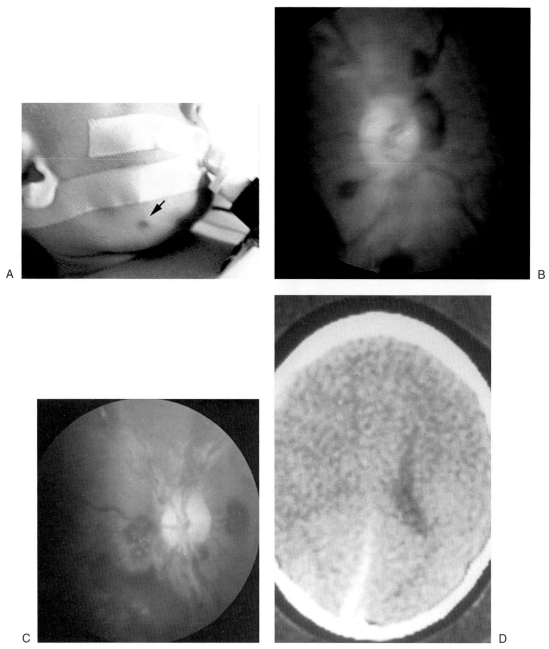

FIG. 26.11. Shaking injuries. **A:** Small bruise of right cheek (*arrow*) in a 6-month-old shaking victim was the only external evidence of injury. The photograph was taken shortly after admission to the hospital to document that the injury was not iatrogenic. The child died the following day and at autopsy had typical findings of shaken baby syndrome. Manifestation of whiplash shaking injury. (From Reece RM, Ludwig S. *Child abuse: medical diagnosis and management*, 2nd ed. Philadelphia: Lippincott Williams & Wilkins, 2001:470, with permission.). **B:** Retinal hemorrhage. **C:** Retinal hemorrhages as seen on funduscopic examination. **D:** Computed tomography shows intrahemispheric subdural bleeding and right cortical brain swelling.

Gastrointestinal System

Gastrointestinal injuries are relatively uncommon abuse manifestations but, similar to central nervous system injuries, account for a significant percentage of fatal injuries. Of all gastrointestinal injuries, mouth trauma is perhaps the most common. Small infants may sustain a tear of the frenu-

lum resulting from "bottle jamming" (Fig. 26.12A). In the older child, dental trauma may be a sign of abuse (Fig. 26.12B).

Other gastrointestinal system manifestations are more medically serious and generally result from blunt trauma to the abdominal contents (Fig. 26.13). Rupture of the spleen or laceration of the liver causes the child to present with

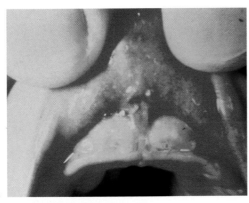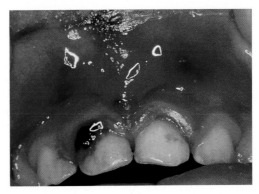

FIG. 26.12. Mouth traumas. **A:** A 2-month-old baby with a laceration of the labial frenum from forced feeding. **B:** A 10-year-old child with multiple oral injuries from an open-handed slap to the face, including laceration of the upper lip, contusions of the vestibule, laceration of the labial frenum, and subluxation of the right central incisor. (From Reece RM, Ludwig S. *Child abuse: medical diagnosis and management*, 2nd ed. Philadelphia: Lippincott Williams & Wilkins, 2001:115–116, with permission.)

elevated liver enzymes, with an acute abdomen, or in shock, with no external source of bleeding and with absent or only minor bruising of the abdominal wall. A less acute presentation is the afebrile child with persistent bilious vomiting from a duodenal hematoma with small bowel obstruction. Documenting an elevated serum amylase or lipase or in-

creased liver enzymes is important in providing tangible evidence of abdominal trauma in cases that lack any radiographic finding or abdominal wall bruising. Elevation of the serum amylase may also identify those cases that should be followed for possible development of a pancreatic pseudocyst.

Cardiopulmonary System

Abuse may be manifested in cardiac or pulmonary trauma with no injuries that are characteristically induced by abuse. Pulmonary contusion, pneumothorax, hemothorax, cardiac tamponade, and myocardial contusion may all occur occasionally.

Genitourinary Systems

Common genitourinary complaints, such as hematuria, dyssuria, urgency, frequency, and enuresis, may be the initial sign of abuse. These problems may result from direct trauma, sexually transmitted infections, or emotional abuse. As for direct trauma, any part of the genitourinary system may be involved, from the renal parenchyma to the urethral meatus. Penile trauma that does not have an adequate explanation may be an alerting sign of abuse.

Sensory

All the sensory organs are vulnerable to physical abuse, including ocular, nasal, and otic injuries. The eye may sustain several different forms of injury (Fig. 26.14), including periorbital ecchymosis, corneal abrasion, subconjunctival hemorrhage, hyphema, dislocated lens, retinal hemorrhages, or detached retina. A careful history of injury is important when treating any of these conditions. Injury to the nose may result in simple hemorrhage or fracture and disfigurement of the

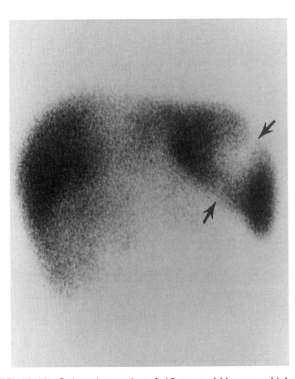

FIG. 26.13. Spleen laceration. A 12-year-old boy was kicked in the abdomen by his father. Liver spleen scintigram reveals a transverse laceration of the mid spleen (*arrows*). (From Reece RM, Ludwig S. *Child abuse: medical diagnosis and management*, 2nd ed. Philadelphia: Lippincott Williams & Wilkins, 2001:164, with permission.)

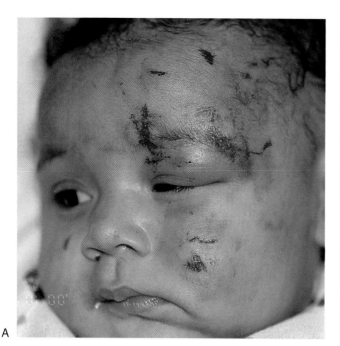

A

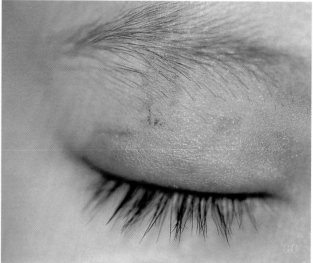

B

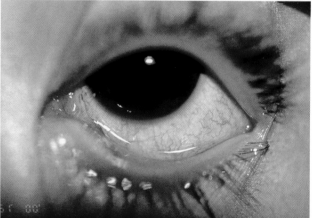

C

FIG. 26.14. A: This 3-month-old infant was evaluated for head trauma after falling out of her infant swing onto a wooden floor. Although her initial trauma evaluation revealed no life-threatening injuries, her facial injuries did not seem consistent with her trauma history. A subsequent investigation pointed to child abuse. (Courtesy of Dr. Mark Neuman.) **B, C:** Sensory organ injuries. Eye injury.

nasal structures (Fig. 26.15). The external ear may show evidence of contusion. In particular, ecchymosis on the internal surface of the pinna may result from "boxing" the ear and crushing it against the skull (Fig. 26.16).

A direct blow to the ear may also cause hemotympanum and perforation of the tympanic membrane. In such cases, hemotympanum on the basis of basilar skull fracture should also be considered. The presence of discoloration behind the

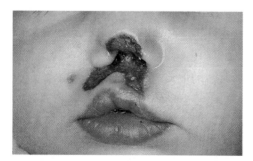

FIG. 26.15. Nasal destruction in a 6-month-old infant. (From Reece RM, Ludwig S. *Child abuse: medical diagnosis and management*, 2nd ed. Philadelphia: Lippincott Williams & Wilkins, 2001:459, with permission.)

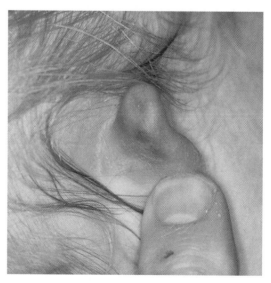

FIG. 26.16. Ear injury: ecchymosis.

ear (Battle sign) may be a further indication of a basilar skull fracture (see also Chapter 24, Trauma: Head and Neck).

Failure to Thrive

The term failure to thrive has been used as a diagnostic term to group several diseases and disorders that result in growth failure. Growth failure is generally measured in weight, length, and head circumference and compared with standard growth curves for these parameters. Growth failure may be defined as measurements that fall below 2 standard deviations for age or patterns that cross percentile lines (i.e., 2 standard deviations) and do not follow the normal lines of growth (Fig. 26.17). Patients diagnosed with failure to thrive

may be subcategorized into three groups: organic, nonorganic, and mixed. Organic refers to children whose failure to thrive is based on a physical cause such as congenital heart disease, renal disease, or a genetic abnormality. Nonorganic refers to those whose growth failure is environmentally related. When these children are hospitalized and fed standard diets, they grow rapidly and thrive. The group of patients with nonorganic failure to thrive includes a substantial number of neglected children who may be brought to the ED for care. The mixed group refers to patients who have a combination of physical and environmental factors. An example might be a physical condition that so overstresses a family that they cannot function and thus neglect the child in some aspect of the feeding process.

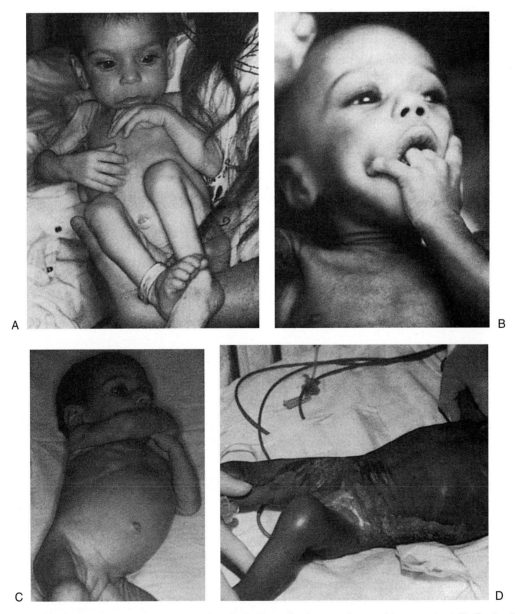

FIG. 26.17. Physical signs of failure to thrive. **A:** Dull, apathetic eyes that avoid eye contact. **B:** Oral self-stimulatory behavior. **C:** Wasted extremities and protuberant abdomen. **D:** Severe diaper rash as a sign of overall neglect.

In recognizing the patients with nonorganic failure to thrive, the following factors are suggestive:

1. History: an idealized feeding history; a chief complaint and history that do not identify the child's growth pattern as a problem; no description of losses such as vomiting or diarrhea; and failure to give a history of a schedule or scheduled pattern of feeding (e.g., baby eats approximately every 4 hours)
2. Physical examination: measurements in which weight is more depressed than length, which is more depressed than head circumference; other signs of neglect such as poor hygiene, diaper rash, and flat and balding occiput; dull, apathetic facies; body posture of an understimulated child; excessive oral self-stimulation; and developmental delay, particularly in the social adaptive and language areas
3. Parental observation: the parent who has an uninterested attitude; does not respond to child's needs (e.g., does not react to crying); lacks concern about health issues; and appears to be a drug or alcohol abuser

Unusual Manifestations

Rarely, the emergency physician is confronted by one of the unusual abuse manifestations. Cases of toxic and nontoxic ingestions, electrolyte disorders such as hyponatremia and hypernatremia, foreign bodies, bathtub drowning, and multiple serious infections may be the result of abuse. In all these situations, the parent actively abuses the child by feeding, instilling, or injecting harmful substances or objects into the child's body. Some children with a toxic ingestion reveal that their parents forced them to ingest the substance. The most common toxic ingestants of this type are alcoholic beverages that are given to or forced on the child to either quiet the child or to demonstrate "manly" qualities. Other drugs may be used to poison the child. The most recent reports are of cocaine ingestions.

Several cases of parents who have placed their children on high-salt, water-only, or pepper diets as a form of punishment have been reported. Such children may present with signs of hypernatremia or hyponatremia, possibly with seizures. Foreign bodies have been found in every orifice as well as under the skin and in fingernail beds. Several cases of Munchausen syndrome by proxy have occurred in which a parent has inflicted illness on the child rather than feigning or inducing illness (Table 26.3). Cases of fictitious fever, hematuria, and even sepsis have resulted from this form of abuse. Although rare, the unusual manifestations of abuse should be considered when more common causes of these problems cannot be identified.

Management

The management of a child abuse case is difficult unless the emergency physician has a previously prepared, well-structured protocol. If reports of abuse are not a daily occurrence, an institutional policy serves as an important guide to the

TABLE 26.3. *Characteristics of Munchausen syndrome by proxy*

Difficult to understand medical situation with recurrent episodes
Failure of other centers to arrive at diagnosis; doctor shopping
Unsupportive or "absent" marital relationship
Compliant, cooperative, overinvolved mother
Medical knowledge in parent's background
Findings abort with surveillance of child
Findings correlate to presence of parent
Extensive medical care in parent's background

mechanics of management. Consultants from different disciplines, such as nursing and social work, provide invaluable assistance. A multidisciplinary approach simplifies the initial decision making and subsequent case management. The steps in the protocol are shown in Figure 26.18.

Suspect Abuse

The first step is to decide whether a reasonable likelihood of abuse exists. Many shades of suspicion make the term abuse imprecise. Although every traumatic injury should be

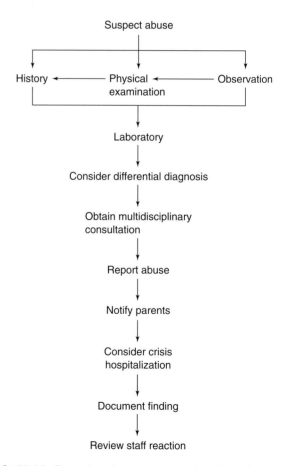

FIG. 26.18. Procedure for emergency department management of suspected physical abuse.

TABLE 26.4. *Historical indicators of abuse*

Is the history one of inflicted injury?
Is there an absence of history, a "magical" injury?
Could the injury have been avoided by better care and supervision?
Are there inconsistencies or changes in the history?
Is there a history of repeated injury or hospitalization?
Was there a delay in seeking medical care?
Does the history overestimate or underestimate the injury?
Is there a medical history of prematurity, failure to thrive, failure to receive adequate medical care such as immunization?

suspected as abuse, the physician has the onerous task of deciding how much suspicion is necessary to take some action (i.e., report). To establish the level of suspicion, data are gathered by obtaining a complete history, performing a thorough physical examination, comparing the history and physical examination, observing interactions, and obtaining laboratory studies and/or radiographs. Then, the physician can formulate a differential diagnosis and assign a rank to abuse. Indications of abuse in the history and physical examination and observational data must be used like building blocks that are added until they achieve a particular threshold of suspicion. When the threshold is reached, a report of suspected abuse must follow.

A detailed history is always important. As in many other medical situations, this process is initiated by asking some general open-ended questions about what happened. If the child has sufficient verbal skills, the first questions are directed at him or her. General inquiries must then be followed with specific requests for information; however, a harsh interrogation only alienates the family. Some specific historical are listed in Table 26.4.

Laboratory data and radiographs are another source of indicators of abuse. The laboratory studies obtained are few and, for the most part, document the obvious or rule out other disease states. Biochemical, hematologic, and urinary studies that are used appear in Table 26.5 along with their indications. Radiographs document a specific bony or soft-tissue injury. They may provide a comprehensive and longitudinal record of osseous injury at any site in the skeletal system. Although no precise indications for ordering a skeletal survey in cases of suspected abuse exist, some relative indications are (1) any child younger than 1 year old presenting with a fracture, (2) any child with severe or extensive fractures, (3) any child who has a history of more than one fracture, and (4) a history in the child or the family of "soft" or easily broken bones.

During the time occupied by the history, physical examination, and performance of laboratory studies, the physician should be cognizant of the interactions among family members and between the parents, the child, and the ED staff. Such an awareness often uncovers subtle indicators of abuse. The observation of parents arguing vehemently on the way to the radiology department may be a clue. The parent who appears to be distant from both the child and the physician is also suspect. Although the parent who is intoxicated or incoherent never fails to gain staff attention, such individuals are in the minority of abusive parents. Observation of the child

TABLE 26.5. *Laboratory/diagnostic evaluation of the physically abused child*

Radiographic skeletal survey	Blood tests for easy bruising/bleeding
Method of choice for screening abused children for bony injury	Complete blood count
For all children younger than 2 years old with suspected physical abuse	Prothrombin time
Of limited use in children older than 5 years	Partial thromboplastin time
For children 2 to 5 years old, use clinical findings	Bleeding time
Radionuclide bone scan	Screening tests for evidence of abdominal trauma
Adjunct to skeletal survey	Liver
Most useful if there is high suspicion of bony injury and skeletal survey is negative	Alanine aminotransferase (SGPT)
CT scan	Aspartate aminotransferase (SGOT)
Provides sliced views through internal organs, such as brain and abdominal organs	Pancreas
Essential part of the evaluation of seriously injured children	Amylase
Initial test used for children with suspected shaking impact syndrome	Lipase
Abdominal trauma	Kidney
Magnetic resonance imaging	Urinalysis
More sensitive than CT for many injuries	Toxicology screens
Can provide images in multiple planes	For children with unexplained neurologic symptoms or symptoms compatible with ingestion
Generally used as an adjunct to CT in the acute care setting	Variance among laboratories in drugs tested in a toxicology screen
	Screening of urine and blood and/or gastric contents
	Consideration of blood alcohol levels for children with altered mental status

CT, computed tomography; SGOT, serum glutamic-oxaloacetic transaminase.
From the U.S. Advisory Board on Child Abuse and Neglect. *A nation's shame: fatal child abuse and neglect in the United States.* Washington, DC: U.S. Department of Health and Human Services, 1995.

is important as well. All abused children are not withdrawn, passive, and depressed. On the contrary, some are competent, outgoing, or "pseudomature."

The final step in establishing a threshold level of suspicion is to review the differential diagnosis. At this point in the management scheme, the physician must add up the indicators and arrive at a judgment. If the process does not lead to a clear determination, most state laws imply that reporting suspected abuse is more prudent than not. Physicians are asked to report suspected, not proven, abuse. The major differentiation is between accidental and nonaccidental trauma. The other elements of the differential diagnosis are all uncommon diseases, including (1) bone diseases such as osteogenesis imperfecta, osteoid osteoma, and hypophosphatasia; (2) hematologic disorders such as idiopathic thrombocytopenic purpura and hemophilia; (3) neoplasms; (4) metabolic disorders such as rickets or scurvy; (5) infections such as syphilis or osteomyelitis; and (6) syndromes in which pain sensation is absent such as spina bifida or congenital indifference to pain. All these diseases occur with much less frequency than abuse, but deserve consideration; simple laboratory and radiographic studies confirm or deny these diagnoses.

Multidisciplinary Consultation

If consultation with a nurse, social worker, or physician with more extensive experience in the management of child abuse is available, it should be obtained. The advantages of consultations are many. They allow information sharing, joint decision making, planning, and mutual support. Planning an approach to the family and subsequent case management is useful. This brief consultation enables the physician to be more secure in making decisions about matters that are generally unfamiliar and often value laden. Joint interviewing is not only time efficient, but it gives the family a uniform approach from the professional staff.

Reporting

Once the suspicion of abuse has been established and consultations obtained, the next step is reporting. Although laws vary from state to state, most have common elements. The emergency physician should become familiar with his or her current state law.

Notifying the Parents

An important, but often avoided, step in case management is notification of the parents. This step is often forgotten because it is a difficult interpersonal task; nonetheless, it must be done. Nothing makes parents more resistant to change than completing a "routine" ED visit, only to later receive notification that the physician has filed a suspected child abuse report. Some specific guidelines are helpful in avoiding this breech of trust. The overall approach to the parents must be based on concern for the child. Concern for the

child, not accusation, should be stressed.

Crisis Hospitalization

In some cases of abuse, the family crisis is at such an acute level that hospitalization is necessary. The physician must ask, "Is the home safe?" If the child's environment poses a potential danger, the child should be admitted, no matter what the extent of injury. Some state laws have included protective custody sections that allow physicians virtual police powers in detaining a child for protection. In other states, the physician may need to obtain parental consent for admission.

Documentation

Throughout each step of case management, documentation is important. The record of this visit is both a medical and a legal document. A precise description of the injuries enhances the document's value, and small sketches are also helpful. Photographs are invaluable in documenting extensive injuries. Some states require parental permission for photographs, whereas other jurisdictions allow photographs to be taken without parental consent.

SEXUAL ABUSE

The sexually abused child is another difficult psychosocial emergency for the emergency physician. The state-of-the-art method of identifying and managing cases of sexual abuse has developed rapidly in the past decade. The number of sexual abuse cases reported now equals the number of physical abuse cases. Of all societal taboos, those that prohibit incest are the strongest. This belief leads to denial and makes even basic recognition of the problem more difficult.

As with the physically abused, the sexually abused child engenders a great deal of emotion from the health care professionals in the ED. Treatment issues for both the child and the perpetrator are more complex. Working in a multidisciplinary fashion with nursing and social work staff is important. The effects of this form of abuse may clearly be profound but may not be expressed as symptoms for many years. Prompt diagnosis, humane emergency management, and referral to long-term treatment resources are the goals of the emergency physician. Many centers have adopted strategies to use the ED for recognition and screening of acute (less than 72 hours) episodes of sexual abuse as well as developing programs for comprehensive evaluation outside the ED.

Background

National Center for Child Abuse and Neglect defines sexual abuse as (1) employment, use, persuasion, inducement, enticement, or coercion of any child to engage in, or assist any other person to engage in, any sexually explicit conduct or any simulation of such conduct for the purpose of producing any visual depiction of such conduct or (2) rape and, in cases

TABLE 26.6. *Identification of sexual abuse*

Physical complaints	Behavioral complaints
Specific	Specific
Genital injury	Explicit descriptions of sexual contact
Bruises	Inappropriate knowledge of adult sexual behavior
Lacerations	Compulsive masturbation
Rectal laceration, fissures	Excessive sexual curiosity, sexual acting out
Sexually transmitted disease	Nonspecific
Pregnancy	Excessive fears, phobias
Nonspecific	Refusal to sleep alone, nightmares
Anorexia	Runaways
Abdominal pain	Aggressive behavior
Enuresis	Attempted suicide
Dysuria	Any abrupt change in behavior
Encopresis	
Evidence of physical abuse in genital area	
Vaginal discharge	
Urethral discharge	
Rectal pain	

of caretaker or interfamilial relationships, statutory rape, molestation, prostitution, or other form of sexual exploitation of children or incest with children. Sexual abuse includes fondling a child's genitals, intercourse, incest, rape, sodomy, exhibitionism, and commercial exploitation through prostitution or the production of pornographic materials. Many experts believe that sexual abuse is the most underreported form of child maltreatment because of the secrecy or "conspiracy of silence" that so often characterizes these cases. Sexual abuse has traditionally been more the domain of police and other law enforcement personnel.

Clinical Manifestations

The manifestations of sexual abuse may occur at a time shortly after the abuse has occurred or at a time more distant from the event. The manifestations may be influenced by a single episode or by a pattern of repeated encounters. Finally, the manifestations may depend on the child's age and maturity. The manifestations may be divided into four categories, as shown in Table 26.6. These categories are specific physical findings, specific behavioral manifestations, nonspecific physical complaints, and nonspecific behavioral complaints.

Management

The primary goals in case management of the sexually abused child are to identify and report the abuse and to avoid

the secondary abuse phenomenon. Secondary abuse phenomenon refers to the physical examination that is so overzealous that it assumes a rapelike quality in the mind of the child. Also to be avoided are parental or staff reactions that make the child feel responsible or blamed for the abuse. Many centers have moved to performing a screening function. If the child has been abused in the past 72 hours or more and no acute symptoms [e.g., bleeding, signs of sexually transmitted disease (Table 26.7)] are present, the child is referred to a sexual assault center, provided such a community service exists. In places where no center is functioning, the entire evaluation must be done in the ED. The following sections offer techniques in management to identify suspected sexual abuse and to gather enough documentation for legal purposes in a manner that is humane for the child and supportive for the family.

Interviewing the Parent

Parents may present the problem of sexual abuse either directly or indirectly. For the parent who is direct (i.e., "My child's been abused"), it is important to provide a controlled, quiet environment because he or she will be upset and angry. It may be necessary to limit what is said in front of the child. With such parents, the interviewer's tasks are calming, limiting, and clarifying. In an example of the indirect presentation, the parent brings the child for complaints such as those detailed in the sections on nonspecific physical or behavioral

TABLE 26.7. *Sexually transmitted diseases and their probability of being caused by child sexual abuse*

Always	Usually	Possibly
Neisseria gonorrhoeae	Herpes simplex	Condylomata
Syphilis	*Chlamydia trachomatis*	Scabies
	Trichomoniasis	Pediculosis
		Gardnerella vaginalis

manifestations. With this parent, the task of the interviewer is to bring the possibility of sexual abuse into the open. After the topic is nominally broached, it becomes apparent that the parent has often already given it consideration. With both types of parents, exploring both their concerns and their information in detail is important.

Interviewing the Child

Beyond standard history taking from the parents, the emergency physician must always obtain a history from the child. This task is difficult for several reasons: (1) the child's level of language development, (2) the child's level of psychosexual development, (3) the desire not to contaminate what may be important evidence, (4) the apprehension of the child and the parent, and (5) the awkwardness and apprehension felt by the interviewer in discussing sexual matters with a child. The first steps are for the physician to obtain a quiet, private place and to decide whether he or she wishes the parent to be present. If possible, the physician may wish to defer the comprehensive examination to a more appropriate time and place. Based on history taking from the parent, the physician can gauge the parent's level of emotional composure. This criterion is useful to decide whether parents should be present. If the parents are excluded, another third party (e.g., a nurse or social worker) should be present. An initial discussion of topics, other than the alleged abuse, comforts the child and encourages him or her to talk to the interviewer. Information about school, peers, and family adjustment is important in looking for nonspecific behavioral manifestations, and this preliminary conversation helps to evaluate the child's developmental level.

Emotional Support

Throughout the interview and in all contacts with the child, the rightness of his or her decision to discuss the abuse should be stressed. A child experiences conflict about revealing a secret, especially a long-standing secret. The patient may also feel conflict in sensing that his or her actions may be provoking a great deal of emotional turmoil. Often, the child has a relationship with the perpetrator and realizes that this admission may alter or end the relationship. At times, the child is aware or is made aware of getting the perpetrator "in trouble." Reaffirm the importance of what the child has revealed and focus the wrongdoing on the perpetrator. The child may have been threatened not to tell. Thus, bringing the nature of the threats into the open and offering to protect the child are important concerns. Finally, many children have fears about the abuse. The physician may anticipate and address these fears based on the child's development.

Physical Examination

The physical examination may be a point of significant trauma for the child. The examination should be conducted in a standard fashion with all parts of the body examined. The position of the child depends on age and comfort. Many young children want to be examined while sitting in their parent's lap. In examining the genitalia of young girls, two positions are recommended. One is a frog-leg posture while sitting on an adult lap. Alternatively, the child can lie prone with knees tucked under the thorax (i.e., the knee–chest position).

In the prepubertal girl, only the external genitalia need be examined (Figs. 26.19 and 11.53). If even minimal vaginal bleed-

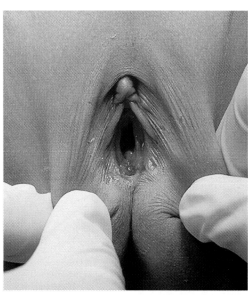

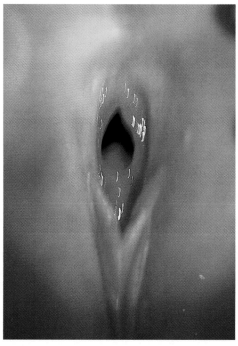

FIG. 26.19. External genitalia examination. **A:** Vaginal laceration. **B:** Hymeneal notch normal variant comparison.

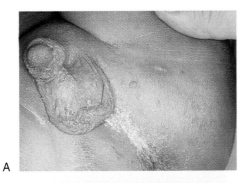

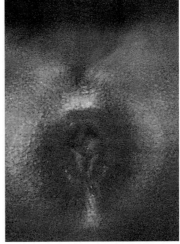

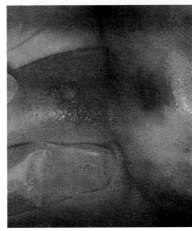

FIG. 26.20. Rectum and oropharynx examination. **A:** Perirectal Condyloma. **B:** Rectal dilation and multiple lacerations after sodomy. **C:** Herpes virus infection in perirectal area.

ing appears to be coming from a more internal source, exploration and possible surgical repair is best done under general anesthesia in the operating room. Examination in the ED should be deferred. In the pubertal child, a full genital examination should be performed. This examination may be modified if it is a girl's first speculum examination and it proves too difficult.

Examination of the rectum and oropharynx needs to be carefully performed (Figs. 26.20), particularly if the history suggests that these were sites of sexual contact. Other physical findings to note carefully are any contusions, abrasions, or lacerations in nongenital areas. Common sites for these signs of trauma are the upper thighs, buttocks, and upper arms.

Evidence Collection

The type of evidence to be collected, the collection methods used, and the procedures for processing the results vary by locale. The specimen-collecting procedures at the Children's Hospital of Philadelphia have been reviewed by the Philadelphia Police Department and District Attorney. The protocol is listed in Table 26.8.

Consider a Differential Diagnosis

In any consideration of abuse, the physician must always consider the question, "What else could it be?" There may be

plausible explanations such as accidental injuries to the genitals as in straddle injuries. Other important alternatives to consider are (1) infections such as streptococcal, *Haemophilus influenzae*, and monilial; (2) congenital anomalies such as hydrometrocolpos, hemangioma, and perineal clefts and pits; (3) foreign bodies of the rectum and vagina; and (4) dermato-

TABLE 26.8. *Evidence for child sexual abuse*

1. Child's history in detail
2. History of observers
3. Documentation of general physical examination; note signs of force (e.g., bruises)
4. Documentation of genital injury (colposcopy)
5. Documentation of sexual contact
   Presence of sperm or semen (e.g., on patient's clothing, linens)
   Sexually transmitted disease
   Pregnancy
   Foreign material
6. Documentation of perpetrator
   Sperm: motile/nonmotile
   Seminal fluid
      Genetic marker (blood group antigens)
      Acid phosphatases
   P30 glycoprotein
   Blood
   Hair analysis
   DNA matching

Adapted from DeJong (*personal communication*).

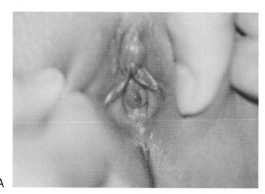
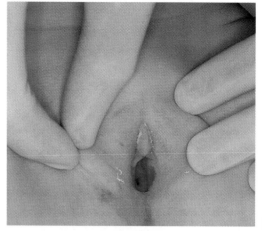

A   B

FIG. 26.21. Differential diagnosis. **A:** Urethral caruncle or partial urethral prolapse in a 3-year-old girl, causing bleeding and concerns about sexual abuse. (From Reece RM, Ludwig S. *Child abuse: medical diagnosis and management*, 2nd ed. Philadelphia: Lippincott Williams & Wilkins, 2001:294, with permission.) **B:** Comparison bruise around introitus: not abusive.

logic conditions such as lichen sclerosus et atrophicus, diaper dermatitis, contact dermatitis, Ehlers–Danlos syndrome, and phytodermatitis. Perhaps the most common mistaken perineal finding is prolapsed urethra, which appears as a hemorrhagic mass covering the upper vaginal area (Fig. 26.21).

Documentation

Careful record keeping cannot be stressed too strongly. As with the collection and processing of evidence, ED records can make or break a case. All the aspects of record keeping mentioned in the section on physical abuse apply. In particular, what the child said in his or her own words should be carefully recorded. Such questions may be the mainstay of any legal actions to be taken. Meticulous records not only help the police and lawyers involved but also help the physician review the case before a hearing that may not take place for 6 months. In some jurisdictions, legal provisions allow videotaping patient interviews. This tool is particularly helpful to the victim in that he or she may not have to repeat the history so many times. It may also be helpful to the physician by serving as another form of documentation. When such tapes are shown during court proceedings, they are most helpful.

Diagnosis

The diagnosis of sexual abuse should be based on a composite of the history, physical examination, and laboratory findings. Many centers have begun to use a four-category classification of assessment developed by Adams and Harper (Table 26.9) using a classification of physician findings noted in Table 26.10.

Reporting

In most jurisdictions, sexual abuse is a criminal offense. Thus, all cases are reported to the police department. In some jurisdictions, when the abuse has occurred in the home or during a time when parental supervision was lax, a civil report to a Child Protection Services agency may also be required. This detail needs to be specified according to local guidelines and included in an ED procedure. In the event of a criminal (police) report, a civil (child abuse) report, or both, the parent needs to be informed that such reports are being made. The physician or social worker must spell out the practical consequences of the reports for the parent.

Preparing the Parent

Beyond notifying the parent about reporting the sexual abuse, additional preparation must be given. Many workers believe that, for the young child, the parental reaction to sexual abuse may have as important a role as the abuse itself in producing subsequent manifestations. Long-term follow-up studies of sexually abused children performed using a case-control methodology show that the sexually abused child is at long-term risk of a variety of psychological and behavioral consequences. Parents need to be aware of this correlation. All parents will be upset. All parents will be angry. Some parents may express disbelief or the feeling that "this could not be happening to me." Parental reactions vary depending on whether the abuse is intrafamilial or extrafamilial. Social worker consultation and collaboration for this aspect of case management are essential.

TABLE 26.9. *Overall assessment of the likelihood of sexual abuse*

Class 1: no evidence of abuse
　Normal examination, no history, no behavioral changes, no witnessed abuse
　Nonspecific findings with another known cause and no history or behavioral changes
　Child considered at risk of sexual but gives no history and has nonspecific behavior changes
Class 2: possible abuse
　Class 1, 2, or 3 findings in combination with significant behavioral changes, especially sexualized behaviors, but child unable to give history of abuse
　Presence of condyloma or herpes 1 (genital) in the absence of a history of abuse and with otherwise normal examination
　Child has made a statement but not detailed or consistent
　Class 3 findings with no disclosure of abuse
Class 3: probable abuse
　Child gives a clear, consistent, detailed description of molestation, with or without other findings present
　Class 4 or 5 findings in a child, with or without a history of abuse, in the absence of any convincing history of accidental penetrating injury
　Culture-proven infection with *Chlamydia frachomatis* in a prepubertal child (child older than 2 years of age). Also culture-proven herpes type 2 infection in a child or documented *Trichomonas* infection
Class 4: definite evidence of abuse or sexual contact
　Finding of sperm or seminal fluid in or on a child's body
　Witnessed episode of sexual molestation (also applies to cases in which pomographic photographs or videotapes are acquired as evidence)
　Intentional, blunt penetrating injury to the vaginal or anal orifice
　Positive, confirmed cultures *Neisseria gonorrhoeae* in a prepubertal child or serologic confirmation of acquired syphilis

From *Adolesc Pediatr Gynecol* 1992;5:73–75, with permission.
Modified from Adams JA, Harper K. Knudson S, "A proposed system for the classification of anogenital findings in children with suspected sexual abuse"

TABLE 26.10. *Proposed classification of anogenital findings in children*

Normal (class I)
　Periurethral bands
　Intravaginal ridges or columns
　Increased erythema in the sulcus
　Hymenal tags, mounds, or bumps
　Elongated hymenal orifice in an obese child
　Ample posterior hymenal rim (1–2 mm wide)
　Estrogen changes (thickened, redundant hymen)
　Diastasis ani/smooth area at the 6 or 12 o'clock position in the perianal area
　Anal tag/thickened fold in the midline
Nonspecific findings (class 2)[a]
　Erythema of vestibule or perianal tissues
　Increased vascularity of the vestibule or hymen
　Labial adhesions
　Rolled hymenal edges in the knee–chest position
　Narrow hymenal rim, but at least 1 mm wide
　Vaginal discharge
　Anal fissures
　Flattened anal folds
　Thickened anal folds
　Anal gaping with stool present
　Venous congestion of the perianal tissues, delayed in examination
　Fecal soiling
Suspicious for abuse (class 3)[b]
　Enlarged hymenal opening, 2 standard deviations from nonabused study (McCann et al.)

Immediate anal dilation of 15 mm with stool not visible or palpable in rectal vault
Immediate, extensive venous congestion of the perianal tissues
Distorted, irregular anal folds
Posterior hymenal rim <1 mm in all views
Condyloma acuminata in a child
Acute abrasions or lacerations in the vestibule or on the labia (not involving the hymen) or perianal lacerations
Suggestive of abuse/penetration (class 4)
　Combination of two or more suspicious anal findings or two or more suspicious findings
　Scar or fresh laceration of the posterior fourchette with sparing of the hymen
　Scar in the perianal area (must take history into consideration)
Clear evidence of penetrating injury (class 5)
　Areas with an absence of hymenal tissue (below the 3 to 9 o'clock position with patient supine), which is confirmed in the knee–chest position
　Hymenal transections or lacerations
　Hymenal laceration extending beyond (deep to) the external anal sphincter
　Laceration of the posterior fourchette, extending to involve hymen
　Scar of posterior fourchette associated with a loss of hymenal tissue between the 5 and 7 o'clock position

[a] Findings that may be caused by sexual abuse but may also be caused by other medical conditions. History is vital in determining significance.
[b] Findings that should prompt the examiner to question the child carefully about possible abuse; may or may not require a report to protective services in the absence of a history.
Modified from Adams JA, Harper K, Knudson S, et al. Examination findings in legally confirmed child sexual abuse: it's normal to be normal. *Pediatrics* 1994;94:310–317, with permission.

Hospitalization

Two indications for hospitalizing the sexually abused child are severe injury requiring treatment and an unsafe home. However, outpatient management of sexual abuse victims is always preferable. The rationale is to avoid victimizing the child twice.

Treatment

Whether the child is hospitalized or discharged from the ED, three additional issues should be considered: (1) gonococcal prophylaxis, (2) human immunodeficiency virus testing, and (3) pregnancy prevention. If the abuse has occurred less than 48 hours before the hospital visit, gonococcal prophylaxis is recommended. Within this time period, cultures for *Neisseria gonorrhoeae* may prove negative, even if a true infection is incubating. In abuse that has occurred more than 48 hours before the visit, the choices are either to treat all children prophylactically or to culture the genitalia, anus, and throat and await culture results. This choice depends in part on the reliability of the microbiology laboratory in recovering *N. gonorrhoeae* (which is a fastidious organism) and the ability to provide follow-up treatment for positive cultures. Recommended treatment regimens are shown in Table 26.11.

TABLE 26.11. *Treatment guidelines: gonorrhea*

Uncomplicated infection such as endocervicitis, urethritis, proctitis or pharyngeal infections: 125 mg ceftriaxone IM × 1 dose or 400 mg cefixime PO × 1 dose or 500 mg ciprofloxacin[a] PO × 1 dose or 400 mg oxfloxacin[a] PO × 1 dose + 100 mg doxycycline[b] PO b.i.d. × 7 days or 1 g azithromycin PO × 1 dose	Uncomplicated vulvoganitis, urethritis, proctitis, or pharyngitis: 125 mg ceftriaxone[c] IM × 1 dose + 40–50 mg/kg erythromycin per day in divided doses × 7 days[d]

[a] Quinolones are not approved for use in children younger than 18 years, pregnant women, or lactating women.

[b] In pregnancy, doxycycline is contraindicated, and safety and efficacy data for the use of azithromycin are lacking. Therefore, replacement with 500 mg amoxicillin orally three times daily for 7 days or 500 mg erythromycin orally four times daily for 7 days is recommended, but efficacy is lower than the standard treatment in nonpregnant women.

[c] May consider 8 mg/kg cefixime orally in one dose, but data are limited.

[d] In those older than 9 years of age, 100 mg doxycycline twice daily for 7 days can be used instead of erythromycin.

IM, intramuscularly; PO, orally; b.i.d., twice daily.

Modified from Sung L, MacDonald NE. Gonorrhea: a pediatric perspective *Pediatr Rev* 1998;19:13–16.

SUGGESTED READINGS

Adams JA, Harper K, Knudson S, et al. Examination findings in legally confirmed child sexual abuse: it's normal to be normal. *Pediatrics* 1994;94: 310–317.

Allard JE. The collection of data from findings in cases of sexual assault and the significance of spermatozoa on vaginal, anal and oral swabs. *Sci Justice* 1997;37:99–108.

Arkovitz MS, Johnson N, Garcia VF. Pancreatic trauma in children: mechanisms of injury. *J Trauma Injury Infect Crit Care* 1997;42:49–53.

Banco L, Lapidus G, Zavoski R, et al. Burn injuries among children in an urban emergency department. *Pediatr Emerg Care* 1994;10:98–101.

Berkowitz CD. Pediatric abuse: new patterns of injury. *Emerg Med Clin North Am* 1995;13:321–341.

Chadwick DL, Chin S, Salerno C, et al. Deaths from falls in children: how far is fatal? *J Trauma* 1991;31:1353–1355.

Cheasty M, Clare AW, Collins C. Relation between sexual abuse in childhood and adult depression: case-control study. *BMJ* 1998;316:198–201.

Coant PN, Kornberg AE, Brody AS, et al. Markers for occult liver injury in cases of physical abuse in children. *Pediatrics* 1992;89:274–278.

Committee on Child Abuse and Neglect, American Academy of Pediatrics. Gonorrhea in prepubertal children. *Pediatrics* 1998;101:134–135.

da Fonseca MA, Feigal RJ, ten Bensel RW. Dental aspects of 1248 cases of child maltreatment on file at a major county hospital. *Pediatr Dent* 1992;14:152–157.

Dailey JC, Bowers CM. Aging of bite marks: a literature review. *J Forensic Sci* 1997;42:792–795.

Duhaime AC, Christian CW, Rorke LB, et al. Nonaccidental head injury in infants—the "shaken-baby syndrome." *N Engl J Med* 1998;338:1822–1829.

Finkel MA, Ricci LR. Documentation and preservation of visual evidence in child abuse. *Child Maltreat* 1997;2:322–330.

Frank DA, Silva M, Needlman R. Failure to thrive: mystery, myth, and method. *Contemp Pediatr* 1993;Feb:114–133.

Friedrich WN, Fisher J, Broughton D, et al. Normative sexual behavior in children: a contemporary sample. *Pediatrics* 1998;101:E9.

Harris VJ, Lorand MA, Fitzpatrick JJ, et al. *Radiographic atlas of child abuse: a case studies approach.* New York: Igaku-Shoin, 1996.

Hodge D, Ludwig S. Child homicide: emergency department recognition. *Pediatr Emerg Care* 1985;1:3–6.

Homer C, Ludwig S. Categorization of etiology of failure to thrive. *Am J Dis Child* 1981;135:848–851.

Hymel KP, Rumack CM, Hay TC, et al. Comparison of intracranial computer tomographic (CT) findings in pediatric abusive and accidental head trauma. *Pediatr Radiol* 1997;27:743–747.

Joffe M, Ludwig S. Stairway injuries in children. *Pediatrics* 1988;82:457–472.

Kleinman PK. *Diagnostic imaging of child abuse*, 2nd ed. Baltimore: Williams & Wilkins, 1998.

Kleinman PK, Schlesinger AE. Mechanical factors associated with posterior rib fractures: laboratory and case studies. *Pediatr Radiol* 1997;27:87–91.

Ludwig S. A multidisciplinary approach to child abuse. *Nurs Clin North Am* 1981;16:161–165.

Ludwig S. Failure to thrive/starvation. In: Ludwig S, Kornberg A, eds. *Child abuse: a medical reference*, 2nd ed. New York: Churchill Livingstone, 1992.

Ludwig S, Kornberg AE. *Child abuse: a medical reference,* 2nd ed. New York: Churchill Livingstone, 1992.

Ludwig S, Rostain A. Family dysfunction. In: Levine MD, Carey WB, Crocker AC, eds. *Developmental behavioral pediatrics*, 2nd ed. Philadelphia: WB Saunders, 1992.

McCann J, Voris J, Simon M, et al. Comparison of genital examination techniques in prepubertal girls. *Pediatrics* 1990;86:182–187.

National Center on Child Abuse and Neglect. *Third national incidence study of child abuse and neglect: final report* (NIS-3). Washington, DC: U.S. Department of Health and Human Services, 1996.

Ng CS, Hall CM, Shaw DG. The range of visceral manifestations of nonaccidental injury. *Arch Dis Child* 1997;77:167–174.

Nichols JS, Elger C, Hemminger L, et al. Magnetic resonance imaging: utilization in the management of central nervous system trauma. *J Trauma* 1997;42:520–524.

Paradise J. The medical evaluation of the sexually abused child. *Pediatr Clin North Am* 1990;39:839–862.

Paradise JE, Finkel MA, Beiser AS, et al. Assessment of girls' genital findings and the likelihood of sexual abuse: agreement among physicians self-rated as skilled. *Arch Pediatr Adolesc Med* 1997;151:883–891.

Reece RM. Unusual manifestations of child abuse. *Pediatr Clin North Am* 1990;34:905–921.

Reece RM, Ludwig S. *Child abuse: medical diagnosis and management*, 2nd ed. New York: Lippincott Williams & Wilkins, 2001.

Schwengel D, Ludwig S. Rhabdomyolysis and myoglobinuria as manifestations of child abuse. *Pediatr Emerg Care* 1985;1:194–197.

Sirotnak AP, Krugman RD. Physical abuse of children: an update. *Pediatr Rev* 1994;15:394–399.

Slosberg E, Ludwig S, Duckett J, et al. Penile trauma as a sign of child abuse. *Am J Dis Child* 1978;132:719–721.

Starling S, Holden JR, Jenny C. Abusive head trauma: the relationship of perpetrators to their victims. *Pediatrics* 1995;95:259–262.

Starling SP. Syphilis in infants and young children. *Pediatr Ann* 1994;23:334–340.

Sung L, MacDonald NE. Gonorrhea: a pediatric perspective. *Pediatr Rev* 1998;19:13–16.

U.S. Advisory Board on Child Abuse and Neglect. *A nation's shame: fatal child abuse and neglect in the United States*. Washington, DC: U.S. Department of Health and Human Services, 1995.

Wyatt JP, McLeod L, Beard D, et al. Timing of paediatric deaths after trauma. *BMJ* 1997;314:868.

Zimmerman RA, Bilaniuk LT. Pediatric head trauma. *Neuroimag Clin North Am* 1994;4:349–366.

SECTION IV

Procedures

CHAPTER 27

Selected Procedures

Editor: Gary R. Fleisher

MAJOR THERAPEUTIC PROCEDURES

Airway Management

Most children with airway compromise can be managed with simple maneuvers and/or an oral or nasal airway, with or without manual ventilation. In some cases, this initial approach proves insufficient or the clinical situation requires a protected airway. Oral endotracheal intubation, usually preceded by rapid sequence induction, is the method of choice. Most operators prefer a straight (Miller) blade for younger children. Proper placement of the endotracheal tube and maintenance of this position requires attention to clinical signs of aeration and is best supplemented by end-tidal carbon dioxide monitoring and secure taping (Fig. 27.1).

Vascular Access

Intraosseous Access

Intraosseous access is most commonly achieved at the flat medial surface of the proximal tibia in children. After lying dormant for many years, emergency physicians reintroduced this technique into clinical practice in the 1980s. Originally, spinal needles were commonly used because they have a stylet (Fig. 27.2). Currently, medical manufacturers provide a variety of devices designed for this specific purpose.

Central Vascular Access

The Seldinger technique (Fig. 27.3) is preferred for central venous access in children and may be facilitated by bedside ultrasonography. After preparation and draping of the field, the physician inserts a narrow-gauge needle into the lumen of the vessel to be cannulated. The flexible end of the guidewire is passed through the needle, which is then removed. The catheter is then advanced into the vessel over the guidewire, which is retracked. Commonly used sites include the external jugular (Fig. 27.3), the femoral (Fig. 27.4), the internal jugular (Fig. 27.5), and the subclavian (Fig. 27.6) veins.

Venotomy (Cutdown)

The most commonly cannulated vein is the lesser saphenous at the ankle (Fig. 27.7), although a myriad of sites exist. To access the lesser saphenous vein, the skin is incised just above and anterior to the medial malleolus, exactly at the point where percutaneous cannulation is performed. The physician then uses a curved hemostat to dissect the vein free of the surrounding tissue and passes a ligature under the vessel. Placing slight tension on the ligature to stabilize the vessel, it is possible to achieve cannulation using a catheter over the needle device.

Closed Thoracostomy (Chest Tube Insertion)

Chest tubes may be inserted via an incision through the chest wall or by the Seldinger technique using a guidewire. In an emergent situation, such as major trauma, or to evacuate a large hemothorax, regardless of the circumstances, a large bore chest tube placed directly by incision offers the best solution. Applications of the Seldinger technique for insertion of relatively small bore chest tubes include relief of pneumothoraces and drainage of nonviscous effusions (Fig. 27.8). After achieving local anesthesia, a narrow-gauge needle is inserted into the chest cavity over the rib. Easy withdrawal of air or fluid confirms entry into the pneumothorax of pleural effusion. The physician then passes the flexible end of the guidewire through the needle, directing the tip upward for evacuation of air and downward for fluid. Sliding the dilator, provided with the kit, back and forth over the guidewire further dilates the passageway through the chest wall. Finally, the chest tube (usually a "pigtail" catheter) is advanced over the guidewire, which is then removed.

MINOR THERAPEUTIC PROCEDURES

Laceration Repair

Repair of a laceration represents one of the most frequent procedures confronting the practitioner. Maximization of

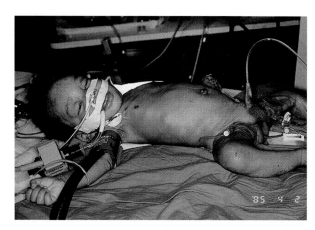

FIG. 27.1. The endotracheal tube in this infant has been well secured and the end-tidal CO_2 concentration is being monitored.

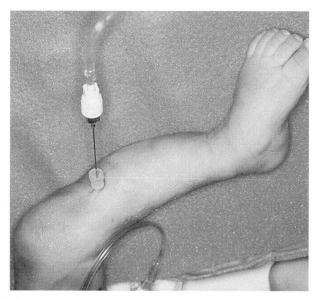

FIG. 27.2. This child has had a spinal needle inserted into the intraosseous cavity of his proximal tibia. Note that the needle lies well below the physis of the bone.

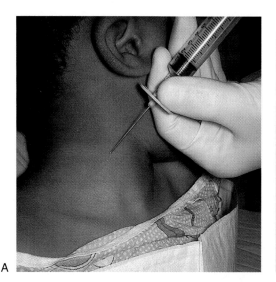

A

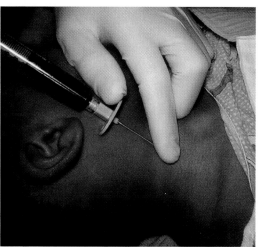

B

FIG. 27.3. This simulation demonstrates the Seldinger technique at the site of the external jugular vein. **A:** While aspirating on a syringe, the vein is cannulated with a needle. **B:** Free flow of blood into the syringe confirms entry into the lumen of the vessel.

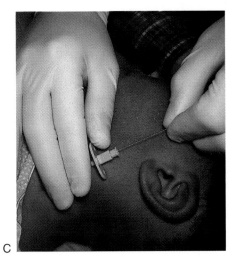

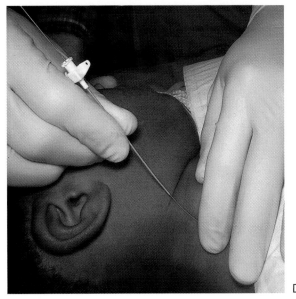

FIG. 27.3. *Continued* **C:** While stabilizing the needle, the operator inserts the guidewire. **D:** After the needle is removed, the operator advances the catheter over the needle.

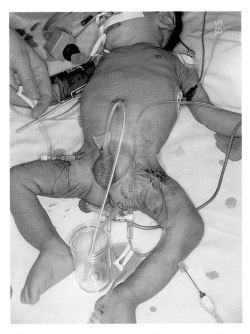

FIG. 27.4. This child has a femoral venous catheter on the left and a femoral arterial catheter on the right.

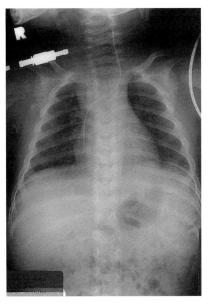

FIG. 27.5. A radiograph of an internal jugular catheter in an infant.

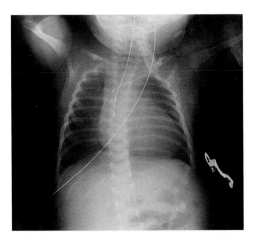

FIG. 27.6. A radiograph of a subclavian catheter in an infant who developed cardiogenic shock secondary to supraventricular tachycardia that responded to administration of adenosine.

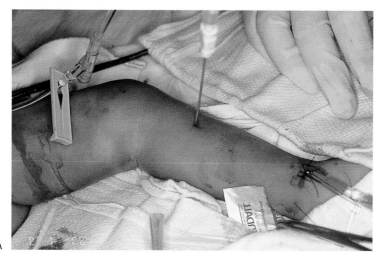

A

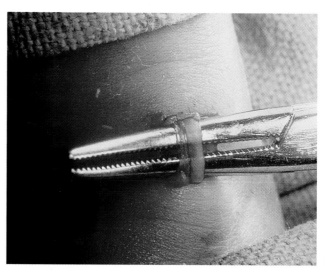

B

FIG. 27.7. A: This child, who presented with severe hypovolemic dehydration, received initial fluid resuscitation via an intraosseous needle and, after a failed attempt to catheterize the femoral vein, had a cutdown, as shown. **B:** Isolation of the saphenous vein during a cutdown procedure.

functional and cosmetic outcome relies on a knowledge of anatomy, an understanding of the mechanisms of wound healing, and technical skills. Before initiating the repair, the physician should prepare for the procedure. Specific steps include

1. Perform a pertinent history and general physical examination.
2. Inspect the wound preliminarily. In some cases, even a cursory examination reveals a complex wound that will require repair with the expertise of a surgical colleague (Fig. 27.9). For instance, visualization of a severed flexor tendon strongly points to the need for operative repair.
3. Test the ligaments and neurovascular function.
4. Evaluate the need for prophylaxis. Potential forms of prophylaxis include rabies immunoglobulin/rabies vaccine, tetanus toxoid, and antibiotic agents.

5. Decide on the type of sedation needed, if any.
6. Discuss the plan with the family.

After the physician has prepared the necessary materials and received approval from the patient and/or family, the actual process of repair begins. Steps in this phase include

1. Provide local anesthesia. Direct injection of 0.5% to 1% lidocaine (unless the patient is allergic) with epinephrine into the margins of the wound provides excellent local anesthesia. Alternatively, a peripheral nerve block can be performed (Fig. 27.10).
2. Prepare the field and drape the wound.
3. Irrigate the wound.

FIG. 27.8. A child with a pleural effusion who had the fluid drained via placement of a pigtail catheter using the Seldinger technique.

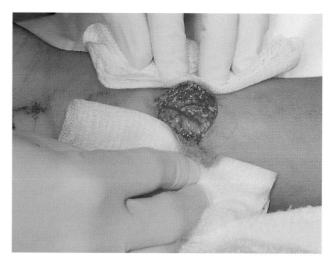

FIG. 27.9. Careful inspection of all lacerations is essential because even seemingly superficial wounds, particularly at the hand and wrist, may sever a tendon, as in this patient with a partial tear of the palmaris longus.

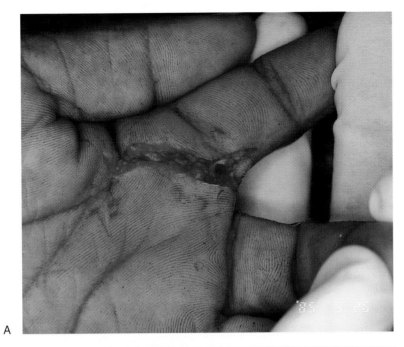

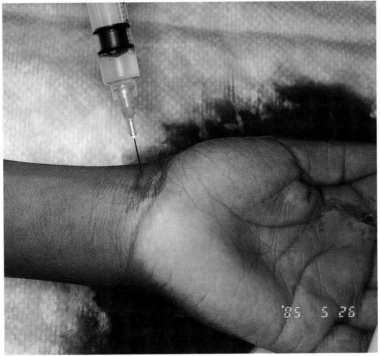

FIG. 27.10. This child sustained a laceration on the palmar surface of his hand at the base of his index finger, which was sufficiently deep **(A)** to require a layered repair. Placement of a median nerve block **(B)** provided excellent anesthesia.

4. Explore the wound. Search diligently for injuries to underlying structures (Fig. 27.11) and nonradiopaque foreign bodies (Fig. 27.12).
5. Debride necrotic tissue as needed. Necrotic tissue contributes to infections and scar formation and should generally be removed (Fig. 27.13), with particular care taken on the face.
6. Perform the repair. Use the smallest possible suture material or other appropriate material (Table 27.1) that will close the wound adequately. Simple wounds that are superficial and not subject to undue tension usually require only interrupted cuticular sutures for repair (Fig. 27.14). Deeper wounds require a layered repair, usually starting with buried subcuticular sutures (Fig. 27.15). The objective of the subcuticular sutures is to eliminate dead space within the wound and to take the tension off the margins. More complex wounds may need debridement, closure of a fascial layer, placement of a drain, or other specialized approaches (Figs. 27.16 and 27.17). A layered repair offers the best cosmetic result and is appropriate for all but the most superficial lacerations, especially on the face.

After the repair, more work remains. The final tasks are as follows:

1. Dressing the wound.
2. Administering and/or prescribing prophylaxis (Table 27.2).
3. Obtaining closure with the family, by discussing issues of wound care, suture removal (Table 27.3), and the expectations in terms of scar formation.

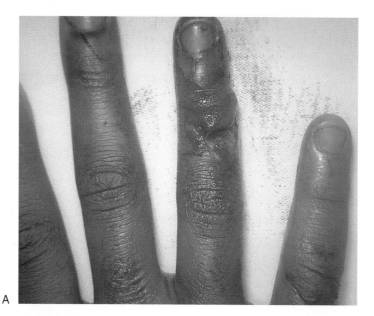

A

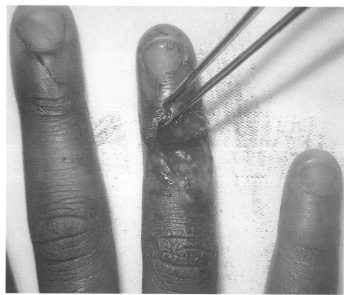

B

FIG. 27.11. This laceration **(A)**, which initially appeared superficial, involved the extensor tendon **(B)** on further exploration.

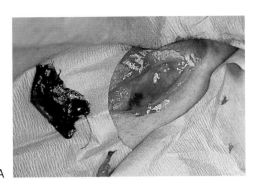

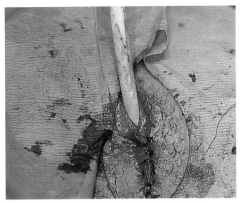

FIG. 27.12. A: This obese boy rode his bicycle into a tree at high speed and was struck in the groin by the end of the handlebar. Although there were no visible foreign bodies on initial inspection, exploration of the depths of the wound uncovered a fragment from his jeans, driven into the tissues by the handlebar **(B)**. Given the contaminated nature of the wound, a drain was placed.

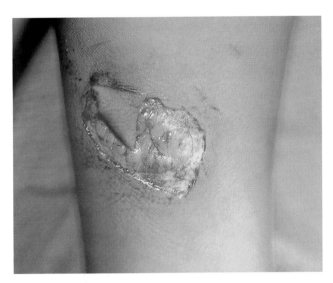

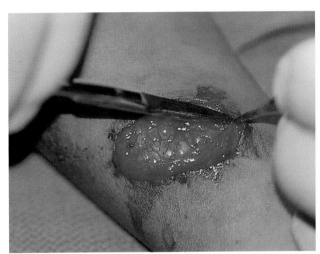

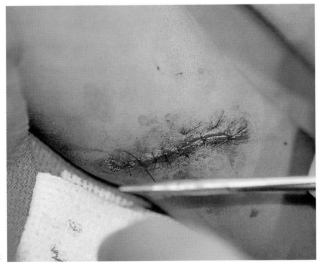

FIG. 27.13. This small flap of tissue **(A)** was deemed to be nonviable and was excised **(B)**. The wound was extended minimally to form an ellipse, undermined, and closed in layers **(C)**, yielding an excellent outcome.

TABLE 27.1. *Common techniques of wound closure*

Technique	Advantages	Disadvantages
Sutures	Greatest tensile strength, meticulous closure, low dehiscence rate	Painful, removal needed, slow application, increased tissue reaction, risk of needle stick (clinician)
Staples	Rapid application, low cost, low tissue reaction	Not for use on face (less meticulous closure)
Tissue adhesive	Rapid application, painless, no removal needed, low cost, no risk of needle stick (clinician)	Lower tensile strength, not for use on joints
Tape strips	Rapid application, painless, low cost, low infection risk, least tissue reaction	High risk of dehiscence, not for use in moist areas or young children

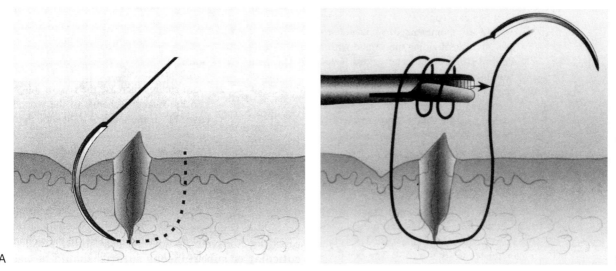

FIG. 27.14. A,B A simple interrupted cuticular suture secured with an instrument tie.

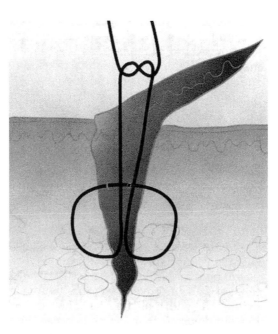

FIG. 27.15. A buried subcutaneous suture.

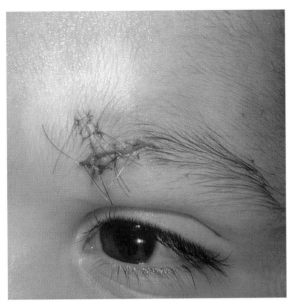
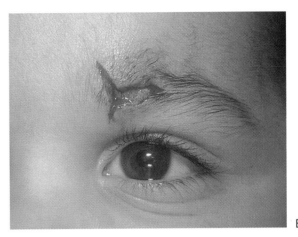

FIG. 27.16. This young girl had a flap type laceration **(A)** of her eyebrow that was repaired using a corner stitch **(B)**.

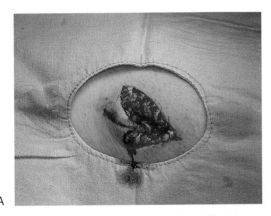
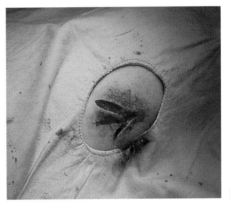
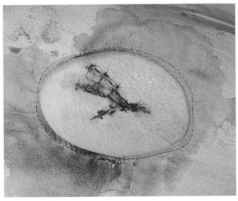

FIG. 27.17. This boy sustained a deep laceration of his abdominal wall **(A)** when he became impaled on a picket fence. After exploration showed no penetration into the abdominal cavity, deep sutures **(B)** were placed to approximate the flap. **C:** A corner stitch was used for the cuticular closure.

TABLE 27.2. *Tetanus prophylaxis*

Prior tetanus toxoid immunization (doses)	Clean minor wound	All other wounds
Uncertain (or <3)	DTP or Td	DTP or Td and TIG or TAT
≥3 (most recent >10 yrs ago)	Td	Td
≥3 (most recent within past 5 yrs)	None	None
≥3 (most recent between 5 and 10 yrs)	None	Td

DTP, diphtheria, tetanus, pertussis toxoid; Td, adult formulation of diphtheria, tetanus toxoid; TIG, tetanus immunoglobulin (dose, 250–500 units intramuscularly); TAT, tetanus antitoxin (should be used only if TIG is not available and after testing; dose, 3,000–5,000 units intramuscularly).

TABLE 27.3 *Timely suture removal*

Wound location	Time of removal (days)
Neck	3–4
Face, scalp	5
Upper extremities, trunk	7–10
Lower extremities	8–10
Joint surface	10–14

Foreign Body Removal

Subcutaneous Foreign Bodies

The decision of whether to remove a foreign body and who should perform the procedure requires clinical judgment. In general, organic material and large, sharp, or painful foreign bodies should be extracted. Very small, asymptomatic, nonorganic objects, such as a speck of glass visualized radiographically, usually cause no problems if left *in situ*. Foreign bodies that are partially visible or easily palpable should be removed in the emergency department. Conversely, even the experienced physician may decline the opportunity to chase a deeper object, such as a sewing needle embedded in the sole of the foot far beneath the cuticular surface (Fig. 25.13).

Hard objects (metal or glass) protruding through the skin may be grasped and removed. Deeper objects and those likely to fragment (splinters) require an incision (Fig. 27.18). The physician should make the smallest possible superficial excision that will allow easy extraction, follow-ing the skin lines and exercising care for adjacent anatomic structures. In many cases, dissection with a curved hemostat is needed to free up the object. Fishhooks, which have a barb at the end, require a unique approach (Fig. 27.19). Generally, the barbed end is advanced until it protrudes through the skin, at which point it is snipped off with a wire cutter. The physician can then simply and painlessly slide the hook back through the track. Occasionally, local anesthesia may be needed.

Rings and Other Encircling Objects

Curiosity has snagged many a finger. Tight rings are the most common offenders, but children manage to find a variety of circular objects in which to entrap their digits. Jewelry usually succumbs to a mechanical ring cutter because the metal is soft (Fig. 27.20). For steel objects, such as washers, a motor-driven device with a diamond-tipped blade is available. At times, the size and consistency of the encircling object may call for a larger instrument, such as a wire cutter, tin snips, or hacksaw (Fig. 27.21).

Tick Removal

The literature offers a potpourri of options for removal of ticks, but only one approach works. Use a forceps to grasp the tick as close to the surface of the skin as possible and remove it directly (See Fig. 3.7).

Nose

Foreign bodies that are visible in the anterior nares can be grasped directly with an alligator forceps, if of appropriate consistency, such as paper, pieces of sponge, and small toys with edges (Fig. 27.22). For harder, smooth foreign bodies, such as beads, either a right-angle hook or curette can often be passed just beyond the object, which is then pulled out. Alternatively, a balloon-tipped catheter serves the same purpose (Fig. 27.23). A nasal speculum, with or without the use of a headlight, facilitates visualization of objects lodged further up in the nares.

Ear

As with the nose, some objects will be visible to the naked eye and readily amenable to extraction, either by grasping them with an alligator forceps or with the use of a right-angle hook. Those lying more proximally require the use of an otoscope with an operating head or an operating microscope.

The recent upsurge in body piercing has led to an increase in the occurrence of an earring being partially submerged within the earlobe or adjacent portions of the ear

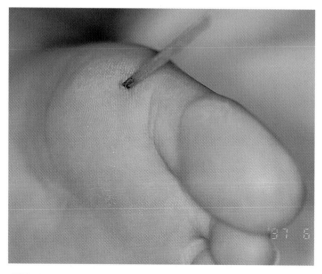

FIG. 27.18. This deeply embedded, but partially visible, splinter was removed through a small incision made to extend the puncture wound. Care must be exercised to not leave any wood fragments because they are likely to cause an infection.

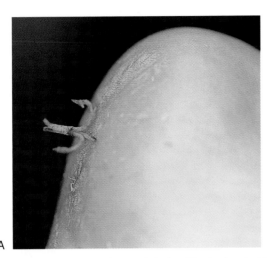

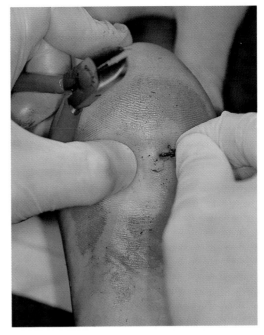

A

B

FIG. 27.19. A: A fishhook lodged in the heel of this child. Lidocaine infiltration of the adjacent skin provided local anesthesia in this very anxious boy. **B:** After advancing the hook through the anesthetized patch of skin and using a wire cutter to remove the barb, the physician was able to remove the hook through the existing track.

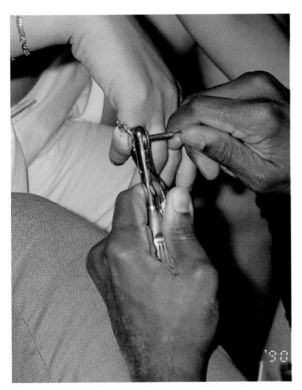

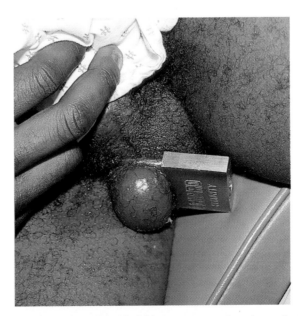

FIG. 27.20. The physician removes a ring using a mechanical ring cutter.

FIG. 27.21. The girlfriend of this young man placed a padlock around his testicle. To the surprise of the couple, they could not locate the key. Attempts to slide the lock off were unsuccessful. After slipping the handle of a scalpel between the bar and the scrotum to protect the skin, the physician cut the lock with a metal cutter.

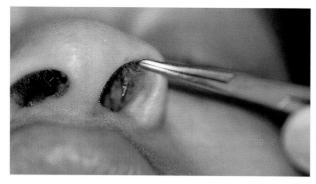

FIG. 27.22. An earring lodged in the nose of this child was easily removed with a curved hemostat under direct visualization.

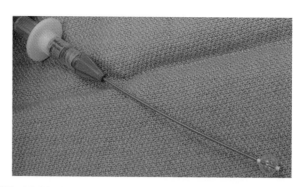

FIG. 27.23. A balloon-tip catheter with the balloon inflated. After the tip is passed beyond the object, the balloon is inflated and the catheter is gently withdrawn.

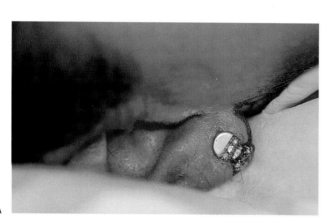

A

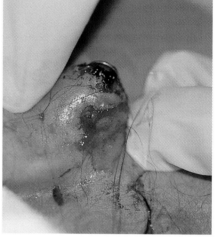

B

FIG. 27.24. A: An earring eroded through the superficial tissues of the earlobe of this child. **B:** Gentle pressure was used to force the submerged clasp to the surface, at which time both the post and the clasp were grasped with hemostats and separated.

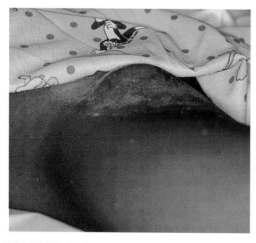

A

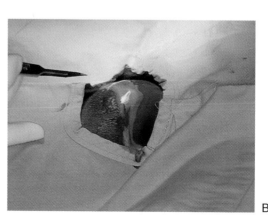

B

FIG. 27.25. A: A large abscess formed in the groin of this child, directly over the femoral vessels and nerve. **B:** A superficial incision produced an immediate return of pus.

(Fig. 27.24). In most cases, gentle digital pressure will force the submerged end to the surface. At that point, both the clasp and the decorative side of the earring can be grasped with hemostats and separated.

Incision and Drainage

Abscess

Treatment of loculated pus mandates drainage. An incision is made over the most fluctuant area, taking care not to injure adjacent structures (Fig. 27.25). Using a curved hemostat to disrupt any loculations within the cavity maximizes drainage; a wick lessens the chance that pus will reaccumulate (See Fig. 11.15).

Subungual Hematoma

Small subungual hematomas produce minimal discomfort, but larger accumulations of pus under the nail may cause significant pain. Drainage is achieved by cauterization of the nail (Fig. 27.26).

Fractures and Dislocations

Clavicle

An older patient with a clavicular fracture often complains of pain at the midshaft of the bone, but the findings may be subtler in young children. As the mechanism of injury usually involves a force applied laterally to medially, a bruise over the deltoid serves as a clue to this injury (Fig. 27.27). Closed fractures of the clavicle, regardless of the degree of angulation or displacement, heal without complications.

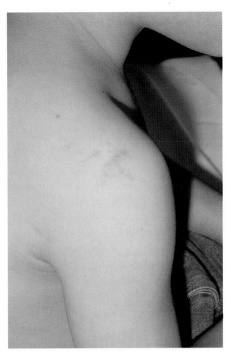

FIG. 27.27. A bruise over the deltoid of this boy, who rolled out of bed onto the floor, suggests a fracture of the clavicle from the force applied laterally to medially along the long axis of the bone.

The physician must make certain, however, that a sternoclavicular dislocation has not occurred because this injury may compromise the great vessels in the mediastinum. A clavicle strap in young children (Fig. 27.28) or a sling in older patients provides immobilization and reduces discomfort.

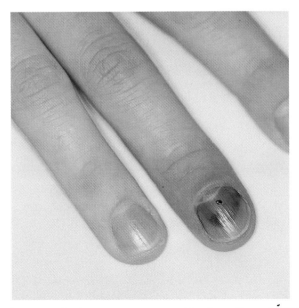

FIG. 27.26. A microcautery was used to pierce the nail of this child and drain a subungual hematoma that was painful.

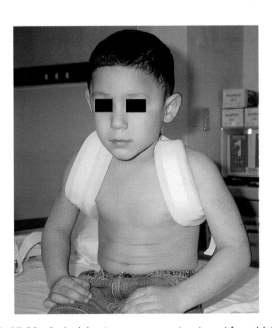

FIG. 27.28. A clavicle strap serves as treatment for midshaft clavicular fractures.

Shoulder

Trauma to the shoulder most often causes a Salter fracture in prepubertal patients, whereas a dislocation occurs commonly in older teenagers. Radiographs generally reveal inferior and anterior displacement of a dislocated humeral head. Reduction is achieved with traction/countertraction or via a number of different maneuvers.

Elbow

True elbow dislocations occur infrequently in pediatrics. More often, young children experience a subluxation of the radial head or nursemaid's elbow, presenting with refusal to use the affected upper extremity. Reduction is achieved with supination and extension, followed by pronation, and is facilitated by slight pressure over the radial head.

Hand

Dislocations involving the metacarpal-phalangeal or interphalangeal joints are frequent (Fig. 27.29), most commonly with dorsal displacement of the distal portion of the finger. Placement of a digital block eases the pain of reduction with an interphalangeal dislocation and is particularly recommended for young children. Reduction is achieved with longitudinal traction, although an initial, brief exaggeration of the deformity by dorsiflexion may be necessary in some cases. A finger splint should be applied after confirmatory radiographs are obtained. Splinting or buddy taping provide adequate immobilization for most nondisplaced phalangeal fractures.

Many fractures of the hand require only immobilization in a splint or by buddy taping. Malalignment, including rotational deformity, must be corrected (Fig. 27.30).

Hip

Hip dislocations occur infrequently, usually after major trauma, such as with a motor vehicle collision. Reduction should be accomplished promptly.

Patella

Compared with the hip, a minor force may dislocate the patella, which usually slides laterally. Patients present in se-

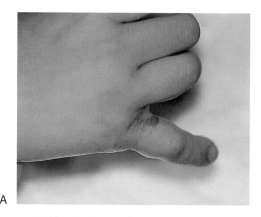

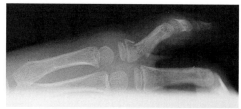

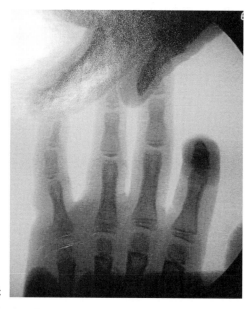

FIG. 27.30. The clinical deformity **(A)** of the finger in this child results from a displaced fracture **(B)** of the proximal phalanx, easily reduced **(C)** under fluoroscopy in the emergency department.

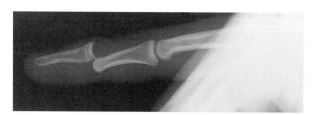

FIG. 27.29. A radiograph of a dislocation at the distal interphalangeal joint of the finger shows the overlap of the phalanges that may make reduction difficult.

vere pain with the extremity held in flexion (Fig. 27.31). Reduction is achieved by extending the leg at the knee while applying pressure to the lateral edge of the patella in a medial direction.

Foot

Dislocations of the metatarsal-phalangeal and interphalangeal joints of the foot are managed in a similar fashion to those of the hand.

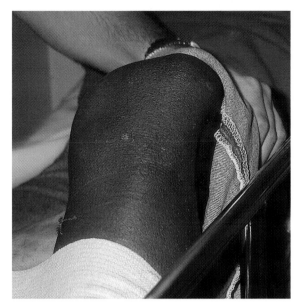

FIG. 27.31. This adolescent sustained a lateral dislocation of his patella.

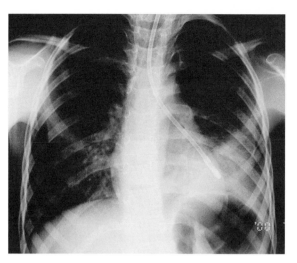

FIG. 27.33. This child consumed an overdose of barbiturates and received a dose of charcoal at a hospital in her community. On transfer to a referral center, she developed decreased breath sounds on the left side. A radiograph revealed a nasogastric tube in the left mainstem bronchus and an early pneumonia. This case illustrates the importance of checking the placement of a gastric tube, particularly in a patient who is or may potentially be neurologically compromised.

Reduction of Rectal Prolapse

Rectal prolapse (Fig. 27.32) occurs most commonly in children with chronic constipation but may be a finding in chronic diseases, such as cystic fibrosis. Inspection confirms the diagnosis. Reduction is accomplished by applying circumferential pressure to the prolapsed tissue, which should be well lubricated.

Gastric Tube Insertion

Insertion of a gastric tube for diagnostic and/or therapeutic purposes is frequently performed. The nasal route is preferred, unless midfacial injury is present or a large bore tube is necessary for lavage. When using the nasal approach, the tube should be directed posteriorly along the floor of the nasal cavity. Proper placement should be checked immedi-

ately by aspiration of gastric contents and by auscultation. Before instilling any substances through the tube, verification by radiography or pH testing of the aspirate is suggested (Fig. 27.33).

DIAGNOSTIC PROCEDURES

Lumbar Puncture

Next to venipuncture, no other procedure occurs as frequently in pediatric practice as lumbar puncture. The usual position for the patient is lying on the left side (for right-handed physicians), with the head bent down and the knees curled up toward the chest, thereby maximizing the distance between the spinous processes (Fig. 27.34). A

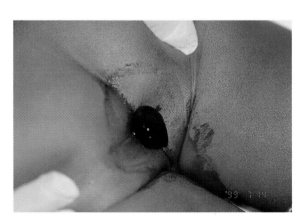

FIG. 27.32. Rectal prolapse.

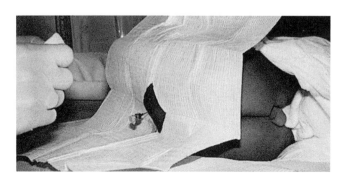

FIG. 27.34. This child in the left lateral recumbent position is having a lumbar puncture in the L4-5 interspace.

22-gauge needle, varying in length from 1.5 in. (for infants) to 3.5 in. or larger (for adolescents) is inserted in the fourth lumbar interspace, directed toward the umbilicus. The physician should advance the needle slowly in infants, withdrawing the stylet periodically to check for cerebrospinal fluid because penetration of the ligamentum flavum does not always produce a distinct "popping" sensation in young children.

SUGGESTED READINGS

Callahan JM, Baker MD. General wound management. In: Henretig FM, King C, eds. *Textbook of pediatric emergency procedures*. Baltimore: Williams & Wilkins, 1997:1125–1139.

Singer AJ, Hollander JE, Quinn JV. Evaluation and management of traumatic lacerations. *N Engl J Med* 1997;337:1142–1148.

Singer AJ, Hollander JE, Valentine SM, et al. Prospective, randomized, controlled trial of tissue adhesive (2-Octylcyanoacrylate) vs. standard wound closure techniques for laceration repair. *Acad Emerg Med* 1998; 5:94–99.

Subject Index

Page numbers followed by f refer to figures; page numbers followed by t refer to tables.